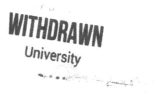

CLINICAL OCULAR TOXICOLOGY
Drugs, Chemicals and Herbs

Commissioning Editor: Russell Gabbedy
Development Editor: Alexandra Mortimer
Associate Editor: Kelly Medler
Project Manager: Bryan Potter
Design: Sarah Russell
Illustration Manager: Merlyn Harvey
Marketing Manager(s): John Canelon/William Veltre

CLINICAL OCULAR TOXICOLOGY
Drugs, Chemicals and Herbs

Frederick T. Fraunfelder, MD
Professor
Department of Ophthalmology
Oregan Health and Science University
Casey Eye Institute
Portland OR

Frederick W. Fraunfelder, MD
Associate Professor
Department of Ophthalmology
Oregan Health and Science University
Casey Eye Institute
Portland OR

Wiley A. Chambers, MD
Clinical Professor of Ophthalmology
Adjunct Assistant Professor of Computer Medicine
George Washington University School of Medicine
Washington, DC

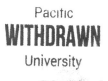
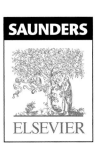

SAUNDERS

ELSEVIER

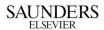

SAUNDERS An imprint of Elsevier Inc
© 2008, Elsevier Inc. All rights reserved.

First published 2008

978-1-4160-4673-8

British Library Cataloguing in Publication Data
A catalogue record for this book is available from the British Library

Library of Congress Cataloging in Publication Data
A catalog record for this book is available from the Library of Congress

Notice
Medical knowledge is constantly changing. Standard safety precautions must be followed, but as new research and clinical experience broaden our knowledge, changes in treatment and drug therapy may become necessary or appropriate. Readers are advised to check the most current product information provided by the manufacturer of each drug to be administered to verify the recommended dose, the method and duration of administration, and contraindications. It is the responsibility of the practitioner, relying on experience and knowledge of the patient, to determine dosages and the best treatment for each individual patient. Neither the Publisher nor the author_assume any liability for any injury and/or damage to persons or property arising from this publication.

The Publisher

Printed in China
Last digit is the print number: 9 8 7 6 5 4 3 2 1

CONTENTS

PREFACE

Clinical Ocular Toxicology - Drugs, Chemicals, and Herbs is a major revision of the 5th edition of Drug-Induced Ocular Side Effects. These changes have come from the requests of the ophthalmic community to include adverse ocular effects from chemicals and herbal medicines, and photographs of ocular toxicities. Further, we have expanded clinical sections with specific recommendations for physicians on how to follow patients taking a certain drug. Seventy new drugs which cause ocular side effects and five new chapters on clinical ocular toxicology have been added. A major feature is an attempt to add the probability of the adverse ocular event being due to the agent, in part, based on the World Health Organization (WHO) classification system (page). Dr. Chambers has not taken part in the WHO classification system due to his affiliation with the U.S. Food and Drug Administration (FDA) and this text has no relationship in any way to the FDA.

Clinical Ocular Toxicology - Drugs, Chemicals, and Herbs incorporates the most recent data from the spontaneous reporting systems of the Food and Drug Administration, Silver Spring, Maryland, the World Health Organization, Uppsala, Sweden, and the National Registry of Drug-Induced Ocular Side Effects, Casey Eye Institute, Oregon Health and Science University, Portland, Oregon. The National Registry contains case reports from clinicians in many countries, and includes the world literature in its database. Data in this book have been accumulated from innumerable physicians and scientists who have suspected adverse drug reactions and reported their suspicions to the FDA, WHO, or the National Registry.

This book is intended as a guide to help the busy clinician decide whether a visual problem is related to a chemical or medication. The clinician's past experience, the known natural course of the disease, the adverse effects of similarly structured compounds, and previous reports, all help physicians make their decision. Unfortunately, there has been only limited attempts to apply rigorous science to the clinical ocular toxicology of marketed products. There are many variables and there have been few research dollars in assessing a cause-and-effect relationship between most drugs, chemicals or herbs and any particular visual adverse event. The clinician needs to keep in mind the marked variability of how each human metabolizes or reacts to the drug or its metabolites. This variability may affect the incidence data. A significant change in the expected course of a disease after starting a drug should heighten the physician's suspicion of a drug-related event. Peer review journals have difficulty in accepting papers on potential visual side effects of drugs, since, causation once the agent is marketed, is usually difficult to prove by scientific parameters. At this stage, medical case reports and spontaneous reporting systems and their inherent pitfalls are left as the backbone of clinical ocular toxicology. While we have made an attempt to classify a suspected adverse event with our "impression" as to causality (i.e. certain, probable, possible, etc.), one needs to remember that this is not based on science. This is only a guide for the busy clinician and will always be a work in progress. We welcome your input.

F. T. Fraunfelder, M.D.
F. W. Fraunfelder, M.D.

Wiley A. Chambers, M.D.

CONTRIBUTORS

Devin Gattey, MD
Assistant Professor of Ophthalmology
Casey Eye Institute
Oregon Health & Science University
Portland, OR

Focke Ziemssen, MD
Senior Ophthalmologist
Centre for Ophthalmology
Eberhard Karls University
Tuebingen, Germany

Manfred Zierhut, MD
Professor of Medicine
Centre for Ophthalmology
Eberhard Karls University
Tuebingen, Germany

Eberhart Zrenner, MD
Professor of Ophthalmology
Centre for Ophthalmology
Eberhard Karls University
Tuebingen, Germany

DEDICATION

Frederick T. Fraunfelder, M.D.

To: Wendee, Mikayla, Jacob, Gracie-anne, and Sara-jane

Frederick W. Fraunfelder, M.D.

To: Yvonne and our grandchildren: Matthew, Kara, Courtney, J.D., Brooke, Mikayla, Nicolette, Jake, Gracie-anne, Rees, Connor, Asher, Sara-jane, Keilan Bree and Ava Grace

Wiley A. Chambers, M.D.

To: Jayne and Wesley

Kelly L. Medler, B.S.

To: Mom, Dad, Sara and Jen

INSTRUCTIONS TO USERS

The basic format used in each section of ocular side effects is:

Class: The general category of the primary action of the drug, chemical or herb is given.

Generic Name: The recommended International Nonproprietary Name (rINN) for each drug is listed, which is designated by the World Health Organization. In parentheses is the United States National Formulary name or other commonly accepted name.

Proprietary Name: The United States trade names are given but this is not an all-inclusive listing. In a group of drugs, the number before a generic name for both the systemic and ophthalmic forms corresponds to the number preceding the proprietary drug. International trade names and multi-ingredient preparations are not listed unless indicated.

Primary Use: The class of medicine and its current use in the management of various conditions are listed.

Ocular Side Effects:

Systemic Administration: Ocular side effects are reported from oral, nasal, intravenous, intramuscular, or intrathecal administration.

Local Ophthalmic Use or Exposure: Ocular side effects are reported from topical ocular application, subconjunctival, retrobulbar, or intracameral injection.

Inadvertent Ocular Exposure: Ocular side effects as reported due to accidental ocular exposure.

Inadvertent Systemic Exposure: Ocular side effects as reported due to accidental systemic exposure from topical ophthalmic medications.

Systemic Absorption from Topical Application to the Skin: Ocular side effects as reported secondary to topical dermatologic application.

The ocular side effects are listed as certain, probable, possible and conditional/unclassified. This classification is based, in part, on the system established by the World Health Organization. There is debatable scientific basis for our opinions. They are only intended as a guide for the clinician and are the results of "educated" conjectures from the authors, F.T. Fraunfelder and F.W. Fraunfelder. The name of a preparation in parentheses adjacent to an adverse reaction indicates that this is the only agent in the group reported to have caused this side effect.

Systemic Side Effects:

Systemic Administration: Systemic side effects as reported from ophthalmic medications administered by an oral, intravenous, or intramuscular route.

Local Ophthalmic Use or Exposure: Systemic side effects as reported from topical ocular application or subconjunctival or retrobulbar injection.

The listing as to certainty of causality is the same as used by systemic medication.

WHO Classification System
Where data is available (i.e., published or submitted for publication), we have classified medication adverse reactions according to the following World Health Organization's Causality Assessment of Suspected Adverse Reactions Guide.

Certain: A clinical event, including laboratory test abnormality, occurring in a plausible time relationship to drug administration, and which cannot be explained by concurrent disease or other drugs or chemicals. The response to withdrawal of the drug (dechallenge) should be clinically plausible. The event must be definitive pharmacologically or phenomenologically, using a satisfactory rechallenge procedure if necessary.

Probable/Likely: A clinical event, including laboratory test abnormality, with a reasonable time sequence to administration of the drug, unlikely to be attributed to concurrent disease or other drugs or chemicals, and which follows a clinically reasonable response on withdrawal (dechallenge). Rechallenge information is not required to fulfill this definition.

Possible: A clinical event, including laboratory test abnormality, with a reasonable time sequence to administration of the drug, but which could also be explained by concurrent disease or other drugs or chemicals. Information on drug withdrawal may be lacking or unclear.

Unlikely: A clinical event, including laboratory test abnormality, with a temporal relationship to drug administration which makes a causal relationship improbable, and in which other drugs, chemicals or underlying disease provide plausible explanations.

Conditional/Unclassified: A clinical event, including laboratory test abnormality, reported as an adverse reaction, about which more data is essential for a proper assessment or the additional data are under examination.

Unassessible/Unclassifiable: A report suggesting an adverse reaction which cannot be judged because information is insufficient or contradictory, and which cannot be supplemented or verified.

Photos: An asterisk placed adjacent to the reaction on the side effects outline corresponds with the photo in that section.

Clinical Significance: A concise overview of the general importance of the ocular side effects produced is given.

References: References have been limited to the most informative articles, the most current, or those with the most complete bibliography.

Recommendations: For specific medications, we make recommendations on following patients for probable related effects on the visual system. This was often done in consultation with other coworkers interested in the specific drug, however this is only intended as a possible guide .

Index of Side Effects: The lists of adverse ocular side effects due to preparations are intended in part to be indexes in themselves. The adverse ocular reactions are not separated in this index as to route of administration; however, this can be obtained by going to the text.

PART

1

Principles of therapy

Focke Ziemssen, MD and Manfred Zierhut, MD

PHARMACODYNAMICS

'Pharmacodynamics' can be defined as the quantitative relationship between the observed tissue concentration of the active drug and its pharmacologic effects. In contrast to pharmacokinetics, which describe how the body interacts with a drug, pharmacodynamic models predict what the drug does to the body. Ocular pharmacodynamics is therefore not just an abstract issue. Knowing how a substance causes the response, which pathways are involved and which cell will be affected is of the utmost importance not only in drug development, but also when applying a drug. Exact understanding of the concentration-dependent response for an individual patient provides more precise information for deciding how to dose. The main challenge in designing a drug dosage regimen is the variability that exists from patient to patient.

Extensive studies and clear specifications have to be made during the approval process of a drug. The effect of a formulation might vary with its dosage, the affected tissue and confounding co-morbidity. Because some of the different reactions to a molecule are not known at the time of approval, caution is important when treating understudied populations such as women, minorities and patients who have multiple health problems or pre-existing medication (Olson 2004).

Initially, the term 'receptor' was introduced as an abstract model, before any molecular structure had been exactly identified (Langley 1904). The leading aspect of the receptor is the quantitative relationship between drug dose and the pharmacological effect.

Where does the drug act?

The target of the active agent is not necessarily the body itself but, for example, a foreign organism, as is the case in antibiotics. The action of the drug can be initiated either by extracellular localization or by intracellular binding. Very often, membrane proteins, forming receptors (beta-blocker) and ion channels (glutamate receptor antagonists), are the target structures of a drug. There are also examples of drugs targeting the structures of the intracellular compartment, e.g. the cytoskeleton (taxanes).

Many drugs make an impact on enzymatic activity (inhibitors of carboanhydrase). However, more and more substances are developed which influence promoter regions of the DNA or directly interfere with transcriptional activity. By binding the messenger RNA, small aptamers can prevent synthesis of new proteins.

Biotechnological engineering enables the design of drugs that are specifically directed against a cytokine, a surface receptor or a key step in signal transduction. The invention of the so-called 'biologicals' has revolutionized the opportunity to intervene more specifically with particular reactions by focusing on single pathophysiological sequences (Meibohm 2006). In terms of toxicity, these treatment modalities bear the risk of antigenicity. When using fully humanized proteins, specific autoantibodies can provoke loss of function. If biotechnological synthesis leaves residuals of different species, anaphylactic reactions can occur during treatment with foreign proteins.

Beside the receptor-mediated effects, mechanisms that are caused by chemical or physical interaction also have to be considered. Ophthalmologic examples are rinsing solutions neutralizing the ocular surface after alkali burn injuries.

In reality some drugs may have several mechanisms of action, for example it is possible to distinguish a fast from a slower effect. The delayed decline in the intraocular pressure by prostaglandins seems to be related to collagen degradation after the activation of metal-matrix proteases. In contrast, the early decrease in intraocular pressure within the first hours was assigned to relaxation of the trabecular meshwork after inhibition of a Ca^{2+}-dependent contraction (Thieme et al 2006).

Non-specific effects are typically mediated through a generalized effect in many organs, and the response observed depends on the distribution of the drug. It must be appreciated that many drugs exist whose sites of action have not been elucidated in detail. Furthermore, many drugs are known to bind to plasma proteins as well as to various cellular compartments without producing any obvious physiological effect.

How does a drug interact with its target?

A variety of different types of drug actions exists. Accordingly, drugs can be classified into specific categories such as agonists, antagonists, partial agonists, inverse agonists, allosteric modulators and enzyme inhibitors or activators.

Agonists bind to a receptor or site of action and produce a conformational change, which mimics the action of the normal physiological binding ligand. At low concentrations, the activity of the drug can be additive to the natural ligand. The affinity of the drug to the receptor ultimately determines the concentration necessary to produce a response. The presence of *spare receptors* becomes an important point when considering changes in the numbers of available receptors resulting from adaptive responses in chronic exposure or irreversible binding. The effect of a drug is thought to be proportional to the number of occupied receptors. Drug antagonists bind either to the receptor itself or to a component of the effector mechanism, which then prevents the agonist's action. If the antagonist-mediated inhibition can be overcome by increasing agonist concentration, ultimately reaching the same maximal effect, the antagonist is termed *competitive* (Fig. 1.1). In contrast, a *non-competitive* agonist will prevent the agonist from producing a maximal effect. If the antagonist is reversible and binds at the active site, the inhibition will be competitive.

1

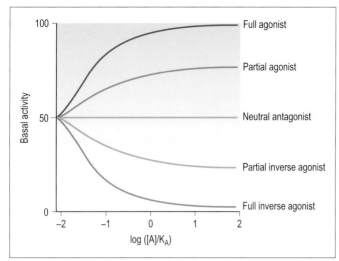

Fig. 1.1 In a constitutively active system, an antagonist modulates the activity and is defined as a full or partial inverse agonist depending on the degree of inhibition.

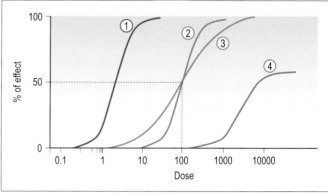

Fig. 1.2 The potency of drug 1 is higher than that of drug 2, according to a superior binding affinity. The efficacy and potency of drugs 2 and 3 are the same, but the mode of action differs. Drug 4 is less effective and less potent.

However, often the rate of binding/dissociation is not so important in determining the onset or termination of the elicited effect because such behavior mostly depends on the delivery and distribution.

Antagonists bind to the receptor without eliciting the necessary conformational changes required to produce the response effect. These drugs block access to the receptor. Most antagonists shift the dose-response curve to the right but do not alter the magnitude of the maximum response. *Functional antagonism* is defined as antagonism of tissue response that is unrelated to blockade at receptors but instead represents blockade at a site distal to receptors. Functional antagonists may affect second messenger production. Non-specific antagonism might depress all cellular excitability, e.g. by energy charge.

Receptors and signal cascades

A receptor is a macromolecule whose biological function changes when a drug binds to it. Most drugs produce their pharmacological effects by binding to specific receptors in target tissues. *Affinity* is the measure of the propensity of a drug to bind a receptor and depends on the force of attraction between drug and receptor. There are different structural and functional classifications of receptors, but generally speaking there are just a few functional families whose members share both common mechanisms of action and similarities in molecular structure. There are at least four main types.

Type 1 receptors are typically located in a membrane and are directly coupled to an ion channel. Receptors for several neurotransmitters send their signals by altering a cell's membrane potential or its ionic composition. This group includes nicotinic cholinergic receptors and γ-aminobuytric acid receptors. These receptors are all multiple subunit proteins arranged symmetrically to form a channel.

Type 2 receptors are also located in a membrane and are coupled by a G protein to an enzyme or channel. There is a large family that utilizes heterotrimeric guanosine 5'-triphosphate (GTP)-binding regulatory proteins. Ligands for G-protein receptors include eicosanoids and biogenic amines. Second messengers include adenyl cyclase, phospholipase C, Ca^{2+} currents and phosphatidyl inositol-3-kinase. G-protein-coupled receptors span the cell membrane and exist as a bundle of seven helices.

Type 3 receptors, usually located in membranes, are directly coupled to an enzyme. Receptors with inherent enzymatic activity are most commonly cell surface protein kinases. These receptors demonstrate their regulatory activity by phosphorylating various effector proteins at the inner face of the cell membrane. Phosphorylation changes the structures, biological properties and hence the biological activity.

Finally, *type 4 receptors* are located in the nucleus or cytoplasm and are coupled via DNA to gene transcription. Receptors for steroid hormones, thyroid hormones, retinoids, vitamin D and other molecules are soluble proteins and can bind DNA. These transcription factors are regulated by phosphorylation, association with other proteins, binding metabolites or regulatory ligands.

Drug-receptor binding triggers a cascade of events known as *signal transduction,* through which the target tissue responds. Within a physiologic entity there are myriad possible chemical signals that can affect multiple different processes. Subsequently, a very important, but not totally understood, property of a receptor is its specificity or the extent to which a receptor can recognize, discriminate and respond to only one signal. Some receptors demonstrate a very high degree of specificity and will bind only a signal endogenous ligand, while other receptors are less specific. In most cases the binding is transient and each binding triggers a signal. Furthermore, there may be different subtypes of a given receptor, each of which recognizes or binds to the same specific ligand but generates different intracellular responses. Spatial organization is one possible explanation why cross-talk between the pathways does not lead to tremendous confusion.

The magnitude of receptor-mediated responses can decrease with repeated drug administration, thus after exposure to catecholamines there is a progressive loss of the ability of the target site to respond. This phenomenon is termed *tachyphylaxis*. The receptor desensitization is usually reversible.

Spare receptors allow maximal response without total receptor occupancy by increasing the sensitivity of the system. Spare receptors can bind extra ligands, preventing an exaggerated response if too much ligand is present.

A question of quantity – dose-response

Characterizing the dose-response relationship in populations often is not informative enough when the inter-subject variation is relatively high. The response can vary across subjects who achieve the same concentration. In the majority of cases, the

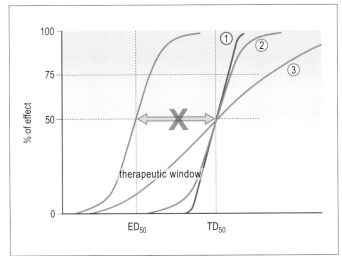

Fig. 1.3 Therapeutic width is characterized by the distance of both sensitivity curves, the therapeutic (ED_{50}, left) vs. toxic (TD_{50}, right) effect. For toxicity, curves 1, 2 and 3 illustrate the different toxic response, shown by the rate of rise. If the ratio of TD_{50}/ED_{50} is used to estimate the therapeutic width, the same value would be wrongly assumed for all three curves. In reality, the therapeutic index TD_5/ED_{95} more exactly represents the safety of a drug. The therapeutic window is sometimes given as the difference $TD_5 - ED_{95}$.

effect of a drug is dependent on the number of bound receptors, although mostly there is no linear relationship.

It is necessary to differentiate between efficacy and potency. From the clinician's point of view, the *efficacy* is more important as it stands for the maximum effect achievable (ED_{max}). ED_{50} indicates the dose of a drug that produces 50% of the maximal response. In contrast, the *potency* is a measure of the affinity and indicates which concentration has to be provided at the site of action (Fig. 1.2).

Graphically, potency is illustrated by the relative position of the dose-effect curve along the dose axis. Because a more potent drug is not necessarily clinically superior, potency has little clinical significance for a given therapeutic effect. However, low potency is a disadvantage only if it is so large that it is awkward to administer. Potency is determined by the affinity and intrinsic activity of a drug.

Pharmacodynamics is very tightly connected with toxicodynamics, both showing a very similar dose-response curve. The curve progression is characterized by the concentration where 50% (95% for LD_{95}) of the effect appears. For many years, the LD_{50} (median lethal dosage) was tested in rodents before approval of new drugs. Since 1991 LD_{50} estimations in animals have become obsolete and are no longer required for regulatory submissions as a part of preclinical development. In addition to the effect level, the relationship between time and response is crucial.

In practice, the therapeutic window is much more relevant than the maximum efficacy (treatment dosage in g or mg). Drugs with a narrow margin are more difficult to dose and administer, and may require therapeutic drug monitoring. The more innocuous a drug is, the higher is its therapeutic width (Fig. 1.3). Side effects can be classified by the dosage or the cause. *Adverse drug reactions* (ADRs) can be seen following overdose or therapeutic dose. The intended pharmacological action, effects which are independent from the primary effect or interactions with other drugs can cause undesired effects. Correspondingly, ADRs can be classified as *type A* (augmented) or *type B* (bizarre) reactions. Withdrawal

reactions, which may occur with abrupt withdrawal of some drugs, and delayed onset were assigned to type A reactions.

In overdose, increased development of the therapeutic effect often occurs. Although the patient may be prescribed a dose within the normal recommended range, impaired organ function affects clearance and may result in adverse effects. However, when the level is accordingly further increased, nearly every drug shows toxicity.

Examples for undesired effects unrelated to the primary effect are hemolytic anemia following sulfonamides, atropine-like effects in the use of tricyclic antidepressives and thrombophilia induced by contraceptives. Some serious side effects do not occur before longer lasting therapy, e.g. osteoporosis in chronic steroid treatment.

Various type B reactions are unexpected because they are unrelated to the known pharmacological action of the drug. Many of these reactions have an immunological basis, e.g. anaphylaxis with antibiotics. Others are due to genetic abnormalities such as drug-induced hemolysis in patients with glucose-6-phosphate dehydrogenase deficiency when given oxidative drugs. Allergic reactions are idiosyncratic and normally unrelated to dosage. Management of such ADRs usually requires stopping the offending drug.

Some ocular reactions (miosis, mydriasis or intraocular pressure) show a very reproducible pattern of the pharmacodynamic response. Ophthalmic pharmacological responses are therefore often used to investigate the administration and pharmacokinetics of a drug with special interest in the quantitative response.

PHARMACOKINETICS

Because a later chapter concentrates on ocular pharmacokinetics and drug delivery in detail, only some general considerations are given here.

The *bioavailability* describes the proportion of the unchanged drug delivered to the site of potential action regardless of the route of administration. To facilitate the calculation of absorption and elimination rates, a compartment is usually postulated as a space where the drug is supposed to be homogeneously distributed. *First-order kinetics* are found when the rates (absorption, elimination) are proportional to the concentration. However, usually *zero-order kinetics* are detectable for most eye drops because the rates are independent of the concentration but proportional to the functional capacity of the body.

It has been estimated that only 1–5% of the active drug enclosed in an eye drop penetrates the eye (Schoenwald 1997). The maximum bioavailability is afforded by a drop size of 20 μl. An increase in volume or number of drops only leads to systemic toxicity due to increased lacrimal outflow and mucosal absorption of the drug. Up to 80% may reach the general circulation. Otherwise, after intraocular penetration there is no first-pass metabolism. Tissue binding has to be taken into consideration, reducing the elimination process by retention.

Barriers of the eye

Despite its apparent easy accessibility, the eye is well protected against the absorption of foreign materials, including therapeutic agents. The corneal epithelium acts as a trilaminar barrier to the penetration of topical drugs. Absorption of drugs depends on their solubility: lipophilic substances seem to penetrate readily in the corneal epithelium.

Drugs administered topically will drain into the nasolacrimal duct and be absorbed through the epithelial mucosa lining into the systemic circulation. One of the reasons for this behavior is that the fornix of the lower eyelid can hold only the volume of one drop of topical medication, that is approximately 40 μl at most. Most ophthalmic drugs are adapted from other therapeutic applications and were not specifically developed for the treatment of eye disease. Hence, they are not well suited to provide eye-specific effects.

For maximal corneal drug penetration a molecule must have an optimized ratio of hydro- and lipophilicity, as non-ionized molecules penetrate the epithelium/endothelium well and ionize the stroma. The clinical state of the eye also strongly determines ocular pharmacokinetics. Transcorneal drug penetration is greater when the epithelium is altered or the corneal stroma is edematous (Ueno et al 1994). Similarly, preservatives improve the penetration of the drug (Ramselaar et al 1982). The blood ocular barrier is based on tight junctions of the non-pigmented ciliary epithelium, the retinal pigment epithelium and the retinal capillary endothelial cells. Intraocular structures are also shielded by these barriers from systemic toxins. However, these natural ocular barriers may also act as drug depots and can play an important role in the pathogenesis of drug-induced ocular toxicity.

The retinal pigment epithelium (RPE) is metabolically very active and can participate in the detoxification of various drugs. As chlorpromazine and chloroquine have an affinity to the melanin of the pigment epithelium, both drugs are metabolized by the RPE and are, therefore, retinotoxic (Koneru et al 1986).

Factors affecting the availability of drugs

Surfactants increase the solubility of hydrophilic drugs by altering the permeability of epithelial membranes. Solutions with high viscosity increase the contact time of a drug on the cornea. The pH determines the degree of ionization of a drug. Since the pH of tears is slightly alkaline (7.4) many ocular drugs are weak bases (alkaloids), existing in both their charged and uncharged forms at that pH. However, if the pH of the solution is made more basic then more uncharged forms of the molecule are present, resulting in increased lipid solubility and epithelial penetration.

After systemic administration, the ability of blood-borne agents to reach the globe depends on the lipid solubility, the plasma protein binding (only the unbound form is bioavailable) and the molecular weight (Worakul and Robinson 1997; Moorthy and Valluri 1999). Calculating the *loading dose* of a drug is similar to calculating the amount of drug required to achieve a desired concentration in a predefined volume. This ratio can also be used to estimate the top-up dose that may be required if the drug is already present but the concentration is too low. Drugs start to be eliminated as soon as they are absorbed. Target drugs can, therefore, only be maintained if doses are given at a rate that balances the clearance rate. *Maintenance dosage* regimens are designed to achieve this balance. The time to reach this steady state depends only on the *half-life* of the drug.

Understanding the reasons for pharmacokinetic variability and adjusting drug doses accordingly can make a major impact on risk management and patient care. Besides the genetic background, we know many sources for variability related to observable clinical characteristics. Age, gender, weight and hormonal status are important. The elimination of the drug and therefore renal and liver function are determinant factors.

When describing the pharmacokinetic properties of a chemical, the four points of absorption, distribution, metabolism and excretion (ADME) are considered. A pharmacokinetic system can be determined to be linear or non-linear, and time-invariant or time-varying with respect to the modeling.

Many of the clinically significant interactions between drugs are pharmacokinetic in origin. Not only can induction/inhibition of metabolizing enzymes occur, but also direct competition for transport mechanisms can influence tissue distribution and accumulation. Drugs competing for albumin are phenylbutazone and warfarine, therefore each affects the distribution of the other. Thyroxine influences the absorption of calcium. Probenecid vies with penicillin for renal excretion.

Important pathways, such as the microsomal cytochrome P_{450} monooxygenase, are known to be inducible, but also genetically determined. These enzymes act on structurally unrelated drugs. In phase I of biotransformation drugs are made more polar by oxidation, reduction and hydrolytic reactions, before phase II reaction results in drug inactivation by conjugation (glucuronidation, sulfation, acetylation). Mutations in the cytochrome P_{450} monooxygenase lead to slower metabolizing of drugs. The application of pharmacogenetics therefore holds great promise for an optimized, individualized therapy. However, there is little clinical impact at present because of the complex variability of the pharmacology (different pathways, active metabolites), leading to a high level of operating expense. The benefits of prospective testing still need to be weighed against the costs.

PHARMACOLOGY PRINCIPLES

When designing drug regimens it is important to consider the risks and limitations of medical treatment. We recommend paying attention to the following 10 reminders of what not to do.

1) Do not be ignorant of the pharmacology

General pharmacology often is not an exciting issue. Complicated and unusual names of agents, difficult schemes of dosages and biochemical pathways do not invite the study of the basics of pharmacologic treatment. However, the effective therapy is intimately connected with the pathophysiology of a disease as designing selective inhibitors to a cytokine or receptor has become feasible. Although it is often not a simple story, the knowledge of the background facilitates the choice of the appropriate therapeutic approach.

In terms of legal advice, a physician's liability is based on negligence, the legal equivalent of malpractice. Professional negligence means that a professional person (physician, pharmacist) acting within the scope of his or her reputation has performed in a substandard fashion, causing a person to suffer damages. Physicians may be negligent in two ways – by failing to do something or by doing something incorrectly (Francisco 1990). When a physician has not been obviously negligent by inappropriately prescribing a drug, many considerations are examined to determine whether a physician's conduct fell below the requisite standard of care.

Some questions are raised before a legal proceeding: Was the physician aware of the risks involved prescribing the medication, and, if the physician was not aware, should he or she have been? Were there warnings included in the pharmaceutical manufacturer's literature that were not followed? Would a physician read the literature in exercising reasonable care? Were the expected benefits of use of that particular drug sufficient to justify exposing the patients to the risks? Were specific tests recommended in the literature that the physician failed to perform before initiating the drug? Should the physician have noticed the adverse effect of the drug when it occurred and taken countermeasures? Could the medication have been stopped in time to avoid injury?

2) Do not mix too many drugs

Maintaining an overview of the situation can be difficult, especially in challenging situations. If the therapeutic benefit is still missing in the presence of psychological strain, the physician is at risk of escalating the therapeutic regimen by just adding further drugs.

Blind polypragmasia ('If a little is good, more is better') rarely achieves an improvement. In combining too many remedies, it is not possible to differentiate between the effects of several drugs and acknowledge the exact agent responsible for the observed side effects or therapeutic response. Do not prescribe any medication unless it is absolutely needed and discontinue use of the drug as soon as possible.

3) Do not forget the aim of treatment

The strategy of the approach should always include a clear definition of the therapeutic target. Even though the therapy sometimes makes the diagnosis, it is important to clarify the suspected problem before looking for the solution. Waiting for a further course of the disease and defining the suspected diagnosis exactly might be wiser in some situations before intensified treatment is considered. For example, in the case of intraocular lymphoma, (steroid) treatment should be stopped before diagnostic vitrectomy in order to harvest enough significant cells.

Controlling the success of therapy is essential. Although only a few drugs need special biomonitoring, the drug concentration has to be assessed if the high variability of bioavailability fails to meet the therapeutic window, e.g. in systemic cyclosporine therapy. Other agents only require additional safety assessment. Because tamoxifen, chloroquine, amiodarone and cetirizin are reported to produce ocular toxicity, clinicians are usually careful to note their particular toxicities.

Control of the outcome is also important in general treatment for several reasons. First, non-responders would otherwise not be detected. Second, it should not be forgotten that most patients expect a final examination giving them positive feedback. Telling patients that their disease has been cured or at least stability has been achieved can give an additional feeling of safety. This may be of major importance in improving individual compliance in chronic diseases. Finally, recognizing potential adverse events (and reporting them to the United States Food and Drug Administration (US FDA) or equivalent) is the physician's liability (Kaufman and Soukides 1994). Without looking for side effects no toxicity would be identified. Systemic adverse effects of topical ocular treatment are not easy to recognize. We need an optimum level of alertness and an interdisciplinary comprehension.

4) Do not taper anti-infective drugs

For many drugs it is mandatory to adjust the dosage in accordance with the development of the disease. Immunosuppressives are a prime example, where tapering reduces side effects, while fine adjustment allows the possibility of inflammatory activity developing over time. If dose reduction is too fast, tapering may lead to recurring activity (rebound phenomena).

To a certain extent, varying the frequency at which eye drops are administered provides an additional tool for adapting dosage. For example, repeated applications are able to achieve the same levels in aqueous humor as a subconjunctival injection. However, in antibiotics the therapeutic range usually is very limited. The width of the therapeutic window is restricted by the required effective dosage (Mattie 1993).

Using antibiotic agents for too long and with an insufficient dosage is not only the reason for ineffective treatment, but can increase the risk of developing resistance (Gaynor et al 2005). Anti-infective drugs should always be stopped abruptly and never tapered.

5) Do not overestimate patient compliance

'Real world' conditions are often very different from theoretical considerations. Although a combination of multiple drugs might be necessary in the advanced stage of a disease and frequent administration can achieve higher drug concentrations, the ability to apply drugs as frequently as prescribed may be restricted for the average patient (Buller 2006).

Blinded prospective studies have evaluated application behavior in detail and have shown that non-compliance is very often the limiting factor (Stewart et al 2004; Herrmann and Diestelhorst 2006). The issue is even more relevant in permanent treatment, e.g. with anti-glaucomatous drugs.

With higher frequency dosing and an increasing number of drugs, a growing number of patients do not comply with drug therapy recommendations. However, there are ways of overcoming these problems. An exact written plan helps the patient to follow the prescription. This should explain how to administer the drug and discuss side effects clearly. Administration is an important issue, especially for older or disabled patients. The dose regimen should be critically optimized for the individual patient to address administration issues. Explaining the background and convincing the patient of the necessity of the planned treatment and its aim can strongly improve the acceptance of the drug (Gardiner and Dvorkin 2006).

6) Do not disregard patients' warnings

Incompatibility and allergic predisposition mostly arise with clear symptoms. Nearly all symptoms related to adverse effects are recognized by the patient. It therefore seems wise to listen carefully to the (sometimes bizarre) reports of the patients' experiences. Depending on what they say, the medication can be adapted.

Drug-induced allergy remains a relatively rare situation, occurring in a small percentage of patients, mostly in the early course of treatment. For the ocular surface, preservatives are major sources of allergic reaction (Baudouin 2005).

Other clinical manifestations may also be related to the toxicity of the drug without the occurrence of allergic reactions. Corneal punctuate staining can occur on account of the agent. Previous studies have illustrated the importance of discriminating early, acute allergic reactions from often more delayed toxic and non-specific inflammatory mechanisms that may require some time to occur or result from indirect inflammatory mechanisms.

7) Do not underestimate drug interactions

Because the tear turnover is 30%/min (following 1 drop, non-irritated eye 15%/min), drops wash out in approximately 5 minutes. This is the minimum time interval between drops. Concurrent use of individual preparations has shown much lower concentrations than achieved with a fixed combination.

In terms of pharmacodynamics, the interaction between different anti-glaucomatous drugs is very well studied. There are many examples where combined treatment does not induce additive or synergistic effects, for example pilocarpin added to prostaglandins seems not to produce an additive decrease in intraocular pressure effect (Toor et al 2005). When the interacting drug has a long elimination half-life, the interaction may persist for some time after the drug has been discontinued. It is important to consider potential interactions not only when two drugs are given together but also when one is stopped.

8) Do not to forget whom to treat

We have to keep in mind that several subgroups of patients are at higher risk of developing side effects. A very important example is treatment during pregnancy, when toxicity and placental transfer must be evaluated in addition to other factors (Chung et al 2004). Data are very limited as large-scale population surveillance is needed to detect individual drug teratogenicity. Researchers are often not willing to invest funds in research that will most likely give a negative association between the two variables studied.

Reasonable care must also be used in children. Besides absolute contraindications (e.g. brimonidine) some drugs have to be weighted in the individual situation (Bowman et al 2004). Topical application offers lower systemic exposure and sometimes enables the use of drugs that are not harmless when applied systemically in children (e.g. chinolones). However, recent FDA warnings for children include some topical medications (e.g. pimecrolimus/tacrolimus ointment because of the potential cancer risk). Changes in clearance vary with age. When there is a special need for dose adjustment, we strongly recommend consultation with pediatricians.

Because of the increasing longevity of the population, a growing number of very old people are exposed to medications. The average number of drugs is five per patient for patients over 65 years old (Labetoulle et al 2005; Wotquenne et al 2006). Geriatric dosing is problematic because of possible drug interactions. Drug therapy in this population is also difficult because changes in body composition, malnutrition and renal failure can cause drug accumulation and toxicity. Liver function and cytochrome P_{450} metabolism can also be affected (Gardiner and Begg 2006). Physicians should therefore always be particularly careful when prescribing drugs to pregnant women, children or elderly patients.

9) Do not mix drops and ointments

Most drugs are available in different formulations, for example as eye drops and ointments at the same time. Different therapies have different advantages and disadvantages. Drops allow faster visual rehabilitation because the effect on the pre-corneal tear film and visual acuity is less pronounced. In the presence of corneal ulcers or erosions, eye drops do not interfere with re-epithelialization. Preservative-free drops can even be used together with bandage contact lenses.

In contrast, ointments have the advantage of increased drug contact time. If the administration is difficult, prolonged concentration can be maintained. Ointments may, however, also act as a barrier to the penetration of other drops. The slow release of some agents from the ointment may result in sub-therapeutic levels of the drug. In contrast, preservatives and antibiotics (e.g. aminoglycosides) can cause damage to the corneal epithelium if contained in the ointment (Napper et al 2003).

10) Do not disregard alternative approaches and recommendations of how to behave in daily life

The acceptance of a drug treatment is much higher if the patient receives the impression that he or she is able to actively fight the disease. In contrast, if they experience a loss of control, patients find it more difficult to cope with the treatment burden. The extent to which any patient adheres to a medical regimen is an essential determinant of clinical success.

Although the perception of disease depends on many different factors, it is possible to satisfy individual demands. A holistic perspective also takes psychosomatic complaints and factors seriously.

There is not a wide base of evidence for the effectiveness of alternative treatment options. Nonetheless, if a patient insists on a treatment attempt, it is important to keep contact and perform control examinations regularly. In terms of toxicity there is not a great difference between approved drugs and homespun remedies (Fraunfelder et al 2003). Because of their widespread use, ophthalmologists should be aware of nutritional supplements and herbal medicines (West et al 2006) and their side effects.

REFERENCES AND FURTHER READING

Baudouin C. Allergic reaction to topical eyedrops. Curr Opin Allergy Clin Immunol 5: 459–463, 2005.

Bowman RJC, Cope J, Nishal KK. Ocular and systemic side effects of brimonidine 0.2% eye drops in children. Eye 18: 24–26, 2004.

Buller A, Hercules BL. Should patients choose their own eyedrops? Acta Ophthalmol Scan 84: 150–151, 2006.

Chung CY, Kwok AKH, Chung KL. Use of ophthalmic medications during pregnancy. Hong Kong Med J 10: 191–195, 2004.

Francisco CJ. Liability for adverse drug reactions. Tex Med 86: 42–46, 1990.

Fraunfelder FW, Fraunfelder FT, Goetsch RA. Adverse effects from over-the-counter lice shampoo. Arch Ophthalmol 121: 1790–1791, 2003.

Gardiner SJ, Begg EJ. Pharmacogenetics, drug-metabolizing enzymes and clinical practice. Pharmacol Rev 58: 521–590, 2006.

Gardiner P, Dvorkin L. Promoting medication adherence in children. Am Fam Physician 74: 793–798, 2006.

Gaynor BD, Chidambaran JD, Cevallos V, et al. Topical ocular antibiotics induce bacterial resistance at extraocular sites. Br J Ophthalmol 89: 1097–1099, 2005.

Herrmann MM, Diestelhorst M. Microprocessor controlled compliance monitor for eye drop medication. Br J Ophthalmol 90: 830–832, 2006.

Kaufman MB, Soukides CA. Physician's liability for adverse drug reactions. South Med J 87: 780–784, 1994.

Koneru PB, Lien EJ, Koda RT. Oculotoxicities of systemically administered drugs. J Ocul Pharmacol 2: 385–404, 1986.

Labetoulle M, Frau E, LeJeune C. Systemic adverse effects of topical ocular treatments. Presse Med 34: 589–595, 2005.

Langley JN. On the sympathetic system of birds, and on the muscles which move the feathers. J Physiol 30: 221–252, 1904.

Mattie H. The importance of pharmacokinetics and pharmacodynamics for effective treatment of infections. Clin Invest 71: 480–482, 1993.

Meibohm B. The role of pharmacokinetics and pharmacodynamics in the development of biotech drugs. In: Meibohm B (ed.). Pharmacokinetics and pharmacokinetics of Biotech Drugs: Principles and Case Studies in Drug Development. Wiley-VSH GmbH & Co, Weinheim, pp 3–13, 2006.

Moorthy RS, Valluri S. Ocular toxicity associated with systemic drug therapy. Curr Opin Ophthalmol 10: 438–446, 1999.

Napper G, Douglass I, Albietz J. Preservative and antibiotic toxicity to the ocular surface. Clin Exp Optom 86: 414–415, 2003.

Olson MK. Are novel drugs more risky for patients than less novel drugs? J Health Econ 23: 1135–1158, 2004.

Ramselaar JA, Boot JP, van Haeringen NJ, et al. Corneal epithelial permeability after instillation of ophthalmic solutions containing anaesthetics and preservatives. Curr Eye Res 7: 947–950, 1982.

Schoenwald RD. Ocular pharmacokinetics. In: Zimmermann TJ, Koonerm KS, Sharir M, Fechtner RD (eds), Textbook of Ocular Pharmacology. 9th edn. Lippincott-Raven, Philadelphia, pp, 119–138, 1997.

Stewart WC, Konstas AG, Pfeiffer N. Patient and ophthalmologist attitudes concerning compliance and dosing in glaucoma treatment. J Ocul Pharmacol 20: 461–469, 2004.

Thieme H, Schimmat C, Munzer G, et al. Endothelin antagonism: effects of FP receptor agonists prostaglandin F2alpha and fluprostenol on trabecular meshwork contractility. Invest Ophthalmol Vis Sci 47: 938–945, 2006.

Toor A, Chanis RA, Polikoff LA, et al. Additivity of pilocarpine to bimatoprost in ocular hypertension and early glaucoma. J Glaucoma 14: 243–248, 2005.

Ueno N, Refojo MF, Abelson MB. Pharmacokinetics. In: Albert DA, Jakobiec FA (eds), Principles and Practice of Ophthalmology 74, Basic Sciences, WB Saunders Company, Philadelphia, pp 916–926, 1994.

West AL, Oren GA, Moroi SE. Evidence for the use of nutritional supplements and herbal medicines in common eye diseases. Am J Ophthalmol 141: 157–166, 2006.

Worakul N, Robinson JR. Ocular pharmacokinetics/pharmacodynamics. Eur J Pharmac Biopharm 44: 71–83, 1997.

Wotquenne P, Petermanns J, Scheen AJ. Drug therapy in the elderly. What should we know? Rev Med Suisse 23: 1878–1883, 2006.

PART 2

Ocular drug delivery and toxicology

Frederick T. Fraunfelder, MD

Drug delivery to the eye is a complex process. As a self-contained system, the eye is unique in the body in many ways that affect pharmacology and toxicology. It includes several different cell types, and functions as a complete, self-contained system. The rate and efficacy of drug delivery differ in healthy and diseased eyes. Variables affecting delivery include age, genetic ancestry and route of administration. The complexities of delivery, toxicology or both are greatly influenced by patient compliance, especially in the management of glaucoma, which requires multiple topical ocular medications given at one sitting each day or multiple times daily. Each method of drug delivery modifies the therapeutic and toxicological response.

Ocular toxicology is dependent on the concentration of the drug, frequency of application, speed of removal, and whether the drug reaches sensitive cells such as the corneal endothelium, lens epithelium or macula in toxic concentrations. Of equal importance is the vehicle for delivery and the pH, buffering systems and preservatives necessary for optimum drug delivery. Each adds its own potentially toxic effect to this complex picture. Originally, much of ocular pharmacology and toxicology was conducted by trial and error, often with local corner pharmacies compounding medications. Today the ocular pharmaceutical industry is acutely aware of potential problems and is continuously researching and producing medications with fewer side effects, delivered by newer and better medications.

TOPICAL OCULAR ADMINISTRATION

This is by far the most commonly used method of drug delivery to the eye. Topically administered medications are convenient, easy to reapply and relatively inexpensive. This method concentrates the pharmacological activity of the drug in the eye while limiting systemic reactions. Local toxic responses are increased, however, especially with lifelong use as with glaucoma medications. Unlike medication given orally, topical ocular medications reach systemic circulation while avoiding the first-order pass effect through the liver. A drug absorbed through the nasal mucosa or conjunctiva 'drains' to the right atrium and ventricle. The blood containing the drug is then pumped to the head before returning to the left atrium and ventricle. The second passage is through the liver, where the primary detoxification occurs before going to the right atrium. When medications are orally administered, the first pass includes absorption from the gut through the liver, where, depending on the drug, up to 90% of the agent is detoxified before going to the right atrium. Thus oral medications are metabolized during the first pass, while ocular or nasally administered drugs are not metabolized until the second pass. This is the reason why therapeutic blood levels, and accompanying systemic side effects, may occur from topical ocular medications. Other factors include racial differences in metabolism, as with timolol. One per cent of people with Japanese or Chinese genetic ancestry, 2.4% of African Americans and 8% of those with European ancestry do not have the p-450 enzyme CYP2D6 that is necessary to metabolize this drug. The lack of this enzyme significantly enhances systemic blood levels of timolol (Edeki et al 1995).

BASIC PHARMACOLOGY AND TOXICOLOGY OF TOPICAL MEDICATIONS

Ocular toxicology is based on pharmacokinetics – how the drug is absorbed, including its distribution, metabolism and elimination – as well as pharmacodynamics, the action of the drug on the body. This bioavailability is influenced by age, body weight, sex and eye pigmentation. It is also affected by the disease process, interactions with other drugs and mode of delivery. Only a small percentage of any topically applied drug enters the eye. At best, 1–10% of topical ocular solutions are absorbed by ocular tissues (Schoenwald 1985). This absorption is governed by ocular contact time, drug concentration, tissue permeability and the characteristics of the cornea and pericorneal tissue. Nearly all solutions will leave the conjunctival sac, or cul-de-sac, within 15 to 30 seconds of application (Shell 1982). The average volume of the cul-de-sac is 7 μL, with 1 additional μL in the precorneal tear film (Mishima et al 1966). The cul-de-sac may hold 25–30 μL of an eyedrop; however, blinking will decrease this volume markedly and rapidly, so that at most only 10 μL remains for longer then a few seconds. The drop size of commercial drugs varies from 25 to more than 56 μL (Mishima et al 1966). In a healthy eye, one not traumatized by disease, lid manipulation to instill the drug will double or triple the normal basal tear flow exchange rate of 16% per minute, thereby decreasing ocular contact time via dilution (Mishima et al 1966).

The cornea is the primary site of intraocular drug absorption from topical drug application. This is a complex process that favors small, moderately lipophilic drugs that are partially non-ionized under physiologic conditions. While the cornea is a five-layer structure, it has significant barriers to absorption into the eye. It can be visualized as three layers, like a sandwich, with a hydrophilic stroma flanked by lipophilic epithelium and endothelial layers (Mishima et al 1966).

Topically administered drugs are also absorbed via the conjunctiva, sclera and lacrimal system. The total surface area of the conjunctiva is 17 times the corneal surface area (Mishima et al 1966). The conjunctiva allows absorption of lipophilic agents to a lesser degree than the cornea, but is relatively permeable to hydrophilic drugs. The sclera is porous via nerve and blood vessel tracts, but otherwise fairly resistant to penetration. Hydrophilic agents may pass through it 80 times faster than through the cornea (Mishima et al 1966); however, the lacrimal system can remove the drug 100 times faster than the cornea and conjunctiva absorb it (Van Ooteghem 1987).

Clearly overflow from every administration of eye drops occurs not only over the eyelid but also in the lacrimal outflow system. Lynch and Brown (1987) showed that 2.5% phenylephrine topically applied to the eyes of newborn babies in 8 or 30 µL aliquots produced no difference in pupillary response. However, neonates who received the 30 µL dosage had double the plasma concentrations of phenylephrine of those who received 8 µL, increasing the potential for systemic complications.

INTRAOCULAR DISTRIBUTION

Once a drug reaches the inside of the eye, anatomical barriers play a major role in where it ends up. Drugs that enter primarily through the cornea seldom penetrate behind the lens. The pattern of aqueous humor flow and the physical barriers of the iris and ciliary body help to keep the drug anterior. It is not uncommon for a drug to be more concentrated in the ciliary body than the aqueous humor due to scleral absorption directly into the ciliary body with less fluid exchange than in the aqueous humor. In addition, pigmented tissue reacts differently to different drugs. For example, lipid-soluble mydriatics that are more slowly absorbed by pigmented cells will dilate dark pupils more slowly, resulting in longer duration but a decrease in maximum dilation (Harris and Galin 1971).

Drug distribution is markedly affected by eye inflammation. Tissue permeability is increased, allowing greater drug availability. However, as Mikkelson et al (1973) have demonstrated, protein binding may decrease drug availability 75–100% in inflamed eyes. The protein-drug complex decreases bioavailability. Increases in aqueous or tear protein, such as mucus, are also factors in bioavailability, as is the increased tearing that may wash away a drug before it can be absorbed (Mikkelson et al 1973).

PRESERVATIVES

Preservatives are an important part of topical ocular medications, not only to prolong shelf life but also to disrupt the corneal and conjunctival epithelium to allow greater drug penetration. Preservatives such as benzalkonium have been shown to have antibacterial properties almost as great as those of topical ocular antibiotics. Even in exceedingly low concentrations benzalkonium causes significant cell damage by emulsification of the cell wall lipids. De Saint Jean et al (1999) report cell growth arrest

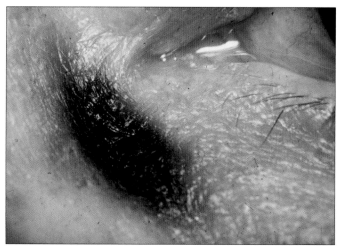

Fig. 2.1 Chronic use of silver nitrate solutions causes staining of the lacrimal sac and surrounding tissue.

and death at concentrations as low as 0.0001%. Short-term use seldom causes clinically significant damage to healthy corneas and conjunctiva other than superficial epithelial changes. However, with long term use, e.g. in patients with glaucoma and dry eye, preservatives in topical eye medication may cause adverse effects. Hong et al (2006) have shown induction of squamous metaplasia by chronic application of glaucoma medications containing preservatives. This may progress to more severe side effects, as shown in Table 2.1.

VEHICLES FOR TOPICAL OCULAR MEDICATION DELIVERY

Aqueous solutions: With aqueous solutions, all ingredients are fully dissolved within a solution. Benefits include easy application and few visual side effects. The main drawback is a short ocular contact time, which leads to poor absorption and limited bioavailability. Nevertheless, this still is the most commonly used means of delivering topical ocular medications. Solutions may congregate in the lacrimal sac (Fig. 2.1).

Suspensions: With this vehicle, the active ingredient is in a fine particulate form suspended in a saturated solution of the same medication. This method allows for longer contact time with greater bioavailability. Its drawbacks include the necessity of vigorously shaking the container prior to application and a possible increase in foreign body sensation after application because of the deposition of particles in the corneal tear film.

Ointments: These consist of a semi-solid lipoid preparation containing a lipid-soluble drug. They are designed to melt at body temperature and are dispersed by the shearing action of blinking. Ointments are frequently entrapped in lashes, fornices and canthal areas, which are capable of acting as reservoirs. They can also become entrapped in corneal defects (Fig. 2.2), for example ointment at the base of the lashes comes in contact with the skin. Since ointment will melt when it comes in contact with the skin, the ointment at the base of the lashes reaches the eye in a continuous process of becoming entrapped in the lashes and re-melting into the eye. Ointments have high bioavailability and require less frequent dosing than other methods, but suffer by being difficult to administer. Other problems include variable dosing (it is difficult to control the amount applied) and possible unacceptability to patients due to blurred vision and cosmetic disfigurement.

Table 2.1 – Preservative Ocular Side Effects	
Eyelids and Conjunctiva	**Cornea**
Allergic reactions	Punctate keratitis
Hyperemia	Edema
Erythema	Pseudomembrane formation
Blepharitis	Decreased epithelial microvilli
Conjunctiva-papillary	Vascularization
Edema	Scarring
Pemphigoid lesion with symblepharon	Delayed wound healing
Squamous metaplasia	Increased transcorneal permeability
Contact allergies	Decreased stability of tear film Squamous metaplasia

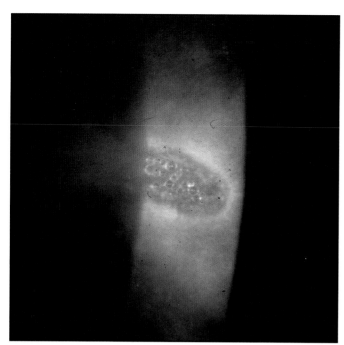

Fig. 2.2 Corneal defects may entrap ointment on the surface, creating ointment globules.

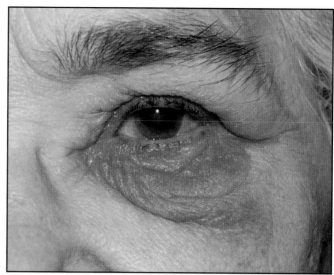

Fig. 2.3 Allergic reaction.

Pledgets: Pledgets, small absorbent pads saturated with medication, may be used to deliver high concentrations of drug directly to the ocular surface for relatively prolonged periods of time. This method of drug delivery to the eye is not US FDA approved. Recently, pledgets of vasoconstrictors to limit bleeding in keratorefractive surgery have been shown to cause significant systemic reactions, including hypertension, cardiac arrest, subarachnoid hemorrhage, convulsions and death (Fraunfelder et al 2002).

Injections: Subconjunctival injections allow low volumes of medication to be concentrated locally, with high bioavailability and limited systemic side effects. Wine et al suggest that the mechanism of drug delivery may in part be simple leakage of the drug through the needle puncture site with subsequent absorption through the cornea. McCartney et al (1965) showed that subconjunctival injections of hydrocortisone did penetrate the overlying sclera and that the injection site should be located directly over the area of pathology.

Intracameral injections are administered directly to the anterior chamber of the eye and are most frequently used to place viscoelastics. While small amounts of antibiotics may also be administered, some of these drugs pose risks to the corneal endothelium, and cataracts, corneal opacities, anterior uveitis or neovascularization are possible.

Intravitreal injections have enjoyed increased popularity due to their efficacy against some forms of macular degeneration, bacterial and fungal enophthalmitis, and viral retinitis. Each drug has its own toxicity profile; however, these injections are so commonly done that the volumes, concentrations and vehicles are well tested and complications are within an acceptable risk-benefit ratio.

Other delivery devices: Ocuserts (small plastic membranes impregnated with medication), collagen corneal shields (biodegradable contact-lens shaped clear films made to dissolve within 12 to 72 hours), contact lenses and various other delivery systems, including nanoparticles, liposomes, emulsions and gels, have either made it to market with limited success or are still in the research pipeline. Other systems that aim to deliver drugs effectively to the anterior segment are in development, including Unidoser, EyeInstill, Optimyst, Visine Pure Tears and intraocular or intravitreal implants of various types.

TOXICITY RESPONSES

Anterior segment: Toxicity produces an inflammatory response without prior exposure to the host, whereas hypersensitivity responses require prior exposure. In general, allergic reactions involve repeated exposure to the antigen and sufficiently elapsed time to allow the immune system to react. Depending on the potency of the sensitizing agent or the strength of the immune system, this may vary from a few days to years (Abelson et al 2005). The clinical diagnosis of a toxic response is usually presumptive, while in allergic reactions conjunctival scraping may reveal esophiles or basophiles. One of the most common signs of ocular toxicity from topical medication is hyperemia. This reaction includes burning and irritation, usually without itching, occurring after starting an offending agent, with classic symptoms of intracanthal eyelid edema and erythema (Fig. 2.3). There are no definitive confirmatory tests. In more severe cases, a papillary hyperemia with a watery mucoid type of discharge is evident. If the cornea is involved this may present as a superficial punctuate keratitis, usually more severe inferiorly or infernasally. Occasionally, intraepithelial microcysts may be seen, although these are more commonly seen with chemical toxicity. If the reaction is severe enough or goes unrecognized, it may become full blown with corneal ulceration, limbal neovascularization, anterior uveitis, cataracts and damage to the lacrimal outflow system. The diagnosis is confirmed if clearing occurs after stopping the offending drug and the eye and adenexa improve markedly.

Drugs can induce a condition such as ocular pemphigoid, a syndrome of non-progressive toxic reactions, which are self-limiting once the drug is discontinued. This condition is clinically and histologically identical to idiopathic ocular pemphigoid and includes a conjunctival cictrical process with scarring of the fornix and tarsal conjunctiva, corneal and conjunctival keratization, corneal vascularization, and lacrimal outflow scarring with occlusion.

Almost any type of pathology can be seen as a result of a toxic response in the anterior segment. Every structure of the anterior segment can be affected by drug toxicity. Frequently, more than one agent in topically applied medications can produce tissue

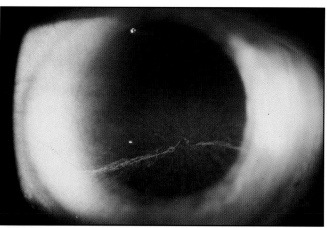

Fig. 2.4 Amiodarone keratopathy, secondary to the drug being secreted in the tears.

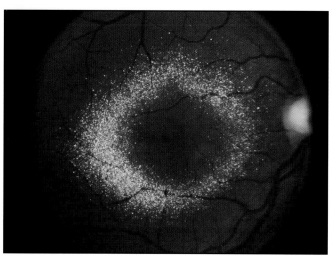

Fig. 2.5 Canthaxantin perimacular deposition.

changes. Systemic medications affect the anterior segment via secretion of the drug into the tears and changes are usually due to the drug or its metabolites (Fig. 2.4). If the drug is secreted in the tears and deposited in the conjunctiva or cornea, it may produce changes in color vision or other visual changes. The key to recognizing a toxic response is a high degree of suspicion that the pattern of symptoms and signs is not characteristic for the clinician's differential diagnosis. A toxic effect is due to a pharmacologic effect from a drug that damages a structure or disturbs its function. An irritation is an inflammatory effect, unrelated to sensitization or cellular immunity.

Ciliary body: Ciliary body ultrasound has shown bilateral choroidal effusions caused by various systemic drugs that may cause bilateral narrow angle glaucoma.

Lens: It is difficult to identify which drugs are weak cataractogenic agents, since these studies require large numbers of patients. Findings are also difficult to confirm, since instrumentation or classification systems are often cumbersome and costly. Some drugs used in the past, such as MER-29 (triparanol), caused acute lens changes, but cataractogenic drugs in current use are slow to cause lens changes, which may take many years to develop. In general, a drug-induced lens change is fairly specific for that drug. For example, both topical and systemic corticosteroid medications produce posterior subcapsular opacities. Early recognition may in some cases reverse these changes, but this is rare for almost all drug-induced cataracts.

Posterior segment: As newer classes of drugs are introduced, we are seeing more adverse retinal and optic nerve abnormalities. While in the past visual acuity, color vision testing and ophthalmoscopy were our primary tools for investigating retinal and optic nerve changes, electrophysiology testing is now being used with improved instrumentation and better standardization of methodology (see Chapter 4). Drugs can cause blood vessels to narrow, dilate, leak, swell and hemorrhage. They can also cause pigmentary changes, photoreceptor damage or inflammation. There can be deposition of the drug or its metabolites into the retina as well as lipidosis. A drug can cause edema of the choroid, exudative detachment or retinal detachment (Fig. 2.5).

Elevation of intraocular pressure: Adverse ocular effects may cause acute glaucoma by dilation of the pupil or ciliary body effusions, by vasodilatation, by affecting the mucopolysaccharides in the trabecula, secondary to uveitis or by means of a substance that interferes with aqueous outflow.

Neurologic disorders: Multiple drugs can affect the extraocular muscles, causing weakness or paralysis, which in turn lead to ptosis, nystagmus, oculogyric crisis or lid retraction. Direct neurotoxicity to the retina or optic nerve can occur, as can secondary optic nerve edema from benign intracranial hypertension.

Miscellaneous: Eyelash, eyebrow and orbital disturbance reactions such as poliosis, madarosis and exopthalmos or enophthalmos can also occur.

Newer methods of delivery and new drugs have brought on side effects and toxicities previously not seen or recognized. The various metabolic pathways of patients and multiple variables such as drug, food or disease interactions make recognition more difficult. Also, the basic incidence is often small, which makes an association difficult to prove.

HOW TO APPLY TOPICAL OCULAR MEDICATION

Applying Medication to Someone Else (Fraunfelder 1999)

1. Tilt the person's head back so he or she is looking up toward the ceiling. Grasp the lower eyelid below the lashes and gently pull it away from the eye (Fig. 2.6a).
2. Apply one drop of solution or a match-head-sized amount of ointment into the pocket between the lid and the eye (Fig. 2.6b). The external eye holds only about one-quarter to one-half of a drop so don't waste medicine by applying two drops.

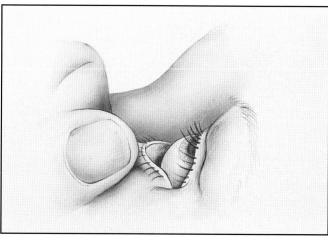

Fig. 2.6a

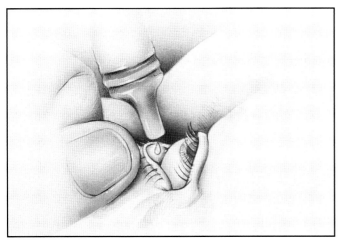

Fig. 2.6b

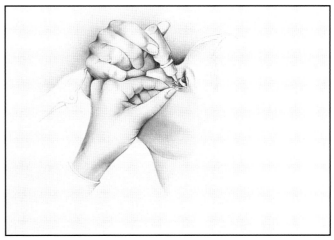

Fig. 2.7a

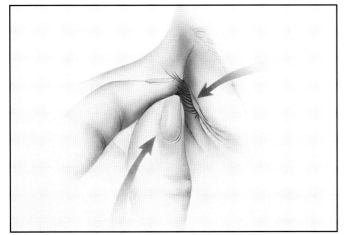

Fig. 2.6c

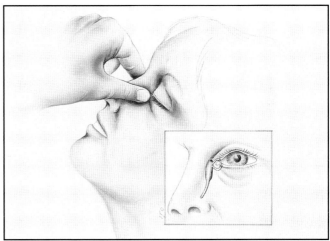

Fig. 2.7b

3. As the person looks down, gently lift the lower eyelid to make contact with the upper lid (Fig. 2.6c). The person should keep their eyelid closed for 3 minutes.

Applying your own medication (Fraunfelder 1999)

1. Tilt your head back. Rest your hand on your cheek and grasp your lower eyelid below the lashes. Gently lift the lid away from your eye. Next, hold the dropper over and as near to your eye as you feel is safe, resting the hand holding the dropper on the hand holding your eyelid (Fig. 2.7a).

2. Look up and apply one drop of the medication into the pocket between the lid and the eye. Close the eyelid and keep it closed for 3 minutes. Blot away any excess medication before opening your eye.

When applying eye medications it is best to ask someone else to apply them for you. It is very important to wash your hands before applying eye medication. The person receiving medication should keep their eyes closed for 3 minutes after application. Blot excess fluid from the inner corner of the lids before opening the eyes. This is especially important with glaucoma medication. Wait 5 to 10 minutes between drug applications when applying more than one eye medication. All medications should be kept at room temperature because cool solutions stimulate tearing. This causes the drug to be diluted and may cause epiphoria.

Lid closure has been well documented as dramatically increasing ocular contact time and decreasing lacrimal drainage (Fraunfelder 1976). Zimmerman et al (1992) demonstrated that merely closing the eyelids for 3 minutes can decrease plasma concentrations of timolol by 65% when measured 60 minutes after topical application. Likewise, the therapeutic benefits of nasolacrimal occlusion are substantial, particularly for drugs absorbed from non-conjunctival routes. Pressure over the lacrimal sac can allow for a decrease in both the frequency and dose of topical ocular agents (Fig. 2.7b). It may be difficult for patients to perform nasolacrimal occlusion routinely, so this technique is not used as frequently as it should be.

REFERENCES AND FURTHER READING

Abelson MB, Torkildsen G, Shapiro A. Thinking outside the eyedropper. Rev Ophthalmol 12: 78–80, 2005.

De Saint Jean M, Brignole F, Bringuier AF, et al. Effects of benzalkonium chloride on growth and survival of change conjunctival cells. Invest Ophthalmol Vis Sci 40: 619–630, 1999.

Edeki T, He H, Wood AJ. Pharmacogenetic explanation for excessive beta-blockage following timolol eye drops. Potential for oral-ophthalmic drug interaction. JAMA 274: 1611–1613, 1995.

Fraunfelder FT. Extraocular fluid dynamics: how best to apply topical ocular medication. Tran Am Ophthalmol Soc 74: 457–487, 1976.

Fraunfelder FT. Ways to diminish systemic side effects. In: Vaughan D, Asbury (eds). General Ophthalmology, 15th edn. Appleton and Lange, Norwalk, CT, pp 68–73, 1999.

Fraunfelder FW, Fraunfelder FT, Jensvold B. Adverse systemic effects from pledgets of topical ocular phenylephrine 10%. Am J Ophthalmol 134: 624–625, 2002.

Harris LS, Galin MA. Effect of ocular pigmentation on hypotensive response to pilocarpine. Am J Ophthalmol 72: 923–925, 1971.

Hong S, Lee CS, Seo KY, et al. Effects of topical antiglaucoma application on conjunctival impression sytology specimens. Am J Ophthalmol 142: 185–186, 2006.

Lynch MG, Brown RH, et al. Reduction of phenylephrine drop size in infants achieves equal dilation with decreased systemic absorption. Arch Opthalmol 105: 1364–1365, 1987.

McCartney HJ, Drysdale IO, Gornall AG, et al. An autoradiographic study of the penetration of subconjunctively injected hydrocortisone into the normal and inflamed rabbit eye. Invest Ophthalmol 4: 297–302, 1965.

Mikkelson TJ, Charai S, Robinson JR. Altered bioavailability of drugs in the system due to drug protein interaction. J Pharmacol Sci 62: 1648–1653, 1973.

Mishima S, Gasset A, Klyce SD Jr, et al. Determination of tear volume and tear flow. Invest Ophthalmol 5: 264–276, 1966.

Schoenwald RD. The control of drug bioavailability from ophthalmic dosage forms. In: Smolen VF, Ball VA (eds). Controlled Drug Bioavailability, Vol. 3: Bioavailability control by drug delivery system design, John Wiley, New York, 257–306, 1985.

Shell JW. Pharmacokinetics of topically applied ophthalmic drugs. Surv Ophthalmol 26: 207–218, 1982.

Van Ootegham MM. Factors influencing the retention of ophthalmic solutions on the eye surface. In Saettone MF, Bucci M, Speiser P (eds). Ophthalmic Drug Delivery. Fidia Research Series, Vol 11, Springer Verlag, Berlin, pp 7–18, 1987.

Wine NA, Gornall AG, Basu PK. The ocular uptake of subconjunctively injected C14 hydrocortisone. Part 1. Time and major route of penetration in a normal eye. Am J Ophthalmol 58: 362–366, 1964.

Zimmerman TJ, Sharir M, Nardin GF, et al. Therapeutic index of epinephrine and dipivefrin with nasolacrimal occlusion. Am J Ophthalmol 114: 8–13, 1992.

PART

3

Methods for evaluating drug-induced visual side effects

Wiley A. Chambers, MD

RISK

All drug products have some risk. If there is any pharmacologic activity due to the drug product, there is also a risk of adverse events from it due to known or unknown pharmacologic activity. Risk is generally best assessed in controlled clinical studies. While risks may also be identified following the commercial marketing of the drug product, it is often difficult to determine the number of people who have been exposed to the drug product after commercial marketing begins. If the number of people exposed cannot be accurately determined, the exact frequency or likelihood of a side effect cannot be accurately determined.

The assessment of risk generally improves as more individuals receive the drug product. While it would be extremely helpful to know the full risk profile of every drug product prior to release into commercial marketing, usually the full risk profile is not completely known until after the drug product is marketed.

SELECTING DIAGNOSTIC TESTS

There are a wide variety of diagnostic testing modalities that may be used to detect and evaluate a suspected ocular toxicity. While it is theoretically possible to perform each of these tests on any individual that is suspected to have an abnormality, the time, expense, resources and ability of the patient to cooperate must be taken into consideration. In broad terms these tests may be divided into two main categories. The first covers methods capable of detecting objective anatomic changes and the second covers methods capable of detecting functional changes. One category of tests is not necessarily better than the other; they simply measure different things.

The number of tests needed to characterize an abnormality or deviation will vary with the deviation being evaluated and the extent to which it needs to be characterized. There should be a justified reason for the selection of each test. Each test should be appropriate for the type of potential event in question. Screening tests may be used to superficially scan for irregularities without fully quantitating the extent of the anomaly.

An important question in assessing the potential for ocular toxicity is which tests, if any, are necessary? As noted above, it may be theoretically possible to perform all possible tests, but consideration of several factors can help to narrow the choice. The questions relevant for deciding which tests to perform include the following:
1. How likely is the test to detect an abnormality?
2. What are the findings from any non-clinical toxicology studies in non-human animals?
3. What abnormalities are expected based on the known pharmacologic action of the drug?
4. How serious is the potential abnormality?
5. How invasive is the test?
6. What is the route of administration of the drug?

When possible, it is recommended that non-clinical toxicology studies be conducted prior to conducting human toxicology studies. Ideally, non-clinical studies should be conducted using higher multiples ($2\times$, $10\times$, $100\times$) of the doses proposed for humans (based on concentration and/or frequency of administration) and the duration of dosing should be at least as long as planned in humans (up to 12 months). It is helpful to compare multiple different dose levels in these studies. The findings of the non-clinical toxicology studies should then be used to help guide the initial tests to be conducted in humans. While the events observed in non-human studies may not be duplicated in human studies, there is frequently some overlap. It is therefore important to assess the potential for these events.

For example, an important characteristic that may be determined by non-clinical studies is whether or not a drug product binds to melanin. Melanin is found widely in the eye and products which bind to melanin may cause ocular toxicities. If a drug product is found to bind to melanin, it would next be important to know whether the non-clinical studies demonstrated abnormalities in electroretinograms (ERGs). If a drug product is found to bind to melanin and demonstrates ERG abnormalities in animals, it would be prudent to monitor best corrected distance visual acuity, ERGs, color vision for acquired defects, automated threshold static visual fields, and dilated photography and/or indirect funduscopy in clinical studies of humans. If a drug product is found to bind to melanin and the results of ERG studies in animals are not known or have not been performed, the same examinations should be performed in clinical studies of humans.

It is important to perform histopathology in the non-clinical studies. If in non-clinical studies a retinal lesion or retinal drug deposit is observed in animals, best corrected distance visual acuity, ERGs, color vision for acquired defects, threshold static visual field, ocular coherence tomography (OCT) and dilated photography and/or indirect funduscopy should be performed in clinical studies of humans. Drug products which cause retinal lesions and ERG changes in non-human animals often cause toxicity in humans as well.

If in non-clinical studies lens opacity is observed in animals, then best corrected distance visual acuity and lens photography or the use of a standardized lens grading system should be included in clinical studies of humans.

The structure of the drug, non-clinical pharmacology studies and clinical pharmacology studies may be helpful in identifying the expected pharmacologic actions of the drug. To the extent that the pharmacologic action potentiates or interferes with ocular functions, ocular tests may be planned to quantitate the enhancement or interference of the function. For example,

15

drug products which affect the sympathomimetic system are likely to affect intraocular pressure and pupil size. It is therefore important to perform tonometry and pupil size measurements to quantitate the expected changes. Drug products that affect the cholinergic system are likely to affect intraocular pressure, pupil size, tear production and the corneal surface. Tests such as tonometry, pupil size measures, Schirmer's tear tests, and rose bengal or lissamine green corneal staining may be useful.

The seriousness of a potential adverse event should influence the effort spent on characterizing the likelihood of the event to occur and any factors which may mitigate or enhance its occurrence. It is most important to be able to predict events that can cause irreversible changes and in particular events that can lead to irreversible blindness. To the extent that they may be predicted, at least some of these events may be preventable. However, some potentially serious events may occur too infrequently to be able to be adequately studied. Taken at the extreme, if an event is so rare that it is expected to occur in one in seven billion patients, even if it results in total blindness the frequency is so low that no-one would expect to ever see another case.

The frequency of a potential adverse event occurring will influence the methods used to characterize the event. For the reasons discussed below, the likelihood of detecting rare events, such as those which occur in less than one per 10 000 subjects, in controlled clinical studies is rare. Other methods must be used to study the events or the frequency of an occurrence of that event must be increased in a monitored setting. In cases where the frequency of events increases with increasing dose, it may be possible study the events in patients receiving higher doses.

The frequency of a potential event occurring in the general population, and more importantly in the population of patients likely to take a particular drug product, may make recognizing an association with that particular drug product difficult. Ocular events such as non-arteritic ischemic optic neuropathy (NAION) occur very rarely. NAION events occur most frequently in patients with known risk factors for NAION events, such as coronary artery disease, diabetes, hyperlipidemia, hypertension, older age and smoking. If patients who have any of these conditions take a drug product and then have a NAION event, it is extremely difficult to determine whether the drug product or the other risk factors, or both, contributed to the NAION event.

The route of administration will affect the particular areas of the eye that are exposed to the drug product. Direct application of a drug product to the eye increases the likelihood that significant concentrations of the drug reach the eye. As a general rule, the following tests are recommended for all subjects of all drug products administered topically to the eye:

1. best corrected distance visual acuity
2. dilated slit lamp of anterior segment
3. dilated indirect fundoscopy or photography
4. pupil diameter
5. applanation tonometry
6. assessment of symptoms in the first minute following topical application.

Additionally, a subset of patients receiving a drug product topically administered to the eye should have corneal endothelial cell counts.

ORDER OF TESTING

The order of conducting the tests is important. A number of tests are capable of producing temporary ocular abnormalities or temporarily masking ocular abnormalities. If the order of the tests is not chosen carefully, some of the temporary ocular abnormalities caused by earlier tests will be detected by later tests and incorrectly attributed to the drug product.

TIMING OF TESTING

Whenever possible, the inclusion of a baseline test before exposure to a drug product is extremely helpful in the interpretation of any suspected abnormalities. It is also helpful to have a post-drug-exposure test to determine whether any abnormality is reversible or permanent. Besides these two time points, additional testing is dependent on the drug and the particular test.

FUNCTIONAL TESTS

Visual acuity

Visual acuity is the most commonly used and universally understood measure of visual function. It is important to measure visual acuity in most circumstances because it provides a simultaneous measurement of central corneal clarity, central lens clarity, central macular function and optic nerve conduction. If it is normal, it provides a quick assessment of this central ocular pathway. If it is abnormal, it does not distinguish between the many causes of an abnormality.

Visual acuity should be measured as best corrected distance visual acuity. A recent refraction is required to obtain the best corrected visual acuity. Although the traditional distance used to measure visual acuity was 20 feet or 6 m, the distance in this case refers to a distance of at least 4 m. The use of a 4-m distance during refraction has the advantage of being one-quarter of a diopter in lens power from testing at a theoretical infinite distance. Each eye should be tested separately. The test should be conducted using a high contrast chart with an equal number of letters per line and equal spacing between lines. The stroke width of the letters should be smaller on each succeeding line such that the visual angle needed to identify the letters is reduced by two-thirds per line.

The result of a visual acuity test should be reported as a log-MAR value (log of the minimum angle of resolution). Normal visual acuity for most adults is approximately –0.1 on this scale, which is equivalent to 20/16 on a Snellen visual acuity chart. A two-line or greater change from one visit to the next in a single patient should suggest additional investigation. A three-line or greater change in a single individual is usually considered clinically significant. In the evaluation of a group of subjects, changes in the mean logMAR score and in shift tables created by categorizing subjects by gains and losses in zero, one, two, three or more lines of visual acuity are often helpful in recognizing changes in visual acuity.

Additional measures of visual acuity such as best corrected near visual acuity, uncorrected distance visual acuity and uncorrected near visual acuity are rarely necessary unless it is not possible to perform a best corrected distance visual acuity. Although abnormalities may occur which alter near visual acuity without affecting best corrected distance visual acuity, these abnormalities are better characterized by measuring the accommodative amplitude together with any observed changes in refractive power in association with the best corrected distance visual acuity. Refractive power can be measured by either a manifest refraction or a cycloplegic refraction. When evaluating the effect of a drug product on refractive power, it is usually best not to perform a cycloplegic refraction as the pharmacologic action of the cycloplegic agent may alter the results.

Color vision

Color vision is a test of macular function since there are relatively few cones outside the macular area. There are a large variety of color vision tests with different degrees of sensitivity and specificity. The different color tests are most commonly distinguished by their ability to screen for color vision defects versus quantitating color defects, and their ability to detect common congenital defects in color vision (red-green confusion) versus typical acquired defects in color vision (blue-yellow confusion). Each eye should be tested separately. The gold standard test of color vision is the Farnsworth Munsell (FM) 100 hue color test. The FM 100 hue color test can be used to detect both red-green and blue-yellow confusion, and to some degree can quantitate the extent of the confusion. The FM 100 hue color test consists of four trays of color caps which are arranged in sequential hue. The test is scored on the basis of caps that are placed out of order and when plotted can provide both the magnitude and type of deviation. The FM 100 hue color test has a learning curve associated with improvements in scores during the first few test administrations.

Subsets of the FM 100 hue color test can also be used to screen for color vision abnormalities. These subsets include 40 and 28 hue tests. The sensitivity of these tests progressively decreases as fewer caps are tested. These tests are also known as the Lanthony 40 hue, Lanthony 28 hue, Roth 28 hue or Farnsworth-Munsell 28-hue desaturated tests.

The 15 hue test, including the desaturated versions of the 15 hue (Farnsworth D15 and Lanthony D15), is not always sensitive enough to detect mild losses in color vision. This test as well as the Hardy Rand and Rittler (HRR) Color Vision Test and the SPP2 color vision test are useful for screening for color vision defects.

The following tests are not useful in testing acquired color vision defects because they do not evaluate blue-yellow confusion: Ishihara test, SPP1 and Dvorine color vision tests. These tests predominantly provide an evaluation of red-green confusion.

Visual fields

Visual field tests can be broadly divided into several categories. These categories include manual versus automated perimetry tests, static versus kinetic perimetry tests, threshold versus suprathreshold perimetry tests, white light target and background tests versus colored targets and background tests, and central field versus peripheral field perimetry tests. When automated, threshold perimetry tests are generally the preferred method for evaluating drug-induced visual field defects; the use of static versus kinetic, central versus peripheral, and white versus color filtered light is dependent on the particular abnormality being investigated. For most drug-induced visual field defects, automated threshold, static, central 24 degree, white object perimetry testing is adequate to detect potential defects. Perimetry programs which meet these criteria include the Humphrey 30-1, 30-2, 24-1, 24-2, SITA Fast, and SITA Standard Visual Field Tests, and the Octopus 30-1 and 30-2 Visual Field Tests.

Reporting of visual fields should always include the actual thresholds determined for each field point and the number of false positives, false negatives and fixation losses. There is a significant learning curve demonstrated by most subjects who take a visual field test. This learning curve should be expected to take place over at least the first three tests completed in each eye. The learning curve most commonly results in a significant increase in mean threshold values for normal individuals.

In cases where there is an expectation that rods will be affected more than cones, an automated peripheral white object perimeter testing program is preferred, for example the Humphrey P-60 and FF-120 Visual Field Tests. In cases where there is an expectation that the cones will be affected more than rods, an automated color filtered, central visual field test is preferred.

The most widely used kinetic test can be performed with a Goldmann perimeter. It is important that the same technician performs the testing with a Goldmann perimeter from visit to visit to reduce the chances of variability in the field due to operator differences.

The Amsler grid test may help to identify central macular changes. It is occasionally useful as a screening test in assessing drug toxicity when there are drug deposits in the macular area.

Contrast sensitivity testing

Contrast sensitivity testing is often not included in toxicity testing because the measurements can overlap with other tests already included. When performed using standardized methodologies, contrast sensitivity testing is capable of measuring aspects of visual function that may not otherwise typically be measured by visual acuity, color vision or visual field. When testing for toxicity purposes, multiple different levels of contrast should be included.

Electroretinography (ERG)

International standards of electroretinography testing are set by the International Society for Clinical Electrophysiology of Vision (ISCEV). These standards provide complete details in the conduct of the testing parameters, including the light stimuli. If ISCEV standards are not followed, an explanation for why they were not should be included. For interpretation purposes, it is important to report full numerical results and graphs when reporting ERG findings.

Testing is expected to measure both rod and cone function in a variety of stimuli. From a toxicology standpoint, amplitudes and/or latent times must usually change by at least 40% to be considered clinically significant.

ERG testing is often the most informative method available for assessing retinal function in non-human animals. It is a mainstay in testing drug products which bind to melanin and/or produce retinal lesions (seen by ophthalmoscopy, OCT or histology). Development of a particular drug product is often stopped if it is shown to cause both retinal lesions and decreased amplitudes on ERG testing.

ERG abnormalities in non-human animal studies alone are not necessarily predictive of human injury, but warrant monitoring in humans with ERG testing unless a more sensitive screening test can be identified.

Photostress tests

Retinal damage may sometimes be manifested in delays in recovery time. Photostress tests may be helpful in identifying this type of injury if the effect is widespread throughout the retina. There is considerable subject-to-subject variability in photostress test evaluations and therefore it is usually difficult to detect unless the injury is great or the number of subjects tested is very large.

Double vision and ocular motility

Complaints of double vision must first be assessed to determine if the double vision is uniocular or binocular. The Worth 4 DOT test can be used to assess this. If the double vision is binocular, assessments of ocular motility in eight fields of gaze should be conducted and cover/uncover tests should be conducted to assess phorias and tropias. This is one of the few times when both eyes should be tested simultaneously.

Pupil measurements

Pupillary measurements provide an opportunity to test ocular responses to ocular stimuli. It is important that pupillary diameters be measured under reproducible controlled settings of light and accommodation. Pupillary responses to light stimuli and to accommodation should be measured separately. Pupillary responses in one eye due to a light stimulus in the other eye should also be measured separately from the pupillary response to a light stimulus in the same eye. Pupillary measurements may be made in a variety of ways. It is rarely necessary to measure pupil responses to a sensitivity of more than a tenth of a millimeter.

Corneal sensitivity

There are relatively few methods to quantitatively measure corneal sensitivity. The most commonly used instrument is the Cochet-Bonnet aesthesiometer. This instrument can discriminate between fairly large changes in corneal sensitivity.

Corneal thickness

The corneal endothelial cells provide an effective pump system and when functioning properly keep the cornea thin. Corneal thickness therefore, while an anatomic measurement, can be a surrogate for corneal endothelial cell function. There are two common corneal pachymetry methods, optical and ultrasonic. For the purposes of assessing corneal endothelial cell function, either can be useful as long as the same instrument is used consistently in a patient.

OBJECTIVE ANATOMICAL METHODS

As described below, for most ocular tissues electronic digital images provide the best method for recording anatomic findings. These electronic photographs generally provide opportunities for more complete analysis and characterization. A large number of different areas of the eye can be well imaged. Theses areas include all five layers of the corneal surface, the corneal surface topography, the corneal thickness, corneal clarity, the anterior chamber depth, anterior chamber inflammation, the lens thickness, lens clarity, the nerve fiber thickness, vitreous inflammation, vitreous traction, retinal surface irregularities, the retinal vascular, the optic nerve size, and optic cup size and contour.

Cornea and conjunctiva

As external, relatively clear structures, the cornea and conjunctiva can be evaluated by direct observation. The direct observation can be aided by the magnification provide by a slit lamp or a confocal microscope. The addition of different stains such as fluorescein, lissamine green or rose bengal can provide assistance by differentially staining different cells or tissues. Fluorescein stain is incorporated when epithelial cells are dead or missing; lissamine green and rose bengal stains are incorporated when epithelial cells are injured and have lost some of their functionality. These stains are useful in assessing corneal or conjunctival epithelial damage.

Corneal endothelial cells, if exposed to a toxic substance, are among the most sensitive in the eye to ocular damage and since they are not regenerated in humans they provide a permanent marker of damage. Endothelial cell counts measure damage to the corneal endothelium.

The best method for recording corneal or conjunctival changes is with electronic images by digitalized photography. This method is generally most useful for future analysis and characterization. When this is not possible, predefined scales may be used to capture a description of any findings.

Tear film

The production of tears may be impacted by different drug products, in both the quantity and quality of the tears produced. The effects on tear quantity may be evaluated by Schirmer's Tear Tests (anesthetized and non-anesthetized conditions). The effects on tear quality may be evaluated by tear breakup time.

Lens

Any evaluation of a lens change should include the type of lens change, and the size and location of the change. Digital photography remains the gold standard for evaluating lens clarity, although a single photograph is rarely capable of capturing all aspects of the lens. Multiple photographs taken on and off the central axis, and including but not limited to retroillumination, are useful in assessing lens clarity and therefore cataract development. If this is not available, a predefined scale system with reference photographs for each point on the scale is useful. It is extremely useful to grade posterior subcapsular changes, cortical changes and nuclear changes separately since they may frequently be independent of one another.

Lens opacities tend to occur slowly. While direct trauma to the lens can cause opacities to develop within minutes or days, most milder injuries take weeks to months or years to develop. Corticosteroid drug products, which are well known to cause cataracts, may often take up to 2 years to cause clinically recognizable lens changes. It is recommended that lens changes, when a drug product is to be administered for a period of 6 weeks or more, be monitored at 6-month intervals for at least 2 years.

At least as important as the size of an opacity in the lens is the location of that opacity in the lens. While all opacities in a lens are important and may spread to other areas of the lens, the initial location may have more impact on the immediate clinical consequences and help characterize a particular toxicity. Opacities that occur in the posterior portion of the lens cause more interference with sight than opacities that occur in the anterior portion of the lens. Opacities that occur in the center of the visual axis cause the most interference with sight. Drug-induced toxicities tend to first occur more commonly in the posterior portion of the lens.

It is not always possible to directly appreciate the impact of a lens change on an individual patient's visual acuity. In some of these cases, visual acuity will change before any lens opacity becomes noticeable. Visual acuity should therefore always be measured when evaluating patients for lens changes.

Anterior chamber

The position of the lens and consequently the size and shape of the anterior chamber can be affected by drug products. This is best assessed by slit lamp examinations and diagnostic ultrasound measurements. It is most commonly identified by cases of elevated intraocular pressure in association with refractive changes.

Retina

Color digital photography together with OCT are the current gold standards for evaluating the retinal surface. Fluorescein angiography (FA) and indocyanine green (ICG) angiography provide separate and additional information on the retinal vasculature. Direct funduscopy and indirect funduscopy, while capable of detecting retinal abnormalities, often provide more limited views with less magnification. Direct funduscopy may include the use of a direct ophthalmoscope or the use of a slit lamp with an additional 78D or 90D lens.

Intraocular pressure

The measurement of intraocular pressure (IOP), for the purposes of toxicology assessments, can be adequately made by applanation tonometry. The invasiveness of more accurate measures is usually not warranted. In the rare cases where a more exact estimate of aqueous production is needed, tonography can be performed.

NUMBER OF PATIENTS TO TEST

Common events are easier to identify and characterize than more unusual ones. It is customary to attempt to identify events which occur at a frequency of 1% or higher. Mathematical principles of probability dictate that when the true event incidence is 1% or higher, in order to have a 95% change of observing at least one event, 300 subjects must be monitored. This is often referred to as the rule of 3 (Hanley and Lippman-Hand 1983).

The rule of 3 states that in order to detect events which would occur at X% or more, you need Y patients where $3/Y = X$. Applying this rule suggests that if an incidence rate of 10% is to be identified, at least 30 patients need to be studied. If an incidence rate of 5% is to be detected, 60 patients must be studied. If an incidence rate of 0.1% is to be detected, 3000 patients must be studied.

SUMMARY

There are many potential ocular toxicity tests. Ocular toxicity tests should be used to investigate potential adverse events that might be either frequent or serious. There should be a justified reason for the selection of each test, and each test should be appropriate for the event in question.

REFERENCES AND FURTHER READING

Hanley JA, Lippman-Hand A. If nothing goes wrong, is everything all right? Interpreting zero numerators. JAMA 249: 1743–1745, 1983.

The role of electrophysiology and psychophysics in ocular toxicology

Eberhart Zrenner, MD

INTRODUCTION

Modern structure-based drug design results increasingly in compounds that act very specifically, e.g. as modulators of the function of channels or enzymes that occur not only in the targeted tissue but also in the eye. Increasingly, therefore, ophthalmological symptoms occur in phases I and II of clinical studies without any ophthalmic signs having been reported in preclinical studies. A well-known case is sildenafil (Viagra®), a selective inhibitor of cGMP-specific phosphodiesterase (PDE) 5 in the corpus cavernosum that, with lower selectivity, also affects the retinal PDE6, and elicits luminous phenomena such as blue-tinged objects and phosphenes, and thus reflects an unexpected pharmacological side effect (for a survey see Laties and Zrenner 2002). In such cases, usually long-term multi-center studies are required to exclude irreversible effects such as retinal degeneration and permanent loss of certain visual functions. As more and more drugs are targeted at specific molecular actions, e.g. specific protein structures or receptor subfamilies with particular ligand abilities that may occur in the eye as well, specifically targeted tests and study designs have to be used to differentiate between effects merely reflecting harmless pharmacological actions at an undesired site from those that lead to irreversible, toxic damage. Moreover, it is still unclear which battery of ophthalmic function tests assesses the safety of specific drug actions best and how one sets the threshold for potential clinical concern and the proper endpoint for safety. In addition, given the complexity and multitude of stimulation and recording conditions of tests such as electroretinography, electrooculography and visually evoked cortical potentials (VEPs), it is not easy to assure comparability and quality of test results in multi-center trials, not to mention the large variations in procedures, devices and methods of evaluation.

This chapter therefore outlines some principles that may help to select proper tests on the basis of their specificity for the function of certain retinal cell subgroups. It gives practical advice for selecting those tests that will enable the investigators to assess the specific functions and morphology of the visual system and it also addresses questions of safety and efficacy, based on hypotheses that stem from preclinical data where the psychophysics of the visual system are not available. Moreover, new developments are pointed out that help to improve the quality of multi-center studies by proper standard operating procedures (SOPs) and stringent case report forms (CRFs), based on the development of international standards and recommendations in ophthalmology (for electrophysiology, e.g. www.iscev.org) as well as the development of international networks of certified centers (http://www.europeanvisioninstitute.org/CT_SE/).

THE VISUAL SYSTEM

Almost half of all neurotoxic chemicals affect some aspect of sensory function (Croft and Sheets 1989), with the visual system being most frequently affected. Grant and Schuhman (1993) in their encyclopsoedic *Toxicology of the Eye* list approximately 3000 substances that produce unwanted side effects in the visual system. Numerous transmitters and mechanisms are involved in processing information in photoreceptors and in the many connected neurons transmitting visual information to perceptual centers whose function can be affected by neurotropic agents, drugs, food and environmental compounds. As shown in Table 4.1, a multitude of transmitters and neuromodulators is found in the various retinal layers, especially in the more than 25 different types of amacrine cells in the inner plexiform layer. Compounds can therefore act specifically on the function and electrophysiological characteristics of these target cells. This specificity often allows the correlation of functional alterations in electrophysiological parameters to the action and adverse reactions of neurotropic compounds. Additionally, there are many non-neuronal cells whose function is important for the integrity of information processing, such as pigment epithelial cells, glial cells and vascular structures, that can be affected by drug action as well. Of further general concern are the factors that determine whether a particular chemical can reach a particular ocular site: concentration and duration of exposure, mode of application and interaction with the various ocular structures as well as integrity of natural barriers. The blood-retinal barrier may be impermeable under normal physiological conditions (Alm 1992). However, in certain areas of the retina, e.g. around the optic disc, the continuous type of capillaries is lacking and hydrophilic molecules may enter the optic nerve head by diffusion from the extra-vascular space.

This chapter aims to convey a basic understanding of toxic mechanisms in the visual system by pointing out cell-specific functional changes and typical symptoms in toxic side effects. In an individual case it is strongly recommended that referenced publications such as Grant and Schuhman (1993) and Fraunfelder (2000) are consulted. These have references on the primary literature concerning the various substances. Additionally, there are very interesting general chapters and books that concern ocular toxicology and may be of help (e.g. Chiou 1992; Potts 1996; Ballantyne 1999; Fox and Boyes 2001; Bartlett and Jaanus 2007).

The retinal pigment epithelium

The retinal pigment epithelium (RPE) has four major functions: phagocytosis, vitamin A transport and storage, potassium metabolism and protection from light damage (see Fig. 4.1). RPE functions can be altered, e.g. by inhibitors of phagocytosis,

Table 4.1 – The various transmitters and modulators present in the retinal layers (modified from Vaney 1990 and Kolb et al 2001)

Neuroactive Substance	Cell Type
Glutamate	Photoreceptors (cones and rods), bipolar cells, ganglion cells
Gamma aminobutyric acid (GABA)	Horizontal cells, amacrine cells
Glycine	Amacrine cells, bipolar cells, ganglion cells
Taurine	Photoreceptors, amacrine cells, bipolar cells
Dopamine	Amacrine cells (including inter-plexiform cells)
Melatonin	Photoreceptors
Serotonin	Amacrine cells, bipolar cells (in non-mammalian vertebrates)
Acetylcholine	Amacrine cells (in the INL and displaced in the GCL)
Substance P	Amacrine cells, ganglion cells
Angiotensin II	Amacrine cells
Nitric oxide	Amacrine cells
Vasoactive intestinal polypeptide (VIP)	Amacrine cells
Somatostatin	Amacrine cells, ganglion cells
ATP	Amacrine cells, ganglion cells
Adenosine	Amacrine cells, ganglion cells
Brain-derived neurotrophic factor (BDNF)	Amacrine cells, ganglion cells
Kynurenic acid	Amacrine cells

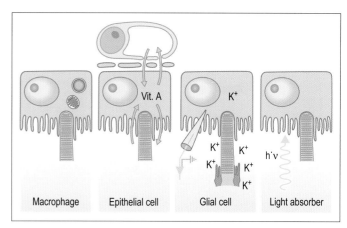

Fig. 4.1 The various roles of the retinal pigment epithelial cells.

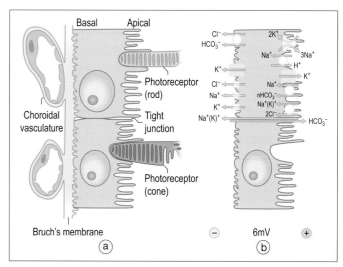

Fig. 4.2 (a) The RPE, with its tight junctions between the cell membranes, forms a cellular monolayer. On its basal side it is attached to Bruch's membrane for its metabolic exchange with the choroidal vasculature; on its apical side it is intrinsically connected to the photoreceptors. (b) A standing potential of 6 mV is obtained across Bruch's membrane, governed by various channels, pumps and exchangers. (Adapted from H. Jaegle, personal communication.)

modulation of potassium metabolism, metabolic alterations in the visual cycle and by the action of melanin-binding substances. Additionally, melanin is found in several different locations, such as the pigmented cells of the iris, the ciliary body and the uveal tract. Melanin has a high binding affinity for polycyclic aromatic carbons, calcium and toxic heavy metals such as aluminum, iron, lead and mercury (Meier-Ruge 1972; Potts and Au 1976; Ulshafer et al 1990; Eichenbaum and Zheng 2000). This may result in excessive accumulation and slow release of numerous drugs and chemicals that bind to melanin granula, such as phenothiazines, glycosides and chloroquine (Alkemade 1968, Bernstein 1967).

The outer retina is supplied by the choriocapillaries and capillaries have loose epithelial junctions, multiple fenestrae and are highly permeable to large proteins (Fig. 4.2a). During systemic exposure to chemicals and drugs by inhalation, transdermally or parenterally, certain compounds can be distributed to all parts of the eye via the bloodstream (Fig. 4.2b). For example, chloroquine phosphate binds strongly to the RPE with a half-life of 5 years, 80 times more strongly than to the liver. This drug is not only used for malarial prophylaxis, but also plays an important role in the treatment of rheumatoid diseases (up to 4 mg/kg, or for

hydroxychloroquine 6 mg/kg, of body weight per day). At these maximal rates, a critical cumulative dose can be reached within 3 to 6 months (Mavrikakis et al 2003).

Signs of chloroquine phosphate retinopathy (typically following a cumulative dose of 100 to 300 g) are:

- a relative paracentral scotoma, usually an annular perifoveal ring-shaped depression in visual fields
- loss of blue/yellow color discrimination
- RPE depigmentation often observed in a pattern matching the ring-shaped visual field depression (most easily seen during fluorescein angiography as window defects)
- reduced light-evoked amplitude rise in the electrooculogram (EOG)
- reduced b-wave amplitudes and prolonged latencies in the electroretinogram (ERG) due to secondary effects on photoreceptor function.

Patients with low body weight and/or poor renal function are particularly susceptible (Ochsendorf et al 1993) therefore care should be taken to avoid over-dosage.

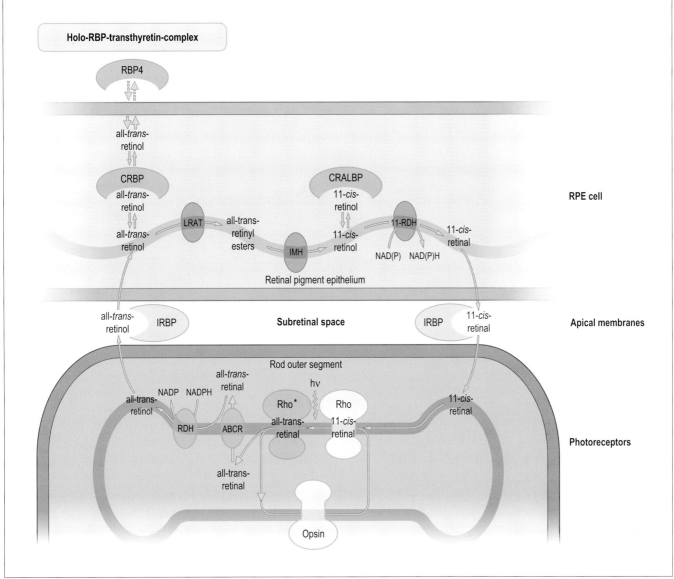

Fig. 4.3 The retinoid metabolism between photoreceptors (below) and RPE cells (above). 11-*cis*-retinal is isomerized into all-*trans*-retinal by light and is dissociated from opsin. The ATP-binding transporter ABCR moves all-*trans*-retinal through the membrane of the photoreceptor disc into the cytoplasma of the outer segment. The all-*trans*-retinol dehydrogenase (RDH) catalyzes the reduction of all-*trans*-retinal into all-*trans*-retinol, which is transported by means of the inter-photoreceptor retinoid binding protein (IRBP) through the subretinal space into the pigment epithelium cell. There it is esterified by means of lecithin retinol acyl transferase (LRAT). Isomerohydrolase (IMH) transforms it into 11-*cis*-retinol and finally by means of 11 LRDH it is transformed into 11-*cis*-retinal. The latter is transported by the interphotoreceptor retinoid binding protein (IRBP) into the photoreceptor and forms a complex with opsin. The visual pigment is thus regenerated and available for another isomerization by light. New all-*trans*-retinol is transported from the liver by means of a retinoid binding protein (RBP), forming a complex with transthyretin. Within the pigment epithelial cells it is transported by the cellular retinol binding protein (CRBP).

Cytostatic agents that disrupt protein metabolism can have an effect similar to the retinal toxicity of the antimalarial drugs. These include vincristine, vinblastine, sparsomycin, triazyquone acting through inhibition of protein synthesis (see Zrenner and Hart 2007) and some neurotoxic antibiotics, such as streptomycin and its associated derivatives as well as phenothiazines and indomethacin (Palimeris et al 1972).

The retinal pigment epithelial cell forms a syncytium with tight junctions that is extremely important for ionic homeostasis of the retina, given the various pumps and channels of the basal as well as of the apical membrane (Fig. 4.2b). This is another source of drug-induced functional alterations by changes in standing potential across Bruch's membrane accessible by electrooculography (see below).

The pigment epithelial cell is intricately connected with the photoreceptor function through the visual cycle (see Fig. 4.3). This includes several transport proteins between photoreceptors and pigment epithelial cells, as well as enzymes that are important for the renewal of rhodopsin. Compounds that affect the transport or metabolism of retinol or retinal can result in functional alteration and retinal toxicity, as seen in oral retinoid therapy. This may influence the dark adaptation of photoreceptors, accessible psychophysically by threshold measurements (Kurtenbach et al 2006) or objectively by monitoring the recovery of electrophysiological signals after bleaching or by measuring contrast vision.

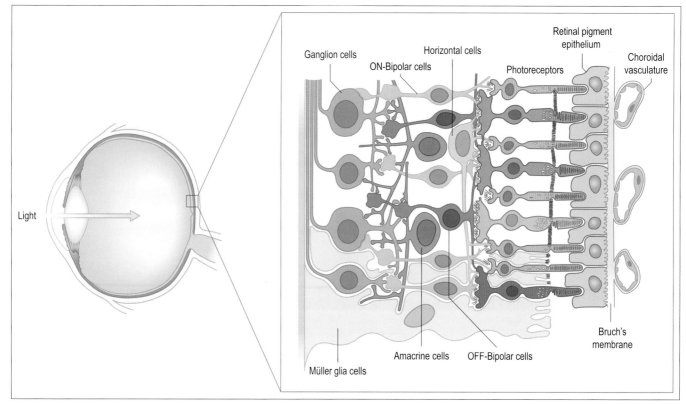

Fig. 4.4 In the retina, rod photoreceptors (grey) and cone photoreceptors (red, green and blue) are contacted by different bipolar cells: invaginating bipolar cells (light blue) form in the outer plexiform layer triade synapses with horizontal cells (violet) and the photoreceptor pedicles or rod spherules. They form the ON-bipolar system, which responds to light by depolarization. Additionally, there are the so-called flat bipolar cells (dark blue), forming the OFF-bipolar system that is hyperpolarized by light and actively responds to the offset of light by depolarization. The synapses of amacrine cells, bipolar cells and ganglion cells form the inner plexiform layer. Magno- and parvo-cellular ganglion cells send their axons via the optic nerve to the lateral geniculate body.

Functional alterations in photoreceptors

Numerous substances can alter visual function by acting on the visual transduction process (lower part of Fig. 4.3). These include, for example, chloramphenicol as well as glycosides such as digoxin and digitoxin. Most frequently the complaints in such drug actions are hazy or blurred vision, flickering lights, colored spots surrounded by a halo and increased glare sensitivity. Color vision problems have been confirmed (Rietbrock and Alken 1980; Haustein and Schmidt 1988; Duncker and Krastel 1990), probably acting through the inhibition of the retinal sodium/potassium ATPase. ERG analysis typically reveals a depressed critical flicker fusion frequency, reduced rod and cone amplitudes and increased implicit times as well as elevated rod and cone thresholds (Robertson et al 1966; Madreperla et al 1994). PDE inhibitors, such as sildenafil (Viagra®) can also affect the photoreceptor transduction process, acting on the retinal PDE (Schneider and Zrenner 1986). In therapeutic doses, sildenafil can lead to reversible color discrimination problems, blurred vision, glare sensitivity, blue-tinged borders between bright and dark areas and ERG changes at higher doses (Laties and Zrenner 2002).

Many drugs can affect the spectrally different cones in the retina in a slightly different manner and even minor imbalances in the excitation of short-, middle- and long-wavelength sensitive cones can produce color vision disturbances (see Lyle 1974a,b; Zrenner 1982; Zrenner et al 1982; Jägle et al 2007; Zrenner and Hart 2007). Alterations of color perception therefore belong to early signs of drug-induced functional alterations of the visual system.

Functional alterations in cells of the inner retina (from outer plexiform to inner plexiform layer)

Approximately 110 million rods and 6 million cones converge through a heavy duty neuronal processor consisting of horizontal cells, several types of bipolar cells and at least 25 types of amacrine cells, the processed signals being forwarded finally onto ganglion cells (see Fig. 4.4). Of special interest is the ON- and OFF-bipolar cell system: ON-bipolar cells that utilize a metabotropic glutamate receptor in order to change their electrical sign are depolarized on light stimulation of the photoreceptors while OFF-bipolar cells with their ionotropic glutamate receptor are hyperpolarized on illumination similar to that of the photoreceptors. A contrast enhancement system is thus established in the retina where ON-bipolar cells actively signal brightness while OFF-bipolar cells actively signal darkness. In the case of function changes in one of the two systems not only does a loss of contrast vision occur but also a selective impact the ON-response in the ERG (b-wave) or of the OFF-response, elicited after switching off a long duration test light. The rod system has only a single bipolar cell system (rod ON-bipolar cell) not directly connected to ganglion cells, but it utilizes a particular glycinergic amacrine cell (AII amacrine cell) as an intermediary to the ganglion cells. Since rod and cone b-waves can nicely be discerned by dark- or light-adapted ERG, drug effects on these systems can be selectively isolated by non-invasive ERG techniques.

The outer and inner layers of the retina have numerous neurotransmitters and modulating substances, e.g. GABA, glycine, acetylcholine, dopamine, serotonin, substance P, vasoactive intestinal peptide, somatostatin, nitric oxide and even angio-tensin-converting enzyme (Zrenner et al 1989). Altering the metabolism, release or uptake of these substances can affect visual function. The following section discusses several more common examples.

GABA and anti-seizure medications

Anti-epileptic drugs act on the GABA metabolism and carbamazepine (Tegretol®), phenytoin (Phenhydan®) and vigabatrin (Sabril®), for example, quite commonly alter visual function (Dyer 1985; Besch et al 2000, 2002; Harding et al 2002). These drugs can cause color vision disturbances. Vigabatrin can produce irreversible concentric visual field defects with incidences between 0.1 and 30% (Miller et al 1999; Schmitz et al 2002). Vigabatrin raises GABA levels by irreversibly binding to GABA transaminase, thus preventing the metabolism of GABA. The earliest report of retinal electrophysiological changes in humans associated with vigabatrin treatment is that of Bayer et al (1990). All patients with visual field defects revealed altered oscillatory potential waveforms in the ERG, especially patients with marked visual field defects (Besch et al 2002), which were also visible in multifocal ERGs (mfERGs; Rüther et al 1998). Such changes are usually irreversible (Schmidt et al 2002). In many patients a delayed cone single flash response was found in the Ganzfeld ERG and a reduced Arden ratio in the EOG. Harding et al (2002) developed a special VEP stimulus with a high sensitivity and specificity for identifying visual field defects.

Agents that modulate GABA can be expected to alter the GABAergic functions of horizontal cells and thereby can alter contrast vision and presumably functions of light adaptation as well.

Dopamine

Drugs such as fluphenazine, haloperidol and sulpiride can affect the dopamine metabolism and thereby modify retinal function (Schneider and Zrenner 1991). In the arterially perfused eye all three dopamine antagonists increased the rod b-wave while b-wave latency and implicit time showed no drug-induced changes. On the other hand, the D1 antagonist fluphenazine increased the fast transient ON-component while simultaneously strongly decreasing the OFF-component. In contrast, concentrations of the D2 antagonist sulpiride that had a comparable effect on the fast transient ON-component of the optic nerve response (ONR) did not influence the OFF-component. These findings indicate that D1 and D2 receptors play different roles in the transmission of rod signals at the border of the middle and inner retina. As reported in patch clamp investigations by Guenther et al (1994), application of the receptor antagonists haloperidole, spiperone and SCH23390 reduces calcium influx by between 8 and 77%, while no effect of dopamine itself was observed. The study of Dawis and Niemeyer (1986) in arterially perfused cat eyes suggests that dopamine itself has an inhibitory effect on the rod visual pathway since the rod b-wave amplitude is reduced after dopamine application (for a review see Witkovsky and Dearry 1991; Witkovsky 2004). The action of these drugs may be based on a particular cell population of dopaminergic neurons, the density of which ranges from 10–80 cells/mm². They surround other amacrine pericaria, probably amacrine cells of the AII type that transmit rod pathway information onto cone bipolar cells.

Other retinal transmitters and modulators

Approximately 20 different transmitter substances and modulators are used by the various types of amacrine cells, as shown in Table 4.1. Consequently, numerous drugs can affect the function of amacrine cells, and individual wavelets of the oscillatory potentials that have their origins in amacrine cells can be affected differently. A good example of this is angiotensinergic amacrine cells (Datum and Zrenner 1991; Jurklies et al 1995; Kohler et al 1997; Wheeler-Schilling et al 2001). Angiotensin II antagonists can considerably alter retinal function, as shown in ERGs and ONRs of the arterially perfused cat eye (Dahlheim et al 1988; Zrenner et al 1989) and by electroretinography in cats (Jacobi et al 1994).

Functional changes in retinal ganglion cells

While the parvocellular system is mainly responsible for coding of fine spatial resolution and color vision, the magnocellular system codes primarily movement and contrast. Drugs that affect ganglion cell function therefore can show different effects on the parvo- and magnocellular systems, e.g. ethambutol.

Ethambutol is widely used for the treatment of tuberculosis. It causes:
- color vision disturbances as early symptoms
- contrast vision changes
- visual field defects, especially central scotomas with loss of visual acuity
- changes in VEPs.

These alterations can occur within a few weeks after starting the treatment. Also, ethambutol may act at different sites. While initially horizontal cell function and thereby color discrimination are altered as seen in VEPs (Zrenner and Krüger 1981) as well as in fish retina single cell recordings (van Dijk and Spekreijse 1983), advanced forms may lead to loss of ganglion cells and degeneration of the optic nerve. After cessation of drug intake color discrimination improves, as can easily be shown by anomaloscopy (Nasemann et al 1989).

Other substances that typically modify ganglion cell functions are methanol and ethanol, chloramphenicol, quinine, thallium and ergotamine derivatives (for references see Zrenner and Hart 2007).

The optic nerve

Several compounds particularly affect axonal fibres of ganglion cells. For example, exposure to acrylamide produces particular damage to the axons of the parvocellular system, while it spares axons of the magnocellular system, leading to specific visual deficits, such as an increase in the threshold for visual acuity and flicker fusion as well as prolonged latency of pattern-VEPs.

Carbon disulfide

The changes induced by carbon disulfide (CS₂) on the visual function are central scotoma, depressed visual sensitivity in the periphery, optic atrophy, pupillary disturbances, disorders of color perception and blurred vision (for a survey see Beauchamp et al 1983). Vasculopathies including the retina were reported as well but histology in animals points primarily to an optic neuropathy (Eskin et al 1988) and alterations in the VEP are expected in such conditions.

Tamoxifen

Kaiser-Kupfer et al (1981) reported widespread axonal degeneration induced by tamoxifen in the macular and perimacular area, accompanied by retinopathy. Clinical symptoms include a permanent decrease in visual acuity and abnormal visual fields (Ah-Song and Sasco 1997). Following cessation of low dose tamoxifen therapy most of the keratopathy accompanying tamoxifen intake and some of the retinal alterations were seen to be reversible (Noureddin et al 1999).

Other toxic optic neuropathies

Other more common drugs that can produce alterations of optic nerve function with concomitant VEP changes are ethambutol (see above), isoniazid, and isonicotinic acid hydrazide, as well as streptomycin and chloramphenicol.

Damage to glial cells

The retina has several types of glial cells: Mueller cells, oligodendrocytes and astrocytes. Mueller cells are important for glutamate metabolism (in the uptake of the transmitter released by photoreceptors), as well as for the storage of calcium ions. Damage to glial cells, e.g. by the ammonia toxicity of alcohol syndrome (caused by severe toxic hepatic damage), produces marked changes in the ERG (Eckstein et al 1997). This arises because of damage to Mueller cells, since the b-wave of the ERG is strongly modulated by the function of the retina's Mueller cells.

CNS damage

As has been outlined for retinal disorders, toxic and pharmacologic disturbances of visual function can also show up in the central nervous system. In addition to neurotropic effects, some drugs can cause an elevation of intracranial pressure, resulting in papillary edema, which is observed, for example, after the treatment with ergotamines and may produce prolonged latency in the pattern-VEP (Heider et al 1986). Since many cortical areas are involved in processing visual information, alteration of vision can also be caused by direct drug action on neurons in higher cortical areas and produce visual hallucinations and neurological deficits.

THE ROLE OF NON-INVASIVE ELECTROPHYSIOLOGY IN DRUG TESTING

Non-invasive tests allow the recording of bio-electric potentials that arise during the neural processing of visual information by the various elements of the afferent visual pathways.

Changes in the various signals allow conclusions about the locations and kinds of functional disturbances in the afferent neurons of the visual system. Electrophysiology, including the EOG, the ERG and VEPs have been standardized by the International Society for Clinical Electrophysiology of Vision (ISCEV, http://www.iscev.org/standards/index.html). This site also provides further guidance for the proper application of electrophysiological tests.

Relationship between anatomy and function

To make valid use of electrophysiology it is necessary to know the anatomic origins of the various potentials, the appropriate stimuli to evoke them, and the methods for recording and measuring their responses.

Table 4.2 shows a survey (modified after Apfelstedt and Zrenner 2007) arranged according to the various anatomic structures of the visual pathway. Nearly every part of the visual pathway can be studied with at least one electrophysiological method.

Electrooculography

The EOG measures a physiological electrical potential difference between the cornea and the posterior pole of the globe, with the cornea by convention being the positive pole. This so-called ocular resting potential is a physiological, transepithelial electrical potential that lies across the RPE, as shown in Fig. 4.2b. Under steady conditions of illumination, the resting potential maintains a constant value called the baseline potential, but it will vary with changes in illumination. An increase in this potential is a response

Table 4.2 – Origin of the various components of the electrophysiological recordings in relation to morphological sites of the retina (modified after Apfelstedt and Zrenner 2007)

Anatomic Structure	Electrophysiological Potential	Clinical Test
Retinal pigment epithelium and photoreceptor outer segments	Ocular resting potential	Electrooculogram (EOG)
Rod outer segments	Rod a-wave	Scotopic flash ERG
Cone outer segments	Cone a-wave	Photopic flash ERG
Rod ON-bipolar cells	Rod b-wave	Scotopic flash ERG
Cone ON-bipolar cells	Cone b-wave	Photopic flash ERG
Rod OFF-bipolar cells	Rod off-effect	Scotopic long duration flash ERG
Cone OFF-bipolar cells	Cone off-effect	Photopic long duration flash ERG
Müller's glial cells	Rod and cone b-wave	Scotopic and photopic flash ERG
Inner plexiform layer and especially amacrine cells	Oscillatory potentials	Scotopic flash ERG, with special filtering
Ganglion cell layer	N 95 potential	Pattern ERG
Posterior pole, cones, bipolar cells and amacrine cells	Local retinal potential tracings	Multifocal ERG
Retinocortical conduction time	Latency	Visually evoked potentials (VEP): pattern VEP
Primary visual cortex and the cone dominated portion of the afferent pathway (central visual field)	P100 amplitude, P2 amplitude	Pattern VEP, flash VEP

of the RPE to light-induced shifts in ion concentrations in the extracellular fluid of the photoreceptor, induced by the activation of the phototransduction process in response to illumination of their outer segments. The light-dependent changes in the ocular resting potential recorded by the EOG require an intact function of the RPE and the photoreceptors.

The EOG is recorded by means of a pair of skin electrodes fixed close to the canthi of the eyelids. The patient is asked to continuously alternate his/her gaze between fixation lights at 1 second intervals for 10 seconds every minute. The fixation lights are separated by a visual angle of 40° from each other and located in a diffusely illuminated Ganzfeld sphere. The gaze-induced change in the eye bulb's angle alters the relative potential difference between the nasal and temporal electrodes. The gaze-induced potential difference is directly related to the size of the ocular resting potential. The gaze-induced modulation of the potential is measured for about 30 minutes.

The EOG procedure is described in the ISCEV Standard by Brown et al (2006).

Dark adaptation of the light-adapted eye results in a decrease in the ocular resting potential, which reaches a minimum value after about 10 minutes, the so-called dark trough (Arden et al 1962).

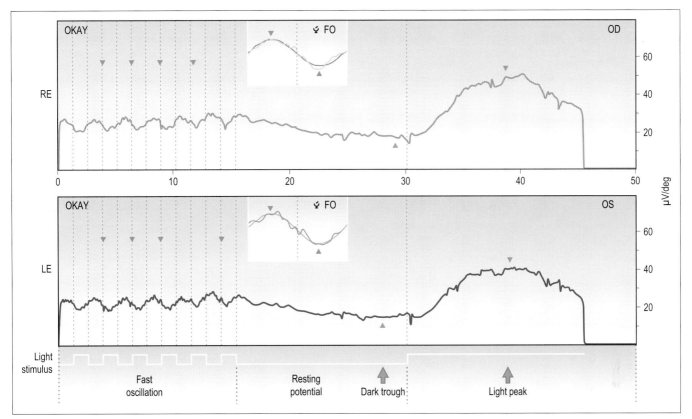

Fig. 4.5 An example of an EOG of the right (RE) and left (LE) eyes. By means of light/dark phases of 75 seconds, fast oscillations (FO) can be elicited, reflecting a change in the potential near the basal membrane of pigment epithelial cells (left third of graph and inset, averaged.) After a dark period of approximately 12 minutes (resting potential), a dark trough is recorded. Approximately 8 minutes after the onset of a light (green trace, right third) an EOG 'light peak' is reached, the so-called slow oscillation (SO).

During subsequent steady illumination of the eye, a continuous rise in the resting potential is evoked, which reaches the so-called 'light peak' 8–10 minutes after light onset (lower line in the right part of Fig. 4.5). The essential measure of the EOG is the ratio between light peak amplitude and dark trough amplitude just before light onset, the Arden ratio, which typically amounts to about 1.5–2.5 (right part of Fig. 4.5). Additionally it is possible to evoke a fast oscillation by setting a light on and off every 75 seconds. This potential is shown on the left of Fig. 4.5 and magnified in the inset figure. It stems from the RPE basal membrane.

Widespread damage to the pigment epithelial/photoreceptor complex results in a diminished light/dark ratio up to a complete loss of the light-induced potential increase.

Due to the origin of the standing potential, the EOG is the test of choice in cases where the primary functional alteration is expected in RPE cells, e.g. in chloroquine retinopathy (Johnson and Vine 1987) or phenothiazine retinopathy (Henkes 1967). Since the light-induced increase in the standing potential is triggered by photoreceptor excitation, an intact function of the neuro-retina is required to identify a pigment epitheliopathy at an early stage. Electroretinographical recordings must therefore accompany the EOG tests as well as careful ophthalmoscopy of the pigment epithelial layer for biomicroscopic alterations. Biomicroscopy is supported by autofluorescence measurements and fluorescence angiography, methods which allow us to assess the state of the RPE layer more accurately.

Ganzfeld Electroretinography

Illumination of the entire retina by a short flash causes all retinal neurons to respond with a change in their electrical potential, triggered by the phototransduction process that finally modulates the glutamate release in the photoreceptor synapses. The sum of light-evoked changes in the membrane potential of retinal cells can be recorded by corneal electrodes, such as contact lenses, gold foils or fibre electrodes, resulting in the ERG. The sketch in Fig. 4.6 points out the light-induced increase in extra-cellular potassium (K^+) in the outer and inner plexiform layers that is picked up by millions of Müller cells. Each Müller cell directs the potassium current towards the vitreous humor, forming a current loop mainly induced by the activity of the depolarizing bipolar cells (blue in Fig. 4.6). While the first event in ERG response to a strong flash is a negative response (the a-wave, shown at the top of Fig. 4.7) that reflects the photoreceptor outer segments at least in the first 10–12 milliseconds, the subsequent positive response (b-wave) is mainly created by the depolarizing bipolar cells, whose excitation is reflected in the Müller cell currents, picked up as b-waves by corneal electrodes.

The various types of amacrine cells contribute to the oscillatory potentials that are visible as little wavelets on the ascending limb of the b-wave and can be made visible by filtering out the slower a- and b-waves electronically or digitally.

While a- and b-waves reflect outer and inner retina layers, respectively, the appropriate choice of the stimulus parameter of the test flash and the ambient light level allows transretinal separation of the rod from the cone system. In a completely dark-adapted condition, achieved after 20 minutes in darkness, rods, stimulated with a weak test light, dominate the ERG response. Under light-adapted conditions (approximately 30 cd/m² of steady white background in a Ganzfeld-bowl), which saturate the rod system, strong test flashes elicit exclusively cone responses. The function of the two systems, rods and cones and the cells in the inner retina connected to the

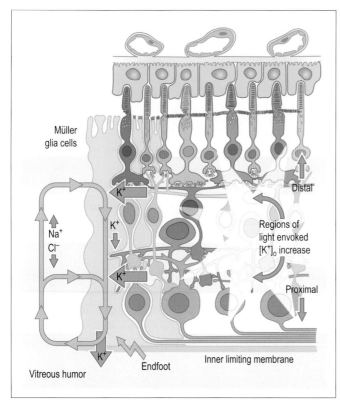

Fig. 4.6 The currents of various retinal neurons are directed perpendicularly to the retina by the Müller glial cells (yellow), forming a potassium-driven, electrical vector towards the anterior pole of the eye by potassium flow from the outer and inner plexiform layers into the vitreous humor through the Müller cell end-foot. The light-evoked current loop is closed by an Na^+/Cl^- driven current loop. The main source of this current loop is the depolarizing ON-bipolar cells (light blue), the primary source for cornea positive b-waves. Pharmacological and toxic effects on retinal neurons as well as Müller cells can therefore change the amplitude and implicit time of the electroretinographic b-wave.

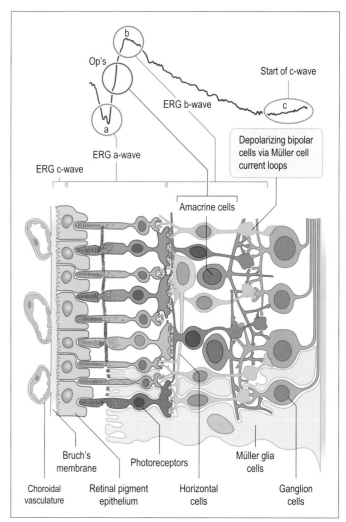

Fig. 4.7 This diagram relates the structures of the retina (lower part) to the response components in the ERG (upper part). The a-wave originates mainly in the outer retina (photoreceptor layer), while the b-wave is driven by depolarizing bipolar cells via Müller cell current loops. Amacrine cells contribute to fast wavelets along the ascending limb of the b-wave, which can be isolated by electronic filtering. The c-wave of the ERG (the beginning of which can be seen at the end of the ERG trace on the right) is a very slow and variable potential originating in the RPE cells. It is rarely used clinically because this function can be better assessed by the ERG and is difficult to record. (Sketch modified from H. Jaegle, personal communication.)

two systems, can therefore be distinguished by means of electroretinographic testing. This is important since certain compounds may predominantly affect cones, which are present everywhere in the retina but in high density in the foveolar region, while rods have a maximum density of distribution at approximately 10° eccentricity. Other compounds may exclusively affect cells in the inner retina such as amacrine cells, whose responses show up in the oscillatory potentials. Ganglion cell activity does not show up in Ganzfeld ERGs because ganglion cells do not produce a transversally directed graded potential in the retina; however, ganglion cell damage can be assessed by pattern ERG (see below).

The ISCEV has developed a Standard for Clinical Electroretinography. Since the first standard (Marmor et al 1989) several updates (Marmor and Zrenner 1999) have been published, the last one in 2004 (Marmor et al 2004). The standard describes the technical requirements in detail. Most importantly, the minimum requirement is to record the responses shown in Fig. 4.8.

1. Rod ERG after 20 minutes of dark adaptation with a dim white flash (the ISCEV standard flash (SF) of 1.5–3 cds/m² attenuated by 2.5 log U), marked by a slow b-wave.
2. Standard combined ERG with large a- and b-waves, elicited by the non-attenuated standard flash in the dark-adapted eye, representing a combination of rod and a minor cone-response.
3. Oscillatory potentials, obtained from the dark-adapted standard combined flash ERG by passing the response through electronic filters that eliminate frequencies below 75 Hz.
4. 30 Hz flicker ERG elicited under the same conditions as the single flash cone response, but at a higher repetition frequency of the stimulus that cannot be resolved by rods.
5. Single flash cone ERG after adaptation to a white background light of 17–34 cd/m², presented at the surface of a full field Ganzfeld bowl for at least 10 minutes. This response represents an isolated cone response because the white Ganzfeld light saturates the rod response.

For further references concerning the principles and practice of the electrophysiology of vision see Fishman et al (2001), Heckenlively and Arden (2006), and Apfelstedt and Zrenner (2007).

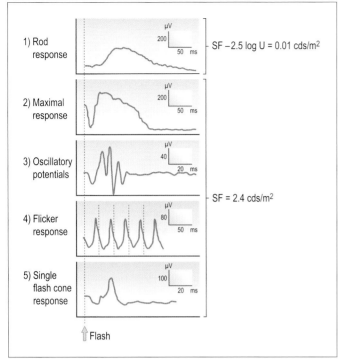

Fig. 4.8 The five ISCEV standard responses of the electroretinogram. The rod response is elicited by a dim light after 20 minutes of dark adaptation. The strength of the light is the ISCEV-defined standard flash (SF) (in this case 2.4 cds/m² attenuated by 2.5 log units, resulting in 0.01 cds/m²). The maximal response is marked by a huge a- and b-wave, representing a mixture of rod and cone responses and is elicited by the ISCEV standard flash (1.5–3 cds/m²). Oscillatory potentials are extracted by electronic filtering of all responses with frequencies of 75 Hz and higher. In the light-adapted state, the cone-driven flicker response is elicited by the standard flash with a repetition rate of 30 Hz. It is also used for the single-flash cone response. This recording reflects the minimum of electroretinographical documentation according to the recommendations of the ISCEV. For clinical trials an extended protocol that is targeted to specific mechanisms is recommended (see below).

Evaluation

In the ERG wave that is elicited by a single flash, typical components of the electrical potentials that correspond to various neuro-anatomic structures can be identified. The two primary components, the a- and b-waves, are particularly clear and easily recognizable in an ERG response that is evoked by a strong flash of light in a fully dark-adapted eye.

- a-wave: A negative component arising at the beginning of the recorded response, produced primarily by the hyperpolarization of the photoreceptor outer segments. This response appears a few milliseconds after a strong light flash stimulus and has its maximum near 16 milliseconds. The a-wave is only the leading edge of the negative potential contributed by the photoreceptors. Its further course is masked by the onset of the b-wave.
- b-wave: The b-wave arises from electrical activity in the inner layers of the retina. On the one hand, the b-wave tests the integrity of the second neuron of the afferent path (the depolarizing bipolar cell) and of Müller cells (see above); on the other hand, it indirectly reflects photoreceptor function, since the activity of the bipolar cells is determined by the strength of the rod and cone signals. A reduction in the ERG a-wave because of photoreceptor degeneration

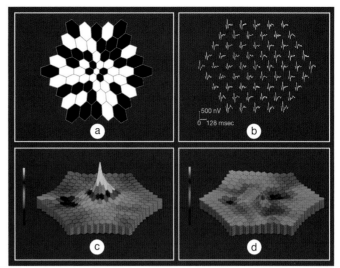

Fig. 4.9 Multifocal ERG. (a) While the Ganzfeld ERG does not allow the assessment of the topography of retinal excitability, a special hexagonal pattern, presented in the so-called m-sequence (Sutter and Tran 1992) allows the recording of multiple small ERGs from individual points (64 locations in this example) of the retina. (b) A three-dimensional plot that shows the excitability of the foveal region in the centre. (c) The amplitude depression near the optic nerve head on the left. (d) In the case of affection of the cone system, the central peak disappears.

therefore also causes a reduction in the b-wave response. Conversely, there are retinal conditions that do not impair photoreceptor function or the a-wave of the ERG, but which selectively depress or delay the b-wave.

In a flash ERG, the following parameters are evaluated:

- the amplitude of the a-wave, measured from the electrical baseline to the negative peak recorded just before the appearance of the b-wave
- the amplitude of the b-wave, measured from the trough of the a-wave to the positive peak of the b-wave
- the implicit time, indicating the time elapsed from the flash stimulus to the peak of the corresponding ERG peak (a- or b-wave)
- amplitude and implicit time of the second oscillatory potential
- amplitude and implicit time of the flicker response or its phase.

It should be noted that the 2004 update of the ISCEV recommendation for full field electroretinography additionally recommends a very strong flash (approx. 12 cds/m²) in order to better isolate the a-wave. In particular the slope of the a-wave during the first 10–12 milliseconds is probably the best parameter for isolating alterations in the photoreceptor response.

All these measurements are a minimum requirement and there are many more possibilities to extend the information on the relationship between structure and function, such as OFF-response, double flash amplitude recovery and others that may be recorded in special situations. These are described in the literature (see Heckenlively and Arden 2006).

Multifocal electroretinography

While Ganzfeld electroretinography only allows the assessment of the function of rod and cone pathways as a whole, multifocal electroretinography, as developed by Sutter and Tran (1992), has made it possible to assess the electrical activity of the retina locally from different regions of the posterior retina. The electrical responses are recorded from the eye with corneal electrodes just as in conventional ERG recording; however, a special stimulation pattern is presented on a computer monitor that consists of many hexagons, each of which has a 50% chance of being bright or dark (Fig. 4.9a). Although a pattern seems to flicker randomly, each element follows a predetermined sequence that ensures that the overall luminance of the screen over time is stable. The focal ERG signal associated with each element is calculated by correlating the continuous ERG signal with the ON or the OFF phase of each stimulus element. The result is a topographic array of many little ERGs (Fig. 4.9b), which reflects the regional response to the corresponding hexagon in Fig. 4.9a.

The waveform of each response resembles the Ganzfeld ERG in shape and origin, although some peculiarities are evident. The preferred designation for labeling these three negative and positive peaks is N1, P1 and N2, respectively, in order to distinguish them from the Ganzfeld ERG.

As shown in Fig. 4.9c, the amplitude of the local potentials can be plotted in terms of the amplitude/area of each hexagon, resulting in a response density plot (Fig. 4.9c). In this three-dimensional representation of the multifocal ERG, the fovea shows the largest response density because of the high cone photoreceptor density in this region. At the left of the peak is a depression in amplitude, indicating the physiologic blind spot. Usually the electrical map of the multifocal ERG represents a retinal area around the foveola with a radius of 25–30°. The amplitude of the pedestal at the borders of the response density array therefore reflects the activities of the retinal eccentricity up to 25–30°. Since multifocal electroretinography is done in a light-adapted state, the responses reflect the cone system's activity only. Diseases or conditions that affect the fovea result in the picture seen in Fig. 4.9d, where the central peak is lost, while generalized cone affection shows an overall loss of amplitude or response density (from Kretschmann et al 1997). Details can be found in the review by Hood (2000). Pharmacological or toxicological drug action which shows local retinal changes, such as vigabatrin (Harding et al 2002) or hydroxychloroquine (Lai et al 2006; Kellner et al 2006), does show up in multifocal ERGs.

The ISCEV has provided guidelines for basic multifocal electroretinography (Marmor et al 2003); a multifocal ERG standard will be finalized by the ISCEV in 2007.

Pattern ERG

The pattern ERG (PERG) is a retinal biopotential that is evoked when a temporary modulated pattern stimuli of constant total luminance, such as a checker-board reversal, is projected onto the retina. While the Ganzfeld ERG does not represent signals from the ganglion cells, the PERG (component P1 vs. N2, also called N95) does reflect the activity of the innermost retina. Its application in dysfunction of the macula is therefore not only strongly correlated to visual acuity (Neveu et al 2006) but also allows the assessment of ganglion cell function (Holder 2001) because its origin is in the ganglion cell level (Baker et al 1988). ISCEV has provided a standard for PERG (Holder et al 2007).

Visually evoked cortical potential

The signals processed in the retina are transmitted to the central nervous system via the axons of the ganglion cells that form the optic nerve, ending in the lateral geniculate body. There the information of both eyes merges and is transmitted to the primary visual cortex at the occipital lobe. The potentials arising in the occipital cortex can be picked up by skin electrodes fixed at the posterior pole, relative to a reference electrode mounted on the cortex. Such VEPs can be elicited by simple flash stimuli;

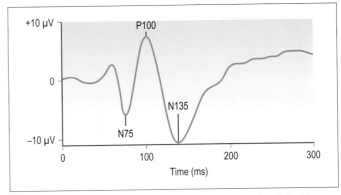

Fig. 4.10 Visually evoked cortical potentials are usually elicited by a checkerboard pattern. Recorded from the posterior pole of the eye, the response to such pattern reversal results in a strong positive deflection near 100 milliseconds (P100) arising from a negative deflection (N75) followed by another negative deflection (N135). Delays in the response properties indicate changes in the transmission velocity of signals in the optic nerve, e.g. in demyelinization.

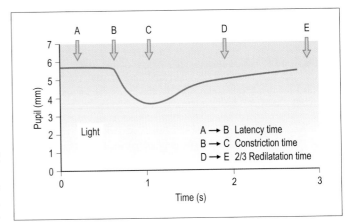

Fig. 4.11 Pupillogram. The efferent visual pathway is most easily assessed by measuring eye motility as well as pupilograms. The pupil diameter starts to decrease after a latency time in response to light and reaches its maximum constriction after approximately 1 second. The pupil usually opens again after approximately 3 seconds. Changes in these temporal dynamics point to alterations in the efferent visual pathway and/or the autonomous nervous system. (From B. Wilhelm, personal communication.)

however, a pattern reversal stimulus is the preferred technique for most clinical purposes because the results obtained with pattern reversal stimuli are less variable in wave form and timing. The patient fixates a visual target on the centre of the black and white reversal pattern; it is important that an adequate optical correction is used. The responses at the occipital lobe are very small and are masked by larger potentials not related to visual function. The stimulus must therefore be presented at least 50–100 times in order to average the stimulus-related potential changes and extract them.

The ISCEV has provided a standard for VEPs (Odom et al 2004). A typical VEP is shown in Fig. 4.10 in response to a pattern reversal stimulus. It has a negative (N75), a positive (P100) and another negative component (N135). In clinical routine testing, the P100 amplitude relative to the N75 trough as well as the implicit time of the P100 peak are determined. The value of the P100 implicit time is a good indicator of retino-cortical response latency. Any condition or compound that affects or destroys the myelin sheets of the ganglion cell axons causes a significant retardation in the velocity of axonal conduction. The prolongation of this component is therefore a good indicator for drug effects on myelin, e.g. in ethambutol.

Pupillography

Pupillography is commonly performed by infrared video systems, providing stable tracking of pupil diameter and automated analysis as an important precondition for objective assessment of visual and autonomous function (Fig. 4.11). The systems available have been listed and characterized by Wilhelm and Wilhelm (2003). For the majority of purposes the light reflex is the focus of attention when toxicological questions arise. The parameters provided during the dynamic recording of pupil size under certain stimulus conditions give selective information about the pharmacological or toxic effects of compounds in either the sympathetic or parasympathetic afferent or efferent pathway (see Wilhelm et al 1998). The exact site of effect – be it central or peripheral, sympathetic or parasympathetic – can be localized in detail if needed by additional pharmacological blocking (eye drops) of the opponent system in the periphery. Principally the constriction of the pupil to a certain light stimulus is influenced predominantly by the parasympathetic system and depends on the afferent visual pathway, while the redilation part of the light reflex is triggered by the sympathetic system.

An additional pupillographic technique (Wilhelm et al 1998) enables the objective assessment of the central nervous activation level and thus can reveal information about sedative or stimulating effects, for example in antidepressants, antihypertensives or amphetamines. This is possible because a decrease in activation level is accompanied by decreasing inhibition of the parasympathetic Edinger-Westphal nuclei in the oculomotor nerve complex. This provokes spontaneous fluctuations of pupil diameter in the dark that are closely correlated to low-frequency bands in electroencephalography. These oscillations can be recorded and analyzed by an automated software system (www.stz-biomed.de), the pupillographic sleepiness test (PST device by AMTech, Weinheim, Germany).

VISUAL ELECTROPHYSIOLOGY IN DRUG DEVELOPMENT

The visual electrophysiological techniques described here can provide useful information on safety, efficacy and proper dosage of novel chemical entities. When a new compound has been selected, preclinical exploratory tests have to be performed. In vitro toxicity tests are available, e.g. in the isolated perfused eye models (Niemeyer 2001).

At this stage whole cell patch clamp recordings from individual neurons, either in culture or in tissues such as isolated retina or retinal slice, also allow direct evaluation of the function of ligand and voltage-gated ion channels (e.g. Guenther et al 1994). This allows an understanding of the targets of the drug, especially in conjunction with immuno-histochemical studies. In order to monitor drug effects on the visual pathway under more natural physiological conditions, in vivo electrophysiological studies have to be performed (typically in rodents, pigs and dogs). As more animal models of diseases of the visual pathway become available, visual electrophysiology in animals will be crucial for questions of efficacy and safety. Preclinical toxicity studies can also help to identify the most sensitive markers for unwanted side effects or potential toxic effects to be used later in clinical studies. Moreover, functional tests can be related to histopathology in animal eyes and there are many instances where electrophysiological alterations are observed well

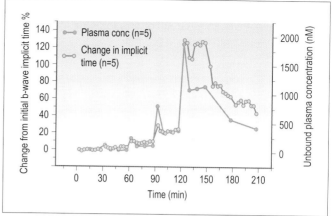

Fig. 4.12 Pharmacodynamic effects of sildenafil (Viagra®) in high doses on the ERG b-wave in dogs. The ERG b-wave implicit time becomes considerably prolonged and closely follows the pharmacokinetic profile with a time lag of approximately 30 minutes. The close relationship between the ERG effects of sildenafil and its pharmacokinetics suggests that the transient visual symptoms experienced by patients taking the drug are related to its binding to PDE6. With long-term exposure to sildenafil the pharmacodynamic effects on the ERG remain constant, with return to pre-exposure baseline following drug wash-out. The absence of any long-term changes in the ERG provides evidence that the effects of sildenafil on PDE are physiological and do not reflect a toxic process. (From Brigell et al 2005.)

ahead of histological changes (see Brigell et al 2005). However, even if an accepted safety margin is present in animal studies, there is no guarantee that this margin will apply across species to humans.

After appropriate preclinical testing, electrophysiological investigations are very important for all phases of the clinical development, as nicely outlined by Brigell et al (2005). In phase I safety studies, usually dose escalation studies, visual electrophysiology can provide variable pharmacodynamic information. It is very important to show reversibility of an effect in order to differentiate a pharmacological drug action from a toxic drug action. An example is shown in Fig. 4.12. The effect of sildenafil (Viagra) in very high doses on the dog ERG b-wave is a prolongation of the implicit time that closely follows the pharmacokinetic profile with a time lag of approximately 30 minutes. Sildenafil increases blood flow by binding PDE5 but it also binds with lower affinity to PDE6, an enzyme needed for phototransduction (for a review see Laties and Zrenner 2002). As outlined by Brigell et al (2005), the long-term exposure to sildenafil in the ERG shows the return to pre-exposure baseline following drug washout that is constant, thus reflecting a physiological and not a toxic process. Electrophysiological measures of this kind can help in differentiating toxic from pharmacological effects at this early stage.

In phase II studies, electrophysiology has successfully been applied to proof of concept trials. As a marker of an effect on the disease progression ERG or VEP is very useful in phase III studies as evidence for regulatory approval. For example, glaucomatous damage to the nerve fiber of the retina has been well characterized in the pattern ERG (Korth et al 1993). Additionally, methods have been developed to detect very tiny ERG amplitudes in patients with retinal degenerations (Birch and Sandberg 1996). In diabetic retinopathy, changes in the oscillatory potentials of the ERG can monitor the disease process (Bresnik and Palta 1987).

In phase III studies, multi-center randomized studies have to be performed, generally involving large numbers of patients. Safety usually must be demonstrated in at least 100 patients

Table 4.3a – Functional 'markers' of the various structures and cell population of the visual system assessed by electrophysiological tests, ordered according to peripheral retina (yellow), central retina (orange) and ascending visual pathways (pink).

Retinal Eccentricity	Structures of the Visual System	Electrophysiology					Clinical Examination
		EOG	Ganzfeld ERG (ISCEV 2004) No Topographic Resolution		Mf ERG and PERG Topographical Map	VEP	
			Dark Adapted Rod ERG	Light Adapted Cone ERG	Light Adapted Cone ERG	Pattern or Flash	
Center and Periphery	**Retinal pigment epithelium**	X					
>30° ecc Peripheral retina: Rod dominated	**Outer** Photoreceptors	X	**a-wave** Combined resp.				Ophthalmoscopy Pigment changes Deposits Vessels etc.
	Inner Bipolar cells		**b-wave** Rod resp.				
	Amacrine cells		Oscillatory potentials				
<30° ecc. Central retina: Cone dominated	**Outer** Photoreceptors	X		**a-wave** Single cone flash resp.	N1	X	Ophthalmoscopy Fovea reflexes Autofluorescence Optic nerve head Pigment changes Deposits Vessels etc.
	Inner Bipolar cells			**b-wave** Flicker resp. Single cone flash resp.	P1	X	
	Amacrine cells			Oscillatory potentials		X	
	Ganglion cells				N2	X	OCT, NFL
Visual pathways	Afferent visual pathway				Maculopapillar nerve fiber bundle	P100	Pupillary reflex
	Efferent visual systems, including autonomous nerve system						Eye motility, tests for diplopia, pupil investigation

OCT, optical coherence tomography; NFL, nerve fiber layer

exposed to the highest dose of the drug for a minimum of 1 year. If a drug has shown preclinical evidence of pharmacological action on the visual system, or toxicity at high doses, electrophysiological testing during clinical trials is usually necessary to provide early signs of problems in humans. It is still often difficult to differentiate the physiological effects of the drug from toxic effects. Since visual toxicity is often dependent on cumulative exposure, it is not unusual for toxicity to show up only in phase III studies.

In phase IV, small studies for the ocular toxicity of drugs are quite often initiated by investigator-driven interests or clinicians not connected to pharmaceutical companies, sometimes triggered by the observation of retinal toxicity or visual side effects reported by patients after long-term use.

The evolution of electrophysiological techniques and standards has led to increased requests for electrophysiological studies by regulatory agencies. Given their power as markers for early non-invasive detection of pharmacological or toxic effects it is likely that the role of electrophysiological ophthalmic techniques will continue to increase in the future.

COMPLEMENTARY TESTS

In clinical studies that involve electrophysiological parameters as a primary or secondary endpoint, it is mandatory to complement these tests with psychophysical testing. The results obtained in psychophysics can help greatly to differentiate between pharmacological and toxicological effects, and to better understand

Table 4.3b – Functional 'markers' of the various structures and cell populations of the visual system assessed by psychophysical tests, ordered according to peripheral retina (yellow), central retina (pink) and ascending visual pathways (pink).

Retinal Eccentricity	Structure of the Visual System	Psychophysics							Clinical Examination
		Visual Acuity	Colour Vision	Glare Sensitivity	Perimetry (visual fields)		Dark Adaptation	Pupillo-graphy	
		ETDRS Chart	D 15/28 Desatu-rated	Nyctometer Mesopto-meter	Kinetic / Cone System	Static / Cone System	Cone and Rod System	Infrared Pupillo-meter	
Center and periphery	Retinal pigment epithelium						X	X	
>30° ecc. Peripheral retina: Rod dominated	Outer Photoreceptors			Rod-cone interaction	Total area per isopter: III4e and I 3e			X	Ophthalmoscopy Pigment changes Deposits Vessels etc.
	Inner Bipolar cells								
	Amacrine cells								
<30° ecc. Central retina: Cone dominated	Outer Photoreceptors	Foveola X	Foveola X	Cone-rod interaction		Threshold method	Threshold method	X	Ophthalmoscopy Fovea reflexes Autofluorescence Optic nerve head Pigment changes Deposits Vessels etc.
	Inner Bipolar cells								
	Amacrine cells								
	Ganglion cells	X	X	X	X	X	X	X	OCT, NFL
Visual pathways	Afferent visual pathway	X	X	X	X	X	X	X	
	Efferent visual systems, including autonomous nerve system							X	Eye motility, tests for diplopia, pupil investigation

OCT, optical coherence tomography; NFL, nerve fiber layer

the site of action. Careful clinical observations of morphological alterations are equally important for this purpose.

Electrophysiology

Tables 4.3a and b summarize the selection of tests in relation to structures and their functional 'markers' of the visual system. It seems important – due to the multitude of electrophysiological and psychophysical rests and parameters – to target the battery of tests and the endpoint of a study to the site of presumed drug action. Table 4.3a relates the various structures of the visual system to the electrophysiological responses that best assess the function of these structures (peripheral retina in yellow shading, central retina in pink shading, ascending visual pathway shown in the last two rows). In Table 4.3b the complementary psychophysical tests are shown on the right-hand side, together with the particular retinal localizations and the structures that they are connected to. On the far right of each table, the clinical examinations that allow judgment on the biomicroscopical morphology and visual functions are listed in relation to the various sites of the visual system. These tables may help in selecting the appropriate tests according the presumed site of drug action.

As shown in Table 4.3a the EOG assesses the global function of the photoreceptor/pigment-epithelial complex of the entire retina. For many other tests, two general retinal areas can be discerned: structures located at eccentricities larger than 30° (upper half of Table 4.3a) and structures, functions and areas within 30° eccentricity from the foveola (lower half of Table 4.3a). Although the peripheral retina is rod-dominated, it contains cones as well, in small numbers, up to the outer periphery. The ERG therefore has to be performed in dark-adapted conditions to isolate rods as well as in light-adapted conditions to isolate cones. The a- and b-waves discern the outer and inner retina for peripheral as well as for central retina, as outlined above. PERGs and multifocal ERGs can assess only the central retina. The VEP tests the integrity of the ascending visual pathway (lowest line).

Psychophysics

The complementary psychophysical tests Table 4.3b complement electrophysiology in many ways:

- Visual acuity assesses the very central foveolar function and, to a certain extent, the patient's ability to resolve fine contrasts.
- Color vision testing with Ishihara plate does not differentiate between spectrally different cones and is therefore not very well suited for screening color vision disturbances in cases of suspected drug side effects.
- Color vision testing with color probe arrangements tests (D15/D28/FM 100 Hue Test) allows the differentiation of the involvement of the different cone mechanisms. This is particularly interesting because the short-wavelength sensitive blue cone system is quite often an early marker of drug toxicity (Pokorny et al 1979). These tests can now easily be evaluated by software available at http://colorvision.belatorok.com/dir_for_use.htm.
- Glare sensitivity is a quite common side effect in drugs that affect the interaction between rods and cones, and can be assessed by nyctometer or mesoptometer.
- Perimetry assesses cone function across visual fields since it is always performed in the presence of bright white backgrounds. Kinetic perimetry is most suited for checking retinal periphery, e.g. in terms of changes of total area/isopter, while static perimetry is most suited for the central retina as a threshold method that detects and monitors changes in local sensitivity, such as glaucoma. There are now perimeters available that perform kinetic and static perimetry in an automatic manner in a single device, e.g. Octopus 101.
- Dark adaptation assesses the time dynamics after switching off a bright light that bleaches cone and rod photopigments. It is most useful in cases where a drug affects steps in the metabolism of the visual cycle that require an intricate interaction between retinal pigment epithelial cells and photoreceptor outer segments. Since the mechanical Goldmann Weekers adaptometer is no longer available, the Roland Consult company has recently provided an alternative full field test for testing dark adaptation function, as has the LKC company with its PS1-device.

All these psychophysical tests do not isolate defects in the horizontal layers of the retina but require the whole chain of the ascending pathway, thus involving photoreceptors, bipolar cells, horizontal cells, amacrine cells, ganglion cells and optic nerve fibers, lateral geniculate function and cortical functions.

Clinical examination

Electrophysiological and psychological tests always have to be complemented by morphological investigations. In the retinal periphery, ophthalmoscopy may reveal pigment changes, deposits and alterations in vessels.

In the central retina, foveal reflexes may be of particular value in the description of pigment changes and deposits as well as alterations in the vascular system. Autofluorescence can be very useful in assessing deposits, especially in the RPE. Optic

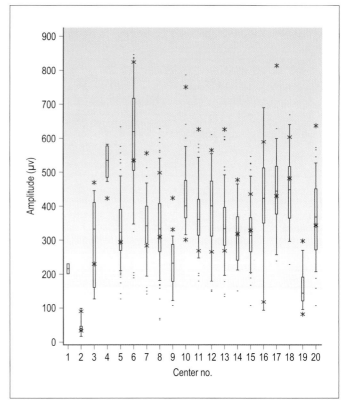

Fig. 4.13 Despite the efforts of ISCEV since 1984 to standardize responses in multi-center studies, great variations in amplitude do occur at various centers (abscissa), even though they claim to adhere to the ISCEV standard (in this case, the response in normal observers to the ISCEV standard flash). It seems necessary to check very strictly the ERG sites in terms of calibration of light and recording conditions before starting a multi-center study with the ERG. (Courtesy of Zrenner et al presentation at the meeting of the International Society of Ocular Toxicology, Lindau, 2002 (see text).)

coherence tomography has been extremely helpful in monitoring retinal edema, deposits and changes in retina thickness. Nerve fiber layer analysers can assess, in particular, ganglion cell integrity. Fundus photography is mandatory in order to document such alterations.

ENSURING QUALITY

Each of the ISCEV standards describes how to correctly perform the individual tests. In addition there is a booklet on calibration and recording published by Brigell et al 1998, which is available at www.iscev.org.

The challenge of multi-center trials

Despite two decades of standardization, unfortunately many electrophysiological laboratories adhere only loosely to the technical requirements of the standard, do not calibrate their light sources sufficiently or do not provide completely light-proof investigation rooms. An example is shown in Fig. 4.13 from a study involving 19 sites that all stated compliance with the ISCEV standard. Fig. 4.13 just shows the combined rod cone response (b-wave amplitude), the single centre normal value of which is typically near to 400 microV. Clearly some centres have lights that are much too strong and far above the ISCEV standard flash (Centre 6); others have lights that have much too weak a flash or lack proper dark adaptation (Centres 2 and 19).

In order to avoid such variation it is very important that electrophysiological laboratories are certified and validated before the study starts. This should not only include a technical description of the site but also submission of the normative values of the laboratory and typical original recordings from which the normative values of the laboratory were derived. Additionally, a copy of the calibration protocol should be requested, as well as a description of the expertise of the technical assistants. It is strongly recommended that an experienced monitor visit the site and that detailed, aim-oriented SOPs and CRFs are provided, as proposed by Zrenner, Holder, Kellner, Koester, Pollentier at the International Society for Ocular Toxicology meeting in Lindau, 2002. More recently, a network of such certified ophthalmic centers has been developed by the European Vision Institute (EVI: www.europeanvisioninstitute.org). The certification of centers, the description of SOPs and assistance with CRFs also maintains the quality of recordings (e.g. by entering calibration tests, pupil size, time and duration of dark adaptation etc.). In particular, the EVI has helped to establish EVI clinical trials sites of excellence (http://europeanvisioninstitute.org/CT_SE/), providing a network of certified centers for clinical multi-center study, including electrophysiology and psychophysiology function testing. In Tübingen, the Steinbeis Transfer Centre for Biomedical Optics and Function Testing has developed SOPs for preclinical and clinical electrophysiology for multi-center trials (www.stz-biomed.de) with electrophysiological endpoints. It is strongly recommended that such certified centers or those that are members of the ISCEV (view these at the ISCEV homepage, www.iscev.org) be selected.

Improving quality by extended protocols and evaluation

The ISCEV standard in the dark-adapted state asks for two responses: the combined rod-cone response, elicited with the standard flash (1.5–3 cds/m²), and the rod response, elicited with the standard flash, attenuated by 2.5 log units. These are just two points that relate the voltage of the amplitude to the luminance of the Ganzfeld bowl. The quality of the recordings is greatly improved if this voltage vs. log intensity function ($V - \log I$) is not only determined by two points but by at least four to six points because each point contributes to this function, as shown in Fig. 4.14. Outliers do not heavily influence the shape of the function in a match when the Naka-Rushton function ($V = V_{max} \times I^n/(k^n \times I^n + I^n)$) is applied, where V_{max} indicates the maximum amplitude, n is the slope of the function as a variable and k is the sensitivity of the half maximal response. The original recordings underlying these two functions (right eye and left eye) are shown on the left of Fig. 4.14. It also can be seen not only that the amplitude increased with luminance but also that the latency of the peak of the b-wave maximum becomes shorter. These recordings were performed in cats but equally well can be performed in humans.

The evaluation of the Naka-Rushton function has additional advantages. Changes in slope and V_{max} indicate changes in gain, while shifts in k (the luminance necessary to evoke a half maximal response) indicate a shift in sensitivity. If V_{max} is unaltered and the $V - \log I$ functions just shift to the right this indicates a change in sensitivity without loss of photoreceptors; in contrast if V_{max} becomes only 50% of a pre-treatment value there is also the possibility of a lost population of photoreceptors.

It is also advisable to record each response in the clinical study twice in order to avoid contamination by artifacts. If the critical parameters of two recordings are not approximately 90% identical, the test should be repeated by the technical assistant.

For assessment of toxic or pharmacological effects an extended targeted protocol should be used, fully exploiting the possibilities of ocular electrophysiology. Proposals for such extended ERG protocols are under development by EVI.CT.SE in close cooperation with the ISCEV (http://www.europeanvisioninsititute.org/CT_SE/).

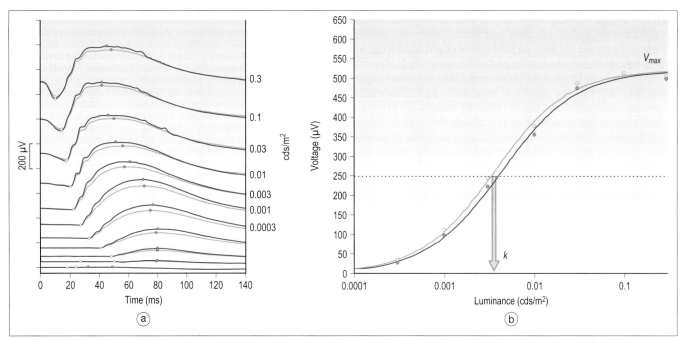

Fig. 4.14 (a) ERG recordings in response to Ganzfeld flashes of increasing intensity (as shown on the right ordinate in cds/m²). The quality of the recording is greatly improved not only if two ISCEV standard recordings are done (rod response to dim light (below) and a mixed rod/cone response to bright light (above)), but a series of responses to stepwise increasing luminance is carried out in between. (b) The amplitudes of the responses on the left side (red is right eye, green is left eye) are plotted against the luminance of the eliciting stimulus. The S-shaped function that matches the individual data points is the Naka-Rushton function. It allows the determination of the sensitivity (k), which is the stimulus luminance necessary to evoke a half-maximal voltage.

Wilhelm H, Wilhelm B, Lüdtke H. Pupillography – principles and applications in basic and clinical research. In: Pupillography: Principles Methods and Applications, Kuhlmann J, Böttcher M (eds), Zuckschwerdt Verlag, München, p 1-10, 1999.

Witkovsky P, Dearry A. Functional roles of dopamine. Prog Retinal Res 11:247-292, 1991.

Witkovsky P. Dopamine and retinal function. Doc Ophthalmol 108:17-39, 2004.

Zrenner E. Electrophysiological characteristics of the blue sensitive mechanism: Test of a model of cone interaction under physiological and pathological conditions. Doc Ophthalmol Proc Series 33:103-125, 1982.

Zrenner E. Tests of retinal function in drug toxicity. In: Manual Oculotoxicity Testing Drugs, Hockwin O, Green K, Rubin LF (eds), Fischer Verlag, Stuttgart, Jena, New York, p 331-361, 1992.

Zrenner E. No cause for alarm over retinal side-effects of sildenafil. Lancet 353:340-341, 1999.

Zrenner E. Drug side effects and toxicology of the visual system. In: Principles and Practice of Clinical Electrophysiology of Vision, 2nd edn, Heckenlively R, Arden GB (eds), MIT Press, Cambridge, London, p 655-663, 2006.

Zrenner E. Hart W. Drug induced and toxic disorders in neuro-ophthalmology. In: Clinical Neuro-Ophthalmology, Schiefer U, Wilhelm H, Hart W (eds), Chapter 17, Springer, Berlin, Heidelberg, New York, pp 223-232, 2007.

Zrenner E, Krüger CJ. Ethambutol mainly affects the function of red/green opponent neurons. Doc Ophthalmol Proc Series 27:13-25, 1981.

Zrenner E, Kramer W, Bittner Ch, et al. Rapid effects on colour vision, following intravenous injection of a new, non glycoside positive inotropic substance (AR-L 115 BS). Doc Ophthalmol Proc Series 33: 493-507, 1982.

Zrenner E, Dahlheim P, Datum KH. A role of the angiotensin-renin system for retinal neurotransmission? In: Neurobiology of the Inner Retina, Weiler R, Osborne NN (eds), Springer-Verlag, Berlin, Heidelberg, p 375-387, 1989.

PART

5 National registry of drug-induced ocular side effects

Frederick W. Fraunfelder, MD and Frederick T. Fraunfelder, MD

RATIONALE

In a specialized area, such as ophthalmology, it is not common for a practitioner or even a group of practitioners to see the patient volume necessary to make a correlation between possible cause and effect of medication-related ocular disease. Postmarketing observational studies from multiple sources permit the evaluation of drug safety in a real-world setting where off-label use and various practice patterns occur. There is no question that this has limited ability to determine causation, but it can detect 'signals' that alert the clinician as to adverse drug events. In subspecialty areas of medicine with comparatively limited markets, sometimes this is all that we have. A national registry specifically interested in a specialized area of medicine has filled a need, as shown by the three-plus decades of the National Registry of Drug-Induced Ocular Side Effects.

The National Registry, which is based at the Casey Eye Institute in Portland, Oregon, USA (www.eyedrugregistry.com), is a clearinghouse of spontaneous reports collected mostly from ophthalmologists from around the world. It is the only database which collects only eye-related ADRs. The Medwatch program run by the US FDA (www.fda.gov/medwatch/index.html) collects ADRs on all organ systems in the USA and is another source to report data to and request data from. The Uppsala Monitoring Center, a branch of the World Health Organization (WHO, Uppsala, Sweden, www.who-umc.org) collects spontaneous reports on all organ systems from around the world and has more than 70 national centers that report to them, including the FDA. Finally, clinicians and patients frequently report an ADR directly to the drug company, who in turn periodically submit these spontaneous reports to the FDA.

Regardless of where an ADR is submitted, the various organizations mentioned above can be contacted with questions about an ADR or how many types of reports exist for specific drug/ADR combinations. The National Registry provides this information free of charge to ophthalmologists and the FDA is required to provide this information to the public through the Freedom of Information Act. The WHO may charge a fee, depending on the type of information requested. The information from pharmaceutical companies should eventually end up in the FDA's Medwatch database.

Recently, spontaneous reporting databases have adopted a statistical analysis method of interpreting ADRs. At the Uppsala Monitoring Center, for instance, a quantitative method for data mining the WHO database is part of the signal detection strategy. Their method is called the Bayesian Confidence Propagation Neural Network (BCPNN) (see references). An Information Component (IC) number is calculated based on a statistical dependency between a drug and an ADR calculated on the frequency of reporting. The IC value does not give evidence of causality between a drug and an ADR, it is only an indication or signal that it may be necessary to study the individual case reports in the WHO database. The IC value calculation is a tool that can guide the WHO to create a hypothesis of association between drugs and ADRs among the over 3 million case reports in the WHO database.

This method of analysis is also being adopted within the pharmaceutical industry and at the FDA. The National Registry is also able to use the IC values as we are consultants to the WHO. If a clinician suspects an ADR, especially if it may be a new drug-induced ocular side effect, he/she is encouraged to report this to the National Registry. Membership on the website is free and it only takes 1–2 minutes to register. Frequent updates are also available on the website, informing clinicians as to what is the latest in ocular pharmacovigilance.

OBJECTIVES OF THE NATIONAL REGISTRY

- To establish a national center where possible drug-, chemical- or herbal-induced ocular side effects can be accumulated.
- To review possible drug-induced ocular side effects data collected through the FDA and the WHO Monitoring Center. To record data submitted by ophthalmologists worldwide to the National Registry.
- To compile data in the world literature on reports of possible drug-, chemical- or herbal-induced ocular side effects.
- To make available these data to physicians who feel they have a possible drug-induced ocular side effect.

HOW TO REPORT A SUSPECTED REACTION

The cases of primary interest are those adverse ocular reactions not previously recognized or those that are rare, severe, serious or unusual. To be of value, data should be complete and follow the basic format shown below.

Age:
Gender:
Suspected drug:
Suspected reaction – date of onset:
Route, dose and when drug started:
Improvement after suspected drug stopped – if restarted, did adverse reaction recur?:
Other drug(s) taken at time of suspected adverse reaction:
Other disease(s) or diagnosis(es) present:
Comments – optional (your opinion if drug-induced, probably related, possibly related or unrelated):
Your name and address (optional):

We are expanding the National Registry from only drugs to include chemicals and herbs, which may have the potential for ocular toxicity.

Send to:
Frederick W. Fraunfelder, Director
National Registry of Drug-Induced Ocular Side Effects
Casey Eye Institute
Oregon Health Sciences University
3375 S.W. Terwilliger Blvd.
Portland, Oregon 97239-4197
http://www.eyedrugregistry.com
E-mail: eyedrug@ohsu.edu

REFERENCES AND FURTHER READING

Bate A, Lindquist M, Edwards IR, et al. A Bayesian neural network method for adverse drug reaction signal generation. Eur J Clin Pharmacol 54: 315–321, 1998.

Bate A, Orre R, Lindquist M, et al. Explanation of data mining methods. BMJ website 2001; http://www.bmj.com/cgi/content/full/322/7296/1207/DC1.html.

Bate A, Lindquist M, Edwards IR, et al. A data mining approach for signal detection and analysis. Drug Saf 25: 393–397, 2002.

Bate A, Lindquist M, Orre R, et al. Data mining analyses of pharmacovigilance signals in relation to relevant comparison drugs. Eur J Clin Pharmacol 58: 483–490, 2002.

Coulter DM, Bate A, Meyboom RHB, et al. Antipsychotic drugs and heart muscle disorder in international pharmacovigilance: a data mining study. BMJ 322: 1207–1209, 2001.

Lindquist M, Stahl M, Bate A, et al. A retrospective evaluation of a data mining approach to aid finding new adverse drug reaction signals in the WHO international database. Drug Saf 23: 533–542, 2000.

Orre R, Lansener A, Bate A, et al. Bayesian neural networks with confidence estimations applied to data mining. Comput Stat Data Anal 34: 473–493, 2000.

Spigset O, Hagg S, Bate A. Hepatic injury and pancreatitis during treatment with serotonin reuptake inhibitors: data from the World Health Organization (WHO) database of adverse drug reactions. Int Clin Psychopharmacol 18: 157–161, 2003.

Van Puijenbroek EM, Bate A, Leufkens HGM, et al. A comparison of measures of disproportionality for signal detection in spontaneous reporting systems for adverse drug reaction. Pharmacoepidemiol Drug Saf 11: 3–10, 2002.

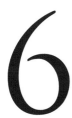

Herbal medicines and dietary supplements – an overview

Frederick W. Fraunfelder, MD

Dietary supplements are prevalent worldwide and play a significant role in the treatment of human disease. In the USA, allopathic physicians are at the early stage of learning how to treat patients with natural remedies and other forms of alternative medicine. Elsewhere, however, alternative remedies have been embraced more fully. In Germany, for example, the German Federal Health Agency created a Commission E, which has allowed for a more sophisticated approach to assessing the efficacy and safety of dietary supplements and herbal medicines, and health insurance in Germany frequently covers costs for doctor-prescribed herbal remedies. Approximately 50% of the population in the USA takes herbal products compared to 70% of the population of Germany. From published studies, only half of patients report supplement use to their physician as many consider naturally occurring products to be safe (Eisenberg 1998).

Dietary supplements represent a $US60 billion industry worldwide. While strong arguments can be made by the natural product industry that the majority of dietary supplements are safe, especially when taken in proper doses, severe toxic reactions can and do occur. Physicians and patients need to be aware of these side effects, especially as many herbal products interact with prescription medications (Coxeter et al 2004).

Frequently, ophthalmologists are the first to identify dietary supplement adverse reactions as loss of vision and eye side effects can be the first symptoms noted by patients (Fraunfelder 2004, 2005a). Systemic adverse events may not be recognized until much later, i.e. urinary tract cancer from aristolochia fangi (Nortier 2000) or death from chronic liver damage from comfrey (symphytum officinale) (Anderson and McLean 1989).

REGULATORY ISSUES AND CLASSIFICATION

Regulation and classification of dietary supplements is a confusing subject and standards vary from country to country. In the USA it is estimated that dietary supplements represent a $20 billion industry. The US Dietary Supplement Health Education Act of 1994 (DSHEA) allows herbal product companies to make 'structure or function' claims and disallows 'disease' claims. In other words, herb A can claim to maintain healthy eyes but herb A cannot make a claim that it treats glaucoma. While this seems straightforward, the FDA is unable to keep up with erroneous and sometimes illegal disease treatment claims made by the dietary supplement industry. Unlike prescription drugs, which fall under the US Food, Drug, and Cosmetic Act, dietary supplements do not have to prove pre-marketing safety or efficacy and only need to conform to the DSHEA to be legal. This creates a particularly difficult situation in which the FDA must prove a medication is dangerous after it is marketed before it can withdraw it from the market. For example, ephedra was withdrawn after causing adverse cardiovascular effects and death (Ling 2004). Even with the DSHEA, many supplements

Table 6.1 – Dietary Supplements Used to Treat Eye Disease	
Condition	**Herb or Supplement Used**
Conjunctivitis, unspecified	California peppertree (*Schinus molle*) Catechu (*Acacia catechu*) Cornflower (*Centaurea cyanus*) Eyebright (*Euphrasia officinalis*) Hibiscus (*Hibiscus sabdariffa*) Holly (*Ilex aquifolium*) Jequirity (*Abrus precatorius*) Lily-of-the-valley (*Convallaria majalis*) Marigold (*Calendula officinalis*) Turmeric (*Curcuma domestica*)
Eyes, infections of	Vinpocetine
Eye, inflammation of	Jack-in-the-pulpit (*Arisaema atrorubens*)
Night blindness	Guar gum (*Cyamopsis tetragonoloba*) Vitamin A
Night vision enhancer	Bilberry (*Vaccinium myrtillus*)
Nystagmus	Fish berry (*Anamirta cocculus*)
Ophthalmia	Asarum (*Asarum europaeum*) California peppertree (*Schinus molle*) Cape aloe (*Aloe ferox*) Chickweed (*Stellaria media*) Corydalis (*Corydalis cava*) Cornflower (*Centaurea cyanus*) Eyebright (*Euphrasia officinalis*) Jimson weed (*Datura stramonium*) Poison ivy (*Rhus toxicodendron*)
Ophthalmic disorders	Black catnip (*Phyllanthus amarus*) Black nightshade (*Solanum nigrum*) Chinese motherwort (*Leonurus japonicus*) Clove (*Syzygium aromaticum*) Dusty miller (*Senecio bicolor*) Horseradish (*Armoracia rusticana*) Licorice (*Glycyrrhiza glabra*) Male fern (*Dryopteris filix-mas*) Northern prickly ash (*Zanthoxylum americanum*) Oleander (*Nerium oleander*) Pasque flower (*Pulsatilla pratensis*) Red sandalwood (*Pterocarpus santalinus*) Scurvy grass (*Cochlearia officinalis*) Stavesacre (*Delphinium staphisagria*)
Retinopathy, diabetic	Bilberry (*Vaccinium myrtillus*)
Styes	Eyebright (*Euphrasia officinalis*)
Uveitis, chronic anterior	Curcuminoids
Visual disturbances	Nutmeg (*Myristica fragrans*)

Table 6.2 – Ocular Side Effects Associated With Dietary Supplements

Ocular Side Effect	Associated Herb or Supplement
Accommodation, impaired	Henbane (*Hyoscyamus niger*) Kava kava (*Piper methysticum*) Scopolia (*Scopolia carniolica*)
Color perception, disturbed	Lily-of-the-valley (*Convallaria majalis*) Strophanthus (*Strophanthus Kombé*)
Conjunctivitis	Chamomile (*Matricaria chamomilla*) Cypress spurge (*Euphorbia cyparissias*) Goa powder (*Andira araroba*) Propolis Psyllium (*Plantago ovata*) Psyllium seed (*Plantago afra*)
Conjunctivitis, allergic	German chamomile (*Matricaria chamomilla*)
Corneal defects	Cypress spurge (*Euphorbia cyparissias*)
Crystalline retinopathy	Canthaxanthine
Cystoid macular edema	Niacin
Diplopia	Yellow jassamine (*Gelsemium sempervirens*)
Dry eyes	Niacin
Eyes, burning of	Dimethyl sulfoxide (DMSO)
Eye movements, abnormal	Yellow jassamine (*Gelsemium sempervirens*)
Eyelid swelling	Cypress spurge (*Euphorbia cyparissias*)
Eyelids, heavy	Yellow jassamine (*Gelsemium sempervirens*)
Eyes, irritation of	Black mustard (*Brassica nigra*)
Hyphema	Ginkgo (*Ginkgo biloba*)
Intracranial hypertension	Vitamin A
Keratitis	Pyrethrum (*Chrysanthemum cinerarifolium*) Not Nice to Lice Shampoo
Miosis	Herb Paris (*Paris quadrifolia*)
Mydriasis	5-Hydroxytryptophan Henbane (*Hyoscyamus niger*) Mandrake (*Mandragora officinarum*) Valerian (*Valeriana officinalis*) Datura (*Datura Wrightii*)
Photosensitivity	Chlorella Parsnip (*Pastinaca sativa*) Pimpinella (*Pimpinella major*) Rue (*Ruta graveolens*) St. John's wort (*Hypericum perforatum*)

Ocular Side Effect	Associated Herb or Supplement
Phototoxicity	Bishop's weed (*Ammi visnaga*) Bitter orange (*Citrus aurantium*) Burning bush (*Dictamnus albus*) Celery (*Apium graveolens*) Contrayerva (*Dorstenia contrayerva*) Haronga (*Haronga madagascariensis*) Hogweed (*Heracleum sphondylium*) Lovage (*Levisticum officinale*) Masterwort (*Peucedanum ostruthium*) Parsnip (*Pastinaca sativa*) Tolu balsam (*Myroxylon balsamum*) Wafer ash (*Ptelea trifoliate*)
Retinal hemorrhage	Ginkgo (*Ginkgo biloba*)
Retrobulbar hemorrhage	Ginkgo (*Ginkgo biloba*)
Vision blurred	5-Hydroxytryptophan Huperzine A Niacin
Vision, temporary loss of	Mountain laurel (*Kalmia latifolia*)
Visual disturbances	Chaulmoogra (*Hydnocarpus* species) Horse chestnut (*Aesculus hippocastanum*) Wormseed (*Artemisia cina*) Licorice (*Glycyrrhiza glabra*)

are marketed illegally, as evidenced by a study in the *Journal of the American Medical Association,* which researched the marketing practices of dietary supplement companies. This study showed that 55% of retailers make illegal disease claims of the treatment, prevention, diagnosis and cure of specific diseases through self treatment with various herbal medicines and nutritional supplements (Morris and Avorn 2003).

Classification of dietary supplements is also a difficult issue. In many countries, including the USA, different parts of the plant are harvested, and the collection and extraction of ingredients vary from company to company. Is the root, the flower, the stem or the seed being used for therapeutic benefit? How much of a herb is in the marketed product? Ginseng was evaluated by the American Botanical Council in 2001 and it was found that only 52% of marketed ginseng products actually contained any ginseng (Dharmananda 2002). Because of issues such as these, the World Health Organization (WHO) has published guidelines on cultivating, collecting, classification, quality control, storage, labeling, distribution and post-marketing surveillance of herbal medicines, which if adhered to worldwide would simplify the classification process (WHO Guidelines 2004).

The following herbal medicines and dietary supplements are described in this book as the ocular side effects are significant and well-documented: *Canthaxanthine, Chamomile, Chrysanthenemum, Datura, Echinacea purpurea, Ginkgo biloba,* licorice, niacin, vitamin A and vitamin D (Fraunfelder 2004, 2005a). There are many other herbs and supplements used to treat eye disease and many are associated with adverse ocular events; these are summarized in Tables 6.1 and 6.2.

REFERENCES AND FURTHER READING

Anderson PC, McLean AEM. Comfrey and liver damage. Hum Toxicol 8: 68–69, 1989.

Coxeter PD, et al. Herb-drug interactions: An evidence based approach. Curr Med Chem 11: 1513–1525, 2004.

Dharmananda S. The nature of ginseng: traditional use, modern research and the question of dosage. Herbal Gram 54: 34–51, 2002.

Eisenberg DM. Trends in alternative medicine use in the United States, 1990-1997: results of a follow-up national survey. JAMA 289(18): 1569–1575, 1998.

Fraunfelder FW. Ocular side effects from herbal medicines and nutritional supplements. Am J Ophthalmol 138(4): 639–647, 2004.

Fraunfelder FW. The science and marketing of dietary supplements. Am J Ophthalmol 140: 302–304, 2005a.

Fraunfelder FW. Ocular side effects associated with dietary supplements and herbal medicines. Drugs Today 41: 537–545, 2005b.

Ling AM. FDA to ban sales of dietary supplements containing ephedra. J Law Med Ethics 32(1): 184–186, 2004.

Morris CA, Avorn J. Internet marketing of herbal products. JAMA 290(11): 1505–1509, 2003.

Nortier JL. Urothelial carcinoma associated with the use of a Chinese herb. N Engl J Med 342: 1686–1692, 2000.

WHO Guidelines on Good Agricultural and Collection Practices for Medicinal Plants. Marketing and Dissemination. World Health Organization, Geneva, Switzerland, 2004.

CLASS: AIDS-RELATED AGENTS

Generic name: Didanosine.

Proprietary name: Videx.

Primary use
A purine analogue with antiretrovirus activity used in HIV infections.

Ocular side effects

Systemic administration
Certain
1. Retina – choroid
   a. RPE mottling
   b. RPE atrophy
   c. RPE hypertrophy
   d. Abnormality of neurosensory retina
   e. Loss of choriocapillaris
2. EOGs – reduced Arden ratio
3. Visual field defects
   a. Scotoma
   b. Constriction
4. Night blindness
5. Optic neuritis

Clinical significance
Didanosine is somewhat unique in that significant neurosensory retinal problems may occur without visual funduscopic changes. Whitcup et al (1992, 1994) described retinal lesions that first appear as patches of RPE mottling and atrophy in the midperiphery of the fundi in children taking didanosine. In time, these lesions became more circumscribed and developed a border of RPE hypertrophy. Cobo et al (1996) described similar changes in adults. Electrophysiological and ophthalmalogical findings suggest diffuse dysfunction of the RPE. Histological findings confirm multiple areas of RPE loss. Electron microscopic findings show normal mitochondria, but with membranous lamellar inclusions and cytoplasmic bodies in the RPE, which resemble the inclusion in lysosomal storage diseases. If didanosine therapy continues progression will occur, although there is some improvement once the drug is stopped. Night blindness and EOG changes appear to be reversible once the drug is discontinued. Although the midperiphery is the area first involved, lesions may encroach on the posterior pole if the drug is continued at high dosage. To date, central visual acuity has been preserved. Didanosine's toxic effects on the retina appear related both to peak dosage and accumulated dosage. Toxicity appears to be worse in patients with advanced stages of HIV disease. Patients taking this drug should be monitored for the development and progression of retinal lesions. Cobo et al (1996) contend that retinal toxicity to this drug is under-recognized.

Recommendations
1. Patients on this drug should be questioned as to visual symptoms, including specific questions regarding night vision, scotoma and constriction of visual fields.
2. If any of the above problems occur, visual fields and/or electrophysiologic studies (i.e. EOGs) should be considered.
3. Since many patients are unaware of visual changes, consider a visual field test in patients on didanosine for over 2 years.
4. This drug may need to be stopped in some patients based on retinal changes and the prognosis of some improvement if didanosine is discontinued.

REFERENCES AND FURTHER READING

Cobo J, et al. Retinal toxicity associated with didanosine in HIV-infected adults. AIDS 10: 1297-1300, 1996.
Nguyen BY, et al. A pilot study of sequential therapy with zidovudine plus acyclovir, dideoxyinosine, and dideoxycytidine in patients with severe human immunodeficiency virus infection. J Infect Dis 168: 810-817, 1993.
Whitcup SM, et al. Retinal toxicity in human immunodeficiency virus infected children treated with 2′,3′-dideoxyinosine. Am J Ophthalmol 113: 1-7, 1992.
Whitcup SM, et al. A clinicopathologic report of the retinal lesions associated with didanosine. Arch Ophthalmol 112: 1594-1598, 1994.

Generic name: Zidovudine.

Proprietary name: Retrovir.

Primary use
Zidovudine is used in the management of AIDS and AIDS-related complex.

Ocular side effects

Systemic administration (oral or intravenous)
Certain
1. Hypertrichosis
2. Eyelids
   a. Urticaria

b. Rashes

c. Vasculitis

3. Hyperpigmentation eyelids and conjunctiva

Probable

1. Cystoid macular edema
2. Color vision abnormalities
3. Visual hallucinations

Conditional/Unclassified

1. Diplopia (only with generalized myopathy)
2. Nystagmus (overdose)

Clinical significance

This drug is usually used in combination with many other drugs, so it is often difficult to put a direct cause-and-effect relationship between the drug and an ocular side effect. There have, however, been a number of reports of cystoid macular edema while on this agent that have resolved when the drug was discontinued. Lalonde et al (1991) support this with a case of positive dechallenge/rechallenge data. Geier et al (1993) reported cases of tritan color vision defects secondary to zidovudine. Clearly, hypertrichosis (Klutman and Hinthorn 1991 and National Registry cases) can occur as well as skin rashes secondary to zidovudine. Hyperpigmentation of the eyelids, conjunctiva, fingernails, etc., especially in heavily pigmented people, has been reported. Diplopia may occur secondary to a generalized myopathy. Nystagmus has only been reported in overdose situations.

REFERENCES AND FURTHER READING

Geier SA, Held M, Bogner J, et al. Impairment of tritan colour vision after initiation of treatment with zidovudine in patients with HIV disease or AIDS. Br J Ophthal 77: 315–316, 1993.

Klutman NE, Hinthorn DR. Excessive growth of eyelashes in a patient with AIDS being treated with zidovudine. N Engl J Med 324(26): 1896, 1991.

Lalonde RG, Deschênes JG, Seamone C. Zidovudine-induced macular edema. Ann Int Med 114(4): 297–298, 1991.

Luchi M, Warren KA, Saverhagen C, Hinthorn D. Transient visual loss due to severe anemia in a patient with AIDS. J La State Med Soc 151(2): 82-85, 1999.

Merenich JA, et al. Azidothymidine-induced hyperpigmentation mimicking primary adrenal insufficiency. Am J Med 86: 469–470, 1989.

Spear JB, Kessler HA, Nusinoff Lehrman S, de Miranda P. Zidovudine overdose. First report of ataxia and nystagmus: case report. Ann Int Med 109: 76–77, 1988.

Steinfeld SD, Demols P, Van Vooren JP, et al. Zidovudine in primary Sjogren's syndrome. Rheumatol 38(9): 814–817, 1999.

Strominger MB, Sachs R, Engel HM. Macular edema from zidovudine? Ann Int Med 115(1): 67, 1991.

Wilde MI, Langtry HD. Zidovudine: an update of its pharmacodynamic and pharmacokinetic properties, and therapeutic efficacy. Drugs 46(3): 515–578, 1993.

CLASS: AMEBICIDES

Generic names: 1. Broxyquinoline; 2. diiodohydroxyquinoline (iodoquinol).

Proprietary names: 1. Starogyn, 2. Sebaquin, Yodoxin.

Primary use

These amebicidal agents are effective against *Entamoeba histolytica*.

Ocular side effects

Systemic administration
Certain

1. Decreased vision
2. Optic atrophy
3. Optic neuritis – subacute myelo-optic neuropathy (SMON)
4. Nystagmus
5. Toxic amblyopia
6. Macular edema
7. Macular degeneration
8. Diplopia
9. Absence of foveal reflex
10. Problems with color vision
    a. Color vision defect
    b. Purple spots on white background

Clinical significance

Major toxic ocular effects may occur with long-term oral administration of these amebicidal agents, especially in children. Since they are given orally for *Entamoeba histolytica*, most reports are from the Far East. Data suggest that these amebicides may cause SMON. This neurologic disease has a 19% incidence of decreased vision and a 2.5% incidence of toxic amblyopia. It has been suggested that in patients being treated for acrodermatitis enteropathica, a disease of inherited zinc deficiency, optic atrophy may be secondary to zinc deficiency instead of diiodohydroxyquinoline. Since long-term quinolone exposure has been shown to result in accumulation of the drug in pigmented tissues, retinal degenerative changes may be observed. The best overall review of this subject is in Grant and Schuman (1993).

REFERENCES AND FURTHER READING

Baumgartner G, et al. Neurotoxicity of halogenated hydroxyquinolines: clinical analysis of cases reported outside Japan. J Neurol Neurosurg Psychiatry 42: 1073, 1979.

Committee on Drugs, 1989–1990. Clioquinol (iodochlorhydroxyquin, vioform) and iodquinol (diiodohydroxyquin): blindness and neuropathy. Pediatrics 86(5): 797–798, 1990.

Grant WM, Schuman JS. Toxicology of the Eye. 4th edn. Charles C Thomas, Springfield, IL, pp 282–283 and 842–843, 1993.

Guy-Grand B, Basdevant A, Soffer M. Oxyquinoline neurotoxicity. Lancet I 993, 1983.

Hanakago R, Uono M. Clioquinol intoxication occurring in the treatment of acrodermatitis enteropathica with reference to SMON outside of Japan. Clin Toxicol 18: 1427, 1981.

Hansson O, Herxheimer A. Neurotoxicity of oxyquinolines. Lancet 2: 1253, 1980.

Kauffman ER, et al. Clioquinol (iodochlorhydroxyquin, vioform) and iodoquinol (diiodohydroxyquin): blindness and neuropathy. Pediatrics 86: 978-979, 1990.

Kono R. Review of subacute myelo-optic neuropathy (SMON) and studies done by the SMON research commission. Jpn J Med Sci Biol 28(suppl): 121, 1975.

Oakley GP. The neurotoxicity of the halogenated hydroxyquinolines. JAMA 225: 395–397, 1973.

Ricoy JR, Ortega A, Cabello A. Subacute myelo-optic neuropathy (SMON). First Neuro-pathological report outside Japan. J Neurol Sci 53: 241, 1982.

Rose FC, Gawel M. Clioquinol neurotoxicity: an overview. Acta Neurol Scand 70(suppl 100): 137–145, 1984.

Shibasaki H, et al: Peripheral and central nerve conduction in subacute myelo-optic neuropathy. Neurology 32: 1186, 1982.

Shigematsu I. Subacute myelo-optic neuropathy (SMON) and clioquinol. Jpn J Med Sci Biol 28(suppl): 35–55, 1975.

Sturtevant FM. Zinc deficiency Acrodermatitis enteropathica, optic atrophy SMON, and 5,7-dihalo-8-quinolinols. Pediatrics 65: 610, 1980.

Tjalve H. The aetiology of SMON may involve an interaction between Clioquinol and environmental metals. Med Hypotheses 15: 293, 1984.

Generic name: Emetine hydrochloride.

Proprietary name: Multi-ingredient preparations only.

Primary use

This alkaloid is effective in the treatment of acute amebic dysentery, amebic hepatitis and amebic abscesses.

Ocular side effects

Systemic administration (subcutaneous or intramuscular injection near toxic levels)
Certain
1. Non-specific ocular irritation
   a. Lacrimation
   b. Hyperemia
   c. Photophobia
   d. Foreign body sensation
2. Eyelids or conjunctiva
   a. Hyperemia
   b. Edema
   c. Urticaria
   d. Purpura
   e. Eczema
3. Cornea
   a. Superficial punctate keratitis
   b. Erosions
4. Pupils
   a. Mydriasis
   b. Absence of reaction to light
5. Paralysis of accommodation
6. Decreased vision
7. Visual fields
   a. Scotomas – central
   b. Constriction
8. Retinal and optic nerve
   a. Ischemia
   b. Hyperemia optic nerve

Inadvertent ocular exposure
Certain
1. Irritation
   a. Lacrimation
   b. Hyperemia
   c. Photophobia
2. Eyelids or conjunctiva
   a. Allergic reactions
   b. Conjunctivitis – non-specific
   c. Blepharospasm
3. Cornea
   a. Keratitis
   b. Ulceration

Conditional/Unclassified
1. Iritis
2. Secondary glaucoma

Clinical significance

While this is a limited use drug, and most of the data are from the older literature, the basic ingredient in ipecac is emetine hydrochloride, which is used off-label to induce vomiting in patients with anorexia nervosa. Emetine hydrochloride is somewhat unique in that somewhere between 4 and 10 hours after exposure in humans, the drug is probably secreted in the tears to give significant bilateral foreign body sensation, epiphoria, photophobia, lid edema, blepharospasm and conjunctival hyperemia. Since the drug is seldom used for longer than 5 days, these signs and symptoms quickly resolve once the drug is discontinued (Fontana 1948). At normal dosages, these are probably the only ocular side effects, but at higher doses Jacovides (1923) describes optic nerve and retinal ischemic changes with pupillary, accommodation, vision and visual field abnormalities. These are all transitory with complete recovery.

Emetine hydrochloride is highly toxic when inadvertent direct ocular exposure occurs. This rarely causes significant scarring with permanent corneal opacities with or without iritis and secondary glaucoma.

REFERENCES AND FURTHER READING

Fontana G. The effect of emetine on the cornea. Arch Ottalmol Ocu (Italian) 52: 115–132, 1948.
Jacovides O. Troubles visuels a la suite d'injections fortes d'emetine. Arch Ophtalmol (Paris) 40: 657, 1923.
Lasky MA. Corneal response to emetine hydrochloride. Arch Ophthalmol 44: 47, 1950.
Porges N. Tragedy in compounding (Letter). J Am Pharm Assoc Pract Pharm 9: 593, 1948.
Reynolds JEF (ed). Martindale: The Extra Pharmacopoeia, 28th edn, Pharmaceutical Press, London, pp 978–979, 1982.
Torres Estrada A. Ocular lesions caused by emetine. Bol Hosp Oftal NS Luz (Mex) 2: 145, 1944 (Am J Ophthalmol 28: 1060, 1945).

CLASS: ANTHELMINTICS

Generic name: Diethylcarbamazine citrate.

Proprietary name: Hetrazan.

Primary use

This antifilarial agent is particularly effective against *Wuchereria bancrofti*, *Wuchereria malayi*, *Onchocherca volvulus* and *Loa loa*.

Ocular side effects

Systemic administration – secondary to the drug-induced death of the organism
Certain
1. Eyelids or conjunctiva
   a. Allergic reactions
   b. Conjunctivitis – non-specific
   c. Edema
   d. Urticaria
   e. Nodules
2. Uveitis
3. Cornea – probably drug related
   a. Fluffy punctate opacities
   b. Punctate keratitis
4. Chorioretinitis
5. Visual field defects
6. Chorioretinal pigmentary changes

7. Loss of eyelashes or eyebrows
8. Toxic amblyopia

Local ophthalmic use or exposure – topical application
Certain
1. Eyelids or conjunctiva
   a. Allergic reactions
   b. Erythema
   c. Edema
2. Irritation
   a. Lacrimation
   b. Hyperemia
   c. Photophobia
   d. Ocular pain
3. Corneal opacities
4. Cornea – probably drug related
   a. Fluffy punctate opacities
   b. Punctate keratitis

Clinical significance
Adverse ocular reactions to diethylcarbamazine are rare, however severe reactions depend in large part on which organism is being treated. Drug-induced death of the filaria can result in a severe allergic reaction due to the release of foreign protein. Nodules may form in the area of the dead worm from a secondary inflammatory reaction. This reaction in the eye may be so marked that toxic amblyopia follows. Newer drugs that kill the organism more slowly are being used, with fewer ocular side effects. The use of diethylcarbamazine eye drops for treatment of ocular onchocerciasis produces dose-related inflammatory reactions similar to those seen with systemic use of the drug. Local ocular effects may include globular limbal infiltrates, severe vasculitis, itching and erythema.

REFERENCES AND FURTHER READING

Bird AC, et al. Visual loss during oral diethylcarbamazine treatment for onchocerciasis. BMJ 2: 46, 1979.
Bird AC, et al. Changes in visual function and in the posterior segment of the eye during treatment of onchocerciasis with diethylcarbamazine citrate. Br J Ophthalmol 64: 191, 1980.
Dadzie KY, Bird AC. Ocular findings in a double-blind study of ivermectin versus diethylcarbamazapine versus placebo in the treatment of onchocerciasis. Br J Ophthalmol 71: 78–85, 1987.
Hawking F. Diethylcarbamazine and new compounds for treatment of filariasis. Adv Pharmacol Chemother 16: 129–194, 1979.
Jones BR, Anderson J, Fuglsang H. Effects of various concentrations of diethylcarbamazine citrate applied as eye drops in ocular onchocerciasis, and the possibilities of improved therapy from continuous non-pulsed delivery. Br J Ophthalmol 62: 428, 1978.
Taylor HR, Greene BM. Ocular changes with oral and transepidermal diethylcarbamazine therapy of onchocerciasis. Br J Ophthalmol 65: 494, 1981.

Generic name: Mepacrine hydrochloride.

Proprietary name: Atabrine.

Primary use
This methoxyacridine agent is effective in the treatment of tapeworm infestations and in the prophylaxis and treatment of malaria.

Ocular side effects

Systemic administration
Certain
1. Decreased vision
2. Yellow, white, clear, brown, blue or gray punctate deposits
   a. Conjunctiva
   b. Cornea
   c. Nasolacrimal system
   d. Sclera
3. Cornea
   a. Corneal edema
   b. Superficial punctate keratitis
4. Problems with color vision
   a. Color vision defects
   b. Objects have yellow, green, blue or violet tinge
   c. Colored haloes around lights – mainly blue
5. Eyelids or conjunctiva
   a. Blue-black hyperpigmentation
   b. Yellow discoloration
   c. Urticaria
6. Photophobia
7. Visual hallucinations

Probable
1. Posterior subcapsular cataracts

Possible
1. Macula - bull's eye appearance with thinning and clumping of the pigment epithelium
2. Subconjunctival or retinal hemorrhages secondary to drug-induced anemia
3. Eyelids or conjunctiva
   a. Exfoliative dermatitis
   b. Eczema

Inadvertent direct ocular exposure
Certain
1. Irritation
   a. Lacrimation
   b. Ocular pain
2. Eyelids, conjunctiva or cornea
   a. Edema
   b. Yellow or yellow green discoloration
3. Blue haloes around lights

Clinical significance
Adverse ocular reactions due to mepacrine are common but most are reversible and fairly asymptomatic. Systemic mepacrine can stain eyelids, conjunctiva, cornea and sclera yellow, and the basal layers of the conjunctival epithelium blue-gray. This is probably due to the drug being present in the tears. The pigmentary deposition and/or corneal edema may cause complaints of decreased vision, as well as yellow, blue, green or violet vision. These changes are reversible once the drug is discontinued. This may or may not be associated with a superficial keratitis. Drug-induced corneal edema may be precipitated in sensitive individuals, especially those with hepatic dysfunction. This can occur on dosages as low as 0.10 g per day and may take several weeks of therapy to occur. If the drug is discontinued this will resolve, but if the drug is restarted the edema occurs again in a few days. Cumming and Mitchell (1998) in the Blue Mountain Eye Study found an association between mepacrine and posterior subcapsular cataracts. Reports

of optic neuritis, scotoma and enlarged blind spots are usually single case reports over 50 years ago and are not substantiated as a cause-and-effect relationship.

Direct ocular exposure mepacrine occurs either from those exposed to the dust during its manufacture (Mann 1947) or those self-infected (Somerville-Large 1947). This drug can stain the eyelids, cornea and conjunctiva. Significant corneal changes, including severe edema and folds in Descemet's membrane, may occur. Color vision changes can also occur. These changes are reversible.

REFERENCES AND FURTHER READING

Abbey EA, Lawrence EA. The effect of atabrine suppressive therapy on eyesight in pilots. JAMA 130: 786, 1946.

Ansdell VE, Common JD. Corneal changes induced by mepacrine. J Trop Med Hyg 82: 206–207, 1979.

Blumenfeld NE. Staining of the conjunctiva and cornea. Vestn Oftalmol 25: 39, 1946.

Carr RE, Henkind P, Rothfield N, et al. Ocular toxicity of antimalarial drugs: long term follow-up. Am J Ophthalmol 66: 738–744, 1968.

Chamberlain WP, Boles DJ. Edema of cornea precipitated by quinacrine (Atabrine). Arch Ophthalmol 35: 120–134, 1946.

Cumming RG, Mitchell P. Medications and cataract – The Blue Mountains Eye Study. Ophthalmol 105(9): 1751–1757, 1998.

Dame LR. Effects of atabrine on the visual system. Am J Ophthalmol 29: 1432–1434, 1946.

Evans RL, et al. Antimalarial psychosis revisited. Arch Dermatol 120: 765, 1984.

Ferrera A. Optic neuritis from high doses of atebrin. Rass Intal Ottalmol 12: 123, 1943.

Granstein RD, Sober AJ. Drug- and heavy metal-induced hyperpigmentation. J Am Acad Dermatol 5: 1, 1981.

Koranda FC. Antimalarials. J Am Acad Dermatol 4: 650, 1981.

Mann I. 'Blue haloes' in atebrin workers. Br J Ophthalmol 31: 40–46, 1947.

Sokol RJ, Lichenstein PK, Farrell MK. Quinacrine hydrochloride yellow discoloration of the skin in children. Pediatrics 69: 232, 1982.

Somerville-Large LB. Mepicrine and the eye. Br J Ophthalmol 31: 191–192, 1947.

Generic name: Piperazine.

Proprietary name: Piperazine.

Primary use
This anthelmintic agent is used in the treatment of ascariasis and enterobiasis.

Ocular side effects

Systemic administration
Probable
1. Decreased vision
2. Problems with color vision – color vision defect
3. Paralysis of accommodation
4. Miosis
5. Nystagmus
6. Visual hallucinations
7. Paralysis of extraocular muscles
8. Visual sensations
   a. Flashing lights
   b. Entopic light flashes
9. Eyelids or conjunctiva
   a. Allergic reactions
   b. Edema
   c. Photosensitivity
   d. Urticaria
   e. Purpura
   h. Angioedema
10. Lacrimation

Possible
1. Subconjunctival or retinal hemorrhages secondary to drug-induced anemia
2. Eyelids or conjunctiva
   a. Erythema multiforme
   b. Eczema

Conditional/Unclassified
1. Cataract

Clinical significance
While a number of ocular side effects have been attributed to piperazine, they are rare, reversible and usually of little clinical importance. Adverse ocular reactions generally occur only in instances of overdose or in cases of impaired renal function or in systemic neurotoxic states. A few cases of well-documented extraocular muscle paralysis have been reported. There are suggestions that this is a cataractogenic agent, but this is unproven.

REFERENCES AND FURTHER READING

Bomb BS, Bebi HK. Neurotoxic side-effects of piperazine. Trans R Soc Trop Med Hyg 70: 358, 1976.

Brown HW, Chan KF, Hussey KL. Treatment of enterobiasis and ascariasis with piperazine. JAMA 161: 515, 1956.

Combes B, Damon A, Gottfried E. Piperazine (Antepar) neurotoxicity report of a case probably due to renal insuffciency. N Engl J Med 254: 223, 1956.

Mezey P. The role of piperazine derivates in the pathogenesis of cataract. Klin Monatsbl Augenheilkd 151: 885, 1967.

Mossmer A. On the effectiveness, dosage, and toxic effects of piperazine preparations. Med Mschr 10: 517–526, 1956.

Neff L. Another severe psychological reaction to side effect of medication in an adolescent. JAMA 197: 218–219, 1966.

Rouher F, Cantat MA. Instructive observation of an ocular paralysis after taking piperazine. Bull Soc Franc Ophthalmol 75: 460–465, 1962.

Generic name: Thiabendazole.

Proprietary name: Mintezol.

Primary use
This benzimidazole compound is used in the treatment of enterobiasis, strongyloidiasis, ascariasis, uncinariasis, trichuriasis and cutaneous larva migrans. It has been advocated as an antimycotic in corneal ulcers.

Ocular side effects

Systemic administration
Probable
1. Decreased vision
2. Problems with color vision
   a. Color vision defect
   b. Objects have yellow tinge
3. Abnormal visual sensations

4. Eyelids or conjunctiva
   a. Allergic reactions
   b. Hyperemia
   c. Angioneurotic edema
   d. Urticaria
5. Visual hallucinations

Possible
1. Keratoconjunctivitis sicca
2. Subconjunctival or retinal hemorrhages secondary to drug-induced anemia
3. Eyelids of conjunctiva
   a. Erythema multiforme
   b. Stevens-Johnson syndrome
   c. Exfoliative dermatitis
   d. Lyell's syndrome

Clinical significance

While thiabendazole is a potent therapeutic agent, it has surprisingly few reported ocular or systemic toxic side effects. Ocular side effects that occur are transitory, reversible, and seldom of clinical importance. However, a mother and daughter after only a few doses developed keratoconjunctivitis sicca, xerostomia, cholangiostatic hepatitis and pancreatic dysfunction. Rex et al (1983) and Davidson et al (1988) reported a case similar to this. Some feel these reactions may represent an allergic response to the dead parasites rather than a direct drug effect. This agent may induce ocular pemphigoid-like syndrome.

REFERENCES AND FURTHER READING

Drugs for parasitic infections. Med Lett Drugs Ther 24: 12, 1982.

Davidson RN, Weir WRC, Kaye GL, McIntyre N. Intrahepatic cholestasis after thiabendazole. Trans R Soc Trop Med Hyg 82: 620, 1988.

Fink AI, MacKay CJ, Cutler SS. Sicca complex and cholestatic jaundice in two members of a family caused by thiabendazole. Trans Am Ophthalmol Soc 76: 108, 1978.

Fraunfelder FT. Interim report: national registry of drug-induced ocular side effects. Ophthalmology 86: 126, 1979.

Fraunfelder FT, Meyer SM. Ocular toxicology update. Aust J Ophthalmol 12: 391–394, 1984.

Rex D, Lumeng L, Eble J, et al. Intrahepatic cholestasis and sicca complex after thiabendazole. Gastroenterology 85: 718–721, 1983.

Robinson HJ, Stoerk HC, Graessle O. Studies on the toxicologic and pharmacologic properties of thiabendazole. Toxicol Appl Pharmacol 7: 53–63, 1965.

CLASS: ANTIBIOTICS

Generic name: Amikacin.

Proprietary name: Amikin.

Primary use

This systemically administered aminoglycoside is primarily used for Gram-negative infections.

Ocular side effects

Systemic administration
Certain
1. Decreased vision
2. Eyelids or conjunctiva
   a. Urticaria
   b. Purpura

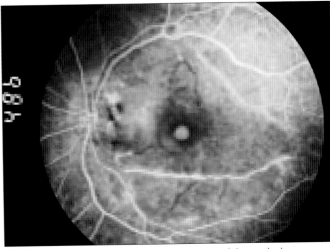

Fig. 7.1a Amikacan retinal toxicity: diffuse arteriolar occlusion as seen on fluroescein angiography. Photo courtesy of the British Journal of Ophthalmology.

Local ophthalmic use or exposure – intravitreal injection
Certain
1. Macular infarcts
2. Retinal toxicity (Fig. 7.1a)
3. Retinal degneration

Clinical significance

This aminoglycoside rarely causes ocular side effects when given orally. Ophthalmologists' interest in this antibiotic is primarily for intravitreal injections, usually in combination with a cephalosporin for management of endophthalmitis. Gentamicin has been the aminoglycoside of choice for intravitreal injections until reports of macular infarcts occurred. Amikacin was shown to be less toxic to the retina than gentamicin, so many surgeons started using it intravitreally. However, now cases of retinal infarcts have been reported with this agent, with perifoveal capillaries becoming occluded, as per fluorescein angiography. Recently, D'Amico et al (1985) found lysomal inclusions in the retinal pigment epithelium secondary to amikacin. Campochiaro (Campochiaro and Conway 1991; Campochiaro and Green 1992; Campochiaro and Lim 1994) pointed out the role of the dependent position of the macula at the time of intravitreal injection with the resultant potential increased concentration of this drug over the macula. Aminoglycosides have a known toxic effect on ganglion and other neural cells of the retina. Doft and Barza (1994, 2004), from the Endophthalmitis Vitreous Study Group, feel that the data are not compelling enough to suggest a different antibiotic, and still continue to recommend amikacin as the empirical standard to date. The National Registry is aware of more than 30 cases of macular infarct associated with amikacin use. However, based on risk/benefit ratios, along with the available clinical data, Doft and Barza's recommendation seems reasonable. This is, however, an area of controversy among retinal specialists shown by Galloway et al (2002, 2004).

REFERENCES AND FURTHER READING

Campochiaro PA, Conway BP. Aminoglycoside toxicity – A survey of retinal specialists: implications for ocular use. Arch Ophthalmol 109: 946–950, 1991.

Campochiaro PA, Green WR. Toxicity of intravitreous ceftazidime in primate retina. Arch Ophthalmol 110: 1625–1629, 1992.

Campochiaro PA, Lim JI. The Aminoglycoside Toxicity Study Group. Aminoglycoside toxicity in the treatment of endophthalmitis. Arch Ophthalmol 112: 48–53, 1994.

D'Amico DJ, Caspers-Velu L, et al. Comparative toxicity of intravitreal aminoglycoside antibiotics. Am J Ophthalmol 100: 264–275, 1985.

Doft BH, Barza M. Ceftazidime or amikacin: choice of intravitreal anti-microbials in the treatment of postoperative endophthalmitis. Arch Ophthalmol 112: 17–18, 1994.

Doft BH, Barza M. Macular infarction after intravitreal amikacin. Br J Ophthalmol 88: 850, 2004.

Galloway G, Ramsay A, Jordan K. Macular infarction after intravitreal amikacin: mounting evidence against amikacin. Br J Ophthalmol 86: 359–360, 2002.

Galloway G, Ramsay A, Jordan K, Vivian A. Macular infarction after intravitreal amikacin: authors' reply. Br J Ophthalmol 88: 1228, 2004.

Jackson TL, Williamson TH. Amikacin retinal toxicity. Br J Ophthalmol 83: 1199–1200, 1999.

Piguet B, Chobaz C, Grounauer PA. Toxic retinopathy caused by intravitreal injection of amikacin and vancomycin. Klinische Monatsblatter fur Augenheilkunde 208: 358–359, 1996.

Seawright AA, Bourke RD, Cooling RJ. Macula toxicity after intravitreal amikacin. Austral New Zealand J Ophth 24: 143–146, 1996.

Verma L, Arora R, Sachdev MS. Macular infarction after intravitreal injection of amikacin. Can J Ophthalmol 28: 241–243, 1993.

Generic names: 1. Amoxicillin; 2. ampicillin; 3. nafcillin sodium; 4. piperacillin; 5. ticarcillin monosodium.

Proprietary names: 1. Amoxil, Augmentin, DisperMox, Trimox; 2. Principen, Unasyn; 3. Nafcil; 4. Pipracil, Zosyn; 5. Timentin.

Primary use

Semisynthetic penicillins are primarily effective against staphylococci, streptococci, pneumococci and various other Gram-positive and Gram-negative bacteria.

Ocular side effects

Systemic administration
Certain
1. Eyelids or conjunctiva
   a. Allergic reactions
   b. Blepharoconjunctivitis
   c. Edema
   d. Photosensitivity
   e. Angioedema
   f. Urticaria

Probable
1. Myasthenia gravis (aggravates)
   a. Diplopia
   b. Ptosis
   c. Paresis of extraocular muscles

Possible
1. Eyelids or conjunctiva
   a. Erythema multiforme
   b. Stevens-Johnson syndrome
   c. Exfoliative dermatitis
   d. Lyell's syndrome

Local ophthalmic use or exposure – topical application or subconjunctival injection
Certain
1. Irritation – primarily with subconjunctival injection
   a. Hyperemia
   b. Ocular pain
   c. Edema
2. Eyelids or conjunctiva
   a. Allergic reactions
   b. Angioedema
3. Overgrowth of non-susceptible organisms
4. Conjunctival necrosis (nafcillin) – subconjunctival injection

Clinical significance

Surprisingly few ocular side effects other than dermatologic- or hematologic-related conditions have been reported with the semisynthetic penicillins. The incidence of allergic skin reactions due to ampicillin, however, may be high. Ampicillin and other semisynthetic penicillins may unmask or aggravate ocular signs of myasthenia gravis. Nafcillin has been reported to cause conjunctival necrosis with subconjunctival injections. Many, and maybe all, of these agents can be found in the tears in therapeutic levels and can cause local reactions if the patients are sensitive to the drug.

REFERENCES AND FURTHER READING

Argov Z, et al. Ampicillin may aggravate clinical and experimental myasthenia gravis. Arch Neurol 43: 255, 1986.

Brick DC, West C, Ostler HB. Ocular toxicity of subconjunctival nafcillin. Invest Ophthalmol Vis Sci 18(Suppl): 132, 1979.

Drug Evaluations, 6th edn, American Medical Association, Chicago, pp 1312–1328, 1986.

Ellis PP. Handbook of Ocular Therapeutics and Pharmacology. 6th edn. Mosby, St Louis, CV, 1981pp 42–45, 165–169, 1981.

Kaeser HE. Drug-induced myasthenic syndromes. Acta Neurol Scand 70(Suppl 100): 39, 1984.

Johnson AP, Scoper SV, Woo FL, et al. Azlocillin levels in human tears and aqueous humor. Am J Ophthalmol 99: 469–472, 1985.

Generic names: 1. Azithromycin; 2. clarithromycin; 3. clindamycin; 4. erythromycin.

Proprietary names: 1. Zithromax; 2. Biaxin; 3. Cleocin, Cleocin T, Clindagel, ClindaMax, Clindets; 4. AkneMycin, ATS, Del-mycin, E-Base, E-Mycin, EES, Emgal, Eramycin, Ery-Ped, Ery-Tab, Eryc, Erycette, Eryderm, Erygel, Erymax, Erythrocin, Ilosone, Ilotycin, PCE, Robimycin Robitabs, Staticin, T-Stat.

Primary use

Azithromycin, clarithromycin and erythromycin are macrolides, while clindamycin is an antibiotic with similar properties. These bactericidal antibiotics are effective against Gram-positive or Gram-negative organisms.

Ocular side effects

Systemic administration
Certain
1. Problems with color vision – color vision defect, blue yellow defect (erythromycin)

2. Eyelids or conjunctiva
   a. Allergic reactions
   b. Hyperemia
   c. Photosensitivity
   d. Angioedema
   e. Urticaria
3. Visual hallucinations (clarithromycin)

Probable

1. Myasthenia gravis – aggravates (erythromycin)
   a. Diplopia
   b. Ptosis
   c. Paresis of extraocular muscles

Possible

1. Cornea – subepithelial deposits (clarithromycin)
2. Subconjunctival or retinal hemorrhages secondary to drug-induced anemia
3. Eyelids or conjunctiva
   a. Stevens-Johnson sydrome
   b. Exfoliative dermatitis
   c. Lyell's syndrome (erythromycin)

Local ophthalmic use or exposure – topical application or subconjunctival injection

Certain

1. Irritation
   a. Hyperemia
   b. Ocular pain
   c. Edema
2. Eyelids or conjunctiva
   a. Allergic reactions
   b. Angioedema
3. Overgrowth of non-susceptible organisms

Possible

1. Mydriasis (erythromycin)
2. Corneas – subepithelial deposits (clarithromycin)
3. Eyelids of conjuncticva – Stevens-Johnson syndrome (erythromycin)

Local ophthalmic use or exposure – intracameral injection

Certain

1. Uveitis (erythromycin)
2. Corneal edema (erythromycin)
3. Lens damage (erythromycin)

Local ophthalmic use or exposure – retrobulbar or subtenon injection

Possible

1. Irritation (clindamycin)
2. Optic neuritis (clindamycin)
3. Optic atrophy (clindamycin)
4. Diplopia (clindamycin)

Clinical significance

Few adverse ocular reactions due to either systemic or topical ocular use of these antibiotics are seen. Nearly all ocular side effects are transitory and reversible after the drug is discontinued. Most adverse ocular reactions are secondary to dermatologic or hematologic conditions. A well-documented rechallenged idiosyncratic response to topical ocular application of erythromycin causing mydriasis has been reported to the National Registry. An interaction of erythromycin with carbamazepine causing mydriasis and gaze evoked nystagmus has been reported. The National Registry has also received a case of Stevens-Johnson syndrome following topical ophthalmic erythromycin ointment. Clarithromycin, with both oral and topical ocular exposure, has been associated with subepithelial infiltrate when treating mycobacterium avium complex. When the drug was stopped the deposits were absorbed. Visual hallucinations due to clarithromycin have only been seen when the drug was used in peritoneal dialysis.

REFERENCES AND FURTHER READING

Birch J, et al. Acquired color vision defects. In: Congenital and Acquired Color Vision Defects, Pokorny J, et al (eds), Grune & Stratton, New York, pp 243–350, 1979.

Dorrell L, Ellerton C, Cottrell DG, Snow MH. Toxicity of clarithromycin in the treatment of *Mycobacterium avium* complex infection in a patient with AIDS. J Antimicrob Chemother 34: 605–606, 1994.

Kaeser HE. Drug-induced myasthenic syndromes. Acta Neurol Scand 70(Suppl 100): 39, 1984.

Lund Kofoed M, Oxholm A. Toxic epidermal necrolysis due to erythromycin. Contact Dermatitis 13: 273, 1985.

May EF, Calvert PC. Aggravation of myasthenia gravis by erythromycin. Ann Neurol 28: 577–579, 1990.

Oral erythromycins. Med Lett Drugs Ther 27: 1, 1985.

Tate GW Jr., Martin RG. Clindamycin in the treatment of human ocular toxoplasmosis. Canad J Ophthalmol 12: 188, 1977.

Tyagi AK, Kayarkar VV, McDonnell PJ. An unreported side effect of topical clarithromycin when used successfully to treat *Mycobacterium avium-intracellulare* keratitis. Cornea 18: 606–607, 1999.

Zitelli BJ, et al. Erythromycin-induced drug interactions. An illustrative case and review of the literature. Clin Pediat 26: 117–119, 1987.

Generic name: Bacitracin.

Proprietary names: Ak-Tracin, Baci-IM.

Primary use

This polypeptide bactericidal agent is primarily effective against Gram-positive cocci, *Neisseria* and organisms causing gas gangrene.

Ocular side effects

Systemic administration

Certain

1. Decreased vision
2. Eyelids or conjunctiva
   a. Allergic reactions
   b. Angioneurotic edema
   c. Urticaria

Probable

1. Myasthenia gravis (aggravates)
   a. Diplopia
   b. Ptosis
   c. Paralysis of extraocular muscles

Local ophthalmic use or exposure – topical application or subconjunctival injection

Certain

1. Irritation
2. Eyelids or conjunctiva
   a. Allergic reactions
   b. Blepharoconjunctivitis
   c. Edema
   d. Urticaria
3. Keratitis
4. Overgrowth of non-susceptible organisms
5. Delayed corneal wound healing – toxic states

Local ophthalmic use or exposure – intracameral injection

Certain

1. Uveitis
2. Corneal edema
3. Lens damage

Inadvertent orbital injection (ointment)

Possible

1. Orbital compartment syndrome

Clinical significance

Ocular side effects from either systemic or ocular administration of bacitracin are rare. Myasthenia gravis is more commonly seen if systemic bacitracin is used in combination with neomycin, kanamycin, polymyxin or colistin. With increasing use of 'fortified' bacitracin solution (10 000 units per ml), marked conjunctival irritation and keratitis may occur, especially if the solutions are used frequently. The potential of decreased wound healing with prolonged use of any topical antibiotic, especially fortified solution, may occur. Severe ocular or periocular allergic reactions, while rare, have been seen due to topical ophthalmic bacitracin application. An anaphylactic reaction was reported after the use of bacitracin ointment. Orbital compartment syndrome, acute proptosis, chemosis, increase intraocular pressure, decreased vision and ophthalmoloplegic were reported by Castro et al (2000) immediately after endoscopic sinus surgery secondary to inadvertent bacitracin ointment.

REFERENCES AND FURTHER READING

Castro E, Seeley M, Kosmorsky G, Foster JA. Orbital compartment syndrome caused by intraorbital bacitracin ointment after endoscopic sinus surgery. Am J Ophthalmol 130: 376–378, 2000.

Fisher AA, Adams RM. Anaphylaxis following the use of bacitracin ointment. Am Acad Dermatol 16: 1057, 1987.

Kaeser HE. Drug-induced myasthenic syndromes. Acta Neurol Scand 70(Suppl 100): 39, 1984.

McQuillen MP, Cantor HE, O'Rourke JR. Myasthenic syndrome associated with antibiotics. Arch Neurol 18: 402, 1968.

Petroutsos G, et al. Antibiotics and corneal epithelial wound healing. Arch Ophthalmol 101: 1775, 1983.

Reynolds JEF (ed). Martindale: The Extra Pharmacopoeia. 28th edn, Pharmaceutical Press, London, p 1100, 1982.

Small GA. Respiratory paralysis after a large dose of intraperitoneal polymyxin B and bacitracin. Anesth Analg 43: 137, 1964.

Walsh FB, Hoyt WF. Clinical Neuro-Ophthalmology, Vol. III. 3rd edn. Williams & Wilkins, Baltimore, p 2680, 1969.

Generic names: 1. Benzathine benzylpenicillin (benzathine penicillin G); 2. benzylpenicillin potassium (potassium penicillin G); 3. phenoxymethylpenicillin (potassium penicillin V); 4. procaine benzylpenicillin (procaine penicillin G).

Proprietary names: 1. Bicillin L-A, Permapen; 2. Pfizerpen; 3. Pen-Vee K, Veetids; 4.Crysticillin.

Primary use

These bactericidal penicillins are effective against streptococci, *S. aureus*, gonococci, meningococci, pneumococci, *T. pallidum*, Clostridium, *B. anthracis*, *C. diphtheriae* and several species of Actinomyces.

Ocular side effects

Systemic administration

Certain

1. Mydriasis
2. Decreased accommodation
3. Diplopia
4. Papilledema secondary to intracranial hypertension
5. Decreased vision
6. Visual hallucinations
7. Visual agnosia
8. Eyelids or conjunctiva
   a. Allergic reactions
   b. Erythema
   c. Blepharoconjunctivitis
   d. Edema
   e. Angioedema
   f. Urticaria

Possible

1. Subconjunctival or retinal hemorrhages secondary to drug-induced anemia
2. Eyelids or conjunctiva
   a. Lupoid syndrome
   b. Stevens-Johnson syndrome
   c. Lyell's syndrome

Local ophthalmic use or exposure – topical application or subconjunctival injection

Certain

1. Irritation
2. Eyelids or conjunctiva - allergic reactions
3. Overgrowth of nonsusceptible organisms

Local ophthalmic use or exposure – intracameral injection

Certain

1. Uveitis
2. Corneal edema
3. Lens damage

Clinical significance

Systemic administration of penicillin rarely causes ocular side effects. The most serious adverse reaction is papilledema secondary to elevated intracranial pressure. The incidence of allergic reactions is greater in patients with Sjögren's syndrome or rheumatoid arthritis than in other individuals. Most other ocular side effects due to penicillin are transient and reversible. Kawasaki and Ohnogi (1989) showed ERG changes with intravitreal injections of penicillin. Topical ocular administration results in a high incidence of sensitivity reactions.

REFERENCES AND FURTHER READING

Alarcón-Segovia D. Drug-induced antinuclear antibodies and lupus syndromes. Drugs 12: 69, 1976.

Crews SJ. Ocular adverse reactions to drugs. Practitioner 219: 72, 1977.

Katzman B, et al. Pseudotumor cerebri: an observation and review. Ann Ophthalmol 13: 887, 1981.

Kawasaki K, Ohnogi J. Nontoxic concentration of antibiotics for intravitreal use – evaluated by human in vitro ERG. Doc Ophthalmol 70: 301–308, 1989.

Laroche J. Modification of color vision by certain medications. Ann Oculist 200: 275–286, 1967.

Leopold IH, Wong EK, Jr. The eye: local irritation and topical toxicity. In: Cutaneous Toxicity, Drill VA, Lazar P (eds), Raven Press, New York, pp 99–103, 1984.

Robertson CR Jr. Hallucinations after penicillin injection. Am J Dis Child 139: 1074, 1985.

Schmitt BD, et al. Benign intracranial hypertension associated with a delayed penicillin reaction. Pediatrics 43: 50–53, 1969.

Snavely SR, Hodges GR. The neurotoxicity of antibacterial agents. Ann Intern Med 101: 92, 1984.

Tseng SCG, et al. Topical retinoid treatment for various dry-eye disorders. Ophthalmology 92: 717, 1985.

Generic names: 1. Cefaclor; 2. cefadroxil; 3. cefalexin 4. cefazolin; 5. cefditoren pivoxil; 6. cefoperazone sodium; 7. cefotaxime sodium; 8. cefotetan disodium; 9. cefoxitin sodium; 10. cefradine 11. ceftazidime; 12. ceftizoxime sodium; 13. ceftriaxone sodium; 14. cefuroxime; 15. cefuroxime axetil.

Proprietary names: 1. Ceclor; 2. Duricef; 3. Biocef, Cefanex, Keflex, Keftab; 4. Ancef, Zolicef; 5. Spectracef; 6. Cefobid; 7. Claforan; 8. Generic only; 9. Mefoxin; 10. Velosef; 11. Ceptaz, Fortaz, Tazicef, Tazidime; 12. Cefizox; 13. Rocephin; 14. Zinacef; 15. Ceftin.

Primary use

Cephalosporins are effective against streptococci, staphylococci, pneumococci and strains of *Escheria coli, Pneumococci* mirabilis and *Klebsiella*.

Ocular side effects

Systemic administration
Certain
1. Eyelids or conjunctiva
   a. Allergic reactions
   b. Erythema
   c. Conjunctivitis – non-specific
   d. Edema
   e. Angioedema
   f. Urticaria
2. Visual hallucinations

Possible
1. Nystagmus
2. Subconjunctival or retinal hemorrhages secondary to drug-induced anemia

3. Eyelids or conjunctiva
   a. Erythema multiforme
   b. Stevens-Johnson syndrome
   c. Exfoliative dermatitis

Conditional/Unclassified
1. Corneal edema – peripheral (cefaclor)
2. Acute macular neuroretinopathy

Local ophthalmic use or exposure – topical application or subconjunctival injection
Certain
1. Irritation
   a. Hyperemia
   b. Ocular pain
   c. Edema
2. Eyelids or conjunctiva
   a. Allergic reactions
   b. Angioedema
   c. Urticaria
3. Overgrowth of non-susceptible organisms

Clinical significance

Rarely does this group of drugs given systemically cause ocular side effects. Kraushar et al (1994) reported an anaphylactic reaction to intravitreal cefazolin. There is significant cross-sensitivity within this group, as well as with penicillin. Platt (1990) described a generalized allergic event of Type III hypersensitivity, including reversible limbal hyperemia, mild conjunctivitis and peripheral corneal edema, in a patient taking cefaclor. The National Registry has a case of acute macular neuroretinopathy associated with Type III hypersensitivity response in a patient on cefotetan. Platt's case and the one in the National Registry make one suspicious of a possible association of a Type III hypersensitivity ocular event.

REFERENCES AND FURTHER READING

Ballingall DLK, Turpie AGG. Cephaloridine toxicity. Lancet 2: 835–836, 1967.

Berrocal AM, Schuman JS. Subconjunctival cephalosporin anaphylaxis. Ophthalmic Sug Las 32(1): 79–80, 2001.

Campochiaro PA, Green R. Toxicity of intravitreous ceftazidime in primate retina. Arch Ophthalmol 110: 1625–1629, 1992.

Green ST, Natarajan S, Campbell JC. Erythema multiforme following cefotaxime therapy. Postgrad Med J 62: 415, 1986.

Jenkins CDG, McDonnell PJ, Spalton DJ. Randomized single blind trial to compare the toxicity of subconjunctival gentamicin and cefuroxime in cataract surgery. Br J Ophthalmol 74: 734, 1990.

Kannangara DW, Smith B, Cohen K. Exfoliative dermatitis during cefoxitin therapy. Arch Intern Med 142: 1031, 1982.

Kramann C, Pitz S, Schwenn O, et al. Effects of intraocular cefotaxime on the human corneal endothelium. J Cataract Refract Surg 27: 250–255, 2001.

Kraushar MF, Nussbaum P, Kisch AL. Anaphylactic reaction to intravitreal cefazolin (letter). Retina 14(2): 187–188, 1994.

Murray DL, et al. Cefaclor-A cluster of adverse reactions. N Engl J Med 303: 1003, 1980.

Okumoto M, et al. In vitro and in vivo studies on cefoperazone. Cornea 2: 35, 1983.

Platt LW. Bilateral peripheral corneal edema after cefaclor therapy. Arch Ophthalmol 108: 175, 1990.

Taylor R, et al. Cephaloridine encephalopathy. BMJ 283: 409, 1981.

Villada JR, Ubaldo V, Javaloy J, Alió JL. Severe anaphylactic reaction after intracameral antibiotic administration during cataract surgery. J Refract Surg 31: 620–624, 2005.

Generic name: Chloramphenicol.

Proprietary names: Ak-Chlor, Chloromycetin, Chloroptic.

Primary use

This bacteriostatic dichloracetic acid derivative is particularly effective against *Salmonella typhi, H. influenzae* meningitis, rickettsia and the lymphogranuloma-psittacosis group, and is useful in the management of cystic fibrosis.

Ocular side effects

Systemic administration
Certain
1. Decreased vision
2. Retrobulbar or optic neuritis
3. Visual fields
   a. Scotomas – central and paracentral
   b. Constriction
4. Optic atrophy
5. Toxic amblyopia
6. Problems with color vision
   a. Color vision defect
   b. Objects have yellow tinge
7. Eyelids or conjunctiva
   a. Allergic reactions
   b. Conjunctivitis – non-specific
   c. Angioedema
   d. Urticaria
8. Paralysis of accommodation
9. Pupils
   a. Mydriasis
   b. Absence of reaction to light
10. Subconjunctival or retinal hemorrhages secondary to drug-induced anemia
11. Blindness

Local ophthalmic use or exposure – topical application or subconjunctival injection
Certain
1. Irritation
2. Eyelids or conjunctiva
   a. Allergic reactions
   b. Conjunctivitis – non-specific
   c. Depigmentation
3. Keratitis
4. Overgrowth of non-susceptible organisms

Possible
1. Eyelids or conjunctiva – anaphylactic reaction

Local ophthalmic use or exposure – intracameral injection
Certain
1. Uveitis
2. Corneal edema
3. Lens damage

Systemic side effects

Local ophthalmic use or exposure
Possible
1. Aplastic anemia
2. Various blood dyscrasias

Clinical significance

Ocular side effects from systemic chloramphenicol administration are uncommon in adults but may occur more frequently in children, especially if the total dose exceeds 100 g or if therapy lasts more than 6 weeks. Optic neuritis with secondary optic atrophy is the most serious side effect. These are most often of acute onset bilateral, and optic neuritis is much more frequent than retrobulbar neuritis. First signs may be sudden visual loss with cencocentral scotoma.

Topical ophthalmic application causes infrequent ocular side effects. Although chloramphenicol has fewer allergic reactions than neomycin, those due to chloramphenicol are often the more severe. Like other antibiotics, this agent may cause latent hypersensitivity, which may last for many years. Topical ocular chloramphenicol probably has fewer toxic effects on the corneal epithelium than other antibiotics. Berry et al (1995) pointed out, however, that after 14 days this is no longer true, and it is second only to gentamicin in toxicity tested in vitro studies on human corneal epithelium.

Over 40 cases of blood dyscrasia or aplastic anemia following topical ocular chloramphenicol have been reported in the literature or to the National Registry, with 16 fatalities. Whether there is a direct cause-and-effect relationship is unknown. The risk of developing pancytopenia or aplastic anemia after oral chloramphenicol treatment is 13 times greater than the risk of idiopathic aplastic anemia in the general population. Two forms of hemopoietic abnormalities, idiosyncratic and dose-related, may occur following systemic chloramphenicol. Although the latter response is unlikely from topical ophthalmic use of the drug, the incidence of the idiosyncratic response is unknown and indeed is a highly controversial topic. After an editorial by Doona and Walsh (1995) asking for a halt in using topical ocular chloramphenicol in Great Britain, there were a large number of articles written in opposition to this. Wilholm et al (1998), Laporte et al (1998) and Walker et al (1998) support an extremely low incidence, implying no correlation of aplastic anemia and topical ocular chloramphenicol. Diamond and Leeming (1995) suggest limiting topical ocular chloramphenicol to 5 to 7 days. Others feel that since this drug has been rotated out of use in most developed countries for almost two decades, many previously resistant strains of bacteria are now susceptible again to chloramphenicol, and the drug should be reserved for these bacteria. It seems unlikely that a clear-cut answer will be forthcoming. Each physician will have to decide individually on the benefit-risk ratio (Fraunfelder and Fraunfelder 2007). A potential interaction between topical ocular chloramphenicol and warfarin has also been suggested, which led to an increased international normalization ratio.

Recommendations for topical ocular chloramphenicol

1. Topical ocular chloramphenicol should not be used on any patient with a family history of a blood dyscrasia without informed consent.
2. Its use is preferably limited to 7 to 14 days.
3. In some physicians' opinions, the only indication for topical ocular chloramphenicol use is if the organism is resistant to all other antibiotics.
4. Only 1 drop should be used at a time. Consider limiting systemic absorption by closing the lids for 3 minutes after drop application and removing excess drug at the inner canthus with a tissue prior to opening the eyelids.
5. Physicians must make their own judgments as to the risk-benefit ratio in using this drug topically. Informed consent may be prudent.

REFERENCES AND FURTHER READING

Abrams SM, Degnan TJ, Vinciguerra V. Marrow aplasia following topical application of chloramphenicol eye ointment. Arch Intern Med 140: 576, 1980.

Berry M, Gurung A, Easty DL. Toxicity of antibiotics and antifungal on cultured human corneal cells: effect of mixing, exposure and concentration. Eye 9(Pt 1): 110–115, 1995.

Brodsky E, Biger Y, Zeidan Z, Schneider M. Topical application of chloramphenicol eye ointment followed by fatal bone marrow aplasia. Isr J Med Sci. 25: 54, 1989.

Bron AJ, Leber G, Rizk SNM, et al. Ofloxacin compared with chloramphenicol in the management of external ocular infection. Br J Ophthalmol 75(11): 675–679, 1991.

Chalfin J, Putterman AM. Eyelid skin depigmentation. Ophthalmic Surg 11: 194, 1980.

De Sevilla TF, Alegre J, Vallespi T, et al. Adult pure red cell aplasia following topical ocular chloramphenicol. Br J Ophthalmol 74: 640, 1990.

Diamond J, Leeming J. Chloramphenicol eye drops: a dangerous drug? The Practitioner 239: 608–611, 1995.

Doona M, Walsh JB. Use of chloramphenicol as topical eye medication: time to cry halt? BMJ 310: 1217–1218, 1995.

Fraunfelder FW, Fraunfelder FT. Scientific challenges in postmarketing surveillance of ocular adverse drug reactions. Am J Ophthalmol 143: 145–149, 2007.

Fraunfelder FT, Bagby GC Jr., Kelly DJ. Fatal aplastic anemia following topical administration of ophthalmic chloramphenicol. Am J Ophthalmol 93: 356, 1982.

Fraunfelder FT, Morgan RL, Yunis AA. Blood dyscrasias and topical ophthalmic chloramphenicol. Am J Ophthalmol 115(6): 812–813, 1993.

Godel V, Nemet P, Lazar M. Chloramphenicol optic neuropathy. Arch Ophthalmol 98: 1417, 1980.

Isenberg SJ. The fall and rise of chloramphenicol. J Am Assoc Pediatr Ophthalmol Strab 7(5): 307–308, 2003.

Issaragrisil S, Piankijagum A. Aplastic anemia following administration of ophthalmic chloramphenicol: report of a case and review of the literature. J Med Assoc Thai 68: 309, 1985.

Lamda PA, Sood NN, Moorthy SS. Retinopathy due to chloramphenicol. Scot Med J 13: 166, 1968.

Laporte JR, Vidal X, Ballarin E, et al. Possible association between ocular chloramphenicol and aplastic anaemia – the absolute risk is very low. Br J Clin Pharm 46(2): 181–184, 1998.

Leone R, Ghiotto E, Conforti A, et al. Potential interaction between warfarin and ocular chloramphenicol (letter). Ann Pharmacother 33(1): 114, 1999.

Liphshitz I, Loewenstein A. Anaphylactic reaction following application of chloramphenicol eye ointment. Br J Ophthalmol 75: 64, 1991.

McGuinness R. Chloramphenicol eye drops and blood dyscrasia. Med J Austral 140: 383, 1984.

McWhae JA, Chang J, Lipton JH. Drug-induced fatal aplastic anemia following cataract surgery. Can J Ophthalmol 27(6): 313–315, 1992.

Walker S, Diaper C, Bowman R, et al. Lack of evidence for systemic toxicity following topical chloramphenicol use. Eye 12: 875–879, 1998.

Wiholm BE, et al. Relation of aplastic anaemia to use of chloramphenicol eye drops in two international case-control studies. BMJ 316: 666, 1998.

Wilson FM III. Adverse external ocular effects of topical ophthalmic medications. Surv Ophthalmol 24: 57, 1979.

Wilson WR, Cockerill FR III. Tetracyclines, chloramphenicol, erythromycin, and clindamycin. Mayo Clin Proc 58: 92, 1983.

Generic name: Ciprofloxacin.

Proprietary names: Ciloxan, Cipro, Cipro XR, Proquin.

Primary use

This fluoroquinolone antibacterial agent is used primarily against most Gram-negative aerobic and many Gram-positive aerobic bacteria.

Ocular side effects

Systemic administration
Certain
1. Visual sensations
   a. Glare phenomenon
   b. Lacrimation
   c. Flashing lights
2. Photosensitivity
3. Abnormal VER

Probable
1. Eyelids
   a. Hyperpigmentation
   b. Angioedema
   c. Urticaria
2. Visual hallucinations
3. Myasthenia gravis (aggravates)
   a. Diplopia
   b. Ptosis
   c. Paresis or extraocular muscles

Possible
1. Papilledema secondary to intracranial hypertension
2. Nystagmus
3. Eyelids or conjunctiva
   a. Erythema multiforme
   b. Erythema nodosum
   c. Exfoliative dermatitis
   d. Lyell's syndrome

Conditional/Unclassified
1. Optic neuropathy (reversible)
2. Acute visual loss

Local ophthalmic use or exposure – topical application
Certain
1. Irritation
   a. Pain
   b. Burning sensation
   c. Lacrimation
   d. Foreign body sensation
2. Eyelids
   a. Crusting – crystalline
   b. Edema
   c. Allergic reactions
   d. Itching
3. Cornea
   a. Precipitates – white (Fig. 7.1b)
   b. Keratitis
   c. Infiltrates
   d. Superficial punctate keratitis
4. Conjunctiva
   a. Hyperemia
   b. Chemosis
5. Decreased vision
6. Photophobia

Systemic reactions from topical ocular medication
Certain
1. Metallic taste
2. Dermatitis
3. Nausea

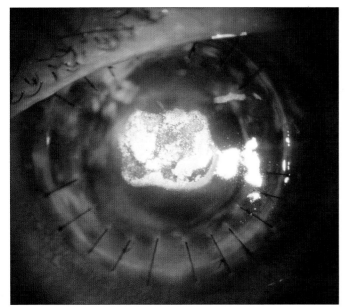

Fig. 7.1b White corneal deposits from topical ocular ciprofloxacin application in corneal transplant. Photo courtesy of Krachmer JH, Palay DA, Cornea Atlas, 2nd edn, Mosby Elsevier, London.

Conditional/Unclassified
1. Psychosis
2. Pediatric warning: arthropathy (theoretically under age 12)

Clinical significance
Ciprofloxacin causes relatively few and minor ocular side effects from systemic use. Of all drug-induced side effects seen with this agent, 12% involve the skin. Exacerbations of myasthenia symptoms involving the eye are well documented, but quite rare. Visual sensations, such as increased glare and increased brightness of color or lights, occur occasionally. From spontaneous reporting systems there are only a few cases of possible optic neuropathy and intracranial hypertension with papilledema. Vrabec et al (1990) described a case of acute bilateral count fingers visual loss associated with ciprofloxacin, which slowly improved after discontinuing the drug.

Ciprofloxacin ophthalmic solutions are generally well tolerated. Transient ocular burning and discomfort, however, occur in approximately 10% of patients. Seldom does this necessitate discontinuation of the drug. The main side effect is the deposition of the drug as a white crystalline deposit on abraded corneal epithelium or stroma. This may occur in approximately 15–20% of patients using either solution or ointment. Leibowitz (1991) as well as Wilhelmus and Abshire (2003) showed this is pure ciprofloxacin deposit with continued antibacterial properties. Patients under 40 years old and those above 70 years old, have a four times increased deposition rate compared to those 40–70 years of age. pH affects the precipitation of the antibiotic as well as sicca and more alkaline surface in the elderly. Precipitates may start as early as 24 hours after starting therapy, and may resolve while on full therapy and can be irrigated off. These deposits may last even a few weeks after the drug is discontinued. Other than a foreign body sensation, these deposits are usually well tolerated. The precipitates do not alter the rate of infection, but may impede epitheliazation. Patwardhan and Khan (2005) reported delay from recovery from viral ocular surface infections secondary to topical ocular ciprofloxacin. Other ocular side effects secondary to topical ocular application occur in less than 1% of patients. Systemic reactions may occur from topical ocular ciprofloxacin.

The primary ones are a metallic or foul taste occurring in 5% of patients and nausea in 1%. There is a warning based on animal work to not use this drug in patients 12 years and younger for fear of causing degenerative articular changes in weight-bearing joints. There is no human data to support this. Temporary hearing disorders have been seen with oral ciprofloxacin, but this has not been reported from topical ocular application. Tripathi and Chen (2002) reported an acute psychosis following topical ocular ciprofloxacin with supporting data that oral ciprofloxacin can cause the same.

REFERENCES AND FURTHER READING
Cokingtin CD, Hyndiuk RA. Insights from experimental data on ciprofloxacin in the treatment of bacterial keratitis and ocular infections. Am J Ophthalmol 112: 255–285, 1991.

Diamond JP, White L, Leeming JP, et al: Topical 0.3% ciprofloxacin, norfloxacin, and ofloxacin in treatment of bacterial keratitis: a new method for comparative evaluation of ocular drug penetration. Br J Ophthalmol 79: 606–609, 1995.

Eiferman RA, Snyder JP, Nordquist RE. Ciprofloxacin microprecipitates and macroprecipitates in human corneal epithelium. J Cataract Refract Surg 27: 1701–1702, 2001.

Kanellopoulos AJ, Miller F, Wittpenn JR. Deposition of topical ciprofloxacin to prevent re-epithelialization of a corneal defect. Am J Ophthalmol 117: 258–259, 1994.

Leibowitz HW. Clinical evaluation of ciprofloxacin 0.3% ophthalmic solution for treatment of bacterial keratitis. Am J Ophthalmol 112: 34S–47S, 1991.

Moore B, Safani M, Keesey J. Ciprofloxacin exacerbation of myasthenia gravis? Case report. Lancet 1: 882, 1988.

Motolese E, D'Aniello B, Addabbo G. Toxic optic neuropathy after administration of quinolone derivative. Boll Oculist 69: 1011–1013, 1990.

Patwardhan A, Khan M. Topical ciprofloxacin can delay recovery from viral ocular surface infection. J Roy Soc Med 98: 274–275, 2005.

Stevens D, Samples JR. Fluoroquinolones for the treatment of microbial infections. J Toxicol Cut Ocular Toxicol 13(4): 275–277, 1994.

Tripathi A, Chen SI. Acute psychosis following the use of topical ciprofloxacin. Arch Ophthalmol 120: 665–666, 2002.

Vrabec TR, Sergott RC, Jaeger EA, et al: Reversible visual loss in a patient receiving high-dose ciprofloxacin hydrochloride. Ophthalmology 97(6): 707–710, 1990.

Wilhelmus KR, Hyndiuk RA, Caldwell DR, et al. 0.3% Ciprofloxacin ophthalmic ointment in the treatment of bacterial keratitis. Arch Ophthalmol 111: 1210–1218, 1993.

Wilhelmus KR, Abshire RL. Corneal ciprofloxacin precipitation during bacterial keratitis. Am J Ophthalmol 136: 1032–1037, 2003.

Winrow AP, Supramaniam G. Benign intracranial hypertension after ciprofloxacin administration. Arch Dis Child 65: 1165–1166, 1990.

Generic names: 1. Demeclocycline; 2. doxycycline; 3. minocycline; 4. oxytetracycline; 5. tetracycline.

Proprietary names: 1. Declomycin; 2. Adoxa, Atridox, Doryx, Doxy 200, Monodox, Oracea, Periostat, Vibra-Tabs, Vibramycin; 3. Arestin, Dynacin, Minocin; 4. Terramycin; 5. Achromycin V, Actisite, Sumycin.

Primary use
These bacteriostatic derivatives of polycyclic naphthacene carboxamide are effective against a wide range of Gram-negative and Gram-positive organisms, mycoplasms and members of the lymphogranuloma-psittacosis group.

Ocular side effects

Systemic administration
Certain
1. Myopia
2. Photophobia
3. Blurred vision
4. Eyelids or conjunctiva
    a. Erythema
    b. Edema
    c. Yellow or green discoloration or deposits (doxycycline, tetracycline, minocycline)
    d. Angioedema
    e. Urticaria
5. Sclera – blue-gray dark blue, or brownish scleral pigmentation (minocycline) (Fig. 7.1c)
6. Enlarged blind spot
7. Visual hallucinations
8. Aggravates keratitis sicca
9. Contact lens intolerance

Probable
1. Intracranial hypertension
    a. Pupil signs
    b. Extraocular muscle paresis and paralysis
    c. Papilledema
    d. Decreased vision
    e. Enlarged blind spot
2. Myasthenia gravis (aggravates)
    a. Diplopia
    b. Ptosis
    c. Paresis of extraocular muscles

Possible
1. Subconjunctival or retinal hemorrhages secondary to drug-induced anemia
2. Eyelids or conjunctiva
    a. Lupoid syndrome
    b. Erythema multiforme
    c. Stevens-Johnson syndrome
    d. Lyell's syndrome

Conditional/Unclassified
1. Retinal pigmentation (minocycline)

Local ophthalmic use or exposure – topical application or subconjunctival injection
Certain
1. Irritation
2. Eyelids or conjunctiva
    a. Allergic reactions
    b. Conjunctivitis – non-specific
3. Overgrowth of non-susceptible organisms
4. Keratitis
5. Yellow-brown corneal discoloration (with drug-soaked hydrophilic lenses)

Local ophthalmic use or exposure – intracameral injection
Certain
1. Uveitis
2. Corneal edema
3. Lens damage

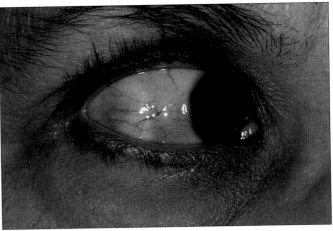

Fig. 7.1c Minocycline blue pigmentation of the sclera.

Ocular teratogenic effects
Probable
1. Corneal pigmentation – permanent

Clinical significance

Systemic or ocular use of the tetracyclines rarely causes significant ocular side effects. While a large variety of drug-induced ocular side effects have been attributed to tetracyclines, most are reversible. This group of drugs can cause intracranial hypertension. This is most commonly reported with tetracycline and minocycline. Minocycline possibly possesses greater lipid solubility as it passes into cerebral spinal fluid, therefore it may cause this side effect more readily. Increased intracranial pressure is not dose related and may occur as early as 4 hours after first taking the drug or may occur after many years of drug usage. While the papilledema may resolve once the drug is discontinued, the visual loss may be permanent (Chiu et al 1998). Paresis or paralysis of extraocular muscles may occur secondary to intracranial hypertension. This can occur in any age group. Gardner et al (1995) feel that this side effect may be related to an underlying genetic susceptibility. Many patients are obese, which is a risk factor for intracranial hypertension and clouds the picture of the role of causation of this drug in this disease. However, most who work in this area feel that tetracycline can cause intracranial hypertension. The tetracyclines have been implicated in aggravating or unmasking myasthenia gravis with its own associated ocular findings. Tetracycline has caused hyperpigmentation in light-exposed skin and yellow-brown pigmentation of light-exposed conjunctiva after long-term therapy. This occurs in about 3% of patients taking 400 to 1600 g. Oral minocycline can cause scleral pigmentation. The pigmentation is most prominent in sun-exposed areas. However, minocycline can cause hyperpigmentation in non-sun-exposed areas, i.e. the roof of the mouth (Fraunfelder and Randall 1997). The pigmentation may resolve over a number of years if the drug is discontinued, or the stain may be permanent. This side effect may be an indication to stop the drug for cosmetic reasons (Fraunfelder and Randall 1997). Yellow-brown discoloration of the cornea can occur if hydrophilic contact lenses are presoaked in tetracycline prior to ocular application. Bradfield et al (2003) described retinal pigmentation after oral minocycline in one case. All tetracycline agents are photosensitizers and they may enhance any or all light-induced ocular changes.

Doxycycline may be the greatest photosensitizer in this group, with minocycline being the least. However, even with minocycline, in susceptible patients significant ocular and periocular photosensitivity reactions may occur. Shah and De Cock (1999) described three cases of ocular and periocular photosensitivity, one occurring after only one exposure and another after 2 weeks of therapy. The latter was the most severe and had the clinical appearance of an arc-welding injury. This includes intense bilateral photophobia, blepharospasm, lid angioedema, marked papillary conjunctivitis and superficial punctate keratitis. This cleared within 2 days after stopping the drug. These drugs are secreted in a crystalline form in the tear film, often in therapeutic concentration. Therefore, oral intake may cause or increase ocular irritation in patients with sicca or contact lenses. Long-term therapy may allow the drug or its metabolites to mix with calcium concretions, which may take on characteristics of the drug, such as yellow color and fluorescence. Permanent discoloration of the cornea has been seen in infants whose mothers received high doses of tetracycline during pregnancy.

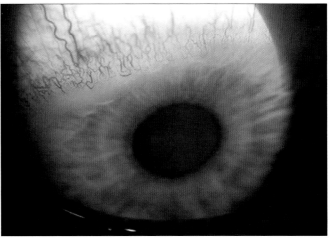

Fig. 7.1d Marginal peripheral ulcerative keratitis (non-staining) from systemic filgrastim treatment.

REFERENCES AND FURTHER READING

Bradfield YS, Robertson DM, Salomao DR, et al: Minocycline-induced ocular pigmentation. Arch Ophthalmol 121: 114–145, 2003.
Brothers DM, Hidayat AA. Conjunctival pigmentation associated with tetracycline medication. Ophthalmology 88: 1212, 1981.
Chiu AM, Cheunkongkaew WL, Cornblath WT, et al. Minocycline treatment and pseudotumor cerebri syndrome. Am J Ophthalmol 126(1): 116–121, 1998.
Edwards TS. Transient myopia due to tetracycline. JAMA 186: 175–176, 1963.
Fraunfelder FT, Randall JA. Minocycline-induced scleral pigmentation. Ophthalmology 104(6): 936–938, 1997.
Friedman DI, Gordon LK, Egan RA, et al. Doxycycline and intracranial hypertension. Neurology 62: 2297–2298, 2004.
Gardner K, Cox T, Digre KB. Idiopathic intracranial hypertension associated with tetracycline use in fraternal twins: case reports and review. Neurology 45: 6–10, 1995; Am J Ophthalmol 119: 536, 1995.
Kaeser HE. Drug-induced myasthenic syndromes. Acta Neurol Scand 70(Suppl 100): 39, 1984.
Krejci L, Brettschneider I, Triska J. Eye changes due to systemic use of tetracycline in pregnancy. Ophthalmic Res 12: 73, 1980.
Messmer E, et al. Pigmented conjunctival cysts following tetracycline/minocycline therapy. Histochemical and electron microscopic observations. Ophthalmology 90: 1462, 1983.
Morrison VL, Herndier BG, Kikkawa DO. Tetracycline induced green conjunctival pigment deposits. Br J Ophthalmol 89: 1372–1373, 2005.
Salamon SM. Tetracycline in ophthalmology. Surv Ophthalmol 29: 265, 1985.
Shah W, De Cock R. Actinic keratoconjunctivitis and minocycline (letter). Eye 13(Pt 1): 119–120, 1999.
Tabbara KF, Cooper H. Minocycline levels in tears of patients with active trachoma. Arch Ophthalmol 107: 93–95, 1989.
Weese-mayer DE, Yang RJ, Mayer JR, Zaparackas Z. Minocycline and pseudotumor cerebri: the well-known but well-kept secret 108: 519–520, 2001.
Wilson FM III. Adverse external ocular effects of topical ophthalmic medications. Surv Ophthalmol 24: 57, 1979.

Generic name: Filgrastim.

Proprietary name: Neupogen.

Primary use

A 175 amino acid protein used to prevent infection in neutropenic patients who are receiving myelosuppresive therapy for non-myeloid malignancies.

Ocular side effect

Systemic administration – intravenous
Possible
1. Non-specific ocular irritation
   a. Hyperemia
   b. Eye pain
   c. Foreign body sensation
2. Cornea
   a. Peripheral marginal subepithelial infiltrates
   b. Ulceration without staining
3. Marginal peripheral ulcerative keratitis (non-staining) (Fig. 7.1d)
4. Photophobia
5. Anterior uveitis – mild

Clinical significance

There are two reports (Esmaeli et al 2002; Fraunfelder and Harrison 2006) in which 2–4 days after receiving IV filgrastim, bilateral marginal ulcerative keratitis occurred. There were subepithelial infiltrates similar to those connected to connective tissue disorders such as Wegener's granulomatosus. This is associated with ocular hyperemia, foreign body sensation and significant ocular irritation. There are only two such reports for the many thousands of patients who have been exposed to this drug so this is a rare event or may not even be drug related. One case resolved with the only treatment being artificial tears after the drug was discontinued. In the other case the patient continued the drug and the eyes were treated with topical ocular steroids and the infiltrate cleared within 24 hours.

REFERENCES AND FURTHER READING

Esmaeli B, et al. Marginal keratitis associated with administration of filgrastim and sargramostim in a healthy peripheral blood progenitor cell donor. Cornea 21: 621–622, 2002.
Fraunfelder FW, Harrison D. Peripheral ulcerative keratitis associated with filgrastim. Arch Ophthalmol. February 2006. MS# OPH06-0177.

Generic names: 1. Gatifloxacin; 2. levofloxacin; 3. moxifloxacin; 4. norfloxacin; 5. ofloxacin.

Proprietary names: 1. Tequin, Zymar; 2. Iquix, Levaquin, Quixin; 3. Avelox, Vigamox 4. Noroxin; 5. Floxin, Ocuflox.

Primary use

These quinolone antibacterial agents are used primarily against most Gram-negative aerobic and many Gram-positive aerobic bacteria.

Ocular side effects

Systemic administration
Probable
1. Eyelids
   a. Hyperpigmentation
   b. Angioedema
   c. Urticaria
2. Conjunctiva
   a. Hyperemia
   b. Hypersensitivity
3. Visual sensations
   a. Blurred vision
   b. Glare phenomenon (norfloxacin)
   c. Lacrimation
4. Photosensitivity (ofloxacin)
5. Ocular pain

Possible
1. Visual hallucinations (ofloxacin)
2. Nystagmus (ofloxacin)
3. Papilledema secondary to intracranial hypertension
4. Eyelids or conjunctiva
   a. Erythema multiforme
   b. Erythema nodosum
   c. Exfoliative dermatitis
   d. Lyell's syndrome
   e. Stevens-Johnson syndrome

Conditional/Unclassified
1. Toxic optic neuropathy (moxifloxacin)
2. Uveitis (moxifloxacin)

Local ophthalmic use or exposure – topical application
Certain
1. Irritation
   a. Pain
   b. Burning sensation
   c. Lacrimation
   d. Foreign body sensation
2. Eyelids
   a. Edema
   b. Allergic reactions
   c. Itching
3. Cornea
   a. Precipitates – white (rare)
   b. Keratitis
   c. Infiltrates
   d. Superficial punctate keratitis
4. Conjunctiva
   a. Hyperemia
   b. Chemosis
   c. Papillary conjunctivitis

5. Decreased vision
6. Photophobia
7. Miosis (moxifloxacin)

Systemic reactions from topical ocular medication
Certain
1. Dermatitis
2. Nausea

Possible
1. Pediatric warning: arthropathy (theoretically under age 12)

Clinical significance

There are surprisingly few and seldom severe adverse systemic effects from these quinolones. While hypersensitivity reactions occur, they are uncommon. Photosensitivity may occur rarely, but appears to be seen most frequently with ofloxacin. Visual sensations are more common with ciprofloxacin and occasionally with norfloxacin. Rare reports of uveitis (Bringas-Clavo and Iglesias-Cortinas 2004; Cano-Parra and Diaz-Llopis 2005) or drug-related optic neuropathy (Gallelli et al 2004) have been reported along with a few cases in the National Registry with moxifloxacin. This data is patchy at best.

Topical ocular quinolones are generally well tolerated. Ocular pain, erythema, pruritis, photophobia and epiphora occur in a small percentage of patients. Seldom is corneal precipitation of these drugs seen as with ciprofloxacin; however, there are reports with ofloxacin (Desai et al 1999; Claerhout et al 2003) and norfloxacin (Castillo et al 1997). Awwad et al (2004) reported corneal intrastromal gatifloxacin crystal deposits after pentrating keratoplasty, with follow-up discussion of pro and cons by Wittpenn (2005) and by Cavanaugh (2005). Donnenfeld et al (2004) reported that topical ocular moxifloxacin can cause pupillary miosis, possibly due to prostaglandin release into the anterior chamber. Since moxifloxacin does not contain the preservative benzalkonium chloride, topical ocular toxicity may be less overall. The Medical Letter still does not generally recommend quinolones in the pediatric age group or in pregnancy.

REFERENCES AND FURTHER READING

Awwad ST, Haddad W, Wang MX, et al. Corneal intrastromal gatifloxacin crystal deposits after penetrating keratoplasty. Eye Contact Lens 30: 169–172, 2004.

Bringas-Calva R, Iglesias-Cortinas D. Acute and bilateral uveitis secondary to moxifloxacin. Arch Soc Esp Oftalmol (Spain) 79: 357–359, 2004.

Burka JM, Bower KS, Vanroekel C, et al. The effect of fourth-generation fluoroquinolones gatifloxacin and moxifloxacin on epithelial healing following photorefractive keratectomy. Am J Ophthalmol 140: 83–87, 2005.

Cano-Parra J, Diaz-Llopis M. Drug induced uveitis. Arch Soc Esp Oftalmol (Spain) 80: 137–149, 2005.

Castillo A, Benitez del Castillo JM, Toledano N, et al. Deposits of topical norfloxacin in the treatment of bacterial keratitis. Cornea 16: 420–423, 1997.

Cavanagh HD. Response: crystallization of gatifloxacin after penetrating keratoplasty. Eye Contact Lens 31: 93, 2005.

Claerhout I, Kestelyn PH, Meire F, et al. Corneal deposits after the topical use of ofloxacin in two children with vernal keratoconjunctivitis. Br J Ophthalmol 87: 646, 2003.

Desai C, Desai KJ, Shah UH. Ofloxacin induced hypersensitivity reaction. J Assoc Physicians India 47: 349, 1999.

Donnenfeld EP, Chruscicki DA, Bitterman A, et al. A comparison of fourth-generation fluoroquinolones gatifloxacin 0.3% and moxifloxacin 0.5% in terms of ocular tolerability. Curr Med Res Opin 20: 1753–1758, 2004.

Gallelli L, Del Negro S, Naty S, et al. Levofloxacin-induced taste perversion, blurred vision and dyspnoea in a young woman. Clin Drug Invest 24: 487–489, 2004.

Konishi M, Yamada M, Mashima Y. Corneal ulcer associated with deposits of norfloxacin. Am J Ophthalmol 125(2): 258–260, 1998.

Kovoor TA, Kim AS, McCulley JP, et al. Evaluation of the corneal effects of topical ophthalmic fluoroquinolones using in vivo confocal microscopy. Eye Contact Lens 30: 90-94, 2004.

Moxifloxacin (Avelox). Can Adverse Reaction Newslett 12: 3, 2002.

Nettis E, Giordana D, Pierluigi T, et al. Erythema multiforme-like rash in patient sensitive to ofloxacin. Acta Derm Venereol 82: 395-396, 2002.

Ophthalmic moxifloxacin (vigamox) and Gatifloxacin (zymar). Med Lett Drugs Ther 46: 25–27, 2004.

Schwab IR, Friedlaender M, McCulley J, et al. A phase III clinical trial of 0.5% levofloxacin in ophthalmic solution versus 0.3% ofloxacin ophthalmic solution for the treatment of bacterial conjunctivitis. Ophthalmology 110: 457-465, 2003.

Silver LH, Woodside AM, Montgomery DB. Clinical safety of moxifloxacin ophthalmic solution 0.5% (Vigamox) in pediatric and nonpediatric patients with bacterial conjunctivitis. Surv Ophthalmol 50(Suppl 1): S55-S61, 2005.

Wittpenn JR. Crystallization of gatifloxacin after penetrating keratoplasty. Eye Contact Lens 31: 93, 2005.

Generic name: Gentamicin sulfate.

Proprietary names: Garamycin, Genoptic, Gentacidin, Gentak, Gentasol, Ocu-Mycin.

Primary use

This aminoglycoside is effective against *Ps. aeruginosa*, Aerobacter, *E. coli*, *K. pneumoniae* and Proteus.

Ocular side effects

Systemic administration
Probable
1. Decreased vision
2. Papilledema secondary to intracranial hypertension
3. Loss of eyelashes or eyebrows
4. Eyelids
   a. Photosensitivity
   b. Urticaria
5. Myasthenia gravis (aggravates)
   a. Diplopia
   b. Ptosis
   c. Paresis of extraocular muscles
6. Visual hallucinations
7. Oscillopsia

Possible
1. Subconjunctival or retinal hemorrhages secondary to drug-induced anemia

Local ophthalmic use or exposure – topical application or subconjunctival injection
Certain
1. Conjunctiva
   a. Hyperemia
   b. Mucopurulent discharge
   c. Chemosis
   d. Ulceration – necrosis
   e. Mild papillary hypertrophy
   f. Delayed healing
   g. Localized pallor
   h. Pseudomembranous conjunctivitis
2. Eyelids
   a. Allergic reactions
      b. Blepharoconjunctivitis
      c. Depigmentation
3. Cornea
   a. Superficial punctate keratitis
   b. Ulceration
   c. Delayed healing
4. Overgrowth of nonsusceptible organisms

Probable – subconjunctival injection
1. Scleral-retinal toxicity and necrosis
2. Extraocular and periocular muscle myopathy
3. Pupil dilation

Local ophthalmic use or exposure – intravitreal or intraocular injection
Certain
1. Retina
   a. Infarcts
   b. Retinal edema
   c. Hemorrhages
   d. Opacities
   e. Pigmentary changes
   f. Degeneration
2. Vitreous opacities
3. Optic nerve changes including atrophy
   a. Retinal edema
   b. Occlusion
   c. Hemorrhages
   d. Ischemia

Clinical significance

Surprisingly few drug-induced ocular side effects from systemic administration of gentamicin have been reported. Intracranial hypertension with secondary papilledema and visual loss following systemic use of gentamicin are the most clinically significant. Other adverse ocular effects are reversible and transitory after discontinued use of the drug. Marra et al (1988) described two cases of self-limiting oscillopsia, probably secondary to gentamicin-induced ototoxicity.

Topical ocular gentamicin may cause significant local side effects, the most common being a superficial punctate keratitis. Chronic use can also cause keratinization of the lid margin and blepharitis. Skin depigmentation in blacks, primarily when topical ocular gentamicin was associated with eye pad use, has been reported. Conjunctival necrosis, especially with fortified solutions, may occur. This usually is found in the inferior nasal conjunctiva, and starts as a localized area of hyperemia or pallor that usually stains with fluorescein. The lesions start after 5–7 days on either gentamicin solution or ointment and resolve after discontinuing the drug within 2 weeks. Bullard and O'Day (1997) reported four cases of pseudomembranous conjunctivitis after topical ocular gentamicin. These also occurred inferiorly and started with an intense focal bulbar conjunctival hyperemia, mucopurulent discharge and palpebral conjunctival papillae. The membranes appeared 4–7 days after starting therapy and resolved 4–5 days after the drug was stopped. Libert et al (1979) and D'Amico and Kenyon (1981) described lamellated cytoplasmic storage inclusion containing lipid material in the conjunctiva secondary to gentamicin injections. Awan (1985) described paresthesia of the eyes from topical ocular gentamicin and pupillary dilation from subconjunctival injections. Chapman et al (1992) showed that subconjunctival injections of gentamicin could cause muscle fiber degeneration with myopathy causing ocular motility impairment.

Intraocular gentamicin has caused severe retinal ischemia, rubeosis, iritis, neovascular glaucoma, optic atrophy and blindness. A number of cases of inadvertent intraocular injections have been reported in the literature and to the National Registry. The degree of ocular damage is primarily dependent on trauma of the injection, volume of the injection, location of the injection and toxicity of the drug. Injections into the anterior chamber are rarely devastating, in part due to early recognition, small volume and immediate irrigation. Inadvertent posterior injection may result in elevated intraocular pressure with secondary vascular occlusions. The trauma of the injection itself may in addition cause intraocular bleeding and retinal detachment.

While there are prior publications outlining posterior gentamicin toxicity from intravitreal injections, Campochiaro and Lim (1994), along with the follow-up Letter to the Editor by Grizzard (1995), give the most complete picture. In essence, even 0.1 mg of gentamicin may cause significant changes since gravity allows the drug to concentrate in a dependent area for an indefinite period of time. If this dependent area is in the fovea, permanent visual changes have occurred. Fluorescein angiograms show discrete geographic involvement with the non-perfusion not corresponding to the vascular pattern. The topography and the abrupt 'cookie cutter' margins, Campochiaro, Lim and Grizzard point out, suggest an event mediated by the drug in contact with the retinal surface. These findings show that a localized infarct is the end result of the gentamicin toxicity. Visual acuity loss has included cases of blindness. Additional findings have included retinal opacities, retinal hemorrhages and edema, neovascular glaucoma, retinal pigmentary degeneration, and optic atrophy.

REFERENCES AND FURTHER READING

Awan KJ. Mydriasis and conjunctival paresthesia from local gentamicin. Am J Ophthalmol 99: 723, 1985.

Bullard SR, O'Day DM. Pseudomembranous conjunctivitis following topical gentamicin therapy. Arch Ophthalmol 115: 1591–1592, 1997.

Campochiaro PA. Aminoglycoside toxicity in the treatment of endophthalmitis (letter). Arch 113: 262–263, 1995.

Campochiaro PA, Lim JI. Aminoglycoside toxicity in the treatment of endophthalmitis. Arch Ophthalmol 112: 48–53, 1994.

Chapman JM, Abdelatif OMA, Cheeks L, Green K. Subconjunctival gentamicin induction of extraocular toxic muscle myopathy. Ophthalmic Res 24: 189–196, 1992.

Conway BP, Campochiaro PA. Macular infarction after endophthalmitis treated with vitrectomy and intravitreal gentamicin. Arch Ophthalmol 104: 367, 1986.

D'Amico DJ, Kenyon KP. Drug-induced lipidoses of the cornea and conjunctiva. Int Ophthalmol 4: 67–76, 1981.

Davison CR, Tuft SJ, Dart JKG. Conjunctival necrosis after administration of topical fortified aminoglycosides. Am J Ophthalmol 111: 690–693, 1991.

De Maio R, Oliver GL. Recovery of useful vision after presumed retinal and choroidal toxic effects from gentamicin administration. Arch Ophthalmol 112(6): 736–738, 1994.

Grizzard WS. Aminoglycoside toxicity in the treatment of endophthalmitis (letter). Arch Ophthalmol 113: 262–263, 1995.

Libert J, Ketelbant-Balasse PE, et al: Cellular toxicity of gentamicin. Am J Ophthalmol 87(405): 411, 1979.

Lowenstein A, Esther Z, Yafa V, et al: Retinal toxicity of gentamicin after subconjunctival injection performed adjacent to thinned sclera. Ophthalmology 108: 759–764, 2001.

Marra TR, Reynolds NC Jr., Stoddard JJ. Subjective oscillopsia ('Jiggling vision') presumably due to aminoglycoside ototoxicity. J Clin Neuroophthalmol 8: 3538, 1988.

Minor LB. Gentamicin-induced bilateral vestibular hypofunction. JAMA 279(7): 541–544, 1998.

Nauheim R, Nauheim J, Merrick NY. Bulbar conjunctival defects associated with gentamicin. Arch Ophthalmol 105: 1321, 1987.

Schatz H, McDonald HR. Acute ischemic retinopathy due to gentamicin injection. JAMA 256: 1725, 1986.

Stern GA, et al: Effect of topical antibiotic solutions on corneal epithelial wound healing. Arch Ophthalmol 101: 644, 1983.

Waltz K. Intraocular gentamicin toxicity. Arch Ophthalmol 109: 911, 1991.

Generic name: Kanamycin sulfate.

Proprietary name: Kantrex.

Primary use

This aminoglycoside is effective against Gram-negative organisms and in drug-resistant staphylococcus.

Ocular side effects

Systemic administration
Certain
1. Decreased vision
2. Eyelids or conjunctiva – allergic reactions

Probable
1. Myasthenia gravis (aggravates)
   a. Diplopia
   b. Ptosis
   c. Paresis of extraocular muscles

Possible
1. Eyelids or conjunctiva - Lyell's syndrome

Conditional/Unclassified
1. Optic neuritis

Local ophthalmic use or exposure – subconjunctival injection
Certain
1. Irritation
2. Eyelids or conjunctiva – allergic reactions
3. Overgrowth of non-susceptible organisms

Clinical significance

Systemic and ocular side effects due to kanamycin are quite rare, partially due to its poor gastrointestinal absorption. Myasthenia gravis occurs more frequently if kanamycin is given in combination with other antibiotics, such as neomycin, gentamicin, polymyxin B, colistin or streptomycin. Allergic reactions with cross-sensitivity have been reported for gentomycin but not for neomycin (Sanchez-Perez et al 2001). Adverse ocular reactions to this agent are reversible, transitory and seldom have residual complications. While optic neuritis has been reported to be associated with this drug, it has not been proven.

REFERENCES AND FURTHER READING

D'Amico DJ, et al: Comparative toxicity of intravitreal aminoglycoside antibiotics. Am J Ophthalmol 100: 264, 1985.

Finegold SM. Kanamycin. Arch Intern Med 104: 15, 1959.

Finegold SM. Toxicity of kanamycin in adults. Ann NY Acad Sci 132: 942, 1966.

Freemon FR, Parker RL Jr., Greer M. Unusual neurotoxicity of kanamycin. JAMA 200: 410, 1967.

Kaeser HE. Drug-induced myasthenic syndromes. Acta Neurol Scand 70(Suppl 100): 9, 1984.

Sanchez-Perez J, Lopez MP, De Vega Haro JM, Garcia-Diez A. Allergic contact dermatitis from gentamicin in eyedrops, with cross-reactivity to kanamycin but not neomycin. Contact Dermatitis 44(1): 54, 2001.

Walsh FB, Hoyt WF. Clinical Neuro-Ophthalmology, Vol. III. 3rd edn. Williams & Wilkins, Baltimore, pp 2655, 2680, 1969.

Generic name: Linezolid.

Proprietary name: Zyvox.

Primary use

A new class of synthetic antibiotics, oxazolidinones, for use in drug-resistant Gram-positive bacterial infections.

Ocular side effects

Systemic administration
Probable
1. Blurred or decreased vision
2. Decreased color vision
3. Visual field defects
   a. Central scotomas
   b. Centrocecal scotomas
4. Optic neuropathy (Fig. 7.1e)
   a. Edema
   b. Micro-hemorrhages
   c. Atrophy
5. Blindness

Clinical significance

The use of this antibiotic is primarily in patients who have a drug-resistant Gram-positive organism, often in a life-threatening circumstance. Ocular symptoms, while rare, are seldom seen in the first 28 days of therapy other than blurred vision. In patients requiring extended treatment, unrecognized drug-induced optic neuropathy could lead to bilateral blindness. To prevent this requires regular examinations, which include visual acuity, amsler grid testing, color vision and visual field tests. To date it appears that stopping the drug can prevent progression to blindness, and in some cases regression. Efforts are underway to find which patients are most susceptible to the neuropathy, how to diagnose it early and possible ways to prevent this side effect.

Recommendations

1. If any visual changes occur, i.e. decreased or blurred vision, color vision abnormalities or any visual field change, the patient should see an ophthalmologist.
2. Perform an ophthalmic evaluation every 3 months if the patient remains on the drug for an extended period of time.
3. If diagnosis of optic neuropathy is suspected, a risk-benefit ratio is needed to determine if it is appropriate to continue the medication. Permanent visual loss, including legal blindness, has occurred if the drug is continued therefore informed consent is recommended.
4. Baseline ophthalmic examinations before starting this drug, including visual acuity, amsler grids, color vision testing and visual fields, while ideal, are probably not cost-effective.

REFERENCES AND FURTHER READING

Carallo CE, Paull AE. Linezolid-induced optic neuropathy. Med J Aust 177: 332, 2002.

De Vriese AS, Van Coster R, Smet J, et al. Linezolid-induced inhibition of mitochondrial protein sytnthesis. Clin Infect Dis 42: 1111–1117, 2006.

Ferr T, Pnceau B, Simon M, et al. Possibly linezolid-induced peripheral and central neurotoxicity: report of four cases. Infection 33(3): 151–154, 2005.

Frippiat F, Derue G. Causal relationship between neuropathy and prolonged linezolid use. Clin Infect Dis 39(3): 439, 2004.

Frippiat F, Bergiers C, Michel C, et al. Severe bilateral neuritis associated with prolonged linezolid therapy. J Antimicrob Chemother 53(6): 1114–1115, 2004.

Hernandez PC, Llinarea TF, Climent GE, Fernandez AC. Peripheral and optic neuropathy associated to linezolid in multidrug resistant Mycobacterium bovis infections. Medicinia Clinica 124(20): 797–798, 2005.

Mckinley SH, Foroozan R. Optic neuropathy associated with linezolid treatment. J Neuroophthalmol 25: 18–21, 2005.

Rucker JC, Hamilton SR, Bardenstein D, et al. Linezolid-associated toxic optic neuropathy. Neurology 66: 595–598, 2006.

Saijio T, Hayashi K, Yamada H, Wakakura M. Linezolid-induced optic neuropathy. Am J Ophthalmol 139(6): 1114–1116, 2005.

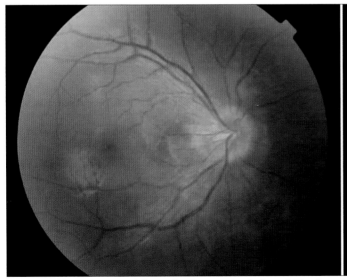
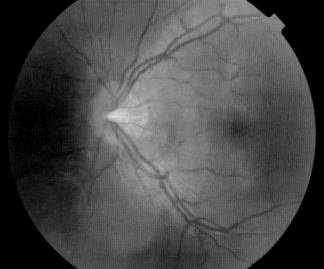

Fig. 7.1e Bilateral temporal disc pallor from systemic linezolid treatment. Photo courtesy of Saijo T, et al: Linezolid-induced optic neuropathy. Am J Ophthalmol 139: 1114-1116, 2005.

Generic name: Nalidixic acid.

Proprietary names: None.

Primary use

This bactericidal naphthyridine derivative is effective against *E. coli*, Aerobacter and Klebsiella. Its primary clinical use is against Proteus.

Ocular side effects

Systemic administration
Certain
1. Visual sensations
   a. Glare phenomenon
   b. Flashing lights – white or colored
   c. Scintillating scotomas – may be colored
2. Problems with color vision
   a. Color vision defect
   b. Objects have green, yellow, blue or violet tinge
3. Photophobia
4. Paresis of extraocular muscles
5. Papilledema secondary to intracranial hypertension
6. Decreased vision
7. Decreased accommodation
8. Nystagmus
9. Eyelids or conjunctiva
   a. Photosensitivity
   b. Angioedema
   c. Urticaria
10. Visual hallucinations

Possible
1. Subconjunctival or retinal hemorrhages secondary to drug-induced anemia
2. Eyelids or conjunctiva – lupoid syndrome

Clinical significance

Numerous ocular side effects due to nalidixic acid have been reported. The most common adverse ocular reaction is a curious visual disturbance, which includes brightly colored appearances of objects as the main feature. This often appears soon after the drug is taken. Temporary visual loss has also occurred and lasted from half an hour to 72 hours. Probably the most serious ocular reaction is papilledema secondary to elevated intracranial pressure. Most of the reports concerning intracranial hypertension deal with children and adolescents, the oldest being 20 years of age. A large series of intracranial hypertension occurred in infants below 6 months of age given 100–150 mg/kg/day for acute bacillary dysentery (Van Dyk and Swan 1969). Use of nalidixic acid during pregnancy carries the possible prenatal risk of increased intracranial pressure. Most adverse ocular reactions due to nalidixic acid are transitory and reversible if the dosage is decreased or the drug is discontinued.

REFERENCES AND FURTHER READING

Birch J, et al. Acquired color vision defects. In: Congenital and Acquired Color Vision Defects, Pokorny J, et al (eds), Grune & Stratton, New York, pp 243–350, 1979.

Drugs that cause psychiatric symptoms. Med Lett Drugs Ther 28: 81, 1986.

Gedroyc W, Shorvon SD. Acute intracranial hypertension and nalidixic acid therapy. Neurology 32: 212, 1982.

Granstrom G, Santesson B. Unconsciousness after one therapeutic dose of nalidixic acid. Acta Med Scand 216: 237, 1984.

Haut J, Haye C, et al. Disturbances of color perception after taking nalidixic acid. Bull Soc Ophthalmol France 72: 147–149, 1972.

Katzman B, et al. Pseudotumor cerebri: an observation and review. Ann Ophthalmol 13: 887, 1981.

Kilpatrick C, Ebeling P. Intracranial hypertension in nalidixic acid therapy. Med J Aust 1: 252, 1982.

Lane RJM, Routledge PA. Drug-induced neurological disorders. Drugs 26: 124, 1983.

Mukherjee A, Dutta P, Lahiri M, et al. Benign intracranial hypertension after nalidixic acid overdose in infants. Lancet 335: 1602, 1990.

Riyaz A, Abbobacker CM, Streelatha PR. Nalidixic acid induced pseudotumor cerebri in children. J Indian Med Assoc 96(10): 308–314, 1998.

Rubinstein A. LE-like disease caused by nalidixic acid. N Engl J Med 301: 1288, 1979.

Safety of antimicrobial drugs in pregnancy. Med Lett Drugs Ther 27: 93, 1985.

Van Dyk HJL, Swan KC. Drug-induced pseudotumor cerebri. In: Symposium on Ocular Therapy, Vol. 4, Leopold IH (ed), Mosby, St Louis, pp 71–77, 1969.

Wall M. Idiopathic intracranial hypertension. Neurol Clin 9: 73, 1991.

Generic name: Neomycin.

Proprietary names: Mycifradin, Neo-fradin.

Primary use

These bactericidal aminoglycosidic agents are effective against *Ps. aeruginosa*, Aerobacter, *K. pneumoniae*, *P. vulgaris*, *E. coli*, Salmonella, Shigella and most strains of *S. aureus*.

Ocular side effects

Systemic administration (neomycin powder to mucus membranes)
Probable
1. Myasthenia gravis (aggravates)
   a. Diplopia
   b. Ptosis
   c. Paresis of extraocular muscles
2. Decreased or absent pupillary reaction to light

Local ophthalmic use or exposure – topical application or subconjunctival injection
Certain
1. Irritation
   a. Hyperemia
   b. Ocular pain
   c. Edema
   d. Burning sensation
2. Eyelids or conjunctiva
   a. Allergic reactions
   b. Erythema
   c. Blepharoconjunctivitis – follicular
   d. Urticaria
3. Punctate keratitis
4. Overgrowth of non-susceptible organisms

Local ophthalmic use or exposure – intracameral injection
Certain
1. Uveitis
2. Corneal edema
3. Lens damage

Clinical significance

These drugs are not used parenterally because of nephro- and oto-toxicity. There are well-documented reports of decreased or absent pupillary reactions due to application of neomycin to the pleural or peritoneal cavities during a thoracic or abdominal operation.

Topical ocular application of neomycin has been reported to cause allergic conjunctival or lid reactions in 4% of patients using this drug. If neomycin is used topically for longer than 7–10 days on inflammatory dermatosis, the incidence of allergic reaction is increased 13-fold over matched controls. Neomycin preparations for minor infections should rarely be used over 7–10 days. Also, if the patient has been previously exposed to neomycin there is a significantly higher chance of an allergic response. In one study neomycin was found to be one of the three most common drugs causing periocular allergic contact dermatitis. Rarely will neomycin be given alone in topical ocular medication. Often a steroid is added, which may mask the incidence of hypersensitivity reactions. Additional antibiotics are frequently added to increase the antimicrobial spectrum. Some feel that, of the more commonly used antibiotics, topical neomycin has the greatest toxicity to the corneal epithelium. It probably produces plasma membrane injury and cell death primarily of the superficial cell layers with chronic topical exposure. Dohlman (1966) describes tiny snowflakes on the corneal epithelial surface, along with superficial punctate keratitis persisting for weeks after topical ocular neomycin use. After long-term ocular exposure to neomycin, fungi superinfections have been reported. Nystagmus has been reported in a 9-year-old child following topical treatment of the skin with 1% neomycin in 11% dimethyl sulfoxide ointment.

REFERENCES AND FURTHER READING

Baldinger J, Weiter JJ. Diffuse cutaneous hypersensitivity reaction after dexamethasone/polymyxin B/neomycin combination eyedrops. Ann Ophthalmol 18: 95, 1986.

Dohlman CH. (Reply to Query). Arch Ophthalmol 76: 902, 1966.

Fisher AA, Adams RM. Alternative for sensitizing neomycin topical medications. Cutis 28: 491, 1981.

Fisher AA. Topical medications which are common sensitizers. Ann Allergy 49: 97, 1982.

Kaeser HE. Drug-induced myasthenic syndromes. Acta Neurol Scand 70(Suppl 100): 39, 1984.

Kaufman HE. Chemical blepharitis following drug treatment. Am J Ophthalmol 95: 703, 1983.

Kruyswijk MRJ, et al. Contact allergy following administration of eyedrops and eye ointments. Doc Ophthalmol 48: 251, 1979.

Wilson FM II. Adverse external ocular effects of topical ophthalmic medications. Surv Ophthalmol 24: 57, 1979.

Generic name: Nitrofurantoin.

Proprietary names: Furadantin, Macrodantin, Macrobid.

Primary use

This bactericidal furan derivative is effective against specific organisms that cause urinary tract infections, especially *E. coli*, enterococci and *S. aureus*.

Ocular side effects

Systemic administration
Certain
1. Non-specific ocular irritation
   a. Lacrimation
   b. Burning sensation
   c. Epiphoria

2. Decreased vision
3. Eyelids or conjunctiva
   a. Allergic reactions
   b. Photosensitivity
   c. Angioedema
   d. Urticaria
   e. Loss of eyelashes or eyebrows
4. Problems with color vision
   a. Color vision defect
   b. Objects have yellow tinge

Probable
1. Papilledema secondary to intracranial hypertension
2. Myasthenia gravis (aggravates)
   a. Diplopia
   b. Ptosis – unilateral or bilateral
   c. Paresis of extraocular muscle

Possible
1. Subconjunctival or retinal hemorrhages secondary to drug-induced anemia
2. Retinal – crystalline retinopathy
3. Eyelids or conjunctiva
   a. Lupoid syndrome
   b. Erythema multiforme
   c. Lyell's syndrome
   d. Stevens-Johnson syndrome

Clinical significance

A unique ocular side effect secondary to nitrofurantoin is a severe itching, burning and tearing reaction, which may persist long after discontinuing the drug. Aggravating or causing an ocular myasthenia has been well documented with nitrofurantoin. This is probably due to interference in the transmission of the neuro impulse pharmacologically to the resting muscle (Wittbrodt 1997). In addition, various degrees of polyneuropathies with demyelination and degeneration of sensory and motor nerves have occurred with long-term use of nitrofurantoin, probably on a toxic basis. Intracranial hypertension associated with nitrofurantoin therapy has been reported (Mushet 1980). A report by Ibanez et al (1994) suggests an intraretinal crystalline deposit in both eyes of a 69-year-old male who for 19 years received nitrofurantoin daily for a chronic urinary tract infection.

REFERENCES AND FURTHER READING

Ibanez HE, Williams DF, Boniuk I. Crystalline retinopathy associated with long-term nitrofurantoin therapy. Case report. Arch Ophthalmol 112: 304–305, 1994.

Mesaros MP, Seymour J, Sadjadpour K. Lateral rectus muscle palsy associated with nitrofurantoin (Macrodantoin). Am J Ophthalmol 94: 816, 1982.

Mushet GR. Pseudotumor and nitrofurantoin therapy. Arch Neurol 34: 257, 1977.

Nitrofurantoin. Med Lett Drugs Ther 22: 36, 1980.

Penn RG, Griffin JP. Adverse reactions to nitrofurantoin in the United Kingdom, Sweden. Holland. BMJ 284: 1440, 1982.

Sharma DB, James A. Benign intracranial hypertension associated with nitrofurantoin therapy. BMJ 4: 771, 1974.

Toole JF, Parrish MD. Nitrofurantoin polyneuropathy. Neurology 23: 554–559, 1973.

Wasserman BN, Chronister TE, Stark BI, Saran BR. Ocular myasthenia and nitrofurantoin. Am J Ophthalmol 130: 531–533, 2000.

Wittbrodt ET. Drugs and myasthenia gravis: an update. Arch Intern Med 157(4): 399–408, 1997.

Generic name: Polymyxin B sulfate.

Proprietary names: Multi-ingredient preparations only.

Primary use
This bactericidal polypeptide is effective against Gram-negative bacilli, especially *Ps. aeruginosa*.

Ocular side effects

Systemic administration
Probable
1. Myasthenia gravis (aggravates)
    a. Diplopia
    b. Ptosis
    c. Paresis of extraocular muscles
2. Decreased vision
3. Diplopia
4. Nystagmus
5. Mydriasis

Local ophthalmic use or exposure – topical application or subconjunctival
1. Injection

Certain
1. Irritation – ocular pain
2. Eyelids or conjunctiva – allergic reactions
    a. Itching
    b. Edema
    c. Erythema

Probable
1. Myasthenia gravis (aggravates)
    a. Diplopia
    b. Ptosis
    c. Paresis
2. Overgrowth of non-susceptible organisms
3. Anaphylactic reaction

Local ophthalmic use or exposure – intracameral injection
Certain
1. Uveitis
2. Corneal edema
3. Lens damage

Clinical significance
Although ocular side effects due to polymyxin B sulfate are well documented, they are quite rare and seldom of major clinical importance. The drug is rarely used by itself as a topical ocular medication, so the true incidence of side effects is difficult to determine. Myasthenia gravis is transitory and does occur from topical ocular administration. To date, we are unaware of systemic polymyxin B sulfate toxicity from topical ocular medication other than transitory neuromuscular transmission defects, such as myasthenia gravis-type clinical syndrome. Some systemic absorption may occur, for example if the drug is given every hour for corneal ulcers. There are reports of anaphylactic reactions from topical polymyxin B-bacitracin applications. The clinically important side effects are secondary to intracameral injections where permanent changes to the cornea and lens have occurred.

REFERENCES AND FURTHER READING
Baldinger J, Weiter JJ. Diffuse cutaneous hypersensitivity reaction after dexamethasone/polymyxin B/neomycin combination eyedrops. Ann Ophthalmol 18: 95, 1986.
Francois J, Mortiers P. The injurious effects of locally and generally applied antibiotics on the eye. T Geneeskd 32: 139, 1976.
Hudgson P. Adverse drug reactions in the neuromuscular apparatus. Adverse Drug React Acute Poisoning Rev 1: 35, 1982.
Kaeser HE. Drug-induced myasthenic syndromes. Acta Neurol Scand 70(Suppl 100): 39, 1984.
Koenig A, Ohrloff C. Influence of local application of Isoptomax eye drops on neuromuscular transmission. Klin Monatsbl Augenheilkd 179: 109, 1981.
Lane RJM, Routledge PA. Drug-induced neurological disorders. Drugs 26: 124, 1983.
Stern GA, et al. Effect of topical antibiotic solutions on corneal epithelial wound healing. Arch Ophthalmol 101: 644, 1983.

Generic names: 1. Sulfacetamide; 2. sulfafurazole (sulfisoxazole); 3. sulfamethizole; 4. sulfamethoxazole; 5. sulfanilamide; 6. sulfasalazine; 7. sulfathiazole.

Proprietary names: 1. Ak-Sulf, Bleph-10, Centamide, Isopto Cetamide, Klaron, Ocusulf-10, Sodium Sulamyd, Sulf-10, Sulfac, Vanocin; 2. Gantrisin; 3. Multi-ingredient preparation only; 4. Multi-ingredient preparation only; 5. Multi-ingredient preparation only; 6. Azulfidine; 7. Multi-ingredient preparation only.

Primary use
The sulfonamides are bacteriostatic agents effective against most Gram-positive and some Gram-negative organisms.

Ocular side effects

Systemic administration
Certain
1. Decreased vision
2. Myopia – transitory
3. Non-specific ocular irritation
    a. Lacrimation
    b. Photophobia
4. Keratitis
5. Problems with color vision
    a. Color vision defect
    b. Objects have yellow or red tinge
6. Periorbital edema
7. Visual hallucinations
8. Decreased anterior chamber depth – may precipitate angle-closure glaucoma
9. Eyelids or conjunctiva
    a. Allergic reactions
    b. Conjunctivitis – non-specific
    c. Photosensitivity
    d. Urticaria
    e. Purpura
    f. Pemphigoid lesion with or without symblepharon
    g. Loss of eyelashes or eyebrows
10. Contact lenses stained yellow
11. Uveitis

Possible

1. Optic neuritis
2. Myasthenia gravis (aggravates)
   a. Diplopia
   b. Ptosis
   c. Paresis of extraocular muscles
3. Papilledema (intracranial hypertension)
4. Vivid light lavender-colored retinal vascular tree
5. Eyelids or conjunctiva
   a. Lupoid syndrome
   b. Erythema multiforme
   c. Stevens-Johnson syndrome
   d. Exfoliative dermatitis
   e. Lyell's syndrome

Local ophthalmic use or exposure – topical application
Certain

1. Irritation
2. Eyelids or conjunctiva
   a. Allergic reactions
   b. Conjunctivitis – follicular
   c. Deposits
   d. Photosensitivity
   e. Hyperemia
3. Overgrowth of non-susceptible organisms
4. Delayed corneal wound healing

Possible

1. Eyelids or conjunctiva
   a. Lupoid syndrome
   b. Erythema multiforme
   c. Stevens-Johnson syndrome

Conditional/Unclassified
1. Cornea – peripheral immune ring

Clinical significance

While there are numerous reported ocular side effects from systemic sulfa medication, most are rare and reversible. Probably the most common ocular side effect seen in patients on systemic therapy is myopia. This is transient, with or without induced astigmatism, usually bilateral and may exceed several diopters. This is most likely due to an increased anterior-posterior lens diameter secondary to ciliary body edema. In rare instances, this may decrease the depth of the anterior chamber or possibly cause a choroidal effusion, inducing angle-closure glaucoma (Waheep et al 2003). Tilden et al (1991) reported 12 cases of uveitis attributed to systemic use of sulfonamide derivatives. Most of the cases were bilateral occurring within 24 hours to as long as 8 days after first exposure to the sulfonamide. Three patients had a positive rechallenged with a recurrence of bilateral uveitis within 24 hours. Some of the patients had systemic findings of Stevens-Johnson syndrome, erythema multiforme, diffuse macular-vesicular rashes, stomatitis, glossitis and granulomatous hepatitis. Optic neuritis has been reported even in low oral dosages and is usually reversible with full recovery of vision (Lane and Routledge 1983).

The ophthalmologist should be aware that anaphylactic reactions, Stevens-Johnson syndrome and exfoliative dermatitis have all been reported, although rarely from topical ocular administration of sulfa preparations. Ocular irritation from crystalline sulfa in the tears may occur. Recently Gutt et al (1988) reported immune rings in the peripheral cornea, associated with topical ocular sulfamethoxazole.

REFERENCES AND FURTHER READING

Bovino JA, Marcus DF. The mechanism of transient myopia induced by sulfonamide therapy. Am J Ophthalmol 94: 99, 1982.

Chirls IA, Norris JW. Transient myopia associated with vaginal sulfanilamide suppositories. Am J Ophthalmol 98: 120, 1984.

Fajardo RV. Acute bilateral anterior uveitis caused by sulfa drugs. In Saari KM, Uveitis Update. Excerpta Medica, Amsterdam, 1984, p 115–118.

Flach AJ, Peterson JS, Mathias CGT. Photosensitivity to topically applied sulfisoxazole ointment. Evidence for a phototoxic reaction. Arch Ophthalmol 100: 1286, 1982.

Genvert GI, et al. Erythema multiforme after use of topical sulfacetamide. Am J Ophthalmol 99: 465, 1985.

Gutt L, Feder JM, Feder RS, et al. Corneal ring formation after exposure to sulfamethoxazole. Arch Ophthalmol 106: 726–727, 1988.

Hook SR, et al. Transient myopia induced by sulfonamides. Am J Ophthalmol 101: 495, 1986.

Lane RJM, Routledge PA. Drug-induced neurological disorders. Drugs 26: 124, 1983.

Mackie BS, Mackie LE. Systemic lupus erythematosus – Dermatomyositis induced by sulphacetamide eyedrops. Aust J Dermatol 20: 49, 1979.

Riley SA, Flagg PJ, Mandal BK. Contact lens staining due to sulphasalazine. Lancet 1: 972, 1986.

Tilden ME, Rosenbaum JT, Fraunfelder FT. Systemic sulfonamides as a cause of bilateral, anterior uveitis. Arch Ophthalmol 109: 67–69, 1991.

Vanheule BA, Carswell F. Sulphasalazine-induced systemic lupus erythematosus in a child. Eur J Pediatr 140: 66, 1983.

Waheep S, Feldman F, Velos P, Pavlin CJ. Ultrasound biomicroscopic analysis of drug-induced bilateral angle-closure glaucoma associated with supraciliary choroidal effusion. Can J Ophthalmol 38: 299–302, 2003.

Generic name: Telithromycin.

Proprietary name: Ketek.

Primary use

A new class of antibacterial agents, ketolides, used in the management of community-acquired pneumonia, acute exacerbation of chronic bronchitis or acute bacterial sinusitis.

Ocular side effects

Systemic administration
Certain

1. Blurred vision
2. Difficulty focusing
3. Delayed accommodation

Probable

1. Visual field disturbance (various scotomas)
2. Myasthenia gravis (aggravates)
   a. Diplopia
   b. Ptosis
   c. Paresis or extraocular muscles

Clinical significance

Telithromycin causes a reversible bilateral central blurred vision and a delay in accommodation, most frequently described as a delay in focusing when adjusting from near to far vision. This occurs in approximately 0.8% of patients and is twice as frequently in women than men. Typically, it first occurs within 1–3 days after starting therapy and at the time of peak blood levels of the drug. The effect occurs within 1–2 hours after dosing and lasts a mean of 2 hours. In some patients this may happen after each dose, but in some patients the visual side effects no longer occur after 1–3 days. The visual side effects may or may not occur if the patient retakes the drug at a later date. Visual field changes or diplopia are very rare events. Most patients with visual symptoms maintain normal visual acuities, but some patients should modify their activities such as driving and operating machinery. Telithromycin has the potential to exacerbate myasthenia gravis in patients who have a pre-existing myasthenia.

REFERENCES AND FURTHER READING

Nieman RB, Sharma K, Edelber H, Caffe SE. Telithromycin and myasthenia gravis. Clin Infect Dis 37: 1579, 2003.
Physicians' Desk Reference, 60th edn, Thomson PDR, Montevale NJ, pp 2920–2925, 2006.
Shi J, Montay G, Bhargava VO. Clinical pharmacokinetics of telithromycin, the first ketolide antibacterial. Clin Pharmacokinet 44(9): 915–934, 2005.
Wellington K, Noble S. Telithromycin. Drugs 64(15): 1683–1694, 2004.

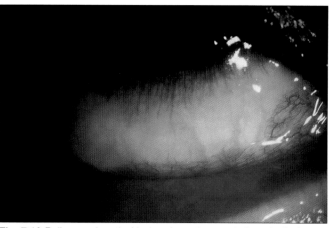

Fig. 7.1f Bulbar conjunctival ischemia and necrosis from topical tobramycin. Photo courtesy of Spalton DJ, Hitchings RA, Hunter PA. Atlas of Clinical Ophthalmology, 3rd edn, Mosby Elsevier, London, 2005.

Generic name: Tobramycin.

Proprietary names: TOBI, Tobradex, Zylet.

Primary use

This aminoglycoside is effective against many Gram-negative organisms, including *Ps. aeruginosa*, *E. coli*, *K. pneumoniae*, Proteus and Enterobacter, and some Gram-positive organisms, including staphylococci and streptococci.

Ocular side effects

Systemic administration
Certain
1. Decreased vision
2. Nystagmus

Probable
1. Myasthenia gravis (aggravates)
   a. Diplopia
   b. Ptosis
   c. Paresis or paralysis of extraocular muscles

Conditional/Unclassified
1. Problems with color vision – color vision defect
2. Visual hallucinations

Local ophthalmic use or exposure – topical application
Certain
1. Eyelids and conjunctiva
   a. Hyperemia
   b. Edema
   c. Burning sensation – pain
   d. Itching
   e. Allergic reactions
   f. Conjunctival necrosis (fortified solutions) (Fig. 7.1f)
2. Epiphora
3. Superficial punctate keratitis
4. Overgrowth of non-susceptible organisms
5. Photophobia

Probable
1. Myasthenia gravis (aggravates)
   a. Diplopia
   b. Ptosis
   c. Paresis or paralysis of extraocular muscles

Tobramycin-soaked collagen shield
Certain
1. Cornea
   a. Keratitis
   b. Edema
   c. Endothelial damage

Inadvertent ocular exposure – intraocular injection
Certain
1. Optic atrophy
2. Retinal degeneration

Inadvertent ocular exposure – subconjunctival injection
Probable
1. Macular infarction

Inadvertent ocular exposure – ointment in anterior chamber
Probable
1. Uveitis
2. Glaucoma

Clinical significance

Few drug-induced ocular side effects from systemic administration of tobramycin have been reported. Decreased vision is rare and transitory. Nystagmus occurs secondary to tobramycin-induced vestibular toxicity. This drug can induce or aggravate myasthenia gravis by interfering with neuromuscular transmission (Kaeser 1984). Other findings are so rare it is difficult to prove they are drug related.

Topical ocular toxicity of tobramycin is totally dependent on concentration, frequency and the integrity of the corneal epithelium and stoma. In non-fortified solutions, the incidences of hypersensitivity reactions occur in about 3–4% of patients. Superficial punctate keratitis is rare, seen primarily with frequent dosing or with fortified solutions. By stopping the drug, ocular tissues return to normal in a few days but occasionally it may require over a month. Systemic absorption from topical ocular application is minimal with normal anterior segments, however with ulcerated corneas or with fortified solutions, absorption can occur. There is a case report by Kella and Kozart (1997) of exacerbation of myasthenia gravis by topical ocular tobramycin, betoxal and dexamethasone. There are two cases in the National Registry where topical ocular tobramycin alone or in a steroid combination was implicated in causing or enhancing myasthenia gravis. Both patients had chronic renal disease. One of these cases, at an academic center, resulted in a lawsuit. A case of anaphylaxis after topical ocular combination of tobramycin, steroid and Naplicon A has been reported to the National Registry.

Systemic absorption and local toxicity significantly increases in collagen-soaked tobramycin shields. Grazozi et al (1999) reported a case of inadvertent tobramycin ophthalmic ointment entering the anterior chamber through a microperforation after radial keratocomy. This was followed by three attacks of uveitis and glaucoma. The endothelial cell count was a third less and the iris texture was slightly atrophic compared to the fellow eye. Animal studies confirm the toxicity of tobramycin to the corneal endothelial cell. Retinal degeneration and optic atrophy have followed inadvertent intraocular injection of tobramycin (Balian 1983). Intraocular complications have possibly occurred from subconjunctival injection, with the drug entering the eye through the cataract wound (Judson 1989). Campochiaro and Conway (1991) reported three cases of macular infarctions after subconjunctival injections or tobramycin.

REFERENCES AND FURTHER READING

American Academy of Ophthalmology. Corneal toxicity with antibiotic/steroid-soaked collagen shields. Clinical Alert 11: 1, 1990.
Balian JV. Accidental intraocular tobramycin injection: a case report. Ophthalmic Surg 14: 353, 1983.
Campochiaro PA, Conway BP. Aminoglycoside toxicity – a survey of retinal specialists. Arch Ophthalmol 109: 946–950, 1991.
Caraffini S, Assalve D, Stingeni L, et al. Allergic contact conjunctivitis and blepharitis from tobramycin. Contact Dermatitis 32(3): 186–187, 1995.
Davison CR, Tuft SJ, Dart KG. Conjunctival necrosis after administration of topical fortified aminoglycosides. Am J Ophthalmol 111: 690–693, 1991.
Garzozi HJ, Muallem MS, Harris A. Recurrent anterior uveitis and glaucoma associated with inadvertent entry of ointment into the anterior chamber after radial keratotomy. J Cataract Refract Surg 25: 1685–1687, 1999.
Judson PH. Aminoglycoside macular toxicity after subconjunctival injection. Arch Ophthalmol 107: 1282–1283, 1989.
Kaeser HE. Drug-induced myasthenic syndromes. Acta Neurol Scand 70(Suppl 100): 39, 1984.
Khella SL, Kozart D. Unmasking and exacerbation of myasthenia gravis by ophthalmic solutions: betoxolol, tobramycin, and desamethasone. A case report (letter). Muscle & Nerve 20(5): 631, 1997.
McCartney CF, Hatley LH, Kessler JM. Possible tobramycin delirium. JAMA 247: 1319, 1982.
Pflugfelder SC, Murchison JF. Corneal toxicity with an antibiotic/steroid-soaked collagen shield (letter). Arch Ophthalmol 111(1): 18, 1993.
Wilhelmus KR, Gilbert ML, Osato MS. Tobramycin in ophthalmology. Surv Ophthalmol 32(2): 111–122, 1987.

CLASS: ANTIFUNGAL AGENTS

Generic name: Amphotericin B.

Proprietary names: Abelcet, AmBisome, Amphotec, Fungizone.

Primary use

This polyene fungistatic agent is effective against Blastomyces, Histoplasma, Cryptococcus, Coccidioides, Candida and Aspergillus.

Ocular side effects

Systemic administration
Probable
1. Decreased vision – transitory

Possible
1. Subconjunctival or retinal hemorrhages secondary to drug-induced anemia

Conditional/Unclassified
1. Paresis of extraocular muscles
2. Retinal exudates
3. Diplopia
4. Blindness (IV)

Local ophthalmic use or exposure – topical application or subconjunctival injection
Certain
1. Irritation
   a. Ocular pain
   b. Burning sensation
2. Punctate keratitis
3. Eyelids or conjunctiva
   a. Allergic reactions
   b. Ulceration
   c. Conjunctivitis – follicular
   d. Necrosis – subconjunctival injection
   e. Nodules – subconjunctival injection
   f. Yellow discoloration – subconjunctival injection
4. Overgrowth of non-susceptible organisms
5. Uveitis
6. Hyphema
7. Delayed wound healing

Local ophthalmic use or exposure – intracameral injection
Certain
1. Uveitis
2. Corneal edema
3. Lens damage

Clinical significance

Seldom are significant ocular side effects seen from systemic administration of amphotericin B, except with intrathecal injections. In general, transitory blurred vision is the most common ocular side effect. Allergic reactions are so rare that initially it was felt they did not even occur. Li and Lai (1989) reported that after IV amphotericin B, a patient with previously bilateral normal vision went to irreversible light perception within 10 hours and optic atrophy within 10 weeks.

Topical ocular administration of amphotericin B can produce significant conjunctival and corneal irritative responses. This agent can affect cell membranes and allow increased penetration of other drugs through the cornea. There have been rare reports of marked iridocyclitis with small hyphemas occurring after each exposure of topical ocular amphotericin B. The formation of salmon-colored raised nodules can occur secondary to subconjunctival injection, especially if the dosage exceeds 5 mg (Bell and Ritchey 1973). These regress somewhat with time. The injection of this agent subconjunctivally or subcutaneously can cause permanent yellowing. Some clinicians feel that amphotericin B is too toxic to the tissue to be given subconjunctivally. However, in extreme circumstances, even intracorneal injections have been done (Garcia-Vlaenzuela and Song 2005).

REFERENCES AND FURTHER READING

Bell RW, Ritchey JP. Subconjunctival nodules after amphotericin B injection. Arch Ophthalmol 90: 402–404, 1973.

Brod RD, Flynn HW, Clarkson JG, et al. Endogenous candida endophthalmitis. Management without intravenous amphotericin B. Ophthalmology 97: 666–674, 1990.

Doft BH, et al. Amphotericin clearance in vitrectomized versus nonvitrectomized eyes. Ophthalmology 92: 1601, 1985.

Foster CS, et al. Ocular toxicity of topical antifungal agents. Arch Ophthalmol 99: 1081, 1981.

Garcia-Valenzuela E, Song D. Intracorneal injection of amphotericin B for recurrent fungal keratitis and endophthalmitis. Arch Ophthalmol 123: 1721–1723, 2005.

Li PKT, Lai KN. Amphotericin B-induced ocular toxicity in cryptococcal meningitis. Br J Ophthalmol 73: 397–398, 1989.

Lavine JB, Binder PS, Wickham MG. Antimicrobials and the corneal endothelium. Ann Ophthalmol 11: 1517, 1979.

O'Day DM, et al. Intraocular penetration of systemically administered antifungal agents. Curr Eye Res 4: 131, 1985.

O'Day DM, Smith R, Stevens JB. Toxicity and pharmacokinetics of subconjunctival amphotericin B. Cornea 10(5): 411–417, 1991.

Generic name: Griseofulvin.

Proprietary name: Gris-PEG, Grisfulvin V.

Primary use

This oral antifungal agent is effective against tinea infections of the nails, skin and hair.

Ocular side effects

Systemic administration

Certain

1. Decreased vision
2. Visual hallucinations
3. Eyelids or conjunctiva
   a. Allergic reactions
   b. Hyperemia
   c. Edema
   d. Photosensitivity
   e. Angioedema
   f. Urticaria

Probable

1. Papilledema secondary to intracranial hypertension

Possible

1. Subconjunctival or retinal hemorrhages secondary to drug-induced anemia
2. Eyelids or conjunctiva
   a. Lupoid syndrome
   b. Exfoliative dermatitis
   c. Erythema multiforme

Conditional/Unclassified

1. Macular edema (transient)
2. Systemic lupus erythematosis
3. Superficial corneal opacities
4. Color vision defect

Clinical significance

Systemic griseofulvin rarely causes ocular side effects, but severe allergic reactions with secondary ocular involvement may occur. Decreased vision rarely occurs and seldom requires stopping the drug except in cases of intracranial hypertension. Delman and Leubuscher (1963) reported a single case of unilateral, greenish vision with transient macular edema possibly secondary to this agent. There is a case of bilateral superficial corneal deposits resembling Meesman's corneal dystrophy with ocular injection and superficial punctate keratitis which was reported to the National Registry that resolved within 1 week after discontinuation of the drug. This agent is a photosensitizing drug, and increased light exposure increases the prevalence of eyelid and conjunctival reactions.

REFERENCES AND FURTHER READING

Alarcón-Segovia D. Drug-induced antinuclear antibodies and lupus syndromes. Drugs 12: 69, 1976.

Delman M, Leubuscher K. Transient macular edema due to griseofulvin. Am J Ophthalmol 56: 658, 1963.

Epstein JH, Wintroub BU. Photosensitivity due to drugs. Drugs 30: 41, 1985.

Madhok R, et al. Fatal exacerbation of systemic lupus erythematosus after treatment with griseofulvin. BMJ 291: 249, 1985.

Spaeth GL, Nelson LB, Beaudoin AR. Ocular teratology. in Jakobiec FA, Ocular Anatomy, Embryology and Teratology. JB Lippincott, Philadelphia, 1982, p 955-975.

Generic name: Voriconazole.

Proprietary name: Vfend.

Primary use

This is a new triazole antifungal agent given both orally and intravenously. Its greatest use is in aspergillosis infections.

Ocular side effects

Systemic administration

Certain

1. Altered or enhanced visual perception
2. Blurred vision
3. Photophobia
4. Decreased color vision
5. Visual hallucinations
6. ERG abnormalities
7. Eyelids or conjunctiva
   a. Photosensitivity reactions

Possible

1. Eyelids or conjunctiva
   a. Erythema multiforme
   b. Stevens-Johnson syndrome
   c. Toxic epidermal necrolysis

Conditional/Unclassified

1. Visual field changes
   a. Cecocentral scotomas
   b. Arcuate scotoma
2. Optic neuropathy

Clinical significance

Voriconazole has unique ocular side effects. The most common visual complaints are altered or enhanced visual perception, 'enhanced perception of light', 'brighter lights and objects', blurred or 'hazy' vision and photophobia 'dazzle' or 'glare'. The onset of these symptoms occurs within 15–30 minutes after exposure (more rapid with IV than oral) with a mean duration of 30–60 minutes (IV more prolonged than oral). In rare instances these visual phenomena may last 1–2 weeks. With repeat exposure, the incidence and severity of the visual reaction decreases in most patients. The altered visual perceptions are reversible and seldom cause a patient to discontinue using the drug. This reaction occurs in up to 38% of patients, most frequently in the very young and the elderly, and is more pronounced when given IV. Humphrey visual field testing showed overall a slight drop in mean sensitivity, resolving in a few days after the drug was discontinued. Patients are most often unaware of decreased color vision and/or any changes in their visual field. Hallucinations occurred in 4.7% of patients exposed to voriconazole.

The certainty of these visual effects due to voriconazole is a combination of positive rechallenges, high incidences, typical pattern of onset and course, and data to show peaks associated with peak serum levels. The mechanism of voriconazole on the visual system probably is a retinal effect. Possibly, voriconazole may keep the retinal receptors in an artificially 'light adapted' state, acting on the mechanism of the phototransductor cascade and/or horizontal cell coupling. The importance of these studies to the ophthalmologist is that all findings to date are reversible and nearly always of short duration. There have been scattered spontaneous reports of optic neuropathy and retinal vascular disturbances but most patients who receive this drug have systemic fungal diseases and are on multiple medications. To date there is no data to prove that these findings are drug related. This is a new drug and long-term follow-up is necessary.

REFERENCES

Denning DW, Griffiths CEM. Muco-cutaneous retinoid – effects and facial erythema related to the novel triazole agent voriconazole. Clin Exp Dermatol 26: 648–653, 2001.

FDA Antiviral Drugs Advisory Committee, Briefing document for voriconazole (oral and intravenous formulations), 4 October 2001.

Hariprasad SM, Mieler WF, Holz ER, et al. Determination of vitreous, aqueous, and plasma concentration of orally administered voriconazole in humans. Arch Ophthalmol 122: 42–47, 2004.

Herbrecht R, Denning DW, Patterson TF, et al. Open randomized comparision of voriconazole and amphotericin-B followed by other licensed antifungal therapy for primary therapy of invasive aspergillosis. Presented at the 4th Interscience Conference on Antimicrobial Agents and Chemotherapy, Chicago, IL, December 2001.

Martindale: The Complete Drug Reference, 34th edn, Pharmaceutical Press, London, 2005.

Physicians' Desk Reference, 60th edn, Thomson PDR, Montvale, NJ, pp 2543–2552, 2006.

Rubenstein M, Levy ML, Metry D. Voriconazole-induced retinoid-like photosensitivity in children. Pediatr Dermatol 21: 675–678, 2004.

CLASS: ANTILEPROSY AGENTS

Generic name: Clofazimine.

Proprietary name: Lamprene.

Primary use

This phenazine derivative is used in the treatment of leprosy and also as an anti-inflammatory in psoriasis, discoid lupus and pyoderma gangrenosum.

Ocular side effects

Systemic administration

Certain

1. Ocular irritation
2. Decreased vision
3. Eyelids or conjunctiva
   a. Pigmentation (red-brown)
   b. Discoloration of lashes
   c. Perilimbal crystalline deposits
4. Tears
   a. Discoloration
   b. Crystalline drug in tears
   c. Aggravation of keratoconjunctivitis sicca
5. Cornea – polychromatic crystalline deposits
6. Photosensitivity
7. Retina
   a. Variable macular pigmentary changes
   b. Bull's-eye maculopathy
   c. Abnormal ERG
8. Iris – crystalline deposits

Possible

1. Lens – bluish discoloration

Clinical significance

This phenazine derivative can cause dose-related ocular changes mimicking those of choloroquine. Reversible reddish pigmentation of the skin, conjunctiva and cornea can be seen. Polychromatic crystals have been found in the tear film, giving it a reddish appearance. Findings include fine, reddish-brown subepithelial corneal lines and perilimbal crystalline deposits seen on biomicroscopy. These crystals have been seen on the iris and possibly the lens. This rarely interferes with vision, and the crystalline deposits can disappear within a few months to many years after clofazimine has been discontinued. It is unclear if this drug can cause keratoconjunctivitis sicca. It is more likely that the crystals act as an aggravation in patients with clinical or subclinical ocular sicca. These crystals may give a foreign body sensation and symptomatology consistent with a sicca-like syndrome. In one series, up to 50% of patients had some form of conjunctival pigmentation, 12% had variable changes in their vision, 25% had ocular irritation and 32% had crystals in their tears (Kaur et al 1990). Craythorn et al (1986), Cunningham et al (1990) and Forester et al (1992) reported that this drug can produce bull's-eye maculopathy. Visual loss can be permanent, even if the drug is discontinued.

REFERENCES AND FURTHER READING

Craythorn JM, Swartz M, Creel DJ. Clofazimine-induced bull's-eye retinopathy. Retina 6: 50, 1986.

Cunningham CA, Friedberg DN, Carr RE. Clofazamine-induced generalized retinal degeneration. Retina 10(2): 131–134, 1990.

Font RL, Sobol W, Matoba A. Polychromatic corneal and conjunctival crystals secondary to clofazimine therapy in a leper. Ophthalmology 96(3): 311–315, 1989.

Forester DJ, Causey DM, Rao NA. Bull's eye retinopathy and clofazamine (letter). Ann Int Med 116(10): 876–877, 1992.

Granstein RD, Sober AJ. Drug and heavy metal-induced hyperpigmentation. J Am Acad Dermatol 5: 1, 1981.

Kaur I, Ram J, Kumar B, Sharma VK. Effect of clofazimine on eye in multi-bacillary leprosy. Indian J Lepr 62(1): 87–90, 1990.

Mieler WF, Williams GA, Williams DF, Sneed SR. Systemic therapeutic agents retinal toxicity. American Academy of Ophthalmology Instruction Course, New Orleans, LA, 26 October 2004.

Moore VJ. A review of side effects experienced by patients taking clofazimine. Lepr Rev 54: 327–335, 1983.

Ohman L, Wahlberg I. Ocular side effects of clofazimine. Lancet 2: 933, 1975.

Walinder PE, Gip L, Stempa M. Corneal changes in patients treated with clofazimine. Br J Ophthalmol 60: 526, 1976.

Generic name: Dapsone.

Proprietary names: Generic only.

Primary use

This sulfone is used in the treatment of leprosy and ocular phemigoid.

Ocular side effects

Systemic administration
Certain
1. Decreased vision
2. Eyelids or conjunctiva
   a. Edema
   b. Hyperpigmentation
   c. Urticaria
   d. Purpura
   e. Hypersensitivity reaction
3. Retina
   a. Necrosis
   b. Macular exudates
   c. Intra-retinal hemorrhages
   d. Peripheral powdery deposits
4. Optic nerve
   a. Optic neuritis
   b. Optic atrophy – toxic states
5. Photosensitivity
6. Visual hallucinations

Possible
1. Subconjunctival or retinal hemorrhages secondary to drug-induced anemia
2. Eyelids or conjunctiva
   a. Erythema multiforme
   b. Exfoliative dermatitis
   c. Lyell's syndrome

Clinical significance

Dapsone has few ocular side effects except in massive doses or in the presence of a glucose-6-phosphate dehydrogenase deficiency. Daneshmend and Homeida (1981), Kenner et al (1980) and Alexander et al (1989) described retinal and optic nerve findings in overdosed patients. These include massive retinal necrosis, yellow-white lesions in the macula, intra-retinal hemorrhages and varying degrees of optic nerve damage. Alexander et al (1989) described two cases, one with long-term therapy of dapsone and another case of overdose in an attempted suicide. There was massive deposition of grayish-white material in the macula with a relatively clear fovea. Scattered powdery deposits were seen in the peripheral retina. They felt that the drug or its metabolites were in the inner layers of the retina. This cleared over time. Permanent blindness has occurred in some cases. These findings, at lower doses, may be seen in patients with glucose 6-phosphate

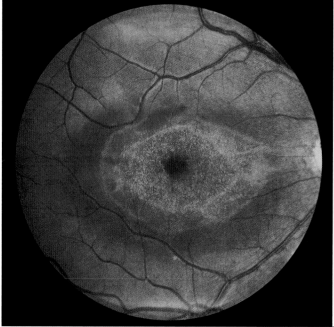 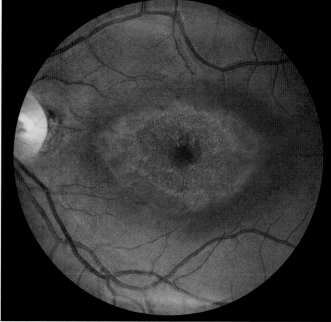

Fig. 7.1g Chloroquine bull's eye maculopathy. Photo courtesy of Spalton DJ, Hitchings RA, Hunter PA, Atlas of Clinical Ophthalmology, 3rd edn, Tan JCH (ed.), Elsevier Mosby, London.

dehydrogenase deficiency (Chakrabarti et al 1999). Darkening of skin color may be due to iatrogenic cyanosis, as a slate gray discoloration characteristic of drug-induced methemoglobinemia. Some patients under treatment with dapsone for leprosy have been known to develop lagophthalmos and posterior synechiae, but these effects are probably due to the disease rather than to the drug (Brandt et al 1984).

REFERENCES AND FURTHER READING

Alexander TA, et al. Presumed DDS ocular toxicity. Indian J Ophthalmol 37: 150–151, 1989.
Brandt F, Adiga RB, Pradhan H. Lagophthalmos and posterior synechias during treatment of leprosy with diaminodiphenylsulfone. Klin Monatsbl Augenheilkd 184: 28, 1984.
Chakrabarti M, Suresh PN, Namperumalsamy P. Bilateral macular infarction due to diaminodiphenyl sulfone (4,4' DDS) toxicity. Retina 19(1): 83–84, 1999.
Daneshmend TK. The neurotoxicity of dapsone. Adverse Drug React. Acute Poisoning Rev 3: 43–58, 1984.
Daneshmend TK, Homeida M. Dapsone-induced optic atrophy and motor neuropathy. BMJ 283: 311, 1981.
Homeida M, Babikr A, Daneshmend TK. Dapsone-induced optic atrophy and motor neuropathy. BMJ 281: 1180, 1980.
Kenner DJ, et al. Permanent retinal damage following massive dapsone overdose. Br J Ophthalmol 64: 741, 1980.
Leonard JN, et al. Dapsone and the retina. Lancet 1: 453, 1982.
Seo MS, et al. Dapson maculopathy. Korean J Ophthalmol 11: 70–73, 1997.

CLASS: ANTIMALARIAL AGENTS

Generic names: 1. Chloroquine; 2. hydroxychloroquine.

Proprietary names: 1. Aralen; 2. Plaquenil.

Primary use
These aminoquinolines are used in the treatment of malaria, extraintestinal amebiasis, rheumatoid arthritis and lupus erythematosus.

Ocular side effects

Systemic administration
Certain
1. Decreased vision
2. Cornea
   a. Punctate – yellowish to white opacities
   b. Lineal – whorl-like pattern, primarily in palpebral aperture
   c. Enhanced Hudson-Stähli line
   d. Transient edema
   e. Decreased sensitivity
3. Retina and/or macula
   a. Perifoveal granularity of retinal pigment epithelium (early)
   b. Bull's-eye appearance of the macula, with thinning and clumping of pigment epithelium (Fig. 7.1g)
   c. Attenuation of vascular tree
   d. Peripheral fine granular pigmentary changes
   e. Prominent choroidal pattern
   f. Angiography changes
4. Parafoveal retinal pigment epithithelium window defects (early)
5. Window defects in annular pattern
6. Choroidal filling defects (late)
7. Decreased or absent foveal reflex (rare)
8. Abnormal sensory testing
   a. Critical flicker fusion
   b. Macular recovery times
   c. Decreased dark adaptation
   d. EOG and ERG changes
9. Tear film
   a. Drugs found in tear film
   b. Aggravates sicca
   c. Decreased contact lens tolerance
10. Decreased accommodation
11. Visual fields
    a. Scotoma – annular, central, paracentral
    b. Constriction
    c. Hemianopsia
12. Eyelids and conjunctiva
    a. Pigmentary changes – hyper or hypo effects
    b. Yellow, bluish or blackish deposits
    c. Photosensitivity reactions
    d. Blepharospasm or clonus
13. Optic atrophy (late)
14. Color vision defect
    a. Blue-yellow defects (early)
    b. Red-green defects (late)
    c. Objects have yellow, green or blue tinge
    d. Colored haloes around lights

Probable
1. Oculogyric crisis
2. Myasthenia gravis (aggravates)
   a. Diplopia
   b. Ptosis
   c. Paresis of extraocular muscle

Clinical significance
Although hydroxychloroquine is widely used in Britain, North America and Australia, chloroquine may be more common in Europe, South America and Asia. Hydroxychloroquine use has markedly increased because it has become a first-line drug for some forms of arthritis and lupus erythematosus. Probably all side effects seen with chloroquine can also be seen with hydroxychloroquine, but serious ones are primarily seen with chloroquine in long-term usage or large dose situations. Toxicity to the retina due to these drugs is dose related.

Corneal deposits due to chloroquine have no direct relationship to posterior segment disease and may be seen as early as 3 weeks after starting the medication. Corneal changes may first appear as a Hudson-Stähli line or an increase in a pre-existing Hudson-Stähli line. Probably more common is a whorl-like pattern known as 'cornea verticillata'. It is known that a number of drugs and diseases can cause this pattern, in which morphological, histological and electron microscopic findings are identical. 'Amphophilic' drugs, such as chloroquine, amiodarone and chlorpromazine, form complexes with cellular phospholipids, which cannot be metabolized by lysosomal phospholipases therefore these intracellular deposits occur and are visible in the superficial portion of the cornea.

Corneal deposits due to hydroxychloroquine are of more clinical importance as an indication to hunt more aggressively for retinal toxicity. These are best seen with a dilated pupil and retroillumination. These deposits are finer and less extensive than with chloroquine. Easterbrook (1990, 1999) has found these corneal deposits to be a possible indicator of hydroxychloroquine macular toxicity. Corneal deposits occasionally cause haloes around lights. All corneal deposits are reversible. Hydroxychloroquine crystals have been found in the tear film, which may aggravate some sicca patients and contact lens wearers.

Toxic maculopathy is usually reversible only in its earliest phases. If these drugs have caused skin, eyelid, corneal (hydroxychloroquine) or hair changes, this may be an indicator of possible drug-induced retinopathy. Since the aminoquinolines are concentrated in pigmented tissue, macular changes have been thought to progress long after the drug is stopped. (This is now being questioned by some investigators as not being true for hydroxychloroquine.) The bull's-eye macula is not diagnostic for aminoquinoline-induced disease since a number of other entities can cause this same clinical picture. While retinal toxicity occurs in patients taking hydroxychloroquine, the incidence is much lower than with chloroquine.

Recommendations for hydroxychloroquine

The goal for the clinician is to find early, relative scotomas. Disease in patients with early paracentral relative scotomas seldom advances when the drug is discontinued. Later findings include retinal changes, color vision loss, absolute scotoma or decreased vision. Even if the drug is stopped, once these changes occur they are often irreversible and some patients may continue to lose some vision and/or peripheral fields.

Patients at greatest risk are those who are on hydroxychloroquine for longer than 5 years and those with renal or liver disease (this drug is metabolized via kidney and liver). Elderly, thin patients may also be overdosed, as may obese patients. Editorial articles by Marmor (Marmor et al 2002; Marmor 2005) and another by Lee (2005) explain the dilemma of the diagnosis of macular toxicity and to date there is no clear-cut answer on how best to detect toxicity. The multifocal ERG may be an effective clinical screening test, but this remains to be resolved. Neubauer et al (2003, 2004) have found a computerized color vision test that is effective in screening. Disturbances on the tritan axis appear to occur first. How best to follow patients on hydroxychloroquine was summarized in an article in the July 2002 issue of *Ophthalmology* (Marmor et al 2002).

1. Baseline examination: We recommend a baseline eye exam within 4–8 weeks after starting hydroxychloroquine and yearly thereafter including a dilated ophthalmic examination, including the informed consent, warning of possible permanent visual problems in rare instances. This baseline exam should include visual acuity, Amsler grids (with instructions for monthly home use) and optional color vision testing (preferably including the blue-yellow axis, such as the pseudo-isochromatic plates for color by the American Optical Corporation). If macular abnormalities are evident, it would be ideal to obtain fundus photographs. If any progressive ocular abnormality is suspected, consider a baseline Humphrey 10-2 or other automated perimetry. Multifocal ERG is optional.
2. Follow-up examinations: For patients who are not obese, frail, elderly, extremely thin, are without significant renal of hepatic disease or macular disease of any type, and who are younger than 40, exams should be completed yearly thereafter. Patients should be seen sooner if they experience any persistent visual symptoms or if their dosage exceeds 6.5 mg/kg.
3. Eye examinations more than once a year should be considered if patients have been on hydroxychloroquine therapy for longer than 5 years, if they are obese, or lean and small (especially in the case of elderly patients), or if they have progressive macular disease of any type, significant renal or liver disease, or their dosage exceeds 6.5 mg/kg/day.
4. Follow-up examination procedures:
   a. Repeat baseline examination.
   b. Fundus photography if any macular abnormality is noted.
   c. Consider fluorescein angiography only in the presence of suspicious pigmentary changes.
   d. Automated central visual fields (optional).
   e. Multifocal ERG (selected cases).
5. Recommendations by Don C Bienfang, MD, are available on www.eyedrugregistry.com. Baseline testing consists of a complete eye exam, including HVF-10, amsler and color vision screeing. Record height and weight at baseline and on each returning visit. During baseline examination, ask the patient if he or she is having problems with color vision, vision in dim illumination (movie theaters) or if parts of the TV screen are missing.

Toxicity can occur on low doses and once the toxicity appears, even if the drug is stopped, the toxicity can get worse. If caught early, patients tend to do better in recovery and the clinician feels often the first clue is found in the more subjective parts of the examination, i.e. asking about even minimal changes in color vision, night vision and missing parts of vision.

Recommendations for chloroquine

For patients taking chloroquine, perform the tests listed above. See patients at least annually if dosage is less than 3.0 mg/kg of ideal body weight. See every 6 months if dosage is greater than 3.0 mg/kg body weight, or if patients are short, obese or have renal and/or liver impairment.

Caution

To date, there are no data to show hydroxychloroquine toxicity worsening pre-existing macular degeneration. Common sense in a litigious society that has to find blame somewhere may make informed consent and explanation of risk-benefit ratios necessary on an individualized basis. A recent preliminary paper by Shroyer et al (2001) suggests that individuals with an ABCR mutation (Stargardt's disease) may be predisposed to develop retinal toxicity when exposed to chloroquine or hydroxychloroquine.

REFERENCES AND FURTHER READING

Almony A, Garg S, Peters RK, et al. Threshold amsler grid as screening tool for asymptomatic patients on hydroxychloroquine therapy. Br J Ophthalmol 89: 569–574, 2004.

Beebe WE, Abbott RL, Fung WE. Hydroxychloroquine crystals in the tear film of a patient with rheumatoid arthritis. Am J Ophthalmol 101: 377, 1986.

Easterbrook M. Is corneal decompensation of antimalarial any indication of retinal toxicity? Can J Ophthalmol 25(5): 249–251, 1990.

Easterbrook M. An ophthalmological view on the efficacy and safety of chloroquine hydroxychloroquine. (Editorial). J Rheumatol 26(9): 1866–1868, 1999.

Ehrenfeld M, Nesher R, Merin S. Delayed-onset chloroquine retinopathy. Br J Ophthalmol 70: 281, 1986.

Elder M, Rahman AM, McLay J. Early paracentral visual field loss in patients taking hydroxychloroquine. Arch Ophthalmol 124:1729–1733, 2006.

Fraunfelder FW, Fraunfelder FT. Scientific challenges in postmarketing surveillance of ocular adverse drug reactions. Am J Ophthalmol 143: 145–149, 2007.

Johnson MW, Vine AK. Hydroxychloroquine therapy in massive total doses without retinal toxicity. Am J Ophthalmol 104: 139, 1987.

Kellner U, Kraus H, Foerster MH. Multifocal ERG in chloroquine retinopathy: regional variance of retinal dysfunction. Graefe's Arch Clin Exp Ophthalmol 238: 94–97, 2000.

Lai TYY, Chan W-M, Li H, et al: Multifocal electroretinographic changes in patients receiving hydroxychloroquine therapy. Am J Ophthalmol 140: 794–807, 2005.

Lee AG. Hydroxychloroquine screening: who needs it, when, how and why? Br J Ophthalmol 89: 521–522, 2005.

Levy GD. Hydroxychloroquine ocular toxicity. J Rheumatol 25: 1030–1031, 1998.

Levy GD, Munz SJ, Paschal J, et al. Incidence of hydroxychloroquine retinopathy in 1207 patients in a large multicenter outpatient practice. Arthritis Rheum 40: 1482–1486, 1997.

Marks JS. Chloroquine retinopathy: Is there a safe daily dose? Ann Rheum Dis 41: 52, 1982.

Marmor MF, Carr RE, Easterbrook M, et al. Recommendations on screening for chloroquine and hydroxychloroquine retinopathy. Ophthalmology 109: 1377–1382, 2002.

Marmor MF. The dilemma of hydroxychloroquine screening: new information from the multifocal ERG. Am J Ophthalmol 140: 894–895, 2005.

Maturi RK, Minzhong Y, Weleber RG. Multifocal electroretinographic evaluation of long-term hydroxychloroquine users. Arch Opthalmol 122: 973–981, 2004.

Mavrikakis I, Sfikakis PP, Mavrikakis E, et al. The incidence of irreversible retinal toxicity in patients treated with hydroxychloroquine. Ophthalmology 110: 1321–1326, 2003.

Moon SJ, Park P, Mieler WF. Screening for chloroquine and hydroxychloroquine retinopathy. Contemp Ophthalmol 2: 1–5, 2003.

Morand EF, McCloud PI, Littlejohn GO. Continuation of long term treatment with hydroxychloquine in systemic lupus erythematosus and rheumatoid arthritis. Ann Rheum Dis 51: 1318–1321, 1992.

Morsman CDG, Liversey SJ, Richards IM, et al. Screening for hydroxychloroquine retinal toxicity: is it necessary? Eye 4: 572–576, 1990.

Motta M, et al. Follow-up of infants exposed to hydoxychloroquine given to mothers during pregnancy and lactation. J Pernatol 25: 86–89, 2005.

Neubauer AS, Samari-Kermani K, Schaller U, et al. Detecting chloroquine retinopathy: electro-oculogram versus colour vision. Br J Ophthalmol 87: 902–908, 2003.

Neubauer AS, Stiefelmeyer S, Berninger T, et al. The multifocal pattern electroretinogram in chloroquine retinopathy. Ophthalmic Res 36: 106–113, 2004.

Penrose PJ, Tzekov RT, Sutter EE, et al. Multifocal electroretinography evaluation for early detection of retinal dysfunction in patients taking hydroxychloroquine. Retina 23: 503–512, 2003.

Razeghinejad MR, Torkaman F, Amini H. Blue-yellow perimetry can be an early detector of hydroxychloroquine and chloroquine retinopathy. Med Hypotheses 65: 629–630, 2005.

Robertson JE, Fraunfelder FT. Hydroxychloroquine retinopathy. JAMA 255: 403, 1986.

Selvaag E. Vitiligolike depigmentation: possible side effect during chloroquine antimalarial therapy. J Toxicol Cut Ocular Toxicol 16: 5–8, 1997.

Shroyer NF, Lewis RA, Lupski JR. Analysis of the ABCR (ABCA4) gene in 4-aminoquinoline retinopathy: is retinal toxicity by chloroquine and hydroxychloroquine related to Stargardt disease? Am J Ophthalmol 131: 761–766, 2001.

Spalton DJ. Retinopathy and antimalarial drugs – the British. Lupus S1: 570–572, 1996.

Tobin DR, Krohel GB, Rynes RI. Hydroxychloroquine. Seven-year experience. Arch Ophthalmol 100: 81, 1982.

Wei LC, Chen SN, Ho CL, et al. Progression of hydroxychloroquine retinopathy after discontinuation of therapy: case report. Chung Gung Med J 24: 329–334, 2001.

Weiner A, Sandberg MA, Gaudio AR, et al. Hydroxychloroquine retinopathy. Am J Ophthalmol 112: 528–534, 1991.

Wittbrodt ET. Drugs and myasthenia gravis. Arch Int Med 157: 399–408, 1997.

Generic name: Mefloquine hydrochloride.

Proprietary name: Lariam.

Primary use

This agent is primarily used in the treatment of malaria.

Ocular side effects

Systemic administration
Certain
1. Blurred vision
2. Diplopia

3. Eyelids or conjunctiva
   a. Urticaria
   b. Rash
   c. Pruritus
4. Visual hallucinations

Possible
1. Eyelids of conjunctiva
   a. Stevens-Johnson syndrome
   b. Erythema multiforme
   c. Exfoliative dermatitis
   d. Toxic epidermal necrolysis

Clinical significance

This agent was developed for resistant malaria but has become a favorite for malaria prevention. It does not cause deposits in the cornea, retina, etc., which are seen with other commonly used antimalarial agents. Palmer et al (1993) point out that at least 20% of patients taking this drug complain of diplopia. This figure is much higher than reported by others. Around 1% of patients taking prophylactic dosages have had visual hallucinations lasting a few seconds or up to 1 hour. This occurs after each dosage. There does not appear to be a relationship between total dosage of mefloquine and the onset of neuropsychiatric side effects.

REFERENCES AND FURTHER READING

Borruat F-X, Nater B, Robyn L, Genton B. Prolonged visual illusions induced by mefloquine (lariam): a case report. J Travel Med 8: 148–149, 2001.

Croft AMJ, World MJ. Neuropsychiatric reactions with mefloquine chemoprophylaxis. Lancet 347: 326, 1996.

Lobel HO, Bernard KW, Williams SL, et al. Effectiveness and tolerance of long-term malaria prophylaxis with mefloquine. JAMA 3: 361–364, 1991.

Palmer KJ, Holliday SM, Brogden RN. Mefloquine: a review of its antimalarial activity pharmacokinetic properties and therapeutic efficacy. Drugs 45(3): 430–475, 1993.

Shlim DR. Severe facial rash associated with mefloquine. Correspondence. JAMA 13: 2560, 1991.

Suriyamongkol V, Timsaad S, Shanks GD. Mefloquine chemoprophylaxis of soldiers on the Thai-Cambodian border. Southeast Asian J Trop Med Pub Health 22: 515–518, 1991.

Van den Enden E, Van Gompel A, Colebunders R, Van den Ende J. Mefloquine-induced Stevens-Johnson syndrome (letter). Lancet 337(8742): 683, 1991.

Weinke T, Trautmann M, Held T, et al. Neuropsychiatric effects after the use of mefloquine. Am J Trop Med Hyg 45: 86–91, 1991.

Generic name: Quinine.

Proprietary names: Generic only.

Primary use

This alkaloid is effective in the management of nocturnal leg cramps, myotonia congenita, and in resistant *P. falciparum*. It is also used in attempted abortions. Ophthalmologically it is useful in the treatment of eyelid myokymia.

Ocular side effects

Systemic administration
Certain
1. Decreased vision – all gradations of visual loss, including toxic amblyopia

2. Pupils
   a. Mydriasis
   b. Decreased or absent reaction to light
3. Retinal or macular
   a. Edema
   b. Degeneration
   c. Pigmentary changes (Fig. 7.1h)
   d. Exudates
   e. Vasodilatation followed by vasoconstriction
   f. Absence of foveal reflex
   g. Abnormal ERG, EOG, VEP or critical flicker fusion
4. Visual sensations
   a. Distortion due to flashing lights
   b. Distortion of images secondary to sensations of wave
5. Optic nerve
   a. Papilledema
   b. Atrophy
6. Problems with color vision
   a. Color vision defect, red-green or blue-yellow defect
   b. Objects have red or green tinge
7. Visual fields
   a. Scotomas
   b. Constriction
8. Eyelids or conjunctiva
   a. Allergic reactions
   b. Edema
   c. Photosensitivity
   d. Angioedema
   e. Purpura
   f. Urticaria
9. Night blindness
10. Visual hallucinations

Probable

1. Myasthenia gravis (aggravates)
   a. Diplopia
   b. Ptosis
   c. Paresis of extraocular muscle

Possible

1. Subconjunctival or retinal hemorrhages secondary to drug-induced anemia
2. Eyelids or conjunctiva
   a. Erythema multiforme
   b. Stevens-Johnson syndrome

Conditional/Unclassified

1. Myopia – transitory
2. ERG changes
3. Granulamatous uveitis
4. Angle-closure glaucoma
5. Iris atrophy
6. Vertical nystagmus

Ocular teratogenic effects
Conditional/Unclassified

1. Optic nerve hypoplasia

Clinical significance

Quinine has been used for centuries and serious ocular side effects occur mainly in deliberate self-harm situations. It is also used as a diluent for many 'street drugs' and as a method of terminating a pregnancy. An excellent overview of almost 300 articles on this subject can be found in Grant's *Toxicology of the Eye*. Quinine seldom causes ocular side effects except in overdose situations. Waddell (1996) reports two cases of blindness occurring on routine therapy. In rare instances, hypersensitivity reactions or long-term low dosages can cause significant ocular effects. In cases of massive exposure, visual loss may be sudden or progressive over a number of hours or days. In the worst cases, retinal arteriolar constriction, venous congestion, and retinal and papillary edema are pronounced. Complete, irreversible loss of vision may occur, but most patients have some return of vision. In severe cases there is often permanent loss of the peripheral visual field. Boland et al (1974) give an excellent overview of 165 patients hospitalized with quinine poisoning, of which 42% had significant visual

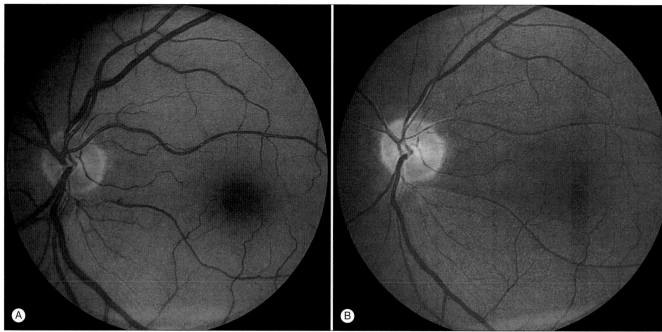

Fig. 7.1h Quinine retinopathy with palish opalescent retina (A) and quinine retinopathy with fibrotic sheathing, pale disc and aterial attenuation (B). Photo courtesy of Spalton DJ, Hitchings RA, Hunter PA. Atlas of Clinical Ophthalmology, 3rd edn, Mosby Elsevier, London, 2005.

side effects. Mild cases may show only minimal macular changes by Amsler grid, blurred vision or some constriction of the visual field. Zahn et al (1981) showed that early ERG may be normal, however in late ERG, scotopic b-wave and a-waves are altered. Hustead (1991) has shown that in individuals hypersensitive to quinine, a granulomatous uveitis may occur. Segal et al (1983) reported shallowing of the anterior chamber precipitating narrow-angle glaucoma. Schuman (1997) reported a case of acute bilateral transitory myopia. Worden et al (1987) and others have noted that chronic overuse of tonic water (which contains quinine) can cause toxic quinine effects in the eye.

According to the evidence presently available, the etiology of the toxic effect of quinine seems to involve not only an early effect on the outer layers of the retina and pigment epithelium, but also probably a direct effect on retinal ganglion cells and optic nerve fibers.

Quinine can cause optic nerve hypoplasia and decreased vision, including blindness, in the offspring secondary to prenatal maternal ingestion.

REFERENCES AND FURTHER READING

Birch J, et al. Acquired color vision defects. In Pokorny J Congenital and Acquired Color Vision Defects. Grune & Stratton, New York, 1979, p 243–350.

Boland MD, Roper SMB, Henry JA. Complications of quinine poisoning. J Ir Med Assoc 67: 46–47, 1974.

Brinton GS, Norton EW, Zahn JR, et al. Ocular quinine toxicity. Am J Ophthalmol 90: 403, 1980.

Dyson EH, Proudfoot AT, Prescott LF, et al. Death and blindness due to overdose of quinine. BMJ 291: 31, 1985.

Dyson EH, Proudfoot AT, Bateman DN. Quinine amblyopia: is current management appropriate? Clin Toxicol 23: 571, 1985–1986.

Fisher CM. Visual disturbances associated with quinidine and quinine. Neurology 31: 1569, 1981.

Fong LP, Kaufman DV, Galbraith JEK. Ocular toxicity of quinine. Med J Austr 141: 528, 1984.

Friedman L, Rothkoff L, Zaks U. Clinical observations on quinine toxicity. Ann Ophthalmol 12: 641, 1980.

Gangitano JL, Keltner JL. Abnormalities of the pupil and visual-evoked potential in quinine amblyopia. Am J Ophthalmol 89: 425, 1980.

Grant WM, Schuman JS. Effects on the eyes and visual system from chemicals, drugs, metals and minerals, plants, toxins and venoms; Systemic side effects from eye medications. Toxicology of the Eye. 4th edn. Charles C. Thomas, Springfield, IL, 1993.

Horgan SE, Williams RW. Chronic retinal toxicity due to quinine in Indian tonic water (letter). Eye 9(Pt.5): 637–638, 1995.

Hustead JD. Granulomatous uveitis and quinidine hypersensitivity. Am J Ophthalmol 112(4): 461–462, 1991.

Kaeser HE. Drug-induced myasthenic syndromes. Acta Neurol Scand 70(Suppl 100): 39, 1984.

Rheeder P, Sieling WL. Acute, persistent quinine-induced blindness. A case report. So Afr Med J 79: 563–564, 4 May 1991.

Schuman JS. Acute bilateral transitory myopia associated with open angle glaucoma. Chandler and Grant's Glaucoma. 4th edn. Epstein DL, Allingham RR, Schuman JS (eds), Williams and Wilkens, Baltimore, p 341, 1997.

Segal A, Aisemberg A, Ducasse A. Quinine transitory myopia, and angle-closure glaucoma. Bull Soc Ophtalmol Fr 83: 247–249, 1983.

Waddell K. Blindness from quinine as an antimalarial (letter). Trans Roy Soc Trop Med Hygiene 89(4): 331–332, 1996.

Worden AN, Frape DL, Shephard NW. Consumption of quinine hydrochloride in tonic water. Lancet 1: 271–272, 1987.

Zahn JR, Brinton GF, Norton E. Ocular quinine toxicity followed by electro-retinogram, electro-oculogram, and pattern visually evoked potential. Am J Optom Physiol Optics 58: 492, 1981.

CLASS: ANTIPROTOZOAL AGENTS

Generic name: Metronidazole.

Proprietary names: Flagyl, Flagyl ER, Flagyl IV, Metrocream, Metro IV, Metrogel, Metrogel-vaginal 3M, Metrolotion, Noritate, Vandazole.

Primary use
This nitroimidazole derivative is an antibacterial and antiprotozoal agent effective in the treatment of trichomoniasis, amebiasis, giardiasis and anaerobic bacterial infections.

Ocular side effects

Systemic administration
Certain
1. Decreased vision
2. Photophobia
3. Visual field changes – scotoma
4. Eyelids or conjunctiva
   a. Erythema
   b. Conjunctivitis – non-specific
   c. Edema
   d. Photosensitivity
   e. Angioneurotic edema
   f. Urticaria

Probable
1. Retrobulbar or optic neuritis
2. Visual hallucinations
3. Diplopia
4. Myopia – reversible

Possible
1. Subconjunctival or retinal hemorrhages secondary to drug-induced anemia
2. Eyelids or conjunctiva
   a. Stevens-Johnson syndrome
   b. Toxic epidermal necrolysis

Conditional/Unclassified
1. Oculogyric crises
2. Abnormal red-green color vision
3. Abnormal visual evoked potential

Local ophthalmic use or exposure
Certain
1. Irritation
2. Erythema
3. Epiphora

Ocular teratogenic effects

Conditional/Unclassified
1. Telecanthus

Clinical significance
Ocular side effects from systemic use of metronidazole are unusual, and most are reversible on discontinuation of treatment. Putnam et al (1991) reported seven patients on metronidazole who developed optic or retrobulbar neuritis. This is associated with color vision defects, decreased vision and various scotomas. This may

be unilateral initially, but most with time are bilateral. Grinbaum et al (1992) reported a case with rechallenge data showing this agent can cause a reversible myopia. Oculogyric crisis has been reported in one patient who also experienced limb tremors.

While not approved by the FDA, topical periocular application is said to be of value in acne rosacea. Use on the eyelid may cause ocular irritation, but to date no permanent ocular side effects.

A midline facial defect, including telecanthus, has been reported by Cantu and Garcia-Cruz (1982) following maternal use of this drug during the first trimester. Recent articles suggest little to support the concern that this drug used orally has any teratogenic effects.

REFERENCES AND FURTHER READING

Cantu JM, Garcia-Cruz D. Midline facial defect as a teratogenic effect of metronidazole. Birth Defects 18: 85, 1982.
Chen K-T, Twu S-J, Chang H-J, Lin R-S. Outbreak of Stevens-Johnson syndrome/toxic epidermal necrolysis associated with mebendazole and metronidazole use among Filipino laborers in Taiwan. Am J Public Health 93: 489–492, 2003.
Czeizel AE, Rockenbauer M. A population based case-control teratologic study of oral metronidazole treatment during pregnancy. Br J Obstetrics Gyn 105: 322–327, 1998.
DeBleecker JL, Leroy BP, Meire VI. Reversible visual deficit and corpus callosum lesions due to metronidazole toxicity. Eur Neurol 53: 93–95, 2005.
Dunn PM, Stewart-Brown S, Peel R. Metronidazole and the fetal alcohol syndrome. Lancet 2: 144, 1979.
Grinbaum A, Ashkenazi I, Avni I, et al. Transient myopia following metronidazole treatment for trichomonas vaginallis. JAMA 267(4): 511–512, 1992.
Kirkham G, Gott J. Oculogyric crisis associated with metronidazole. BMJ 292: 174, 1986.
Metronidazole hydrochloride (Flagyl IV). Med Lett Drugs Ther 23: 13, 1981.
Putnam D, Fraunfelder FT, Dreis M. Metronidazole and optic neuritis. Am J Ophthalmol 112(6): 737, 1991.
Schentag JJ, et al. Mental confusion in a patient treated with metronidazole – A concentration-related effect? Pharmacotherapy 2: 384, 1982.
Snavely SR, Hodges GR. The neurotoxicity of antibacterial agents. Ann Intern Med 101: 92, 1984.

Generic name: Suramin sodium.

Proprietary names: None.

Primary use

This non-metallic polyanion is effective in the treatment of trypanosomiasis and is used as adjunctive therapy in onchocerciasis and acquired immune deficiency syndrome. Recently this drug has been used in anticancer therapy.

Ocular side effects

Systemic administration
Certain
1. Blurred vision
2. Intraepithelial inclusions
   a. Cornea
   b. Conjunctiva
   c. Anterior lens epithelium
3. Cornea
   a. Keratitis
   b. Superficial punctate keratitis
   c. Erosions
   d. Vortex keratopathy
4. Foreign body sensation
5. Hypermetropia
6. Non-specific ocular irritation
   a. Lacrimation
   b. Photophobia
   c. Conjunctivitis
7. Eyelids or conjunctiva
   a. Edema
   b. Urticaria

Possible
1. Subconjunctival or retinal hemorrhages secondary to drug-induced anemia

Clinical significance

When suramin sodium is used in the management of parasitic disease, it is difficult to differentiate an adverse drug effect from the adverse reaction of the death of the intraocular organism. However, Hemady et al (1996), in a study of 114 patients, reported that suramin sodium for metastatic cancer of the prostate had an incidence of 16.6% of ocular signs and symptoms. These include bilateral, whorl-like corneal deposits, often with foreign body sensation and lacrimation. This was also associated with blurred vision and a hyperopic shift in a range of +0.75 to +2.00 diopters. This refractive change was persistent throughout the course of treatment. No patients showed a decrease in baseline best corrected vision, and the drug was not considered dose limiting due to ocular toxicity. In AIDS patients on high-dose suramin sodium, Teich et al (1986) reported not only vortex keratopathy but fine, cream-colored, deep epithelial or subepithelial deposits. Holland et al (1988) described these as light golden-brown deposits starting on the lower portion of the cornea and progressing into a whorl keratopathy that involved the whole cornea. One patient had these deposits on the anterior lens epithelium. These deposits histologically are identified as membranous lamellar inclusion bodies, the same as with other drug-induced lipid storage diseases produced by lysosomal enzyme inhibition.

REFERENCES AND FURTHER READING

Adverse effects of antiparasitic drugs. Med Lett Drugs Ther 24: 12, 1982.
Hemady RK, Sinibaldi VJ, Eisenberger MA. Ocular symptoms and signs associated with suramin sodium treatment for metastatic cancer of the prostate. Am J Ophthalmol 121(3): 291–296, 1996.
Holland EJ, Stein CA, Palestine AG, et al. Suramin keratopathy. Am J Ophthalmol 106: 216–220, 1988.
Reynolds JEF (ed). Martindale: The Extra Pharmacopoeia, 28th edn. Pharmaceutical Press, London, pp 983–984, 1982.
Teich SA, et al. Toxic keratopathy associated with suramin therapy. N Engl J Med 314: 1455, 1986.
Thylefors B, Rolland A. The risk of optic atrophy following suramin treatment of ocular onchocerciasis. Bull WHO 57: 479, 1979.

Generic name: Tryparsamide.

Proprietary names: None.

Primary use

This organic arsenical is used in the treatment of trypanosomiasis (African sleeping sickness) as back-up to safer drugs.

Ocular side effects

Systemic administration
Certain
1. Constriction of visual fields
2. Decreased vision
3. Visual sensations
    a. Smokeless fog
    b. Shimmering effect
4. Optic neuritis
5. Optic atrophy
6. Toxic amblyopia

Clinical significance

The most serious and common adverse drug reactions due to tryparsamide involve the eye. Incidence of ocular side effects varies from 3 to 20% of cases, with constriction of visual fields followed by decreased vision as the characteristic sequence. Almost 10% of individuals taking tryparsamide experience visual changes consisting of 'shimmering' or 'dazzling', which may persist for days or even weeks. If the medication is not immediately discontinued following these visual changes, the pathologic condition of the optic nerve may become irreversible and progress to blindness. Due to the severity of side effects of this drug on the optic nerve, it has generally been replaced by melarsoprol.

REFERENCES AND FURTHER READING

Doull J, Klaassen CD, Amdur MO (eds). Casarett and Doull's Toxicology: The Basic Science of Poisons, 2nd edn, Macmillan, New York, pp 301–302, 1980.
LeJeune JR. Les oligo-elements et chelateurs. Bull Soc Belge Ophtalmol 160: 241, 1972.
Potts AM. Duality of the optic nerve in toxicology. In: Neurotoxicity of the Visual System. Merigan WH, Weiss B (eds), Raven Press, New York, pp 1–15, 1980.
Sloan LL, Woods AC. Effect of tryparsamide on the eye. Am J Syph 20: 583-613, 1936.
Walsh FB, Hoyt WF. Clinical Neuro-Ophthalmology, Vol. III. 3rd edn. Williams & Wilkins, Baltimore, 2594–2596, 2004.

CLASS: ANTITUBERCULAR AGENTS

Generic name: Cycloserine.

Proprietary name: Seromycin.

Primary use

This isoxazolidone is effective against certain Gram-negative and Gram-positive bacteria and *M. tuberculosis*.

Ocular side effects

Systemic administration
Certain
1. Decreased vision
2. Eyelids or conjunctiva
    a. Allergic reactions
    b. Conjunctivitis – non-specific
    c. Photosensitivity
3. Trichomegaly

Probable
1. Visual hallucinations
2. Flickering vision

Possible
1. Subconjunctival or retinal hemorrhages secondary to drug-induced anemia

Conditional/Unclassified
1. Optic nerve
    a. Neuritis
    b. Atrophy

Clinical significance

Even though ocular complications due to cycloserine are quite rare, this drug is primarily used in combination with other drugs therefore pinpointing cause and effect for an ocular side effect is very difficult. An increased number of eyelashes (hypertrichosis) has been reported (Weaver and Bartley 1990) and may prompt the clinical suspicion of an immune system abnormality. Optic nerve damage (including optic neuritis and atrophy) has been reported, but these data are not conclusive.

REFERENCES AND FURTHER READING

Drug Evaluations, 6th edn, American Medical Association, Chicago, pp 1539–1540, 1986.
Drugs that cause psychiatric symptoms. Med Lett Drugs Ther 28: 81, 1986.
Gilman AG, Goodman LS, Gilman A The Pharmacological Basis of Therapeutics. 6th edn. Macmillan, New York, 1980, p 1210–1211.
Walsh FB, Hoyt WF. Clinical Neuro-Ophthalmology, Vol. III. 3rd edn. Williams & Wilkins, Baltimore, 1969 p 2680.
Weaver DT, Bartley GB. Cyclosporine-induced trichomegaly. Am J Ophthalmol 109(2): 239, 1990.

Generic name: Ethambutol.

Proprietary name: Myambutol.

Primary use

Ethambutol is a tuberculostatic agent that is effective against *M. tuberculosis*.

Ocular side effects

Systemic administration
Certain
1. Problems with color vision – red-green or blue-yellow defect
2. Decreased vision
3. Contrast sensitivity – decreased
4. Visual evoked potential – decreased
5. ERG changes
6. Visual fields
    a. Scotomas – annular, central or centrocecal
    b. Constriction
    c. Hemianopsia
    d. Enlarged blind spot
7. Optic nerve
    a. Retrobulbar or optic neuritis
    b. Papilledema
    c. Peripapillary atrophy
    d. Atrophy (Fig. 7.1i)

Probable
1. Optic nerve
    a. Micro-hemorrhages
    b. Hyperemia

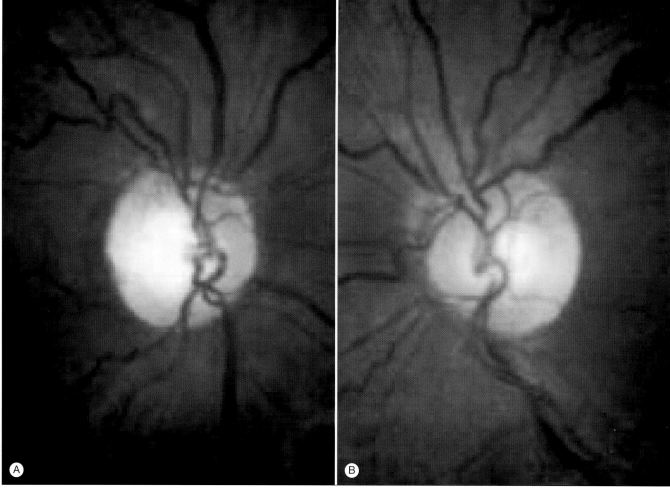

Fig. 7.1i Right (A) and left (B) optic nerve atrophy secondary to ethambutol. Photo courtesy of Melamud A, et al: Ocular ethambutol toxicity. Mayo Clin Proc 78: 1409-1411, 2003.

2. Photophobia
3. Retinal or macular
   a. Retinitis
   b. Vascular disorder
   c. Edema
   d. Pigmentary changes

Possible

1. Hemorrhages
2. Paresis of extraocular muscles
3. Eyelids or conjunctiva
   a. Lyell's syndrome
   b. Erythema multiforme

Unconditional/Unclassified

1. Mydriasis
2. Spasms
3. Visual hallucinations

Clinical significance

Ethambutol is still a first-line agent used in the multidrug treatment of tuberculosis. Its use is on the increase since there are more resistant forms of tuberculosis occurring. The most significant adverse effect of ethambutol is optic neuritis, which is usually bilateral and can be asymmetric. Ethambutol toxicity may affect only the small caliber papillo-macular bundle axons and optic atrophy will not develop until months after the fibers are lost. This means objective findings on the fundus exam are frequently absent. Optic neuropathy may occur, on average, at 2–5 months after starting therapy. The earliest ophthalmologic findings in toxic optic neuropathy from ethambutol may be loss of visual acuity, color vision loss or central scotomas. Ethambutol also has an affinity for the optic chiasm with bitemporal visual field defects manifesting toxicity. Some authors have proposed electrophysiologic tests to screen for toxicity due to ethambutol. A multifocal ERG may be of value to diagnose and monitor patients taking ethambutol, and full field ERGs and EOGs also have demonstrated abnormalities. Contrast sensitivity measurement may also be useful in detecting subclinical ethambutol toxic optic neuropathy. Optical coherence tomography shows promise as a screening tool to detect subclinical optic neuropathy.

Isoniazid is frequently prescribed concomitantly with ethambutol for tuberculosis due to multiple cases of drug resistance to single agent therapy. Isoniazid has also been associated with optic neuropathy, and differentiating toxicity due to ethambutol versus isoniazid can be challenging. In general, the toxicity from isoniazid is less frequent, less severe and is usually reversible. When in doubt, a dechallenge with isoniazid and/or ethambutol may need to be undertaken after consultation with the primary care physician.

Once a defect is found and the ethambutol is discontinued, occasionally the abnormality may continue to progress for 1–2 months. The vast majority will improve over weeks to many months to complete recovery. However, there are over 200 well-documented cases of permanent visual loss, including blindness. Some authors feel that patients with initial severe central visual loss before the drug is stopped have the poorest prognosis for full recovery. While direct toxic effects to the retina are supported by abnormal visual evoked cortical potentials and patterned ERGs (Kakisu et al 1988), the clinical retinal findings are rare but may include macular edema and pigmentary disturbances. Conventional ERG findings remain controversial as to clinical usefulness. Dotti et al (1998) described a case of ethambutol-induced optic neuropathy aggravating a genetic predisposition for optic nerve pathology.

Recommendations

1. Obtain informed consent prior to assuming care for patients taking ethambutol, explaining that optic neuropathy can occur at any dose despite regular ophthalmic exams and that the vision loss can be severe and irreversible.
2. Obtain a baseline exam to include a visual field test, color vision test, dilated fundus and optic nerve exam, and visual acuity.
3. If any visual symptoms occur, discontinue the medication and see an ophthalmologist.
4. Frequency of examination is monthly for doses greater than 15 mg/kg/day (PDR); however, monthly exams at lower doses may be necessary for patients at increased risk for toxicity:
   a. diabetes mellitus
   b. chronic renal failure
   c. alcoholism
   d. elderly
   e. children
   f. other ocular defects
   g. ethambutol-induced peripheral neuropathy.
5. Consider discontinuation of ethambutol after any signs of loss of visual acuity, color vision or for a visual field defect.
6. Consider optical coherence tomography or contrast sensitivy testing as these tests could pick up early ethambutol toxicity not detected with the baseline exam.
7. Some suggest that if no improvement occurs in visual signs after 4 months of being off the drug, hydroxycobalamin therapy should be considered (Guerra and Casu 1981), but this is not proven. If the vision does not improve 10–15 weeks after ethambutol discontinuation, parenteral administration of 40 mg of hydroxocobalamin daily over a 10- to 28-week period has been suggested as a possible treatment. Also consider glutamate antagonists in limiting the ocular side effects of ethambutol during drug therapy (Heng et al 1999). There are also data to suggest that cases of optic nerve toxicity should be treated with 100–250 mg of oral zinc sulfate three times daily. The bottom line is that the best way to treat this entity is unknown.

REFERENCES AND FURTHER READING

Behbehani RS, et al. Multifocal ERG in ethambutol associated visual loss. Br J Ophthalmol 89: 976–982, 2005.
Dette TM, Spitznas M, Gobbels M, et al. Visually evoked cortical potentials for early detection of optic neuritis in ethambutol therapy (German). Fortschritte der Ophthalmologie 88(5): 546–548, 1991.
Dotti MT, Plewnia K, Cardaioli E, et al. A case of ethambutol-induced optic neuropathy harbouring the primary mitochondrial LHON mutation at nt 11778. J Neurol 245(5): 302–303, 1998.
Guerra R, Casu L. Hydroxocobalamin for ethambutol-induced optic neuropathy. Lancet 2: 1176, 1981.
Heng JE, Vorwerk CK, Lessell E, et al. Ethambutol is toxic to retinal ganglion cells via excitotoxic pathway. Invest Ophthalmol Vis Sci 40(1): 190–196, 1999.
Hennekes R. Clinical ERG findings in ethambutol intoxication. Graefe's Arch Clin Exp Ophthalmol 218: 319–321, 1982.
Joubert PH, et al. Subclinical impairment of colour vision in patients receiving ethambutol. Br J Clin Pharmacol 21: 213, 1986.
Kaimbo WK, et al. Color vision in 42 Congolese patients with tuberculosis receiving ethambutol treatment. Bull Soc Belge D Ophthalmol 284: 57–61, 2002.
Kakisu Y, Adachi-Usami E, Mizota A. Pattern of electroretinogram and visual evoked cortical potential in ethambutol optic neuropathy. Doc Ophthalmol 67: 327–334, 1988.
Karmon G. Bilateral optic neuropathy due to combined ethambutol and isoniazid treatment. Ann Ophthalmol 11: 1013, 1979.
Karnik AM, Al-Shamali MA, Fenech FF. A case of ocular toxicity to ethambutol – An idiosyncratic reaction? Postgrad Med J 61: 719, 1985.
Kozak SF, Inderlied CB, Hsu HY, et al. The role of copper on ethambutol's antimicrobial action and implications for ethambutol-induced optic neuropathy. Diagn Microbiol Infect Dis 30(2): 83–87, 1998.
Kumar A, Sandramouli S, Verma L, et al. Ocular ethambutol toxicity: is it reversible? J Clin Neuro-Ophthalmol 13(1): 15–17, 1993.
Leibold JE. The ocular toxicity of ethambutol and its relation to dose. Ann NY Acad Sci 135: 904–909, 1966.
Physicians' Desk Reference, 56th edn, Thompson Healthcare, Montvale NJ, pp 1290–1291, 2002.
Salmon JF, Carmichael TR, Welsh NH. Use of contrast sensitivity measurement in the detection of subclinical ethambutol toxic optic neuropathy. Br J Ophthalmol 71: 192–196, 1987.
Seth V, Khosla PK, Semwal OP, et al. Visual evoked responses in tuberculous children on ethambutol therapy. Indian Pediatrics 28(7): 713–727, 1991.
Sivakumaran P, Harrison AC, Marschner J, et al. Ocular toxicity from ethambutol: a review of four cases and recommended precautions. N Z Med J 111(1077): 428–430, 1998.
Srivastava AK, et al. Visual evoked responses in ethambutol induced optic neuritis. J Assoc Physicians India 45: 847–849, 1997.
Trau R, et al. Early diagnosis of myambutol (ethambutol) ocular toxicity by electrophysiological examination. Bull Soc Belge Ophtalmol 193: 201, 1981.
Tsai RK, Lee YH. Reversibility of ethambutol optic neuropathy. J Ocular Pharm Therap 13(5): 473–477, 1997.
Yen MY. Ethambutol retinal toxicity: an electrophysiologic study. J Formos Med Assoc 99: 630–634, 2000.
Yiannikas C, Walsh JC, McLeod JG. Visual evoked potentials in the detection of subclinical optic toxic effects secondary to ethambutol. Arch Neurol 40: 645, 1983.

Generic name: Ethionamide.

Proprietary name: Trecator-Sc.

Primary use

This isonicotinic acid derivative is effective against *M. tuberculosis* and *M. leprae*. It is indicated in the treatment of patients when resistance to primary tuberculostatic drugs has developed.

Ocular side effects

Systemic administration
Possible
1. Decreased vision
2. Diplopia

3. Eyelids or conjunctiva
   a. Allergic reactions
   b. Erythema
   c. Pellegra-like syndrome
   d. Urticaria
4. Photophobia
5. Problems with color vision
   a. Color vision defect
   b. Heightened color perception
6. Visual hallucinations

Possible

1. Eyelids of conjunctiva – exfoliative dermatitis

Conditional/Unclassified

1. Optic neuropathy

Clinical significance

The incidence of adverse ocular effects due to ethionamide is quite small and seldom of clinical significance. While certain adverse effects occur at low dosage levels, they usually do not continue even if the dosage is increased. Optic neuritis has been reported, but in so few cases that it is difficult to pinpoint a cause-and-effect relationship.

REFERENCES AND FURTHER READING

Argov Z, Mastaglia FL. Drug-induced peripheral neuropathies. BMJ 1: 663–666, 1979.

Drugs that cause psychiatric symptoms. Med Lett Drugs Ther 28: 81, 1986.

Fox W, et al. A study of acute intolerance to ethionamide, including a comparison with prothionamide, and of the influence of a vitamin B-complex additive in prophylaxis. Tubercule 50: 125, 1969.

Michiels J Noxious effects of systemic medications on the visual apparatus. Bull Soc Belge Ophtalmol 160:1972, p 515–516. French.

Reynolds JEF Martindale: The Extra Pharmacopoeia. 30th edn. Pharmaceutical Press, London, 1993, p 166.

Sweetman S Ethionamide. Martindale: The Complete Drug Reference. Pharmaceutical Press, London, 2005.

Zurcher K, Krebs A. Cutaneous side effects of systemic drugs. S Karger, Basel, pp 18–19, 1980.

Generic name: Isoniazid.

Proprietary names: Laniazid, Nydrazid.

Primary use

This hydrazide of isonicotinic acid is effective against *M. tuberculosis*.

Ocular side effects

Systemic administration
Certain

1. Decreased vision
2. Optic nerve
   a. Retrobulbar or optic neuritis
   b. Papilledema
   c. Optic atrophy
3. Visual fields
   a. Scotomas
   b. Constriction
   c. Hemianopsia

4. Eyelids or conjunctiva
   a. Allergic reactions
   b. Angioedema
   c. Urticaria
5. Problems with color vision – color vision defect, red-green defect
6. Paralysis of accommodation
7. Photophobia
8. Visual hallucinations

Possible

1. Eyelids of conjunctiva
   a. Lupoid syndrome
   b. Erythema multiforme
   c. Stevens-Johnson syndrome
   d. Exfoliative dermatitis
   e. Lyell's syndrome

Conditional/Unclassified

1. Cornea
   a. Keratitis
   b. Brownish infiltrates
2. Extraocular muscles
   a. Paresis
   b. Nystagmus

Clinical significance

Isoniazid can induce a peripheral neuritis in 5–20% of patients. The drug interferes with pyridoxine metabolism. This is probably the cause of optic neuritis. There are a large number of cases with a full return of vision without sequelae by giving pryridoxine. The association seems certain. There are cases, however, of optic atrophy and permanent blindness, especially if the side effect goes unrecognized. Rarely (Dompeling et al 2004) extraocular muscles may be involved, possible by the same mechanism.

Honegger and Genee (1969) found that about one-third of patients had some impairment of accommodation. This was transient and reversible. Neff (1971) described a single case with positive rechallenge in which isoniazid caused brownish corneal infiltrates and anterior uveitis.

REFERENCES AND FURTHER READING

Alarcón-Segovia A. Drug-induced antinuclear antibodies and lupus syndromes. Drugs 12: 69, 1976.

Birch J, et al. Acquired color vision defects. In Pokorny J, Congenital and Acquired Color Vision Defects. Grune & Stratton, New York, 1979, pp 243–350.

Bomb BS, Purohit SD, Bedi HK. Stevens-Johnson syndrome caused by isoniazid. Tubercle 57: 229, 1976.

Boulanouar A, Abdallah E, el Bakkali M, et al. Severe toxic optic neuropathies caused by isoniazid. Apropos of 3 cases. J Francais d'Ophtalmologie 18(3): 183–187, 1995.

Dompeling E, Schut E, Vles H, et al. Diplopia and strabismus convergens mimicking symptoms of tuberculous meningitis as side-effects of isoniazid. Eur J Pediatr 163: 503–504, 2004.

Gonzalez-Gay MA, Sanchez-Andrade A, Aguero JJ, et al. Optic neuritis following treatment with isoniazid in a hemodialyzed patient. [Letter]. Nephron 63(3): 360, 1993.

Honegger H, Genee E. Disturbances of accommodation in association with treatment with tuberculostatics. Klin Monatsbl Augenheilkd 155: 361–380. German, 1969.

Karmon G, et al. Bilateral optic neuropathy due to combined ethambutol and isoniazid treatment. Ann Ophthalmol 11: 1013, 1979.

Kass I, Mandel W, et al. Isoniazid as a cause of optic neuritis and atrophy. JAMA 164: 1740–1743, 1957.

Keeping JA, Searle SWA. Optic neuritis following isoniazid therapy. Lancet 2: 278, 1955.

Kiyosawa M, Ishikawa S. A case of isoniazid-induced optic neuropathy. Neuro-Ophthalmology 2: 67, 1981.

Kratka W. Isoniazid and ocular tuberculosis. Arch Ophthalmol 54: 330–334, 1955.

Nair KG. Optic neuritis due to INH complicating tuberculous meningitis. J Assoc Physicians India 24: 263, 1976.

Neff TA. Isoniazid toxicity – lactic acidosis and keratopathy. Chest 59: 245, 1971.

Renard G, Morax PV. Optic neuritis in the course of treatment of tuberculosis. Ann Oculist 210: 53, 1977.

Stratton MA. Drug-induced systemic lupus erythematosus. Clin Pharm 4: 657, 1985.

Sutton PH, Beattie PH. Optic atrophy after administration of isoniazid with PAS. Lancet 1: 650–651, 1955.

Zuckerman BD, Lieberman TW. Corneal rust ring. Arch Ophthalmol 63: 254–265, 1960.

Zurcher K, Krebs A. Cutaneous side effects of systemic drugs. S Karger, Basel, 1980pp 18–21.

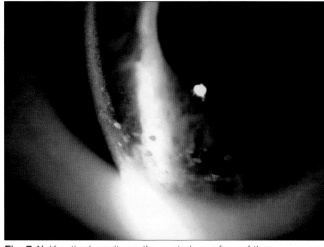

Fig. 7.1j Keratic deposits on the posterior surface of the cornea from systemic rifabutin. Photo courtesy of Ponjavic V, et al: Retinal dysfunction and anterior segment deposits in a patient treated with rifabutin. Acta Ophthalmol Scand 80: 553-556, 2002.

Generic name: Rifabutin.

Proprietary name: Mycobutin.

Primary use

This agent is used in the treatment of *Mycobacterium avium*, leprosy tuberculosis, staphylococcal infections, brucellosis, HIV patients, atypical mycobacteria and Legionnaires' disease. It is also used in the prophylaxis of Haemophilus, meningococcal meningitis and *Mycobacterium avium*.

Ocular side effects

Systemic administration
Certain
1. Uveitis
   a. Anterior (from fine stellate keratic precipitates to large hypopyon)
   b. Posterior
   c. Panuveitis
   d. Hypopyon
2. Blurred vision
3. Photophobia
4. Pain
5. Conjunctiva
   a. Hyperemia
   b. Micro-hemorrhages
6. Vitreous
   a. Vitritis
   b. Yellow-white opacities
7. Contact lens staining
8. Retina
   a. Micro-hemorrhages
   b. Vasculitis
9. Eyelids
   a. Contact dermatitis
   b. Rashes
   c. Orange-tan discoloration
10. Cornea
    a. Endothelial fine or large stellate deposits (Fig. 7.1j)
11. Lacrimation – rose colored

Probable
1. Staining IOL – rose color
2. Macular edema

Conditional/Unclassified
1. Cornea
   a. Opacities
   b. Ulcers

Clinical significance

Uveitis associated with rifabutin is the predominant ocular side effect with this drug. Fraunfelder and Rosenbaum (1997) reported 113 cases of rifabutin-associated uveitis from a spontaneous reporting systems database. Shafran et al (1994) performed a prospective randomized study of 119 patients, 59 of whom received rifabutin in combination with clarithromycin and ethambutol. About 40% of those who received rifabutin developed uveitis, about two thirds bilateral, with an onset mean of 65 days. The uveitis may occur within 2 weeks to 7 months after starting the drug. The inflammatory-like response may involve only the anterior segment or, rarely, the whole uvea. It may be mild, with only fine peripheral endothelial deposits without uveitis, to a fulminating panuveitis with significant posterior corneal and vitreal deposits. It may or may not be associated with hypopyon, significant vitritis, including vitreal opacities (Chaknis et al 1996), or in rare instances, a retinal vasculitis. While it is most commonly associated with HIV-infected patients who are often on other antibiotics concomitantly, this entity is now being reported in immune suppressed patients, patients without AIDS, on rifabutin alone and in immune competent persons. The uveitis is more common in patients on rifabutin along with clarithromycin or fluconazole. These agents may elevate rifabutin serum levels by inhibition of the hepatic microsomal cytochrome P_{450} system, which metabolizes rifabutin. The uveitis is unique, in part because topical ocular steroids, even in fulminating cases, often clear the intraocular inflammation quite rapidly (Jacobs et al 1994). This ocular inflammatory response clears on topical ocular steroids and stopping the drug. There are a few cases where the drug was not discontinued and the uveitis cleared on its own. The etiology of this uveitis is unknown, and some postulate the possibility of interaction of multiple drugs, an altered immune system, underlying infections or drug-related factors contributing to the development of this uveitis syndrome. Smith et al (1999) described bilateral peripheral endothelial stellate-shaped deposits in children with HIV disease on rifabutin. They suggest that these may be enlarged macrophages due to the pseudopod-like components of these refractile lesions. With time, these endothelial keratotic precipitates may become more central. Rifabutin can stain multiple body fluids, including tears and aqueous humor. It has a potential to stain silicone, i.e. contact lenses or intraocular lenses (Jones and Irwin 2002). High doses of rifabutin have also been associated with an orange/tan discoloration of the skin, as well as the sclera and oral mucosa. There are a number of reports in the World Health Organization spontaneous reporting system of corneal ulceration and opacities, but these data are unconfirmed.

REFERENCES AND FURTHER READING

Arevalo JF, Freeman WR. Corneal endothelial deposits in children positive for human immunodeficiency virus reveiving rifabutin prophylaxis for *Mycobacterium avium* complex bacteremia. Am J Ophthalmol 127: 164–169, 1999.

Awotesu O, Missotten T, Pitcher MC, et al. Uveitis in a patient receiving rifabutin for Crohn's disease. J Roy Soc Med 97: 440–441, 2004.

Bhagat N, Read RW, Narsing RA, et al. Rifabutin-associated hypopyon uveitis in human immunodeficiency virus-negative immunocompetent individuals. Ophthalmology 108: 750–752, 2001.

Brogden RN, Fitton A. Rifabutin: a review of its antimicrobial activity pharmacokinetic properties and therapeutic efficacy. Drugs 47(6): 983–1009, 1994.

Chaknis MJ, Brooks SE, Mitchell KT, et al. Inflammatory opacities of the viteous in rifabutin-associated uveitis. Am J Ophthalmol 122(4): 580–582, 1996.

Dunn AM, Tizer K, Cervia JS. Rifabutin-associated uveitis in a pediatric patient. Pediatr Infect Dis J 3(14): 246–247, 1995.

Frank MO, Graham MB, Wispelway B. Rifabutin and uveitis. To the Editor. New Engl J Med March 24: 868, 1994.

Fraunfelder FW, Rosenbaum JT. Drug-induced uveitis. Drug Safety 17(3): 197–207, 1997.

Fuller JD, Stanfield LE, Craven DE. Rifabutin prophylaxis and uveitis (letter). N Engl J Med 330(18): 1315–1316, 1994.

Jacobs DS, Piliero PJ, Kuperwaser MG, et al. Acute uveitis associated with rifabutin use in patients with human immunodeficiency virus infection. Am J Ophthalmol 118: 716–722, 1994.

Jones DF, Irwin AE. Discoloration of intraocular lens subsequent to rifabutin use. Arch Ophthalmol 120: 1211–1212, 2002.

Nichols CW. *Mycobacterium avium* complex infection, rifabutin, and uveitis: is there a connection? Clin Infect Dis 22(Suppl. 1): S43–S49, 1996.

Ponjavic V, Gränse L, Bengtsson-Stigma E, Andréasson S. Retinal dysfunction and anterior segment deposits in a patient treated with rifabutin. Act Ophthalmol Scand 80: 553–556, 2002.

Saran BR, Maguire AM, Nichols C, et al. Hypopyon uveitis in patients with acquired immunodeficiency syndrome treated for systemic *Mycobacterium avium* complex infection with rifabutin. Arch Ophthalmol 112: 1159–1165, 1994.

Shafran SD, Deschênes J, Miller M, et al. for the MAC study group of the Canadian HIV trials network. Uveitis and pseudojaundice during a regimen of clarithromycin, rifabutin, and ethambutol. N Engl J Med 330: 438, 1994.

Skolik S, Willermain F, Caspers LE. Rifabutin-associated panuveitis with retinal vasculitis in pulmonary tuberculosis. Ocul Immunol Inflamm 13: 483–485, 2005.

Smith JA, Mueller BU, Nussenblatt RB, Whitcup SM. Corneal endothelial deposits in children positive for human immunodeficiency virus receiving rifabutin prophylaxis for *Mycobacterium avium* complex bacteremia. Am J Ophthalmol 127(2): 164–169, 1999.

Tseng AL, Walmsley SL. Rifabutin-associated uveitis. Ann Pharmaco Ther 29: 1149–1155, 1995.

Vaudaux JD, Guex-Crosier Y. Rifabutin-induced cystoid macular oedema. J Antimicrob Chemother 49: 421–422, 2002.

Generic name: Rifampicin.

Proprietary names: Rifadin, Rimactane.

Primary use

Systemic
This bactericidal as well as bacteriostatic agent is effective against Mycobacterium, many Gram-positive cocci and some Gram-negative, including Neisseria species and *Haemophilus influenzae*.

Ophthalmic
This agent is used for treatment of ocular chlamydia infections.

Ocular side effects

Systemic administration
Certain
1. Decreased vision
2. Eyelids or conjunctiva
   a. Hyperemia
   b. Erythema
   c. Blepharoconjunctivitis
   d. Edema
   e. Yellow or red discoloration
   f. Angioedema
   g. Urticaria
   h. Purpura
   i. Pemphigoid lesion
   j. Hypersensitivity reactions
3. Lacrimation
4. Problems with color vision
   a. Color vision defect
   b. Red-green defect
5. Tears and/or contact lenses stained orange
   a. Periorbital edema

Possible
1. Subconjunctival or retinal hemorrhages secondary to drug-induced anemia
2. Eyelids of conjunctiva
   a. Lupoid syndrome
   b. Stevens-Johnson syndrome
   c. Exfoliative dermatitis

Local ophthalmic use or exposure (ointment)
Certain
1. Irritation
   a. Lacrimation
   b. Hyperemia
   c. Ocular pain
   d. Edema

Clinical significance

Ocular side effects from systemic rifampicin are quite variable. Reactions may include conjunctival hyperemia, mild blepharoconjunctivitis or painful severe exudative conjunctivitis. The latter includes markedly congested palpebral and bulbar conjunctiva with thick white exudates (Girling 1976). Although not all patients seem to secrete this drug or a by-product in their tears, Lyons (1979), as well as Fraunfelder (1980), reported orange-red staining of contact lenses and the inability to wear lenses while taking this drug. Systemic rifampicin may stain other body fluids as well, but this discoloration disappears once the drug is discontinued. Ocular side effects seen with this drug appear to occur more frequently during intermittent treatment than during daily treatment and are reversible when the drug has been discontinued. In animals this drug accumulates in ocular pigment, but there are no data for this in humans.

Topical ocular use of 1% rifampicin ointment has been reported to cause approximately a 10% incidence of adverse ocular effects, which are primarily due to irritation and include discomfort, tearing, lid edema and conjunctival hyperemia. The irritation, discomfort and tearing usually last only 10–50 minutes after the application of the ointment.

REFERENCES AND FURTHER READING

Birch J, et al. Acquired color vision defects. In Pokorny J, Congenital and Acquired Color Vision Defects. Grune & Stratton, New York, 1979, p 243–350.
Bolan G, Laurie RE, Broome CV. Red man syndrome: Inadvertent administration of an excessive dose of rifampin to children in a day-care center. Pediatrics 77: 633, 1986.
Calissendorff B. Melanotropic drugs and retinal functions. Acta Ophthalmol 54: 118–128, 1976.
Cayley FE, Majumdar SK. Ocular toxicity due to rifampicin. BMJ 1: 199-200, 1976.
Darougar S, et al. Topical therapy of hyperendemic trachoma with rifampicin, oxytetracycline, or spiramycin eye ointments. Br J Ophthalmol 64: 37, 1980.
Fraunfelder FT. Orange tears. Am J Ophthalmol 89: 752, 1980.
Girling DJ. Ocular toxicity due to rifampicin. BMJ 1: 585, 1976.
Grosset J, Leventis S. Adverse effects of rifampin. Rev Infect Dis 5(Suppl 3): 440, 1983.
Lyons RW. Orange contact lenses from rifampin. N Engl J Med 300: 372, 1979.
Mangi RJ. Reactions to rifampin. N Engl J Med 294: 113, 1976.
Nyirenda R, Gill GV. Stevens-Johnson syndrome due to rifampicin. BMJ 2: 1189, 1977.

Generic name: Thioacetazone (Amithiozone).

Proprietary names: Conteben, Tibione.

Primary use
This tuberculostatic agent is effective against *M. tuberculosis* and *M. leprae*. This drug is also used for lupus vulgaris.

Ocular side effects

Systemic administration
Certain
1. Decreased vision
2. Non-specific ocular irritation
   a. Photophobia
   b. Ocular pain
   c. Burning sensation
3. Eyelids or conjunctiva
   a. Allergic reactions
   b. Hyperemia
   c. Blepharoconjunctivitis
   d. Hypertrichosis

Possible
1. Subconjunctival or retinal hemorrhages secondary to drug-induced anemia
2. Eyelids or conjunctiva
   a. Erythema multiforme
   b. Stevens-Johnson syndrome
   c. Exfoliative dermatitis
   d. Lyell syndrome

Conditional/Unclassified
1. Retinal edema
2. Color vision defect
3. Scotoma

Clinical significance
Numerous adverse ocular reactions due to thioacetazone have been seen. Skin manifestations have been the most frequent. Nearly all ocular side effects are reversible and are of minor clinical significance. One instance of irreversible toxic amblyopia with a central scotoma and decreased color vision has been reported; however, the patient was also receiving aminosalicylic acid.

REFERENCES AND FURTHER READING

Mame-Thierna D, On S, Thierno-Nydiaye S, Ndiaye B. Lyell syndrome in Senegal: responsibility of thiacetazone. Ann Dermatol Venereol 128: 1305–1307, 2001.
Ravindran P, Joshi M. Dermatological hypersensitivity to thiacetazone. Indian J Chest Dis 16: 58, 1974.
In Reynolds JEF Martindale: The Extra Pharmacopoeia. 30th edn. Pharmaceutical Press, London, 1993, p 216–217.
Sahi SP, Chandra K. Thiacetazone-induced Stevens-Johnson syndrome: a case report. Indian J Chest Dis 16: 124, 1974.
Sarma OA. Reactions to thiacetazone. Indian J Chest Dis 18: 51, 1976.

SECTION 2
AGENTS AFFECTING THE CNS

CLASS: ANALEPTICS

Generic name: Gabapentin.

Proprietary name: Neurontin.

Primary use
This antiepileptic drug is used in refractory seizure patients.

Ocular side effects

Systemic administration
Certain
1. Decreased or blurred vision
2. Nystagmus
3. Diplopia
4. Visual hallucinations
5. Eyelids or conjunctiva – conjunctivitis

Probable
1. Myasthenia gravis – aggravation
   a. Diplopia
   b. Ptosis
   c. Paresis of extraocular muscles

Possible
1. Eyelids or conjunctiva
   a. Erythema multiforme
   b. Stevens-Johnson syndrome

Clinical significance

Gabapentin's most common ocular side effect is a decrease in central vision. The effect may be zigzag lines, a crowding of central letters on Snellen testing or blurred vision. The median onset of these symptoms is 4 days. While Browne (1993) reported an incidence of nystagmus at 11% and diplopia at 6%, these figures in other trials are lower than this (Physicians' Desk Reference 2006). Conjunctivitis occurs in 1.2% over placebo controls. All Ocular side effects are reversible. This drug may aggravate myasthenia with worsening of ptosis.

REFERENCES AND FURTHER READING

Boneva N, Brenner T, Argov Z. Gabapentin may be hazardous in myasthenia gravis. Muscle Nerve 23: 1204–1208, 2000.
Browne T. Efficacy and safety of gabapentin. In: New Trends in Epilepsy Management: the Role of Gabapentin, Chadwick D (ed), London, Royal Society of Medicine Service, pp 47–58, 1993.
Goa KL, Sorkin EM. Gabapentin. A review of its pharmacological properties and clinical potential in epilepsy. Drugs 46(3): 409–427, 1993.
Scheschonka A, Beuche W. Treatment of post-herpetic pain in myasthenia gravis: exacerbation of weakness due to gabapentin. Pain 104: 423–424, 2003.
Physicians' Drug Reference, 60th edn, Thomson PDR, Montvale NJ, pp 2498–2503, 2006.

Generic name: Lamotrigine.

Proprietary name: Lamictal.

Primary use

This is an antiepileptic drug believed to suppress seizures by inhibiting the release of excitatory neurotransmitters.

Ocular side effects

Systemic administration
Certain
1. Diplopia
2. Blurred vision
3. Nystagmus
4. Eyelids or conjunctiva
   a. Conjunctivitis
   b. Photosensitivity

Probable
1. Angioneurotic edema
2. Visual hallucinations

Possible
1. Eyelids or conjunctiva
   a. Stevens-Johnson syndrome
   b. Toxic epidermal necrolysis

Conditional/Unclassified
1. Visual field changes – primarily generalized constriction
2. Retinal pigmentary change

Clinical significance

Lamotrigine is mainly an add-on drug used when current antiepileptic drugs are ineffective, which confuses its adverse effect profile. In placebo-controlled clinical trials, two of its five most common side effects were ocular (Schachter 1992), with 22% of patients having diplopia and 15% having blurred vision compared to controls. Betts et al (1991) noted that less than 5% had nystagmus. Alkawi et al (2005) reported a case of downbeat nystagmus. Decreasing the dosage may significantly decrease ocular side effects. All ocular side effects appear to be reversible. There are cases of severe bilateral visual loss that returned fully when the drug is discontinued. There have been reports to the National Registry of ptosis, hallucinations and pigmentary retinal defects. These are too few to draw any correlation with lamotrignine.

REFERENCES AND FURTHER READING

Alkawi A, Kattah JC, Wyman K. Downbeat nystagmus as a result of lamotrigine toxicity. Epilepsy Res 63: 85–88, 2005.
Betts T, Goodwin G, Withers RM, Yuen AWC. Human safety of lamotrigine. Epilepsia 32(Suppl. 1): S17–S21, 1991.
Das KB, Harris C, Smyth DP, Cross JH. Unusual side effects of lamotrigine therapy. J Child Neurol 18: 479–480, 2003.
Goa KL, Ross SR, Chrisp P. Lamotrigine. Drugs 46: 152–176, 1993.
Schachter SC. A multicenter, placebo-controlled evaluation of the safety of lamotrigine (Lamictal®) as add-on therapy in outpatients with partial seizures. Presented at the 1992 Annual Meeting of the American Epilepsy Society, Seattle, December 4–10, 1992.

Generic name: Vigabatrin.

Proprietary name: Orphan drug production.

Primary use

Antiepileptic drug effective for refractory epilepsy, generalized tonic-clonic seizures and infantile spasms.

Ocular side effects

Systemic administration
Certain
1. Decreased or blurred vision
2. Visual field defects – may be irreversible
   a. Concentric peripheral constriction
   b. Tunnel vision
   c. Variable visual field defects
   d. Scotoma
3. Retina
   a. Peripheral atrophy
   b. Nerve fiber layer loss (Fig. 7.2a)
   c. Surface wrinkling retinopathy
   d. Hypopigment spots
4. Contrast sensitivity – reduced
5. Optic atrophy
6. Color vision abnormalities
7. Electroretinography
   a. Abnormal ERG
   b. Abnormal EOG

Possible
1. Eyelids – angioneurotic edema

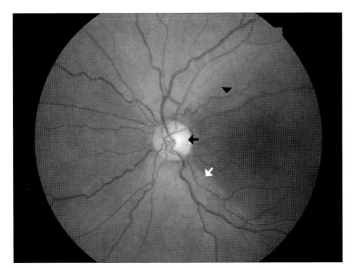

Fig. 7.2a Vigabatrin-induced retinal nerve fiber layer loss. The black arrow indicates temporal disc pallor, the white arrow the demarcation between atrophic and non-affected nerve fiber layer and the black triangle shows the telltale change in superficial light reflex aligning along the course of the exposed small vessel of the atrophic macula. Photo courtesy of Buncic JR. Characteristic retinal atrophy with secondary 'inverse' optic atrophy identifies vigabatrin toxicity in children. Ophthalmology 111: 1935–1942, 2004.

Clinical significance

While vigabatrin has been available for almost two decades, the potential for ocular side effects make it one of the most controversial drugs with regard to ocular safety issues. Some countries have banned its use. This drug may be indispensable for adults with refractory epilepsy, but as many as 30–40% of patients develop significant ocular side effects. The incidence in children is less clear due, in part, to the variability of responses to testing methods in children.

Lawden's recent editorial based on the work of Krauss et al (1998) and others showed that vigabatrin, not epilepsy or other nervous system diseases, causes these ocular changes (Lawden 2003). Visual field defects may occur after a few months to years after starting the drug. They are bilateral and range from a localized nasal defect of 30–40⁰ in eccentricity and may extend to complete concentric contraction. In rare instances, central vision can be involved. Johnson et al (2000) deny reversibility of visual field loss; however, visual acuity, color vision and ERG amplitude loss may be reversible if recognized early in patients with minimal or no field loss. Best and Acheson (2005) studied patients on the drug alone or in combination with other antiepileptic agents for a minimum of 5 years. This was in patients who elected to continue the medication for good seizure control. All patients had unequivocal visual field defects. They found only one in 16 had progression, and the range of follow-up was 18–43 months. Arndt et al (1999) feel that visual field changes are enhanced if the patients are also on valproate. Graniewski-Wijnands and Van Der Torren (2002) showed some recovery of EOG and ERG, but no change in visual fields once the drug was discontinued.

The primary retinal effects are peripheral atrophy and nerve fiber bundles defects. Choi and Kim (2004) have shown retinal nerve fiber layer defects correlating with visual field constriction. Outer retinal dysfunction should be present if visual field changes are present. Banin et al (2003) suggest that vigabatrin not only impairs peripheral cones, but foveal cones based on electroretinographic amplitudes. In the main these changes are irreversible; however there are rare reports of some reversibility (Fledelius 2003). Other retinal effects include abnormal macular light reflexes, surface wrinkling retinopathy and narrowing of the arterial tree.

The incidence of visual field defects varies from a 2% incidence at 6 months (Wilton et al 1999) to 10–20% or more. There is evidence to suggest that this is dose related, but the time of onset varies greatly. Some cases occur as soon as 1 month after starting the drug, and others have occurred after 6 or more years of treatment. The mechanism behind the visual field defects could be related to impairment of the highly GABA-ergic amacrine cells in the retina. Histopathological studies in animals show a microvacuolation in myelin sheaths of white matter when exposed to vigabatrin. How these alterations affect the visual field in patients receiving vigabatrin is not known. Frisén and Malmgren (2003), Viestenz et al (2003), Buncic et al (2004) and Rebolleda et al (2005) have described optic nerve pallor and atrophy secondary to vigabatrin. It is felt that there is a toxic effect on the axons of the retinal ganglion cells resulting in various degrees of optic atrophy. This atrophy occurs most frequently nasally.

The EOG is possibly a more sensitive and specific diagnostic tool than ERG for drug-related retinal effects. Wild et al feel ocular coherence tomography of the retinal nerve fiber layer thickness can efficiently identify this drug's damage in adults and children unable to perform perimetry. It may also be helpful in cases where the question of toxic damage is equivocal.

Recommendations (modified from recommendations by the manufacturer, Hoechst Marion Roussel)

1. Baseline visual field – if patient has a cognitive age of 9 years or more, Goldmann or Humphrey fields. Below the age of 9, there is currently no reliable method available. Possibly, ERG has a role here.
2. Visual field testing every 6 months. If visual fields are abnormal this needs to be confirmed by retesting.
3. Question patients regularly for visual symptoms.
4. If there are any new visual symptoms, consider repeating the visual field testing. If defects are extensive, progressive and reproducible, the risk-benefit ratio needs to be revisited. If the drug is discontinued, this should be done over a 2- to 4-week period.
5. Electroretinography or visual evoked potential have been of minimal value to date, but may be of benefit as more data are accumulated.

REFERENCES AND FURTHER READING

Arndt CF, Derambure P, Defoort-Dhellemmes S, Hache JC. Outer retinal dysfunction in patients treated with vigabatrin. Neurology 52: 1205–1208, 1999.

Banin E, Shclev RS, Obolensky A, et al. Retinal function abnormalities in patients treated with vigabatrin. Arch Ophthalmol 121: 811–816, 2003.

Baulac M, Nordmann JP, Lanoe Y. Severe visual field constriction and side-effects of GABA-mimetic antiepileptic agents (letter). Lancet 352: 546, 1998.

Beck RW. Vigabatrin-associated retinal cone system dysfunction (letter). Neurology 51: 1778–1779, 1998.

Best JL, Acheson JF. The natural history of vigabatrin associated visual field defects in patients electing to continue their medication. Eye 19: 41–44, 2005.

Blackwell N, Hayllar J, Kelly G. Severe persistent visual field constriction associated with vigabatrin. Patients taking vigabatrin should have regular visual field testing (letter, comment). BMJ 314: 180–181, 1997.

Brigell MG. Vigabatrin-associated retinal cone system dysfunction (letter). Neurology 51: 1778–1779, 1998.

Buncic RJ, Westall CA, Panton CM, et al. Characteristic retinal atrophy with secondary 'inverse' optic atrophy identifies vigabatrin toxicity in children. Ophthalmology 111: 1935–1942, 2004.

Choi HJ, Kim DM. Visual field constriction associated with vigabatrin: retinal nerve fiber layer photographic correlation. J Neurol Neurosurg Psychiatry 75: 1395, 2004.

Eke T, et al. Severe persistent visual field constriction associated with vigabatrin. BMJ 314: 180–181, 1997.

Fledelius HC. Vigabatrin-associated visual field constriction in a longitudinal series. Reversibility suggested after drug withdrawal. Acta Ophthalmol Scand 81: 41–45, 2003.

Frisén L, Malmgren K. Characterization of vigabatrin-associated optic atrophy. Acta Ophthalmol Scand 81: 466–473, 2003.

Graniewski-Wijnands HS, Van Der Torren K. Electro-ophthalmological recovery after withdrawal from vigabatrin. Doc Ophthalmol 104: 189–194, 2002.

Harding GFA, et al. Severe persistent visual field constriction associated with vigabatrin. BMJ 316: 232–233, 1998.

Harding GFA, Robertson K, Spence EL, Holliday I. Vigabatrin; its effect on the electrophysiology of vision. Doc Ophthalmol 104: 213–229, 2002.

Johnson MA, Krauss GL, Miller NR, et al. Visual function loss from vigabatrin: effect of stopping the drug. Neurology 55: 40–45, 2000.

Koul R, Chacko A, Ganesh A, et al. Vigabatrin associated retinal dysfunction in children with epilepsy. Arch Dis Child 85: 469–473, 2001.

Krauss GL, et al. Vigabatrin-associated retinal cone system dysfunction. Neurology 50: 614–618, 1998.

Krauss GL, Johnson MA, Miller NR. Vigabatrin-associated retinal cone system dysfunction (reply). Neurology 51: 1779–1781, 1998.

Lawden MC. Vigabatrin, tiagabine, and visual fields. J Neurol Neurosurg Psychiatry 74: 286, 2003.

Lhatoo SD, Sander JW. Infantile spasms and vigabatrin. Visual field defects may be permanent (letter). BMJ 318: 57, 1999.

Mackenzie R, Klistorner A. Severe persistent visual field constriction associated with vigabatrin. Asymptomatic as well as symptomatic defects occur with vigabatrin (letter; comment). BMJ 314: 233, 1998.

Nousiainin I, Kalviainen R, Mantyjarvi M. Color vision in epilepsy patients treated with vigabatrin or carbamazepine monotherapy. Ophthalmology 107: 884–888, 2000.

Rao GP, Fat FA, Kyle G, et al. Study is needed of visual field defects associated with any long term antiepileptic drug (letter). BMJ 317: 206, 1998.

Rebolleda G, García Pérez JL, Muñoz Negrete FJ, Tang RA. Vigabatin toxicity in children. Ophthalmology 112: 1322–1323, 2005.

Roff Hilton EJ, Cubbidge RP, Hosking SL, et al. Patients treated with vigabatrin exhibit central visual function loss. Epilepsia 43: 1351–1359, 2002.

Roubertie A, Bellet H, Echenne B. Vigabatrin-associated retinal cone system dysfunction (letter). Neurology 51: 1779, 1998.

Ruether K, et al. Electrophysiologic evaluation of a patient with peripheral visual field contraction associated with vigabatrin. Arch Ophthalmol 116: 817–819, 1998.

Van Der Torren K, Graniewski-Wijnands HS, Polak BCP. Visual field and electrophysiological abnormalities due to vigabatrin. Doc Ophthalmol 104: 181–188, 2002.

Viestenz A, Viestenz A, Mardin CV. Vigabatrin-associated bilateral simple optic nerve atrophy with visual field constriction. A case report and a survey of the literature. [German]. Ophthalmologe 100: 402–405, 2003.

Wild JM, Robson CR, Jones AL, et al. Detecting vigabatrin toxicity by imaging of the retinal nerve fiber layer. Invest Ophthalmol Vis Sci 47: 917–924, 2006.

Wilson EA, Brodie MJ. Severe persistent visual field constriction associated with vigabatrin. Chronic refractory epilepsy may have role in causing these unusual lesions (letter; comment). BMJ 314: 1693–1695, 1997.

Wilton LV, Stephens MDB, Mann RD. Interim report of the incidence of visual field defects in patients on long term vigabatrin therapy. Pharmacoepidemiol Drug Safety 8: S9–S14, 1999.

CLASS: ANOREXIANTS

Generic names: 1. Amfetamine; 2. dextroamfetamine sulfate (dexamphetamine); 3. methamfetamine hydrochloride.

Proprietary names: 1. Multi-ingredient preparation only; 2. Dexedrine, Dextrostat; 3. Desoxyn.

Street names: 1-3. Crank, Rx Diet Pills, speed, uppers, ups.

Primary use

These sympathomimetic amines are used in the management of exogenous obesity; amfetamine, dextroamfetamine and methamphetamine, and are also effective in narcolepsy and in the management of minimal brain dysfunction in children. They are also used off-label as recreational drugs.

Ocular side effects

Systemic administration
Certain
1. Decreased vision
2. Increase in critical flicker frequency
3. Visual hallucinations
4. Problems with color vision – objects have blue tinge (amfetamine)
5. Pupils (toxic states)
   a. Mydriasis – may precipitate narrow-angle glaucoma
   b. Decreased reaction to light

Possible
1. Ocular teratogenic effects (methamfetamine)
2. Oculogyric crisis (dextroamfetamine sulfate)
3. Eyelids and conjunctiva
   a. Stevens-Johnson syndrome
   b. Toxic epidermal necrolysis

Nasal application – methamphetamine
Certain
1. Decreased vision
2. Cornea
   a. Keratitis
   b. Ulceration
3. Conjunctivitis

Possible
1. Retina
   a. Venous thrombosis
   b. Intraretinal hemorrhages
   c. Ischemic changes
   d. Arterial narrowing
   e. Vasculitis
   f. Central or branch vein occlusion
2. Optic nerve
   a. Ischemic changes
   b. Optic atrophy

Clinical significance

Ocular side effects due to these sympathomimetic amines are seldom of consequence and are mainly seen in recreational use or overdose situations. Chuck et al (1996) describe recurrent corneal ulcers in a patient on chronic methamfetamine abuse, much like the 'crack eye syndrome' resulting from the smoked form of cocaine. This same ocular pattern is evident secondary to the smoked form of methamfetamine, 'ice'. Several hours after methamfetamine was applied to the nose of a young female, she developed blurred vision and intraretinal hemorrhages. This was felt to be due to a sudden increase in blood pressure caused by the drug (Wallace et al 1992). Wijaya et al (1999) described a similar case of methamfetamine applied once nasally to a 35-year-old male with a unilateral acute loss of vision with resultant ischemic optic nerve and optic atrophy. Shaw et al (1985) described a patient who developed amaurosis fugax and retinal vasculitis 36 hours after nasal exposure to methamfetamine on the same side as the nasal drug exposure.

Hertle et al (2001) reported a case of 'paradoxically' improved nystagmus, binocular function and visual acuity in a child with retinal dystrophy and congenital nystagmus while taking Dexedrine (dextroamfetamine sulfate).

REFERENCES AND FURTHER READING

Acute drug abuse reactions. Med Lett Drugs Ther 27: 77, 1985.
Chuck RS, Williams JM, Goldberg MA, Lubniewski AJ. Recurrent corneal ulcerations associated with smokeable methamphetamine abuse. Am J Ophthalmol 121(5): 571–572, 1996.
D'Souza T, Shraberg D. Intracranial hemorrhage associated with amphetamine use. Neurology 31: 922, 1981.
Hertle RW, Maybodi M, Bauer RM, Walker K. Clinical and oculographic response to Dexedrine in a patient with rod-cone dystrophy, exotropia, and congenital aperiodic alternating nystagmus. Binocul Vis Strabismus Q 16: 259–264, 2001.
Limaye SR, Goldberg MH. Septic submacular choroidal embolus associated with intravenous drug abuse. Ann Ophthalmol 14: 518, 1982.
Lowe T, et al. Stimulant medications precipitate Tourette's syndrome. JAMA 247: 1729, 1982.
Rouher F, Cantat MA. Anorexic medications and retinal venous thromboses. Bull Soc Ophtalmol France 62: 65–71, 1962.
Shaw HE Jr., Lawson JG, Stulting RG. Amaurosis fugax and retinal vasculitis associated with methamphetamine inhalation J Clin. Neuro-ophthalmol 5: 169–176, 1985.
Smart JV, Sneddon JM, Turner P. A comparison of the effects of chlorphentermine, diethylpropion, and phenmetrazine on critical flicker frequency. Br J Pharmacol 30: 307–316, 1967.
Spaeth GL, Nelson LB, Beaudoin AR. Ocular teratology. In: Ocular Anatomy, Embryology and Teratology, Jakobiec FA (ed), Philadelphia J.B. Lippincott, 1982, pp 955–975.
Vesterhauge S, Peitersen E. The effects of some drugs on the caloric induced nystagmus. Adv Otorhinolaryngol 25: 173, 1979.
Wallace RT, Brown GC, Benson W, Sivalingham A. Sudden retinal manifestations of intranasal cocaine and methamphetamine abuse. Am. J Ophthalmol 114: 158–160, 1992.
Wijaya J, Salu P, Leblanc A, Bervoets S. Acute unilateral visual loss due to a single intranasal methamphetamine abuse. Bull Soc Belge Opthalmol 271: 19–25, 1999.
Yung A, Agnew K, Snow J, Oliver F. Two unusual cases of toxic epidermal necrolysis. Australas. J Dermatol 43: 35–38, 2002.

Generic names: 1. Benzfetamine hydrochloride; 2. amfepramone hydrochloride (diethylpropion); 3. phendimetrazine tartrate; 4. phentermine.

Proprietary names: 1. Didrex; 2. Tenuate, Tenuate Dospan; 3. Bontril, Bontril PDM, X-Trozine, X-Trozine L.A.; 4. Adipex-p, Ionamin.

Primary use

These sympathomimetic amines are used in the treatment of exogenous obesity.

Ocular side effects

Systemic administration
Certain
1. Decreased vision
2. Decreased accommodation
3. Diplopia
4. Visual hallucinations

5. Non-specific ocular irritation
   a. Photophobia
   b. Ocular pain
   c. Burning sensation
6. Eyelids or conjunctiva
   a. Allergic reactions
   b. Erythema
   c. Urticaria
7. Increased critical flicker fusion frequency (amfepramone)

Conditional/Unclassified
1. Optic neuritis (phentermine)
2. Posterior subcapsular cataracts (phentermine, amfepramone)
3. Vasoplastic amairosis fugax (amfepramone)

Clinical significance

Ocular side effects due to these sympathomimetic amines are rare and seldom of clinical significance. All proven side effects are reversible or resolve even while remaining on the drug. Posterior subcapsular cataracts have been reported in patients receiving phentermine or amfepramone, but a cause-and-effect relationship has not been proven. There are 11 cases of optic neuritis in patients on phentermine in the National Registry, but most occurred during the age that multiple sclerosis may occur. Evans (2000) reported a unilateral reversible ocular migraine type aura with a positive dechallenge but no rechallenge in a patient on amfepramone.

A female adult had 'paradoxical' improvement of her congenital nystagmus and binocular function while taking amfepramone (Hertle et al 2002).

REFERENCES AND FURTHER READING

Chan JW. Acute nonarteritic ischaemic optic neuropathy after phentermine. Eye 19: 1238–1239, 2005.
Evans RW. Monocular visual aura with headache: retinal migraine? Headache 40: 603–604, 2000.
Hertle RW, Maybodi M, Mellow SD, Yang D. Clinical and oculographic response to tenuate dospan (diethylpropionate) in a patient with congenital nystagmus. Am J Ophthalmol 133: 159–160, 2002.
Smart JV, Sneddon JM, Turner P. A comparison of the effects of chlorphentermine, diethylpropion, and phenmetrazine on critical flicker frequency. Br J Pharmacol 30: 307–316, 1967.

CLASS: ANTIANXIETY AGENTS

Generic names: 1. Alprazolam; 2. chlordiazepoxide; 3. clonazepam; 4. clorazepate dipotassium; 5. diazepam; 6. flurazepam; 7. lorazepam; 8. midazolam; 9. oxazepam; 10. temazepam; 11. triazolam.

Proprietary names: 1. Niravam, Xanax; 2. Librium; 3. Klonopin; 4. Gen-xene, Tranxene, Tranxene SD; 5. Acudial, Diastat, Valium; 6. Dalmane; 7. Ativan; 8. Generic only; 10. Generic only; 11. Restoril; 12. Halcion.

Primary use

These benzodiazepine derivatives are effective in the management of psychoneurotic states manifested by anxiety, tension or agitation. They are also used as adjunctive therapy in the relief of skeletal muscle spasms and as preoperative medications.

Ocular side effects

Systemic administration
Certain
1. Decreased or blurred vision
2. Eyelids or conjunctiva
   a. Allergic reactions
   b. Erythema
   c. Conjuctivitis – non-specific
   d. Steven-Johnson syndrome
   e. Angioneurotic edema
   f. Blepharospasm (lorazepam)
3. Diplopia
4. Decreased corneal reflex (clorazepate, diazepam)
5. Extraocular muscles
   a. Nystagmus – horizontal or gaze evoked
   b. Decreased spontaneous movements
   c. Abnormal conjugate deviations
   d. Jerky pursuit movements
   e. Decreased saccadic movements
   f. Oculogyric crises
   g. Paralysis
6. Decreased accommodation
7. Decreased depth perception (chlordiazepoxide)
8. Visual hallucinations
9. Problems with color vision – color vision defect (lorazepam, oxazepam)
10. Photophobia
11. Abnormal EOG (diazepam)

Possible
1. Pupils
   a. Mydrasis – weak
   b. Decreased reaction to light
   c. Miosis (midazolam)
   d. May precipitate narrow angle glaucoma
2. Lacrimation
3. Non-specific ocular irritation
   a. Ocular pain
   b. Burning sensation
5. Subconjunctival or retinal hemorrhages secondary to drug-induced anemia
6. Loss of eyelashes or eyebrows (clonazepam)

Conditional/Unclassified
1. Brown lens opacification (diazepam)
2. Retinopathy (clonazepam)
3. Visual field defects (diazepam)

Ocular teratogenic effects
Probable
1. Increased incidences strabismus (diazepam)
2. Epicanthal folds (oxazepam, diazepam)
3. 'Slant eyes' (oxazepam, diazepam)

Clinical significance

Benzodiazepine derivatives are often used in combination with other drugs, so clear-cut drug-induced ocular side effects are difficult to determine. However, ocular side effects are seldom of clinical importance and most are reversible. At therapeutic dosage levels, these agents may cause decreased corneal reflex, decreased accommodation, decreased depth perception and abnormal extraocular muscle movements. Speeg-Schatz et al (2001) and others have shown that single dosage in susceptible individuals can cause phorias, diplopia and fusional impairment. There are reports in the National Registry that diplopia was severe enough to require discontinuing the drug. All drugs in this class appear to cross-react with allergic conjunctivitis since they have the metabolite desmethyldiazepam, a probably antigen, in common. This may give a type I immune reaction. Typically, the allergic conjunctivitis occurs within 30 minutes of taking the drug, with the peak reaction occurring within 4 hours and subsiding in 1 to 2 days. Symptoms include blurred vision, photophobia, burning, tearing and a foreign body sensation. Contact lens wearers have confused this adverse drug effect with poorly fitted lenses. To what degree these benzodiazepine derivatives cause pupillary dilatation is uncertain. There are cases in the literature (Kadoi et al 2000) and the National Registry of patients who developed a narrow-angle attack after receiving one of these drugs. This may be a chance event since these groups of drugs have minimal pupillary effect. The report of maculopathy secondary to gazing into a bright video camera light in two patients taking triazolam may or may not be a drug-enhanced photophic effect.

Diazepam taken over many years has been reported to cause the lens to become brown (Pau 1985) or in high dosage (100 mg) to cause significant visual field loss (Elder 1992).

REFERENCES AND FURTHER READING

Berlin RM, Conell LJ. Withdrawal symptoms after long-term treatment with therapeutic doses of flurazepam: A case report. Am J Psychiatry 140: 488, 1983.
Elder MJ. Diazepam and its effects on visual fields. Aust NZ J Ophthalmol 20: 267–270, 1992.
Gatzonis Karadimas P, Gatzonis Bouzas EA. Clonazepam associated retinopathy. Eur J Ophthalmol 13: 813–815, 2003.
Kadoi C, Hayasaka S, Tsukamoto E, et al. Bilateral angle closure glaucoma and visual loss precipitated by antidepressant and antianxiety agents in a patient with depression. Ophthalmologica 214: 360–361, 2000.
Laegreid L, et al. Teratogenic effects of benzodiazepine use during pregnancy. J Pediatr 114: 126–131, 1989.
Laroche J, Laroche C. Modification of colour vision. Ann Pharm Francaises 35: 5-6, 173–179, 1977.
Lutz EG. Allergic conjunctivitis due to diazepam. Am J Psychiatry 132(5): 548, 1975.
Marttila JK, et al. Potential untoward effects of long-term use of flurazepam in geriatric patients. J Am Pharm Assoc 17: 692, 1977.
Miyagawa M, Hayasaka S, Noda S. Photic maculopathy resulting from the light of a video camera in patients taking triazolam. Ophthalmologica 208(3): 145–146, 1994.
Nelson LB, et al. Occurrence of strabismus in infants born to drug-dependent women. Am J Dis Child 141: 175–178, 1987.
Noyes R, et al. A withdrawal syndrome after abrupt discontinuation of alprazolam. Am J Psychiatry 142: 114, 985.
Pau H. Braune scheibenförmige einlagerungen in die lines nach langzeitgabe von Diazepam (Valium). Klin Monatsbl Augenheilkd 187: 219–220, 1985.
Sandyk R. Orofacial dyskinesia associated with lorazepam therapy. Clin Pharm 5: 419, 1986.
Speeg-Schatz C, Giersch A, Boucart M, et al. Effects of lorazepam on vision and oculomotor balance. Binocular Vision Strabismus Q 16: 99–104, 2001.
Tyrer PJ, Seivewright N. Identification and management of benzodiazepine dependence. Postgrad Med J 60(Suppl. 2): 41, 1984.
Vital-Herne J, et al. Another case of alprazolam withdrawal syndrome. Am J Psychiatry 142: 1515, 1985.
Watanabe Y, Kawada A, Ohnishi Y, et al. Photosensitivity due to alprazolam with positive oral photochallenge test after 17 days administration. J Am Acad Dermatol 40: 832–833, 1999.

Generic names: 1. Carisoprodol; 2. meprobamate.

Proprietary names: 1. Soma; 2. Miltown, Tranmep.

Primary use
These agents are used to treat skeletal muscle spasms. In addition, meprobamate is used as a psychotherapeutic sedative in the treatment of nervous tension, anxiety and simple insomnia.

Ocular side effects

Systemic administration
Certain
1. Decreased accommodation
2. Decreased vision
3. Diplopia – extraocular muscle paresis
4. Eyelids or conjunctiva
   a. Allergic reactions
   b. Angioneurotic edema
   c. Urticaria
5. Random ocular movements

Possible
1. Decreased corneal reflex
2. Visual fields
   a. Constriction
   b. Enlargement
3. Non-specific ocular irritation
   a. Edema
   b. Burning sensation
4. Nystagmus
5. Subconjunctival or retinal hemorrhages secondary to drug-induced anemia
6. Eyelids or conjunctiva
   a. Erythema multiforme
   b. Stevens-Johnson syndrome
   c. Exfoliative dermatitis

Clinical significance
Significant ocular side effects due to these drugs are uncommon and transitory. At normal dosage levels decreased accommodation, diplopia and paralysis of extraocular muscles may only rarely be found. Carisoprodol has been associated with acute porphyria attacks and this needs to be considered if acute photophobia or eyelid reactions occur.

REFERENCES AND FURTHER READING

Barret LG, et al. Internuclear ophthalmoplegia in patients with toxic coma. Frequency, prognostic value, diagnostic significance. J Toxicol Clin Toxicol 20: 373, 1983.
Edwards JG. Adverse effects of antianxiety drugs. Drugs 22: 495, 1981.
Hermans G. Les Psychotropes. Bull Soc Belge Ophtalmol 160: 15, 1972.
McEvoy GK (ed). American Hospital Formulary Service Drug Information 87, American Society of Hospital Pharmacists, Bethesda, pp 1024–1026, 1146–1153, 1987.
Walsh FB, Hoyt WF. Clinical Neuro-Ophthalmology, 3rd edn, Vol. III, Williams & Wilkins, Baltimore, pp 2633–2634, 1969.

CLASS: ANTICONVULSANTS

Generic names: 1. Ethosuximide; 2. methsuximide.

Proprietary names: 1. Zarontin; 2. Celontin.

Primary use
These succinimides are effective in the management of petit mal seizures.

Ocular side effects

Systemic administration
Certain
1. Decreased vision
2. Photophobia
3. Myopia
4. Periorbital edema
5. Eyelids or conjunctiva
   a. Hyperemia
   b. Allergic reactions
   c. Angioneurotic edema
6. Visual hallucinations

Possible
1. Myasthenia gravis (aggravate)
   a. Diplopia
   b. Paresis of extraocular muscles
   c. Ptosis
2. Eyelids or conjunctiva
   a. Lupoid syndrome
   b. Erythema multiforme
   c. Stevens-Johnson syndrome
   d. Exfoliative dermatitis
3. Subconjunctival or retinal hemorrhages secondary to drug-induced anemia

Clinical significance
Methsuximide induces ocular side effects more frequently than ethosuximide or phensuximide. All adverse ocular reactions other than those due to anemias or dermatologic conditions are reversible after discontinuation of the drug. This group of drugs can trigger systemic lupus erythematosus by producing antinuclear antibodies. They may also aggravate myasthenia gravis.

REFERENCES AND FURTHER READING

Alarcón-Segovia D. Drug-induced antinuclear antibodies and lupus syndrome. Drugs 12: 69, 1976.
Beghi E, DiMascio R, Tognoni G. Adverse effects of anticonvulsant drugs – a critical review. Adverse Drug React Acute Poisoning Rev 5: 63, 1986.
Drug Evaluations, 6th edn, American Medical Association, Chicago, pp 72, 187, 1986.
Drugs for epilepsy. Med Lett Drugs Ther 25: 83, 1983.
Millichap JG. Anticonvulsant drugs. Clinical and electroencephalographic indications, efficacy and toxicity. Postgrad Med 37: 22, 1965.
Taaffe A, O'Brien C. A case of Stevens-Johnson syndrome associated with the anti-convulsants sulthiame and ethosuximide. Br Dent J 138: 172, 1975.
Walsh FB, Hoyt WF. Clinical Neuro-Ophthalmology, 3rd edn, Vol. III, Williams & Wilkins, Baltimore, p 2645, 1969.

Generic name: Ethotoin.

Proprietary name: Peganone.

Primary use
This hydantoins is effective in the management of psychomotor and grand mal seizures.

Ocular side effects

Systemic administration
Certain
1. Nystagmus
2. Photophobia
3. Eyelids or conjunctiva
   a. Allergic reactions
   b. Conjunctivitis – non-specific
   c. Angioneurotic edema
   d. Urticaria

Probable
1. Diplopia

Possible
1. Eyelids or conjunctiva
   a. Lupoid syndrome
   b. Erythema multiforme
   c. Stevens-Johnson syndrome
   d. Exfoliative dermatitis
   e. Lyell's syndrome
2. Subconjunctival or retinal hemorrhages secondary to drug-induced anemia

Clinical significance
Ocular side effects are seen more frequently with mephenytoin than with ethotoin, and are reversible either by decreasing the dosage or discontinuing use of the drug. As with phenytoin, nystagmus may persist for some time after the drug is stopped. Mephenytoin has been implicated in inducing systemic lupus erythematosus by producing antinuclear antibodies. Corneal or lens opacities and myasthenic neuromuscular blocking effect have not been proven as drug related.

REFERENCES AND FURTHER READING

Alarcón-Segovia D. Drug-induced antinuclear antibodies and lupus syndromes. Drugs 12: 69, 1976.
Gilman AG, Goodman LS, Gilman A (eds). The Pharmacological Basis of Therapeutics, 6th edn, Macmillan, New York, pp 455–456 1980.
Hermans G. Les anticonvulsivants. Bull Soc Belge Ophtalmol 160: 89, 1972.
Livingston S. Drug Therapy for Epilepsy. Charles C Thomas, Springfield, 1966.
Walsh FB, Hoyt WF. Clinical Neuro-Ophthalmology, 3rd edn, Vol. III, Williams & Wilkins, Baltimore, p 2644, 1969.

Generic name: Phenytoin.

Proprietary names: Cerebyx, Dilantin, Dilantin-125, Phenytek.

Primary use
This hydantoin is effective in the prophylaxis and treatment of chronic epilepsy.

Ocular side effects

Systemic administration
Certain
1. Nystagmus – downbeat, horizontal, or vertical
2. Decreased vision
3. Pupils
   a. Mydriasis
   b. Decreased reaction to light
4. Decreased accommodation
5. Decreased convergence
6. Visual hallucinations
7. Visual sensations
   a. Glare phenomenon – objects appear to be covered with white snow
   b. Flashing lights
   c. Oscillopsia
   d. Photophobia
8. Orbital or periorbital pain
9. Problems with color vision
   a. Objects have white tinge
   b. Colors appear faded
   c. Color vision abnormalities
10. Eyelids or conjunctiva
    a. Allergic reactions
    b. Ulceration
    c. Purpura
11. External ophthalmoplegia
12. ERG abnormalities

Probable
1. Myasthenia gravis
   a. Diplopia
   b. Ptosis
   c. Paresis of extraocular muscles

Possible
1. Subconjunctival or retinal hemorrhages secondary to drug-induced anemia
2. Papilledema secondary to pseudotumor cerebri
3. Cataracts
4. Eyelids or conjunctiva
   a. Lupoid syndrome
   b. Erythema multiforme
   c. Stevens-Johnson syndrome
   d. Exfoliative dermatitis
   e. Lyell's syndrome

Ocular teratogenic effects (fetal hydantoin syndrome)
Probable
1. Hypertelorism
2. Ptosis
3. Epicanthal fields
4. Strabismus
5. Retinal coloboma

Possible
1. Glaucoma
2. Optic nerve or iris hypoplasia
3. Retinoschisis
4. Trichomegaly
5. Abnormal lacrimal system
6. Congenital glaucoma

Clinical significance
Most ocular side effects due to phenytoin are reversible and often will decrease in extent or disappear with reduction in dosage. Phenytoin toxicity may be manifested as a syndrome of vestibular, cerebellar and/or ocular abnormalities. The ocular findings are most notably nystagmus and diplopia.

Nystagmus-induced phenytoin toxicity is directly related to the blood levels of the drug. Fine nystagmus may occur even at therapeutic dosages, but coarse nystagmus is indicative of toxic states. Downbeat and unidirectional gaze paretic nystagmus have also been reported. Instances of nystagmus persisting for 20 months or longer after discontinued use of phenytoin have been reported. Paralysis of extraocular muscles is uncommon, reversible and primarily found in toxic states. Remler et al (1990) have reported an idiosyncratic response in patients on carbamazepine and phenytoin with an increase in incidences of vertical and horizontal diplopia with or without oscillopsia. This appears to be a central effect on the vergence centers and/or the vestibulo-ocular reflex. A prodrome of ocular or systemic 'discomfort' frequently occurred prior to the onset of the above. Color vision changes are complex with various manifestations, including frosting or white tinges on objects, decreased brightness or specific color loss. Benign intracranial hypertension in a patient with a seizure disorder has been confirmed with phenytoin rechallenge. Bar et al (1983) and Mathers et al (1987) reported cases of presenile cataracts in patients on prolonged hydantoin therapy at toxic levels of phenytoin or with concomitant phenobarbital ingestion.

Phenytoin alone or in combination has a two to three times greater risk for delivering a child with congenital defects. Ocular abnormalities are not unusual in these deformities.

REFERENCES AND FURTHER READING

Bar S, Feller N, Savir N. Presenile cataracts in phenytoin-treated epileptic patients. Arch Ophthalmol 101: 422, 1983.

Bartoshesky LE, et al. Severe cardiac and ophthalmologic malformations in an infant exposed to diphenylhydantoin in utero. Pediatrics 69: 202, 1982.

Bayer A, Zrenner E, Thiel HJ, et al. Retinal disorders induced by anticonvulsant drugs. Third Congress, International Society of Ocular Toxicology, November 15–19, Sedona, Arizona, pp 11, 1992.

Bayer A, Thiel HJ, Zrenner E, et al. Sensitive physiologic perceptual tests for ocular side effects of drugs exempliflied by various anticonvulsants. Pediatrics 92(2): 182–190, 1995.

Boles DM. Phenytoin ophthalmoplegia. S Afr Med J 65: 546, 1984.

Glover SJ, Quinn AG, Barter P, et al. Ophthalmic findings in fetal anticonvulsant syndrome. Ophthalmology 109: 942–947, 2002.

Herishanu Y, Osimani A, Louzoun Z. Unidirectional gaze paretic nystagmus induced by phenytoin intoxication. Am J Ophthalmol 94: 122, 1982.

Kalanie H, et al. Phenytoin-induced intracranial hypertension. Neurology 36: 443, 1986.

Lachapelle P, Blain L, et al. The effect of diphenylhydantoin on the electroretinogram. Doc Ophthalmol 73: 359–368, 1990.

Mathers W, et al. Development of presenile cataracts in association with high serum levels of phenytoin. Ann Ophthalmol 19: 291, 1987.

Puri V, Chaudhry N. Total external ophthalmoplegia induced by phenytoin: a case report and review of literature. Neurol India 52: 386–387, 2004.

Remler BF, Leigh J, Osorio I, Tomsak RL. The characteristics and mechanisms of visual disturbance associated with anticonvulsant therapy. Neurology 40: 791–796, 1990.

Rizzo M, Corbett J. Bilateral internuclear ophthalmoplegia reversed by naloxone. Arch Neurol 40: 242, 1983.

Shores MM, Sloan KL. Phenytoin-induced visual disturbances misdiagnosed as alcohol withdrawal. Psychosomatics 43: 336–355, 2002.

Spaeth GL, Nelson LB, Beaudoin AR. Ocular teratology. In: Ocular Anatomy, Embryology and Teratology, Jakobiec FA (ed), J.B. Lippincott, Philadelphia, pp 955–981, 1982.

Wittbrodt ET. Drugs and myasthenia gravis: an update. Arch Intern Med 157: 399–408, 1997.

Generic names: 1. Sodium valproate; 2. valproate semisodium; 3. valproic acid.

Proprietary names: 1. Depacon; 2. Depakote; 3. Depakene, myproic acid.

Primary use

Valproic acid is a carboxylic acid derivative, and sodium valproate is the sodium salt of valproic acid. Valproate semisodium is a compound comprised of sodium valproate and valproic acid. These antiepileptic agents are used in the prophylactic management of petit mal seizures.

Ocular side effects

Systemic administration
Certain
1. Blurred vision
2. Diplopia
3. Nystagmus
4. Oscillopsia
5. Visual hallucinations

Possible
1. Non-specific ocular irritation
   a. Ocular pain
   b. Photophobia
2. Eyelids or conjunctiva
   a. Stevens-Johnson syndrome
   b. Toxic epidermal necrolysis
   c. Conjunctivitis
3. Subconjunctival or retinal hemorrhages secondary to drug-induced hemopoietic abnormalities

Conditional/Unclassified
1. Intracranial hypertension

Ocular teratogenic effects – fetal anticonvulsant syndrome
Certain
1. Myopia

Probable
1. Hypoplastic front – orbital edges
2. Proptosis
3. Depigmentation of eyelashes and eyebrows
4. Epicanthus
5. Shallow orbitals
6. Septo-optic dysplasia

Clinical significance

All three agents appear to have identical adverse ocular side effects. Compared to placebo, in clinical trials by the manufacturers all three drugs caused diplopia, blurred vision and nystagmus. There may be an idiosyncratic susceptibility in some patients characterized by various forms of diplopia, oscillopsia, impaired vergence mechanisms, vertical nystagmus or abnormalities of the vestibular-ocular reflex due to these drugs. Other side effects include ocular motor abnormalities involving pursuit and gaze holding patterns. Based on animal work, this group of drugs may have some effect on the retinal pigment epithelium. A 14-year-old showed retinal pigment epithelial changes while on valproic acid, but there are no other clinical data to support this. Bayer et al (1997) feel that based on psychophysical testing, valproic acid has no effect on retinal function. There are nine cases in the National Registry of mydriasis being caused by this agent, but this is unproven.

Valproic acid has many ocular teratogenic effects, especially myopia. Glover et al reviewed the 'fetal anticonvulsant syndrome'. Boyle et al (2001) reported decreased corneal sensation and severe dry eyes in a child with a fetal valproate syndrome. While intracranial hypertension has been associated with these drugs, this remains unproven.

REFERENCES AND FURTHER READING

Bayer AU, Thiel HJ, Zrenner E, et al. Color vision tests for early detection of antiepileptic drug toxicity. Neurology 48(5): 1394–1397, 1997.

Bellman MH, Ross EM. Side effects of sodium valproate. BMJ 1: 1662, 1977.

Boyle NJ, Clark MP, Figueiredo F. Reduced corneal sensation and severe dry eyes in a child with fetal valproate syndrome. Eye 15: 661–662, 2001.

Filteau MJ, Leblanc J, Lefrancoise S, Demers MF. Visual and auditory hallucinations with the association of bupropion and valproate. Can J Psychiatry 45: 198–199, 2000.

Glover SJ, Quinn AG, Barter P, et al. Ophthalmic findings in fetal anticonvulsant syndrome. Ophthalmology 109: 942–947, 2002.

McEvoy GK (ed). American Hospital Formulary Service Drug Information 87, American Society of Hospital Pharmacists, Bethesda, pp 1042–1045, 1987.

McMahon CL, Braddock SR. Septo-optic dysplasia as a manifestation of valproic acid embryopathy. Teratology 64: 83–86, 2001.

Remler BF, Leigh RJ, Osoria I, et al. The characteristics and mechanisms of visual disturbances associated with anticonvulsant therapy. Neurology 40: 791–796, 1990.

Scullica L, Trombetta CJ, Tuccari G. Toxic effect of valproic acid on the retina. Clinical and experimental investigation. In: Acta XXV Concilium Opthalmologicum, Blodi F, et al (eds), Proceedings of the XXVth International Congress of Ophthalmology, Vol. 2, Rome, May 4–10, 1986, Kugler & Ghedini Publishers, 1988.

Uddin S. Drug-induced pseudotumor cerebri. Clin Neuropharmacol 26: 236–238, 2003.

Generic name: Topiramate.

Proprietary name: Topamax.

Primary use

Topiramate is a novel agent used to treat patients with various types of epilepsy and migraine headaches. It is used off-label as a 'magic' weight-reduction medication, in bipolar disorder and in clinical depression.

Ocular side effects

Systemic administration
Certain
1. Acute glaucoma (mainly bilateral)
2. Anterior chamber shallowing
3. Ocular hyperemia
4. Increased intraocular pressure
5. Mydriasis
6. Suprachoroidal effusions
7. Visual field defects
8. Non-specific ocular irritation
   a. Ocular pain
9. Decreased vision
10. Acute myopia (up to 6–8.5 diopters)
11. Nystagmus
12. Diplopia
13. Palinopsia

Probable
1. Myokymia
2. Blepharospasm
3. Oculogyric crisis
4. Uveitis

Possible
1. Periorbital edema
2. Scleritis
3. Retinal bleeds

Ocular teratogenic effects
Possible
1. Ocular malformations

Clinical significance

Banta et al first reported a case of uveal effusion and secondary angle closure glaucoma associated with topiramate. This has now developed into a well-recognized syndrome. This usually occurs within the first 2 weeks after starting topiramate therapy. In some cases, it develops within hours after doubling the dosage. Almost all cases are bilateral acute secondary angle-closure glaucoma. The syndrome may include the typical findings of acute glaucoma, including acute ocular pain, headache, nausea and vomiting, papillary changes, hyperemia, corneal edema, cataract, retinal and vascular accidents, visual field defect and, if not recognized soon enough, blindness. A few cases of scleritis have been reported but this may be more common than recognized since the glaucoma-induced hyperemia may mask the signs of scleritis. Suprachoroidal effusions have been reported by Rhee et al (2001) and others and should be looked for as the cause of the glaucoma. These effusions cause a forward rotation of the ciliary processes and therefore angle closure. These effusions along with the acute pressure elevation may cause uveitis.

Topiramate is a sulfa drug, a class that is known to cause transient myopia. Acute myopia up to 8.5 diopters may occur in a matter of hours after starting this drug; however, it may take a number of weeks to resolve once the drug is discontinued. Causation is not fully known, but includes lenticular swelling, forward rotation of the iris and lens diaphragm, cilliary body swelling causing increased curvature of the lens surface, and spasms of accommodation. Evans (2006) reported two well-documented cases with multiple positive rechallenge and clearly a positive dose reponse curve of reversible palinopsia after taking topiramate. Diplopia and nystagmus are seen primarily in high dosages and the mechanism is unknown. However, other neurologic muscular defects such as myokymia, oculogryric chrisis, and blepharospasms have been reported. Foroozan and Buono (2003) reported a single case of homonomous hemianopia. Vaphaiades and Mason (2004) reported a single case of bilateral pigmentary retinopathy due to this drug. There are no cases of either in the National Registry.

Recommendations (Fraunfelder, Fraunfelder and Keates)

1. The patient should stop the medication in concert with the prescribing physician since dropping the drug by as little as 50 mg may exacerbate the preexisting systemic disease.
2. Institute maximum medical therapy for glaucoma, including topical ocular cycloplegic agents along with topical beta-blockers and oral pressure lowering agents.
3. Laser iridotomy or peripheral iridectomy are probably not beneficial as they do not resolve the supra choroidal effusions.
4. Topical ocular miotics are probably contraindicated since they may precipitate a relative papillary block.

REFERENCES AND FURTHER READING

Banta JT, Hoffman K, Budenz DL, et al. Presumed topiramate-induced bilateral acute angle-closure glaucoma. Am J Ophthalmol 132: 112–114, 2001.

Chen TC, Chao CW, Sorkin JA. Topiramate induced myopic shift and angle closure glaucoma. Br J Ophthalmol 87: 648–649, 2003.

Craig JE, Ong TJ, Louis DL, Wells JM. Mechanism of topiramate-induced actue-onset myopia and angle closure glaucoma. Am J Ophthalmol 137: 193–195, 2004.

Evans RW. Reversible palinopsia and the Alice in Wonderland syndrome associated with topiramate use in migraineurs. Headache 46: 815–817, 2006.

Foroozan R, Buono LM. Foggy visual field defect. Survey Ophthalmol 48: 447–451, 2003.

Fraunfelder FW, Fraunfelder FT, Keates EU. Topiramate-associated acute bilateral secondary angle-closure glaucoma. Ophthalmology 111: 109–111, 2004.

Hulihan J. Important drug warning [letter]. Available at: http://www.fda.gov/medwatch/SAFETY/2001/topamax_deardoc.PDF. Accessed April 17, 2003.

Mansoor Q, Jain S. Bilateral angle-closure glaucoma following oral topiramate therapy. Acta Ophthalmol Scand 83: 627–628, 2005.

Medeiros FA, Zhang XY, Bernd AS, Weinreb RN. Angle-closure glaucoma associated with ciliary body detachment in patients using topiramate. Arch Ophthalmol 121: 282–284, 2003.

Rhee DJ, Goldbery MJ, Parrish RK. Bilateral angle-closure glaucoma and ciliary body swelling from topiramate. Arch Ophthalmol 119: 1721–1723, 2001.

Sakai H, Morine-Shiniyo S, Shinzato M, et al. Uveal effusion in primary angle-closure glaucoma. Ophthalmology 112: 413–419, 2005.

Sankar PS, Pasquale LR, Grosskreutz CL. Uveal effusion and secondary angle-closure glaucoma associated with topiramate use. Arch Ophthalmol 119: 1210–1211, 2001.

Sen HA, O'Halloran HS, Lee WB. Topiramate-induced acute myopia and retinal striae. Arch Ophthalmol 119: 775–777, 2001.

Thambi L, Leonard KP, Chambers W, et al. Topiramate-associated secondary angle-closure glaucoma: a case series. Arch Ophthalmol 120: 1108, 2002.

Vaphiades MS, Mason J. Foggy visual field defect [letter]. Survey Ophthalmol 4: 266–297, 2004.

Generic name: Zonisamide.

Proprietary name: Zonegran.

Primary use

This sulfonamide derivative is used as a broad spectrum anti-epileptic medication.

Ocular side effects

Systemic administration
Certain
1. Decreased vision

Probable
1. Nystagmus
2. Diplopia
3. Visual hallucination

Possible
1. Acute glaucoma (mainly bilateral)
2. Decreased anterior chamber
3. Increased ocular pressure
4. Pupils – mydriasis
5. Suprachoroidal effusions
6. Visual field defects – acute glaucoma

7. Non-specific ocular irritation
   a. Ocular pain
   b. Photophobia
8. Acute myopia
9. Eyelids or conjunctiva
   a. Chemosis
   b. Congestion
   c. Stevens-Johnson syndrome
   d. Toxic epidermal necrolysis
10. Subconjunctival or retinal hemorrhages secondary to drug-induced anemia

Clinical significance

This sulfonamide derivative can possibly cause most of the sulfonamide ocular side effects. There are two cases in the National Registry of possible choroidal effusions and secondary narrow-angle glaucoma (see topiramate). The blurred vision may be secondary to the drug being secreted in the tears, which can be associated with hyperemia, chemosis and photophobia. Hypersensitivity and cross-hypersensitivity with other sulfonamides have been reported along with Stevens-Johnson syndrome and toxic epidermal necrolysis. Numerous cases in the National Registry and data in the package insert support the side effects of diplopia and nystagmus secondary to zonisamide. Except for skin and hematological disorders, the ocular side effects are reversible when the drug is discontinued.

REFERENCES AND FURTHER READING

Akman CI, Goodkin HP, Rogers DP, Riviello JJ Jr. Visual hallucinations associated with zonisamide. Pharmacotherapy 23: 93–96, 2003.

Majeres KD, Suppes T. A cautionary note when using zonisamide in youths: a case report of association with toxic epidermal necrolysis. J Clin Psychiatry 65: 1720, 2004.

Physcians' Desk Reference, Thomson PDR, Montevale NJ, pp 1089–1092, 2006.

CLASS: ANTIDEPRESSANTS

Generic names: 1. Amitriptyline; 2. desipramine hydrochloride; 3. nortriptyline hydrochloride.

Proprietary names: 1. Generic only; 2. Norpramin; 3. Aventyl hydrochloride, Pamelor.

Primary use

These tricyclic antidepressants and tranquilizers are effective in the relief of symptoms of mental depression.

Ocular side effects

Systemic administration
Probable
1. Decreased or blurred vision
2. Decreased or paralysis of accommodation
3. Pupils – mydriasis (weak)
4. Photophobia
5. Visual hallucinations
6. Eyelids or conjunctiva
   a. Erythema
   b. Edema
   c. Photosensitivity
   d. Urticaria
   e. Purpura
   f. Increased blink rate

Possible

1. Aggravates keratitis sicca

Conditional/Unclassified

1. Upbeat nystagmus on drug withdrawal (amitriptyline)
2. Precipitate narrow-angle glaucoma
3. Induce phorias

Clinical significance

Adverse ocular reactions due to these tricyclic antidepressants are reversible, transitory and seldom of clinical significance. There are numerous reports of transitory decreased vision, decreased accommodation and slight mydriasis. While spontaneous reporting systems contain a few cases of precipitation of narrow-angle glaucoma (primarily amitriptyline), this may be difficult to sort out from emotionally induced mydriasis. These agents should have no effect on glaucoma except in very shallow anterior chamber angles. In patients with already compromised tear production, these drugs may have the potential to aggravate latent or manifested keratoconjunctivitis sicca. Drugs that cause dry mouth have the potential to aggravate ocular sicca. Drugs that have a sedative effect may exacerbate phoria, but only in overdose situations have tropias been reported. The clinician needs to be aware that tricyclic antidepressants potentiate the systemic blood pressure elevation from topical ocular epinephrine preparations. Osborne and Vivian (2004) reported a case of upbeat nystagmus occurring after stopping amitriptyline.

Recommendations

Roberts et al (1992) recommend sunblocking ocular protection for patients placed on imipramine, since it is a photosensitizer for the lens, with peak absorption above that which the cornea filters out. They recommend that when working ouside the home patients on this drug should consider wearing UV blocking glasses that protect to at least 320 nm.

REFERENCES AND FURTHER READING

Beal MF. Amitriptyline ophthalmoplegia. Neurology 32: 1409, 1982.

Blackwell B, et al. Anticholinergic activity of two tricyclic antidepressants. Am J Psychiatry 135: 722, 1978.

Delaney P, Light R. Gaze paresis in amitriptyline overdose. Ann Neurol 9: 513, 1981.

Hotson JR, Sachdev HS. Amitriptyline: Another cause of internuclear ophthalmoplegia with coma. Ann Neurol 12: 62, 1982.

Karson CN. Oculomotor signs in a psychiatric population: a preliminary report. Am J Psychiatry 136: 1057, 1979.

Osborne SF, Vivian AJ. Primary position upbeat nystagmus associated with amitriptyline use. Eye 18: 106, 2004.

Pulst SM, Lombroso CT. External ophthalmoplegia, alpha and spindle coma in imipramine overdose: case report and review of the literature. Ann Neurol 14: 587, 1983.

Roberts JE, Reme CE, Dillon J, et al. Bright light exposure and the concurrent use of photosensitizing drugs. N Engl J Med 326(22): 1500–1501, 1992.

Spector RH, Schnapper R. Amitriptyline-induced ophthalmoplegia. Neurology 31: 1188, 1981.

Von Knorring K. Changes in saliva secretion and accommodation width during short-term administration of imipramine and zimelidine in healthy volunteers. Int Pharmacopsych 16: 69, 1981.

Vonvoigtlander PF, Kolaja GJ, Block EM. Corneal lesions induced by antidepressants: a selective effect upon young Fischer 344 rats. J Pharmacol Exp Ther 222: 282, 1982.

Walter-Ryan WG, et al. Persistent photoaggravated cutaneous eruption induced by imipramine. JAMA 254: 357, 1985.

Generic names: 1. Amoxapine; 2. clomipramine hydrochloride; 3. doxepin hydrochloride; 4. trimipramine.

Proprietary names: 1. Generic only; 2. Anafranil; 3. Sinequan, Zonalon; 4. Surmontil.

Primary use

These tricyclic antidepressants are used in the treatment of psychoneurotic anxiety or depressive reactions.

Ocular side effects

Systemic administration

Certain

1. Decreased vision
2. Mydriasis
3. Decreased accommodation
4. Suppression of rapid eye movement in sleep (clomipramine)

Possible

1. Eyelids or conjunctiva
   a. Erythema
   b. Edema
   c. Photosensitivity
   d. Urticaria
   e. Pigmentation
   f. Blepharospasm
   g. Lyell's syndrome
2. Extraocular muscles
   a. Oculogyric crises
   b. Nystagmus – horizontal or rotary – toxic states
   c. Paresis or paralysis – toxic states
   d. Abnormal conjugate deviations (amoxapine)
3. Visual hallucinations
4. Aggravates keratitis sicca

Clinical significance

Adverse ocular reactions due to these tricyclic antidepressants are seldom of major clinical importance. Ocular anticholinergic effects are the most frequent and include blurred vision, which may require decreasing the dosage, disturbance of accommodation and mydriasis. There have been reports to the National Registry of keratoconjunctivitis sicca associated with the use of these agents, but this is not proven. Since they do cause a dry mouth, the association may be real. Since these tricyclic antidepressants may be bound to ocular melanin, there is a potential for retinal damage. A few cases of retinal pigment abnormalities have been reported to the National Registry, but no definitive relationship has been established. Kupfer et al (1994) have shown that clomipramine suppresses rapid eye movement (REM) during sleep.

REFERENCES AND FURTHER READING

Barnes FF. Precipitation of mania and visual hallucinations by amoxapine hydrochloride. Compr Psychiatry 23: 590, 1982.

Botter PA, Sunier A. The treatment of depression in geriatrics with Anafranil. J Int Med Res 3: 345, 1975.

D'Arcy PF. Disorders of the eye. In: Iatrogenic Diseases, 2nd edn, D'Arcy PF, Griffin JP (eds), Oxford University Press, Oxford, pp 162–168, 1983.

Donhowe SP. Bilateral internuclear ophthalmoplegia from doxepin overdose. Neurology 34: 259, 1984.

Horstl H, Pohlmann-Eden B. Amplitudes of somatosensory evoked potentials reflect cortical hyperexcitability in antidepressant-induced myoclonus. Neurology 40: 924–926, 1990.

Hughes IW. Adverse reactions in perspective, with special reference to gastrointestinal side-effects of clomipramine (Anafranil). J Int Med Res 1: 440, 1973.

Hunt-Fugate AK, et al. Adverse reactions due to dopamine blockade by amoxapine. Pharmacotherapy 4: 35–39, 1984.

Kupfer DJ, Pollock BG, Perel JM, et al. Effect of pulse loading with clomipramide on EEG sleep. Psychiatry Res 54(2): 161–175, 1994.

LeWitt PA. Transient ophthalmoparesis with doxepin overdosage. Ann Neurol 9: 618, 1981.

Litovitz TL, Troutman WG. Amoxapine overdose. Seizures and fatalities. JAMA 250: 1069, 1983.

Micev V, Marshall WK. Undesired effects in slow intravenous infusion of clomipramine (Anafranil). J Int Med Res 1: 451, 1973.

Schenck CH, Mahowald MW, Kim SW, et al. Prominent eye movements during NREM sleep and REM sleep behavior disorder associated with fluoxetine treatment of depression and obsessive-compulsive disorder. Sleep 15(3): 226–235, 1992.

Steele TE. Adverse reactions suggesting amoxapine-induced dopamine blockade. Am J Psychiatry 139: 1500, 1982.

Generic name: Carbamazepine.

Proprietary names: Carbatrol, Epitol, Equetro, Tegretol, Tegretol-XR, Teril.

Primary use

This iminostilbene derivative is used in the treatment of pain associated with trigeminal neuralgia.

Ocular side effects

Systemic administration
Certain
1. Extraocular muscles
   a. Diplopia
   b. Downbeat or horizontal nystagmus
   c. Oculogyric crises – toxic states
   d. Decreased spontaneous movements
   e. Paralysis – toxic states
   f. Ophthalmoplegia
2. Decreased vision
3. Visual hallucinations
4. Eyelids or conjunctiva
   a. Photosensitivity, increased glare
   b. Allergic reactions
   c. Conjunctivitis – non-specific
   d. Edema
   e. Urticaria
   f. Blepharoclonus
   g. Purpura
5. Color vision – decreased blue perception
6. Decreased accommodation
7. Decreased convergence

Possible
1. Subconjunctival or retinal hemorrhages secondary to drug-induced anemia
2. Myasthenia gravis
   a. Diplopia
   b. Ptosis
   c. Paresis of extraocular muscles

3. Eyelids or conjunctiva
   a. Erythema multiforme
   b. Stevens-Johnson syndrome
   c. Exfoliative dermatitis
   d. Lyell's syndrome
   e. Lupoid syndrome

Conditional/Unclassified
1. Cataracts
   a. Punctate cortical
   b. Anterior and posterior sub-capsular
2. Retinal pigmentary change

Ocular teratogenic effects
Certain
1. Anophthalmos
2. Microphthalmos
3. Optic disc coloboma
4. Optic nerve hypoplasia

Clinical significance

The most common side effects due to carbamazepine are ocular, with transitory diplopia being the most frequent, followed by blurred vision and a 'heavy feeling in the eyes.' Ocular adverse reactions are reversible, usually disappear as the dosage is decreased and may spontaneously clear even without reduction of the drug dosage. A toxic syndrome may occur as an acute phenomenon with downbeat nystagmus, confusion, drowsiness and ataxia. Bayer et al (1995a) pointed out that patients complain of increased glare and have a blue color deficiency. This drug can also cause the ocular effects of lupus erythematosus. Carbamazepine can be recovered in the tears, and this method has been advocated to test for blood levels as a non-invasive technique in the pediatric age group.

The cataractogenic potential of this agent is still open to debate. While Neilsen and Syversen (1986) first postulated this association, this has not been proven. The National Registry, however, has 30+ possible cases. Neilsen and Syversen (1986) reported two patients with retinotoxicity attributed to long-term therapeutic use of carbamazepine and while a few cases have been reported to the National Registry, there is no proven association. This drug interacts with multiple other drugs causing visual side effects. Toxic reactions in overdosage situations possibly cause dilated sluggish or non-reactive pupils and papilledema. There are a number of reports of a fetal carbamazepine syndrome, which may include ocular abnormalities (Glover et al 2002; Sutcliffe et al 1998).

REFERENCES AND FURTHER READING

Bayer A, Thiel HJ, Zrenner E, et al. Sensitive physiologic perceptual tests for ocular side effects of drugs exemplified by various anticonvulsants. [German] ophthalmologe 92: 182–190, 1995a.

Bayer A, Thiel HJ, Zrenner E, et al. Disorders of color perception and increased glare sensitivity in phenytoin and carbamazepine therapy. Ocular side effects of anticonvulsants. [German] Nervenarzt 66: 89–96, 1995b.

Breathnach SM, et al. Carbamazepine ('Tegretol') and toxic epidermal necrolysis: report of three cases with histopathological observations. Clin Exp Dermatol 7: 585, 1982.

Chrousos GA, et al. Two cases of downbeat nystagmus and oscillopsia associated with carbamazepine. Am J Ophthalmol 103: 221, 1987.

Delafuente JC. Drug-induced erythema multiforme: a possible immunologic pathogenesis. Drug Intell Clin Pharm 19: 114, 1985.

Glover SJ, Quinn AG, Barter P, et al. Ophthalmic findings in fetal anticonvulsant syndrome(s). Ophthalmology 109: 942–947, 2002.

Goldman MJ, Shultz-Ross RA. Adverse ocular effects of anticonvulsants. Psychosomatics 34: 154–158, 1993.

Gualtieri CT, Evans RW. Carbamazepine-induced tics. Dev Med Child Neurol 26: 546, 1984.

Kinoshita A, Kitaoka T, Oba K, Amemiya T. Bilateral drug-induced cataract in patient receiving anticonvulsant therapy. Jpn J Ophthalmol 48: 81–82, 2004.

Kurian MA, King MD. Antibody positive myasthenia gravis following treatment with carbamazepine – a chance association? Neuropediatrics 34: 276–277, 2003.

Mullally WJ. Carbamazepine-induced ophthalmoplegia. Arch Neurol 39: 64, 1982.

Neilsen N, Syversen K. Possible retinotoxic effect of carbamazepine. Acta Ophthalmol 64: 287, 1986.

Noda S, Umezaki H. Carbamazepine-induced ophthalmoplegia. Neurology 32: l320, 1982.

Ponte CD. Carbamazepin-induced thrombocytopenia, rash and hepatic dysfunction. Drug Intell Clin Pharm 17: 642–644, 1983.

Rasmussen M. Carbamazepine and myasthenia gravis. Neuropediatrics 35: 259, 2004.

Silverstein FS, Parrish MA, Johnston MV. Adverse behavioral reactions in children treated with carbamazepine (Tegretol). J Pediatr 101: 785, 1982.

Smith H, Newton R. Adverse reactions to carbamazepine managed by desensitization. Lancet 1: 785, 1985.

Sullivan JB, Rumack BH, Peterson RG. Acute carbamazepine toxicity resulting from overdose. Neurology 31: 621, 1981.

Sutcliffe AG, Jones RB, Woodruff G. Eye malformations associated with treatment with carbamazepine during pregnancy. Ophthalmic Genet 19: 59–62, 1998.

Tedeschi G, Gasucci G, Allocca S, et al. Neuro-ocular side effects of carbamazepine and phenobarbital in epileptic patients as measured by saccadic eye movements analysis. Epilepsia 30(1): 62–66, 1989.

West J, Burke JP, Stachan I. Carbamazepine, epilepsy, and optic nerve hypoplasia. Br J Ophthalmol 74: 511, 1990.

Wheller SD, Ramsey RE, Weiss J. Drug-induced downbeat nystagmus. Ann Neurol 12: 227, 1982.

Generic names: 1. Citalopram hydrobromide; 2. fluoxetine hydrochloride; 3. fluvoxamine maleate; 4. paroxetine hydrochloride; 5. sertaline.

Proprietary names: 1. Celexa; 2. Prozac, Sarafem; 3. Generic only; 4. Paxil, Paxil CR; 5. Zoloft.

Primary use

These selective inhibitors of serotonin re-uptake are used as antidepressants. They are chemically unrelated to tricyclic, tetracyclic or other available antidepressant agents, and are reported to cause fewer antimuscarinic side effects than tricyclic antidepressants.

Ocular side effects

Systemic administration
Certain
1. Blurred vision
2. Photophobia
3. Increased eye movement during sleep (NREM) (fluoxetine)
4. Abnormal ocular sensations (paroxetine)

Probable
1. Keratitis sicca
2. Pupil
   a. Mydrasis
   b. Anisocoria
3. Increased intraocular pressure (minimal)

Possible
1. Conjunctivitis – non-specific
2. Diplopia

3. Eyelids
   a. Tics
   b. Rash
   c. Urticaria
   d. Angioneurotic edema

Conditional/Unclassified
1. Activation of ocular herpes (fluoxetine)

Clinical significance

This group of selective serotonin reuptake inhibitors (SSRI) is one of the most commonly prescribed antidepressant drugs in the world because of its favorable safety profile. While ocular side effects are few and rare, they may be of clinical importance. Costagliola et al (1996, 2004) in a 20-patient double-blind crossover study showed that all 20 patients had subclinical intraocular pressure elevations within 2 hours of oral ingestion. Some eyes remained elevated for up to 8 hours. This was also found with other SSRI drugs such as citalopram, fluvoxamine (Jiménez-Jiménez et al 2001), paroxetine (Eke and Carr 1998) and sertraline. While the authors cannot prove an association, they strongly implied causation. Further studies are indicated, but very rare precipitation of narrow-angle glaucoma might occur (Ahmad 1991). Clinical trials against placebo shows that blurred vision and dry mouth are significant. It is probable that all drugs that cause dry mouth can aggravate or possibly cause ocular sicca.

There are a number of positive rechallenge cases of photophobia in the National Registry. Schenck et al (1992) have shown that fluoxetine can cause extensive, prominent eye movements during non-rapid eye movement sleep (NREM). In one case, this continued for 19 months after the drug was discontinued. While diplopia, ptosis and nystagmus have been seen, it is hard to prove a direct cause-and-effect relationship since these patients are often on multiple drugs. Armitage et al (1995) reported that fluoxetine could cause these findings since it causes increased availability of serotonin with secondary dopaminergic effects. Wakeno et al (2006) described three patients who, after discontinuing paroxetine, developed abnormal ocular sensations with eye movement. This occurred within 3–6 days after the drug was stopped and disappeared as soon as the drug was restarted. There are two cases in the National Registry of possible drug-induced myopia of up to 3 diopters. A series of three cases of reactivation of genital herpes has been attributed to fluoxetine; however, no cases of reactivation of ocular herpes have been reported. The SSRIs probably have a weak mydriatic effect. For some unknown reason, this may be unilateral, as Barrett (1994) reports, and we confirm this with three additional cases in the National Registry.

REFERENCES AND FURTHER READING

Ahmad S. Fluoxetine and glaucoma. DICP Ann Pharmacother 25: 436, 1991.

Anonymous. SSRIs and increased intraocular pressure. Aust Adverse Drug React Bull 20: 3, 2001.

Armitage R, Trivedi M, Rush AJ. Fluoxetine and oculomotor activity during sleep in depressed patients. Neuropsychopharmacology 12(2): 159–165, 1995.

Barrett J. Anisocoria associated with selective serotonin reuptake inhibitors. BMJ 309: 1620, 1994.

Beasley CM, Koke SC, Nilsson ME, Gonzales JS. Adverse events and treatment discontinuations in clinical trials of fluoxetine in major depressive disorder: an updated meta-analysis. Clin Ther 22: 1319–1330, 2000.

Costagliola C, et al. Fluoxetine oral administration increases intraocular pressure. Br J Ophthalmol 80: 678, 1996.

Costagliola C, Parmeggiani F, Sebastiani A. SSRIs and intraocular pressure modifications: evidence, therapeutic implications and possible mechanisms. CNS Drugs 18: 475–484, 2004.

Cunningham M, Cunningham K, Lydiard RB. Eye tics and subjective hearing impairment during fluoxetine therapy. Am J Psychiatry 147: 947–948, 1990.

Eke T, Carr S. Acute glaucoma, chronic glaucoma, and serotoninergic drugs. Br J Ophthalmol 82: 976–977, 1998.

Heiligenstein JH, Faries DE, Rush AJ, et al. Latency to rapid eye movement sleep as a predictor of treatment response to fluoxetine and placebo in non-psychotic depressed outpatients. Psychiatry Res 52(3): 327–329, 1994.

Jiménez-Jiménez FJ, Ortí-Pareja M, Zurdo JM. Aggravation of glaucoma with fluvoxamine. Ann Pharmacother 35: 1565–1566, 2001.

Ozkul Y, Bozlar S. Effects of Fluoxetine on habituation of pattern reversal visually evoked potentials in migraine prophylaxis. Headache 42: 582–587, 2002.

Reed SM, Glick GW. Fluoxetine and reactivation of the herpes simplex virus. Am J Psychiatry 148: 949–950, 1991.

Schenck CH, Mahowald MW, Kim SW, et al. Prominent eye movements during NREM sleep and REM sleep behavior disorder associated with fluoxetine treatment of depression and obsessive-compulsive disorder. Sleep 15(3): 226–235, 1992.

Wakeno M, Kato M, Takekita Y, et al. A series of case reports on abnormal sensation on eye movement associated with Paroxetine discontinuation. Inter Clin Psychopharmacol 21: A29–A30, 2006.

drug. Pupillary reactions occur primarily in overdose situations. Nystagmus has been associated with phenelzine or tranylcypromine, and visual hallucinations by phenelzine therapy.

REFERENCES AND FURTHER READING

Drugs for psychiatric disorders. Med Lett Drugs Ther 25: 45, 1983.

Drugs that cause photosensitivity. Med Lett Drugs Ther 28: 51, 1986.

Kaeser HE. Drug-induced myasthenic syndromes. Acta Neurol Scand 70(Suppl. 100): 39, 1984.

Kaplan RF, et al. Phenelzine overdose treated with dantrolene sodium. JAMA 255: 642, 1986.

Shader RI, Greenblatt DJ. The reappearance of a monamine oxidase inhibitor. J Clin Psychopharmacol 19(2): 105–106, 1999.

Thomann P, Hess R. Toxicology of antidepressant drugs. Handbk Exp Pharmacol 55: 527, 1980.

Weaver KEC. Amoxapine overdose. J Clin Psychiatry 46: 545, 1985.

Zaratzian VL. Psychotropic drugs – neurotoxicity. Clin Toxicol 17: 231, 1980.

Generic names: 1. Isocarboxazid; 2. phenelzine; 3. tranylcypromine.

Proprietary names: 1. Marplan; 2. Nardil; 3. Parnate.

Primary use
These monoamine oxidase inhibitors are used in the symptomatic relief of reactive or endogenous depression.

Ocular side effects

Systemic administration
Certain
1. Visual hallucinations (phenelzine)

Probable
1. Decreased vision
2. Mydriasis (primarily overdose)
3. Extraocular muscles
   a. Diplopia
   b. Nystagmus (phenelzine, tranylcypromine)
   c. Strabismus
4. Myasthenia gravis
   a. Diplopia
   b. Ptosis
   c. Paresis of extraocular muscles
5. Photophobia
6. Problems with color vision – color vision defect, red-green defect
7. Eyelids – photosensitivity
8. Visual field defects (tranylcypromine)

Possible
1. Subconjunctival or retinal hemorrhages secondary to drug-induced anemia
2. Eyelids or conjunctiva – lupoid syndrome

Clinical significance
Ocular side effects due to these monoamine oxidase inhibitors are reversible and usually insignificant. All of these drugs may cause blurred vision, which only rarely requires stopping of the

Generic names: Maprotiline.

Proprietary name: Generic only.

Primary use
This tetracyclic antidepressant is used in the treatment of depression.

Ocular side effects

Systemic administration
Certain
1. Decreased vision
2. Decreased accommodation
3. Visual hallucinations
4. Mydriasis – may precipitate narrow-angle glaucoma

Probable
1. Eyelids or conjunctiva
   a. Erythema
   b. Conjunctivitis – non-specific
   c. Edema
   d. Photosensitivity
   e. Angioneurotic edema
   f. Urticaria

Possible
1. Subconjunctival or retinal hemorrhages secondary to drug-induced anemia
2. Eyelids or conjunctiva – erythema multiforme

Conditional/Unclassified
1. Palinopsia
2. Illusory visual spread

Clinical significance
Adverse ocular reactions due to these tetracyclic antidepressants are seldom of major clinical significance. Anticholinergic effects are the most frequent and include blurred vision, disturbance of accommodation and mydriasis. Several instances of increased intraocular pressure have been reported to the National Registry following pupillary dilatation in patients on maprotiline. Visual hallucinations are usually associated with drug overdosage.

Myoclonus can be seen in other muscles, so one can expect to see this in periocular muscles as well. Terao and Nakamura (2000) reported a case of visual perseveration on maprotiline, however the patient was also on levopromethazine, which some feel increases the plasma levels of maprotiline.

REFERENCES AND FURTHER READING

Albala AA, Weinberg N, Allen SM. Maprotiline-induced hypnopompic hallucinations. J Clin Psychiatry 44: 149, 1983.
Forstl H, Pohlmann-Eden B. Amplitudes of somatosensory evoked potentials reflect cortical hyperexcitability in antidepressant-induced myoclonus. Neurology 40: 924–926, 1990.
Oakley AMM, Hodge L. Cutaneous vasculitis from maprotiline. Aust NZ J Med 15: 256, 1985.
Park J, Proudfoot AT. Acute poisoning with maprotiline hydrochloride. BMJ 1: 1573, 1977.
Terao HH, Nakamura J. Visual perseveration: a new side effect of maprotiline. Acta Psychiatr Scand 101: 476–477, 2000.

Generic name: Methylphenidate hydrochloride.

Proprietary names: Concerta, Metadate CD, Metadate ER, Methylin, Methylin ER, Ritalin, Ritalin LA, Ritalin-SR.

Primary use

This piperidine derivative is used in the treatment of mild depression and in the management of children with hyperkinetic syndrome.

Ocular side effects

Systemic administration – oral
Certain
1. Eyelids or conjunctiva – urticaria
2. Visual hallucinations

Probable
1. Mydriasis – weak
2. Blepharoclonus

Possible
1. Subconjunctival or retinal hemorrhages secondary to drug-induced anemia
2. Eyelids or conjunctiva
   a. Erythema multiforme
   b. Stevens-Johnson syndrome
   c. Exfoliative dermatitis

Conditional/Unclassified
1. Diplopia
2. Accommodation abnormal
3. Conjunctivitis

Systemic administration – intravenous
Certain
1. Talc retinopathy
   a. Small yellow-white emboli
   b. Neovascularization – late
   c. Retinal hemorrhages
2. Decreased vision
3. Tractional retinal detachment

Clinical significance

Ocular side effects due to methylphenidate are rare, reversible and seldom clinically significant. Bartlik and Harmon (1997) point out that while the packet insert states that the drug is contraindicated in glaucoma patients, it only has a weak anticholinergic effect. The National Registry has around 30 reports of diplopia, abnormal accommodation and conjunctivitis, but these are unproven side effects.

Methylphenidate tablets intended for oral use have been used by drug addicts who crush the tablets and inject the drug intravenously. The filler in the tablet is insoluble talc, cornstarch or various binders, and lodges in the retina and other tissues as emboli (Atlee 1972). These glistening refractile particles in the retina, which are fairly stationary, may cause visual symptoms and neovascularization may form in time.

REFERENCES AND FURTHER READING

Acute drug abuse reactions. Med Lett Drugs Ther 27: 77, 1985.
Atlee WE Jr. Talc and cornstarch emboli in eyes of drug abusers. JAMA 219: 49, 1972.
Bartlik B, Harmon G. Use of methylphenidate in a patient with glaucoma and attention-deficit hyperactivity disorder; a clinical dilemma. Arch Gen Psychiatry 54: 188–189, 1997.
Bluth LL, Hanscom TA. Retinal detachment and vitreous hemorrhages due to talc emboli. JAMA 246: 980, 1981.
Dukes MNG (ed). Meyler's Side Effects of Drugs, Vol. X, Excerpta Medica, Amsterdam, pp 14–15, 1984.
Gross-Tsur V, Joseph A, Shalev RS. Hallucinations during methylphenidate therapy. Neurology 63: 753–754, 2004.
Gualtieri CT, Evans RW. Carbamazepine-induced tics. Dev Med Child Neurol 26: 546, 1984.
Gunby P. Methylphenidate abuse produces retinopathy. JAMA 241: 546, 1979.
Lederer CM Jr., Sabates FN. Ocular findings in the intravenous drug abuser. Ann Ophthalmol 14: 436, 1982.
McEvoy GK (ed). American Hospital Formulary Service Drug Information 87, American Society of Hospital Pharmacists, Bethesda, pp 1115–1117, 1987.
Methylphenidate (Ritalin) and other drugs for treatment of hyperactive children. Med Lett Drugs Ther 19: 53, 1977.
Tse DT, Ober RR. Talc retinopathy. Am J Ophthalmol 90: 624, 1980.

Generic name: Trazodone.

Proprietary name: Desyrel.

Primary use

This triazolopyridine derivative is used in the treatment of depression.

Ocular side effects

Systemic administration
Certain
1. Decreased vision
2. Visual image
   a. Objects have sheen, metallic ghost images, bright shiny lights
   b. Palinopsia

Probable
1. Non-specific ocular irritation
   a. Hyperemia
   b. Photophobia

c. Ocular pain
d. Burning sensation
2. Diplopia

Possible
1. Visual hallucinations
2. Eyelids or conjunctiva
   a. Allergic reactions
   b. Erythema
   c. Blepharoconjunctivitis
   d. Photosensitivity
   e. Erythema multiforme
3. Subconjunctival or retinal hemorrhages secondary to drug-induced anemia
4. Increased blink rate

Conditional/Unclassified
1. Aggravation of narrow-angle glaucoma

Clinical significance

Ocular side effects due to trazodone occur only occasionally and are reversible with decreased dosage or discontinued drug use. Palinopsia, the persistence or reappearance of an image of a recently viewed object, has been well documented by Hughes and Lessell (1990). Occasionally, patients will complain of a sheen on objects, metallic ghost images, bright shiny lights or strobe-light-type effects. Copper and Dening (1986) reported a case of trazodone causing an increased blink rate. The National Registry has cases of changes in refraction and transient problems with accommodation. A single case of trazodone aggravating angle-closure glaucoma has been reported by Chi-un et al (2003). A cause-and-effect relationship of these findings and this drug has not been established.

REFERENCES AND FURTHER READING

Ban TA, et al. Comprehensive clinical studies with trazodone. Curr Ther Res 15: 540, 1973.

Chi-un P, Chang-uk L, Soo-Jung L, Chul L, In-ho P. Association of low dose trazodone treatment with aggravated angle-closure glaucoma. Psychiatry Clin Neurosci 57: 127–129, 2003.

Copper MD, Dening TR. Excessive blinking associated with combined antidepressants. BMJ 293: 1243, 1986.

Damlouji NF, Ferguson JM. Trazodone-induced delirium in bulemic patients. Am J Psychiatry 141: 434, 1984.

Ford NE, Jenike MA. Erythema multiforme associated with trazodone therapy: case report. J Clin Psychiatry 46: 294, 1985.

Hassan E, Miller DD. Toxicity and elimination of trazodone after overdose. Clin Pharm 4: 97, 1985.

Hughes MS, Lessell S. Trazodone-induced palinopsia. Arch Ophthalmol 108: 399–400, 1990.

Kraft TB. Psychosis following trazodone administration. Am J Psychiatry 140: 1383, 1983.

Rongioletti F, Rebora A. Drug eruption from trazodone. J Am Acad Dermatol 14: 274, 1986.

CLASS: ANTIPSYCHOTIC AGENTS

Generic names: 1. Chlorpromazine; 2. fluphenazine; 3. perphenazine; 4. prochlorperazine; 5. promethazine; 6. thiethylperazine; 7. thioridazine.

Proprietary names: 1. Thorazine, Sonazine; 2. Prolixin; 3. generic only; 4. Comprazine, Compro; 5. Phenergan, Promethegan; 6. Torecan; 7. generic only.

Primary use

These phenothiazines are used in the treatment of depressive, involutional, senile or organic psychoses and various forms of schizophrenia. Some of the phenothiazines are also used as adjuncts to anesthesia, antiemetics and in the treatment of tetanus.

Ocular side effects

Systemic administration

(Not all of the ocular side effects listed have been reported for each phenothiazine.)

Certain
1. Decreased vision
2. Decrease or paralysis of accommodation
3. Night blindness
4. Problems with color vision
   a. Color vision defect, red-green defect
   b. Objects have yellow or brown tinge
   c. Colored haloes around lights
5. Cornea
   a. Pigmentary deposits – epithelium, deep stroma and endothelium
   b. Punctate keratitis
6. Pupils – variable dependent on which drug
   a. Mydriasis
   b. Miosis
   c. Decreased reaction to light
7. Oculogyric crises
8. Lens – chlorpromazine
   a. Subcapsular dust-like granular deposits – whitest to yellowish brown in pupillary area (early)
   b. Stellate anterior cortical changes (late) (Fig. 7.2b)
9. Visual hallucinations
10. Nystagmus
11. Jerky pursuit movements
12. Photophobia
13. Eyelids or conjunctiva
    a. Allergic reactions
    b. Edema
    c. Hyperpigmentation

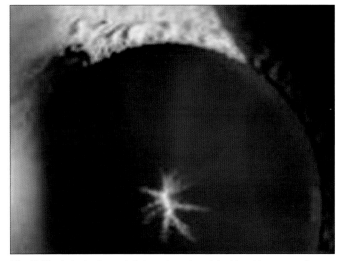

Fig. 7.2b Anterior lens stellate cataracts related to chlorpromazine. Photo courtesy of Kanski JJ. Clinical Diagnosis in Ophthalmology, Mosby Elsevier, London, 2006.

        d. Photosensitivity
        e. Angioneurotic edema
        f. Blepharospasm
 14. Abnormal ERG or EOG

Probable

 1. Retina (rare – long term therapy) (Fig. 7.2c)
        a. Pigmentary changes
        b. Edema
 2. Visual fields
        a. Scotomas – annular, central or paracentral
        b. Constriction
 3. Lacrimation decreased
 4. Horner's syndrome
 5. Toxic amblyopia
 6. Myasthenia gravis
        a. Diplopia
        b. Ptosis
        c. Paresis of extraocular muscles
 7. Ocular teratogenic effects

Possible

 1. Optic atrophy
 2. Papilledema
 3. Myopia
 4. Eyelids or conjunctiva
        a. Lupoid syndrome
        b. Stevens-Johnson syndrome
        c. Exfoliative dermatitis
        d. Erythema multiforme
        e. Lupus erythematosus

Clinical significance

The phenothiazines as a class are one of the most widely used drugs in the practice of medicine. The most commonly prescribed drug in this group is chlorpromazine. This medication has been so thoroughly investigated that over 10 000 publications have been written on this agent alone. Even so, these drugs are remarkably safe. Their overall rate of side effects is estimated at only 3%. However, if patients are on phenothiazine therapy for a number of years, a 30% rate of ocular side effects has been reported. If therapy continues over 10 years,

the rate of ocular side effects increases to nearly 100%. Side effects are dose and drug dependent, with the most significant side effects reported with chlorpromazine, since this agent is the most often prescribed. These drugs in very high dosages can cause significant ocular adverse effects within a few days, while the same reactions usually would take many years to develop in the normal dosage range. Each phenothiazine has the potential to cause ocular side effects, although it is not likely to cause all of those mentioned. Pinpointing the toxic effects to a specific phenothiazine is difficult since most patients are taking more than one drug. The most common adverse ocular effect with this group of drugs is decreased vision, probably due to anticholinergic interference. Chlorpromazine, in chronic therapy, can cause pigmentary deposits in or on the eye, with multiple reports claiming that other phenothiazines can cause this as well. These deposits are first seen on the lens surface in the pupillary aperture, later near Descemet's membrane or corneal endothelium, and only in rare cases in the corneal epithelium. Pigmentary changes in the cornea seem to be reversible, but lens deposits may be permanent. Lens deposits are described as not interfering with vision (pseudocataracts). A report by Isaac et al (1991) clearly showed an increased incidence of cataract surgery in patients taking these agents and in long-term therapy an anterior capsular opacity seems characteristic (Webber et al 2001; Leung et al 1999; Siddal 1966; Rasmussen et al 1976).

Retinopathy, optic nerve disease and blindness are exceedingly rare at the recommended dosage levels, and then they are almost only found in patients on long-term therapy. A phototoxic process has been postulated to be involved in both the increased ocular pigmentary deposits and the retinal degeneration. These groups of drugs with piperidine side chains (thioridazine has been removed from the market) have a greater incidence of causing retinal problems than the phenothiazine derivatives with aliphatic side chains (chlorpromazine), which has had relatively little retinal toxicity reported. Power et al (1991) reported a patient taking fluphenazine for 10 years and developing bilateral maculopathy after 2 minutes of unprotected welding arc exposure. Lee and Fern (2004) described bilateral maculopathy after 10 years of exposure to fluphenazine without increased light exposure.

The phenothiazines combine with ocular and dermal pigment and are only slowly released. This slow release has, in part, been

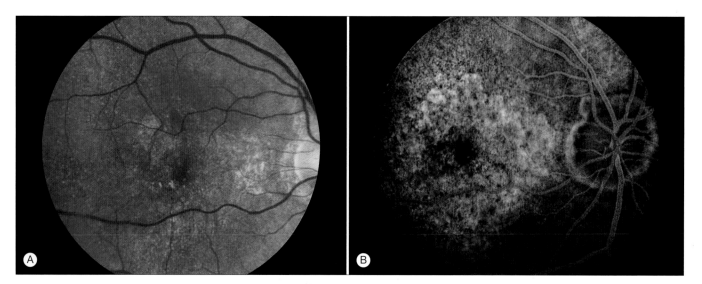

Fig. 7.2c A: Retinal pigment epithelial atrophy from systemic thioridazine. B: Flourescein angiogram of widespread bull's eye changes from systemic thioridazine.

given as the reason for the progression of adverse ocular reactions even after use of the drug is discontinued.

Recommendations
1. Photo-induced skin eruptions are well known, especially with chlorpromazine. Pigmentation-induced photosensitivity can be blocked in part by sunglasses that block out ultraviolet radiation up to 400 nm.
2. The above is also true for possible lens-induced changes.
3. Avoid bright light when possible.

REFERENCES AND FURTHER READING

Ball WA, Caroff SN. Retinopathy, tardive dyskinesia and low-dose thioridazine. Am J Psychiatry 143: 256, 1986.

Cook FF, Davis RG, Russo LS Jr. Internuclear ophthalmoplegia caused by phenothiazine intoxication. Arch Neurol 38: 465, 1981.

Deluise VP, Flynn JT. Asymmetric anterior segment changes induced by chlorpromazine. Ann Ophthalmol 13: 953, 1981.

Eicheubaum JW, D'Amico RA. Corneal injury by a Thorazine spansule. Ann Ophthalmol 13: 199, 1981.

Hamilton J DeV. Thioridazine retinopathy within the upper dosage limit. Psychosomatics 26: 823, 1985.

Isaac NE, Walker AM, et al. Exposure to phenothiazine drugs and risk of cataract. Arch Ophthalmol 109: 256–260, 1991.

Kaeser HE. Drug-induced myasthenic syndromes. Acta Neurol Scand 70(Suppl. 100): 39, 1984.

Lam RW, Remick RA. Pigmentary retinopathy associated with low-dose thioridazine treatment. Can Med Assoc J 132: 737, 1985.

Lee MS, Fern AI. Fluphenazine and its toxic maculopathy. Ophthalmic Res 36: 237–239, 2004.

Leung ATS, Cheng ACK, Chan W, et al. Chlorpromazine-induced refractile corneal deposits and cataract. Arch Ophthalmol 117: 1662–1663, 1999.

Marmor HF. Is thioridazine retinopathy progressive? Relationship of pigmentary changes to visual function. Br J Ophthalmol 74: 739–742, 1990.

Miyata M, et al. Changes in human electroretinography associated with thioridazine administration. Acta Ophthalmol 181: 175, 1980.

Ngen CC, Singh P. Long-term phenothiazine administration and the eye in 100 Malaysians. Br J Psychiatry 152: 278–281, 1988.

Phua YS, Patel DV, McGhee CNJ. In vivo confocal microstructural analysis of corneal endothelial changes in a patient on long-term chlorpromazine therapy. Graefe's Arch Clin Exp Ophthalmol 243: 721–723, 2005.

Power WJ, et al. Welding arc maculopathy and fluphenazine. Br J Ophthalmol 75: 433–455, 1991.

Rasmussen K, Kirk L, Faurbye A. Deposits in the lens and cornea of the eye during long-term chlorpromazine medication. Acta Psychiatr Scand 53: 1–6, 1976.

Siddall JR. Ocular toxic changes associated with chlorpromazine and thioridazine. Can J Opthalmol 1: 190–198, 1966.

Webber SK, Domniz Y, Sutton GL, et al. Corneal deposition after high-dose chlorpromazine hydrochloride therapy. Cornea 20: 217–219, 2001.

Generic names: 1. Droperidol; 2. haloperidol.

Proprietary names: 1. Inapsine; 2. Haldol.

Primary use
These butyrophenone derivatives are used in the management of acute and chronic schizophrenia, and manic depressive, involutional, senile, organic and toxic psychoses. Droperidol is also used as an adjunct to anesthesia and as an antiemetic.

Ocular side effects

Systemic administration
Certain
1. Decreased vision
2. Oculogyric crises
3. Decrease or paralysis of accommodation
4. Pupils
   a. Mydriasis (haloperidol)
   b. Miosis – rare
5. Eyelids or conjunctiva
   a. Allergic reactions
   b. Photosensitivity
   c. Angioneurotic edema
   d. Blepharospasm
6. Visual hallucinations
7. Decreased intraocular pressure
8. Subcapsular cataracts
9. Myopia (haloperidol)

Probable
1. Corneal decompensation (with multiple drugs)
2. Perceptional disorders

Possible
1. Subconjunctival or retinal hemorrhages secondary to drug-induced anemia.

Clinical significance
Most ocular side effects due to these agents are transient and reversible, and most are quite rare. While, on occasion, significant bilateral pupillary dilation occurs due to haloperidol, seldom does this precipitate narrow-angle glaucoma. Myopia is associated with the use of haloperidol, possibly secondary to drug-induced hyponatremia (Mendelis 1981). There is a report by Nishida et al (1992) that in rare individuals, often on multiple tranquilizing agents, including haloperidol, the endothelium may be damaged and give a clinical picture of bilateral bullous keratopathy. Stopping the drugs allows for the corneas to return to normal. The decreased intraocular pressure due to these drugs is not a sufficient amount to be of clinical value. Uchida et al (2003) report a case with positive rechallenge of haloperidol causing the outlines of small objects or patterns to appear increasingly vivid, with the effects lasting for 1 hour after taking the drug. Honda (1974), along with similar case reports received by the National Registry, supports these agents as having been associated with the onset of subcapsular cataracts after long-term therapy. These appear as subepithelial changes near the equator. Histologically, they appear as large, round, balloon cells without proliferation of lens epithelium. An epidemiologic study by Isaac et al supports these agents as causing cataracts.

REFERENCES AND FURTHER READING

Andrus PF. Lithium and carbamazepine. J Clin Psychiatry 45: 525, 1984.

Drugs that cause photosensitivity. Med Lett Drugs Ther 28: 51, 1986.

Honda S. Drug-induced cataract in mentally ill subjects. Jpn J Clin Ophthalmol 28: 521, 1974.

Isaac NE, Walker AM, Jick H, Gorman M. Exposure to phenothiazine drugs and risk of cataract. Arch Ophthalmol 109: 256–260, 1991.

Jhee SS, Zarotsky V, Mohapupt SM, et al. Delayed onset of oculogyric crisis and torticollis with intramuscular haloperidol. Ann Pharmacother 37: 1434–1437, 2003.

Konikoff F, et al. Neuroleptic malignant syndrome induced by a single injection of haloperidol. BMJ 289: 1228, 1984.

Laties AM. Ocular toxicology of haloperidol. In: Symposium on Ocular Therapy, Vol. 9, Leopold IH, Burns RP (eds), John Wiley & Sons, New York, pp 87–95, 1976.

Mendelis PS. Haldol (haloperidol) hyponatremia. ADR Highlights January 12, 1981.

Nishida K, Ohashi Y, Kinoshita S, et al. Endothelial decompensation in a schizophrenic patient receiving long-term treatment with tranquilizers. Cornea 11(5): 475–478, 1992.

Patton CM Jr. Rapid induction of acute dyskinesia by droperidol. Anesthesiology 43: 126, 1975.

Selman FB, McClure RF, Helwig H. Loxapine succinate: a double-blind comparison with haloperidol and placebo in schizophrenics. Curr Ther Res 19: 645–652, 1976.

Shapiro AK. More on drug-induced blurred vision. Am J Psychiatry 134: 1449, 1977.

Uchida H, Suzuki T, Watanabe K, et al. Antipsychotic-induced paroxysmal perceptual alteration. Am J Psychiatr 160: 2243–2244, 2003.

Generic name: Lithium carbonate.

Proprietary names: Eskalith, Eskalith CR.

Primary use

This lithium salt is used in the management of the manic phase of manic depressive psychosis.

Ocular side effects

Systemic administration

Certain

1. Decreased vision
2. Nystagmus
   a. Horizontal
   b. Vertical
   c. Downbeat
3. Extraocular muscles
   a. Oculogyric crises
   b. Decreased spontaneous movements
   c. Lateral conjugate deviations
   d. Jerky pursuit movements
   e. Oscillopsia
4. Eyelids or conjunctiva
   a. Conjunctivitis – non-specific
   b. Edema
   c. Loss of eyelashes or eyebrows
5. Non-specific ocular irritation
   a. Lacrimation
   b. Photophobia
   c. Burning sensation
   d. Decreased lacrimation
6. Decreased accommodation
7. Visual hallucinations
8. Exophthalmos – thyroid eye disease
9. Intracranial hypertension
   a. Papilledema
   b. Visual field defect
10. Abnormal EOG or VEP
11. Decreased dark adaptation

Probable

1. Myasthenia gravis
   a. Diplopia
   b. Ptosis
   c. Paresis of extraocular muscles
2. Aggravates ocular sicca

Possible

1. Subconjunctival or retinal hemorrhages secondary to drug-induced anemia
2. Cornea and conjunctiva – fine lithium deposits

Clinical significance

Lithium salts have been widely used for decades and lithium intoxication is common since therapeutic blood levels have a narrow range before toxicity occurs. Lithium therapy is mainly prophylactic, with therapy lasting years to decades. The review article by Fraunfelder et al (1992) is probably the definitive work on the effects of lithium on the visual system.

Lithium affects many areas of the visual system, including direct effects on the central nervous system and on endocrine glands, which lead to ocular effects. In general, the ocular side effects of lithium are reversible on withdrawal of the drug or lowering of the dosage. However, other side effects, such as downbeat nystagmus, can be permanent. Blurred vision is probably the most common side effect experienced by patients taking lithium, but is seldom significant enough to require the cessation of therapy. Usually with time, even while keeping the same dosage, blurred vision will disappear. Blurred vision, however, can be a signal of pending problems, such as intracranial hypertension. In most cases, patients who develop intracranial hypertension have been taking lithium for many years.

Lithium can cause various forms of nystagmus, the most characteristic being downbeat. This can occur at therapeutic dosage ranges of lithium and may be the only adverse drug effect. While some patients have a full recovery after stopping or reducing the dosage of lithium, it may develop into irreversible downbeat nystagmus. If downbeat nystagmus occurs, one needs to reevaluate the risk-benefit ratio of lithium therapy. Lithium can also cause extraocular muscle abnormalities, especially vertical or lateral far-gaze diplopia. In therapeutic dosages, Gooding et al have shown no effect of lithium on smooth pursuit eye-tracking performance. Diplopia in any patient taking lithium may require a work-up for myasthenia gravis, especially if associated with ptosis. Ptosis can occur alone. Oculogyric crises have been reported primarily in patients also taking haloperidol.

Thyroid-related eye disease in various forms secondary to hypo- or hyperthyroidism has been seen in patients receiving lithium therapy. While this is uncommon, exophthalmos has occurred. Lithium is secreted in the tears and may cause an irritative forum of conjunctivitis, causing epiphora. However, with time many patients complain of a dry mouth and about the same time ocular dryness. Lithium has been reported to cause cornea and the conjunctiva deposits, but the documentation for this is limited. Lithium can cause a decrease in accommodation, which may occur in up to 10% of patients. However, this primarily occurs in young patients and is rare in older patients. In general, this side effect is minimal and usually resolves after a few months, even while taking the drug. Etminan et al (2004), in a case control study, showed that in the elderly lithium increased the risk of injurious motor vehicle accidents.

REFERENCES AND FURTHER READING

Brenner R, et al. Measurement of lithium concentrations in human tears. Am J Psychiatry 139: 678–679, 1982.

Corbett J, et al. Downbeat nystagmus and other ocular motor defects caused by lithium toxicity. Neurology 39: 481–487, 1989.

Deleu D, Ebinger G. Lithium-induced internuclear ophthalmoplegia. Clin Neuropharmacol 12: 224–226, 1989.

Dry J, Aron-Rosa A, Pradalier A. Onset of exophthalmos during treatment with lithium carbonate. Biological hyperthyroidism. Therapie 29: 701–708, 1974.

Emrich H, et al. Reduced dark-adaptation: An indication of lithium's neuronal action in humans. Am J Psychiatry 147: 629–631, 1990.

Etminan M, Hemmelgarn B, Delaney JAC, Suissa S. Use of lithium and the risk of injurious motor vehicle crash in elderly adults: case-control study nested within a cohort. BMJ 328: 895–896, 2004.

Fenwick PBC, Robertson R. Changes in the visual evoked potential to pattern reversal with lithium medication. Electroencephalogr Clin Neurophysiol 55: 538, 1983.

Fraunfelder FT. Lithium carbonate therapy and macular degeneration. JAMA 249: 2389, 1983.

Fraunfelder FT, Meyer S. Ocular toxicity of antineoplastic agents. Ophthalmology 90: 1–3, 1983.

Fraunfelder FT, Fraunfelder FW, Jefferson JW. Monograph: the effects of lithium on the human visual system. J Toxicol Cut Ocular Toxicol 11: 97–169, 1992.

Gooding DC, Iacono WG, Katsanis J, et al. The association between lithium carbonate and smooth pursuit eye tracking among first-episode patients with psychotic affective disorders. Psychophysiology 30: 3–9, 1993.

Halmagyi G, et al. Downbeating nystagmus – a review of 62 cases. Arch Neurol 40: 777–784, 1983.

Halmagyi G, et al. Lithium-induced downbeat nystagmus. Am J Ophthalmol 107: 664–679, 1989.

Levine S, Puchalski C. Pseudotumor cerebri associated with lithium therapy in two patients. J Clin Psychiatry 51: 251–253, 1990.

Levy DL, et al. Pharmacologic evidence for specificity of pursuit dysfunction to schizophrenia. Lithium carbonate associated with abnormal pursuit. Arch Gen Psychiatry 42: 335, 1985.

Pakes G. Eye irritation and lithium carbonate. Arch Ophthalmol 98: 930, 1980.

Sandyk R. Oculogyric crisis induced by lithium carbonate. Eur Neurol 23: 92, 1984.

Saul RF, Hamburger HA, Selhorst JB. Pseudotumor cerebri secondary to lithium carbonate. JAMA 253: 2869–2870, 1985.

Slonim R, McLarty B. Sixth cranial nerve palsy – unusual presenting symptom of lithium toxicity? Can J Psychiatry 30: 443–444, 1985.

Thompson CH, Baylis PH. Asymptomatic Grave's disease during lithium therapy. Postgrad Med J 62: 295, 1986.

Ullrich A, et al. Lithium effects on ophthalmological electrophysiological parameters in young healthy volunteers. Acta Psychiatr Scand 72: 113, 1985.

Possible

1. Subconjunctival or retinal hemorrhages secondary to drug-induced anemia
2. Visual hallucinations

Conditional/Unclassified

1. Lens – pigmentation
2. Retina – pigmentation

Clinical significance

Neuromuscular reactions, including oculogyric crises, are fairly frequently reported, usually during the first few days of treatment with loxapine. These reactions occasionally require reduction or temporary withdrawal of the drug. The anticholinergic effects – blurred vision, mydriasis and decreased accommodation – are more likely to occur with concomitant use of antiParkinsonian agents. The possibility of pigmentary retinopathy and lenticular pigmentation from loxapine cannot be excluded but seems quite rare or unlikely.

REFERENCES AND FURTHER READING

McEvoy GK (ed). American Hospital Formulary Service Drug Information 87, American Society of Hospital Pharmacists, Bethesda, pp 1094–1096, 1987.

Moyano CZ. A double-blind comparison of Loxitane, loxapine succinate and trifluoperazine hydrochloride in chronic schizophrenic patients. Dis Nerv Syst 36: 301, 1975.

Selman FB, McClure RF, Helwig H. Loxapine succinate: a double-blind comparison with haloperidol and placebo in acute schizophrenics. Curr Ther Res 19: 645, 1976.

Sweetmand SC (ed). Martindale: The Complete Drug Reference, 34th edn, Pharmaceutical Press, London, pp 705–706, 2004.

Generic name: Loxapine.

Proprietary name: Loxitane.

Primary use

This dibenzoxazepine derivative represents a subclass of tricyclic antipsychotic agents used in the treatment of schizophrenia.

Ocular side effects

Systemic administration
Certain

1. Oculogyric crises
2. Eyelids or conjunctiva
   a. Edema
   b. Hyperpigmentation
   c. Photosensitivity
   d. Urticaria
3. Ptosis

Probable

1. Decreased vision
2. Mydriasis – may precipitate narrow-angle glaucoma
3. Decreased accommodation

Generic name: Pimozide.

Proprietary name: Orap.

Primary use

This diphenylbutylpiperidine derivative is used for suppression of motor and vocal tics of Tourette's syndrome.

Ocular side effects

Systemic administration
Certain

1. Decreased vision
2. Decreased accommodation
3. Visual hallucinations
4. Oculogyric crises
5. Eyelids
   a. Erythema
   b. Edema

Probable

1. Decreased lacrimation

Clinical significance

Up to 20% of patients on this drug have some form of visual disturbance (Physicians' Desk Reference 2006). This is mainly blurred vision, which is reversible. Decreased accommodation is not uncommon. All ocular side effects are reversible and of little clinical significance. This drug can cause a dry mouth and therefore can probably aggravate ocular sicca.

REFERENCES AND FURTHER READING

McEvoy GK (ed). American Hospital Formulary Service Drug Information 87, American Society of Hospital Pharmacists, Bethesda, pp 1098–1103, 1987.

Morris PA, MacKenzie DH, Masheter HC. A comparative double blind trial of pimozide and fluphenazine in chronic schizophrenia. Br J Psychiatry 117: 683, 1970.

Physicians' Desk Reference, 60th edn, Thomson PDR, Montvale NJ, pp 1220–1222, 2006.

Taub RN, Baker MA. Treatment of metastatic malignant melanoma with pimozide. Lancet 1: 605, 1979.

Generic name: Quetiapine fumarate.

Proprietary name: Seroquel.

Primary use

This drug belongs to a new chemical class, dibenzothiazephine derivatives, used in the management of bipolar mania or in schizophrenia.

Ocular side effects

Systemic administration
Certain
1. Decreased vision

Probable
1. Visual hallucinations
2. Myasthenia gravis
   a. Diplopia
   b. Ptosis
   c. Paresis of extraocular muscles
   d. Aggravates ocular sicca

Possible
1. Cataracts

Clinical significance

Ocular side effects attributed to quetiapine are rare, transitory and infrequent. Ocular sicca is probable, since dry mouth is one of the most frequent systemic side effects of this agent. Since this drug has caused lens changes in dogs and is an inhibitor of cholesterol biosynthesis, there has been interest as to the cataractogenic potential of this agent. Valibhai et al (2001) have reported a clinically suspect case. Large post-marketing surveillance studies have not found a higher incidence of cataracts. The lack of a characteristic pattern led to the conclusion, at worst, that the drug has a very weak cataractogenic potential.

Recommendations

The manufacturer recommends that any patient receiving chronic treatment be examined at the initiation of treatment and then twice yearly for lens changes. Fraunfelder (2004) recommends only having patients examined as per the guidelines established by the American Academy of Ophthalmology, regardless of whether or not the patient is on quetiapine. Gaynes (2005) prefers more frequent examinations in a letter to the editor, but in reply Fraunfelder (2005) did not concur.

REFERENCES AND FURTHER READING

Fraunfelder FW. Twice-yearly exams unnecessary for patients taking quetiapine. Am J Ophthalmol 138: 870–871, 2004.

Fraunfelder FW. Twice-yearly exams unnecessary for patients taking quetiapine [author's reply]. Am J Ophthalmol 140: 349, 2005.

Gaynes BI. Twice-yearly exams unnecessary for patients taking quetiapine [comment]. Am J Ophthalmol 140: 348–349, 2005.

Nasrallah HA, Dev V, Rak I, Raniwalla J. Safety update with quetiapine and lenticular examinations: experience with 300 000 patients [poster]. Presented at the Annual Meeting of the American College of Neuropsychopharmacology, Dec. 12–16, Acapulco, Mexico, 1999.

Shahzad S, Suleman M-I, Shahab H, et al. Cataract occurrence with antipsychotic drugs. Psychosomatics 43: 354–359, 2002.

Valibhai F, Phan NB, Still DJ, True J. Cataracts and quetiapine. Am J Psychiatry 158: 966, 2001.

Generic names: Tiotixene.

Proprietary name: Navane.

Primary use

This thioxanthene derivative is used in the management of schizophrenia.

Ocular side effects

Systemic administration
Certain
1. Decreased vision
2. Decrease or paralysis of accommodation
3. Oculogyric crises
4. Pupils
   a. Mydriasis
   b. Miosis
5. Cornea
   a. Fine particulate deposits
   b. Keratitis
6. Eyelids or conjunctiva
   a. Allergic reactions
   b. Photosensitivity
   c. Angioneurotic edema
   d. Urticaria

Probable
1. Lens
   a. Fine particulate deposits
   b. Stellate cataracts
2. Retinal pigmentary changes

Possible
1. Diplopia
2. Subconjunctival or retinal hemorrhages secondary to drug-induced anemia
3. Aggravate keratitis sicca

Clinical significance

In short-term therapy, ocular side effects due to this drug are reversible and usually insignificant. This drug has antimuscarinic properties, which may account for the occasional patient who gets blurred vision and mydriasis. Dry mouth is not uncommon, so ocular sicca may be aggravated or occur. In long-term therapy, however, cases of corneal or lens deposits or lens pigmentation have been reported. Retinal pigmentary changes are exceedingly rare, and only occur with long-term therapy. These are strong photosensitizing agents.

REFERENCES AND FURTHER READING

Drug Evaluations, 6th edn, American Medical Association, Chicago, pp 126–127, 1986.
Drugs for psychiatric disorders. Med Lett Drugs Ther 25: 45, 1983.
Drugs that cause photosensitivity. Med Lett Drugs Ther 28: 51, 1986.
Eberlein-Konig B, Bindl A, Przybilla B. Phototoxic properties of neuroleptic drugs. Dermatology 194: 131–135, 1997.
McNevin S, MacKay M. Chlorprothixene-induced systemic lupus erythematosus. J Clin Psychopharmacol 2: 411, 1982.
Physician's Desk Reference, 60th edn, Thomson PDR, Montvale NJ, pp 2124–2125, 2006.

CLASS: PSYCHEDELIC AGENTS

Generic names: 1. Dronabinol (tetrahydrocannabinol, THC); 2. hashish; 3. marihuana (marijuana).

Proprietary name: 1. Marinol (Canad.).

Street names: 1. The one; 2. bhang, charas, gram, hash, keif, black Russian; 3. ace, Acapulco gold, baby, Belyando sprue, boo, brown weed, bush, cannabis, charas, dank, dope, gage, ganja, grass, green, gungeon, hay, hemp, herb, home grown, jay, joint, kick sticks, kryptonite, lid, locoweed, Mary Jane, Mexican green, MJ, muggles, OJ (opium joint), Panama red, pot, rainy-day woman, reefer, roach, rope, sinsemilla, stick, tea, twist, weed, wheat.

Primary use

These psychedelic agents are occasionally used as cerebral sedatives and are narcotics commonly available on the illicit drug market. Dronabinol is also medically indicated for the treatment of the nausea and vomiting associated with chemotherapy.

Ocular side effects

Systemic administration
Certain
1. Visual hallucinations
2. Problems with color vision
   a. Color vision defect
   b. Objects have yellow or violet tinge
   c. Colored flashing lights
   d. Heightened color perception
3. Nystagmus
4. Non-specific ocular irritation
   a. Hyperemia
   b. Conjunctivitis
   c. Photophobia (variable)
   d. Burning sensation
5. Decreased accommodation
6. Decreased dark adaptation
7. Decreased vision
8. Blepharospasm

9. Decreased intraocular pressure
10. Decreased lacrimation
11. Pupils
    a. Miosis
    b. Anisocoria
12. Extraocular muscles
    a. Increased phorias
    b. Intermittent tropia
    c. Diplopia
13. Binocular depth inversion – reduced

Clinical significance

Marihuana is the most widely used illicit drug in the USA and one of the oldest recorded medicines in the world. It is almost always smoked. The oral form, dronabinol, is largely unappealing to the addict and therefore has a very low abuse potential. Levi and Miller (1990) as well as Laffi and Safran (1993) found vision disturbances lasting 24 hours after marihuana use. Each report involved only a few patients but included alterations of depth perception, sensorial disconnection when talking with people, intermittent light phenomena, strobe-like effects, bright spots flickering randomly in high frequency and alteration of the sensory perception of one's external environment. Ocular side effects due to these agents are transient and seldom of clinical importance.

Semple et al (2003), using binocular depth inversion testing, discovered persistent sensory visual abnormalities in chronic marihuana users. There is some evidence that marijuana decreases basal lacrimal secretion, decreases photosensitivity, increases dark adaptation, increases color-match limits and increases Snellen visual acuity. Possibly within the first 5–15 minutes some people will get some pupillary constriction; however, most do not and, to date, there is no long-term pupillary effect noted. Conjunctival hyperemia is not uncommon and is more pronounced at 15 minutes after exposure.

The cannabinols found in marihuana can lower intraocular pressure by an average of 25%, but the effect only lasts 3–4 hours. There is significant variation in the individual response to these agents, as well as diminished response with time. Most patients on this agent for glaucoma control cannot use it for prolonged periods due to lack of glaucoma control. Isolated cannabinols, which lower intraocular pressure, have the complicating factor that one cannot separate the central nervous system high from its ocular pressure lowering effect, so their value clinically is quite limited. Few patients are able to use marihuana for long-term control of their glaucoma and remain functional in the workplace.

These drugs are occasionally used medically, but have no long-term value in clinical ophthalmology.

REFERENCES AND FURTHER READING

Flach AJ. Delta-9-tetrahydrocannabinol (THC) in the treatment of end-stage open-angle glaucoma. Trans Am Ophthalmol Soc 100: 215–222, 2002.
Fried PA. Marihuana use by pregnant women and effects on offspring: an update. Neurobehav Toxicol Teratol 4: 451, 1982.
Gaillard MC, Borruat FX. Persisting visual hallucinations and illusions in previously drug-addicted patients. Klin Monatsbl Augenheilkd 220: 176–178, 2003.
Green K. Marijuana and the eye – a review. J Toxicol Cut Ocular Toxicol 1: 3, 1982.
Green K, Roth M. Ocular effects of topical administration of .9-tetrahydrocannabinol in man. Arch Ophthalmol 100: 265, 1982.
Jay WM, Green K. Multiple-drop study of topically applied 1% .9-tetrahydrocannabinol in human eyes. Arch Ophthalmol 101: 591, 1983.
Laffi GL, Safran AB. Persistent visual changes following hashish consumption. Br J Ophthalmol 77: 601–602, 1993.
Levi L, Miller NR. Visual illusions associated with previous drug abuse. F Clin Neuro-ophthalmol 10: 103–110, 1990.

Mazow ML, Garrett CW III. Intermittent esotropia secondary to marihuana smoking. Binocular Vis 3: 219, 1988.

Merritt JC, et al. Topical 9-tetrahydrocannabinol in hypertensive glaucomas. J Pharm Pharmacol 33: 40, 1981.

Poster DS, et al. 9-Tetrahydrocannabinol in clinical oncology. JAMA 245: 2047, 1981.

Qazi QH, et al. Abnormal fetal development linked to intrauterine exposure to marijuana. Dev Pharmacol Ther 8: 141, 1985.

Schwartz RH. Marijuana: a crude drug with a spectrum of underappreciated toxicity. Pediatrics 73: 455, 1984.

Semple DM, Ramsden F, McIntosh AM. Reduced binocular depth inversion in regular cannabis users. Pharmacol Biochem Behav 25: 789–793, 2003.

Tomida I, Pertwee RG, Azuara-Blanco A. Cannabinoids and glaucoma. Br J Ophthalmol 88: 708–713, 2003.

Treffert DA, Joranson DE. .9-Tetrahydrocannabinol and therapeutic research legislation for cancer patients. JAMA 249: 1469, 1983.

Weinberg D, et al. Intoxication from accidental marijuana ingestion. Pediatrics 71: 848, 1983.

Zhan G, Cmaras CB, Palmber PF, Toris CB. Effect of marijuana on aqueous humor dynamics in a glaucoma patient. J Glaucoma 14: 175–177, 2005.

Generic names: 1. Lysergic acid diethylamide (LSD), lysergide; 2. mescaline; 3. psilocybin.

Proprietary name: None.

Street names: 1. Acid, barrels, big d, blotter acid, blue acid, brown dots, California sunshine, crackers, cubes, cupcakes, grape parfait, green domes, Hawaiian sunshine, Lucy in the sky with diamonds, micro dots, purple barrels, purple haze, purple ozolone, sunshine, the animal, the beast, the chief, the hawk, the ticket, trips, twenty-five, yellow dimples, windowpane; 2. buttons, cactus, mesc, peyote, the bad seed, topi; 3. magic mushroom, shrooms.

Primary use

Illicit psychedelic and psychotomimetic agents that may be both natural and synthetic products.

Ocular side effects

Systemic administration
Certain
1. Visual hallucinations
   a. Image distortion
   b. Color intensification
   c. Geometric figure
   d. False perception of movement
   e. Afterimages
2. Spontaneous recurrence of abnormal visual perception following discontinuation of the drug (LSD)
   a. Transitory
   b. Long term
   c. Permanent
3. Palinopsia – visual perversion of recently seen objects (LSD)
   a. Acute
   b. Permanent
4. Problems with color vision
   a. Color vision defect
   b. Heightened color perception
5. Pupils
   a. Mydriasis
   b. Anisocoria
   c. Decreased or absent reaction to light
6. Decreased accommodation
7. Decreased dark adaptation
8. Decreased vision
9. Abnormal ERG, VEP and depressed critical flicker fusion
10. Photophobia

Topical ocular application – liquid LSD
Conditional/Unclassified
1. Cornea
   a. Melting
   b. Scarring
   c. Severe pannus
2. Conjunctiva - scarring

Ocular teratogenic effects
Possible
1. Cataract
2. Iris coloboma
3. Ocular dysplasia
4. Microphthalmos
5. Corneal opacities
6. Persistent hyperplastic primary vitreous
7. Retinal dysplasia
8. Optic disc hypoplasia
9. Optic nerve coloboma
10. Anophthalmia

Clinical significance

Ocular side effects due to these drugs are very common. Some claim true visual hallucinations seldom occur with these drugs, but rather a complicated visual experience results from a drug-induced perceptual disturbance. Perception changes include alterations in colors and shapes. Halpern and Pope (2003) reviewed the literature on 'hallucinogen persisting perception disorder', also known as flashbacks. They are uncommon, but can persist for months or even many years. Some have persisted for 20 years plus. Lysergide (LSD) is 100 times more potent than psilocybin, which in turn is 4000 times more potent than mescaline. The above visual side effects are therefore due to LSD and then to a lesser degree to the other agents. A large number of cases of sun gazing-induced macular damage has been reported in persons using these agents. Abraham (1982) first reported irreversible impairment of color discrimination. Kawasaki and Purvin (1996) reported three patients who had persistent palinopsia after LSD ingestion. These prolonged after-images lasted 3+ years after being off the drug.

A case of liquid LSD splashed into one eye of a 20-year-old has been reported to the National Registry. The cornea had significant melt with a resultant marked pannus. A conjunctival flap was necessary to save the globe. The eye was permanently disabled.

REFERENCES AND FURTHER READING

Abraham HD. A chronic impairment of colour vision in users of LSD. Br J Psychiatry 140: 518, 1982.

Abraham HD. Visual phenomenology of the LSD flashback. Arch Gen Psychiatry 40: 884, 1983.

Abraham HD, Duffy FH. EEG coherence in post-LSD visual hallucinations. Psychiatry Res 107: 151–163, 2001.

Birch J, et al. Acquired color vision defects. In: Congenital and Acquired Color Vision Defects, Pokorny J, et al (eds), Grune & Stratton, New York, pp 243–350, 1979.

Fohlmeister C, Gertsner W, Ritz R, et al. Spontaneous excitations in the visual cortex: stripes, spirals, rings, and collective bursts. Neurol Comput 7: 905–914, 1995.

Gaillard MC, Borruat FX. Persisting visual hallucination and illusion in previously drug-addicted patients. Klin Monatsbl Augenheilkd 220: 176–178, 2003.

Gouzoulis-Mayfrank E, Thelen B, Maier S, et al. Effects of the hallucinogen psilocybin on covert orienting of visual attention in humans. Neuropsychobiology 45: 205–212, 2002.

Halpern JH, Pope HG. Hallucinogen persisting perception disorder: what do we know after 50 years? Drug Alcohol Depend 69: 109–119, 2003.

Kaminer Y, Hrecznyj B. Lysergic acid diethylamide-induced chronic visual disturbances in an adolescent. J Nervous Mental Dis 179: 173–174, 1991.

Kawasaki A, Purvin V. Persistent palinopsia following ingestion of lysergic acid diethylamide (LSD). Arch Ophthalmol 114: 47–50, 1996.

Krill AE, Wieland AM, Ostfeld AM. The effect of two hallucinogenic agents on human retinal function. Arch Ophthalmol 64: 724–733, 1960.

Lerner AG, Sufman E, Kodesh A, et al. Risperidone-associated, benign transient visual disturbances in schizophrenic patients with a past history of LSD abuse. Isr J Psychiatry Relat Sci 39: 57–60, 2002.

Levi L, Miller NR. Visual illusions associated with previous drug abuse. J Clin Neuroophthalmol 10: 103–110, 1990.

Margolis S, Martin L. Anophthalmia in an infant of parents using LSD. Ann Ophthalmol 12: 1378, 1980.

Spaeth GL, Nelson LB, Beaudoin AR. Ocular teratology. In: Ocular Anatomy, Embryology and Teratology, Jakobiec FA (eds), JB Lippincott, Philadelphia, pp 955–975, 1982.

Sunness JS. Persistent afterimages (palinopsia) and photophobia in a patient with a history of LSD use. Retina 24: 805, 2004.

4. Visual hallucinations
5. Ptosis
6. Oculogyric crises
7. Decreased corneal reflex

Conditional/Unclassified
1. Increased intraocular pressure

Clinical significance

Even with relatively low doses (5 mg), phencyclidine may give a characteristic type of nystagmus in which vertical, horizontal and rotary eye movements occur in sudden bursts. In addition, this drug may produce hallucinations and visual defects, including distortion of body image and substitution of fairy-tale characters. Acute toxic reactions can last up to a week after a single dose, although the mental effects can linger for more than a month. These effects may keep recurring in sudden episodes while the patient is apparently recovering. A state of sensory blockade or a blank stare in which the eyes remain conjugate and open but with little or no spontaneous movement is characteristic of phencyclidine coma.

REFERENCES AND FURTHER READING

Acute drug abuse reactions. Med Lett Drugs Ther 27: 77, 1985.

Corales RL, Maull KI, Becker DP. Phencyclidine abuse mimicking head injury. JAMA 243: 2323, 1980.

McCarron MM, et al. Acute phencyclidine intoxication: incidence of clinical findings in 1,000 cases. Ann Emerg Med 10: 237, 1981.

Pearlson GD. Psychiatric and medical syndromes associated with phencyclidine (PCP) abuse. Johns Hopkins Med J 148: 25, 1981.

Sweetman S (ed). Martindale: The Complete Drug Reference, 34th edn, Pharmaceutical Press, London, pp 1730–1733, 2005.

Generic name: Phencyclidine.

Proprietary name: None.

Street names: Angel dust, angel's mist, busy bee, crystal, DOA, goon, hog horse tranquilizer, loveboat, lovely mist, monkey tranquilizer, PCP, peace pill, rocket fuel, sheets, super weed, tac, tic.

Primary use

This non-barbiturate anesthetic was removed from the market because of postoperative psychiatric disturbances; however, it is still commonly available on the illicit drug market.

Ocular side effects

Systemic administration
Certain
1. Extraocular muscles
   a. Nystagmus – horizontal, rotary or vertical
   b. Diplopia
   c. Jerky pursuit movements
2. Pupils
   a. Miosis
   b. Decreased reaction to light
3. Decreased vision

CLASS: SEDATIVES AND HYPNOTICS

Generic names: 1. Amobarbital; 2. butalbital; 3. methohexital; 4. methylphenobarbital (mephobarbital); 5. pentobarbital; 6. phenobarbital; 7. primidone; 8. secbutabarbital; 9. secobarbital.

Proprietary names: 1. Amytal; 2. multi-ingredient preparations only; 3. Brevital sodium; 4. Mebaral; 5. Nembutal; 6. Luminal; 7. Mysoline; 8. Butisol sodium; 9. Seconal sodium.

Street names: 1-9 Barbs, bluebirds, blues, tooies, yellow jackets.

Primary use

These barbituric acid derivatives vary primarily in duration and intensity of action and are used as central nervous system depressants, hypnotics, sedatives and anticonvulsants.

Ocular side effects

Systemic administration (Primarily excessive dosage or chronic use)
Certain
1. Eyelids
   a. Ptosis
   b. Blepharoclonus

2. Pupils
   a. Mydriasis
   b. Miosis (coma)
   c. Decreased reaction to light
   d. Hippus
3. Extraocular muscles
   a. Decreased convergence
   b. Paresis or paralysis
   c. Jerky pursuit movements
   d. Random ocular movements
   e. Vertical gaze palsy
4. Oscillopsia
5. Nystagmus
   a. Downbeat, gaze-evoked, horizontal, jerk or vertical
   b. Depressed or abolished optokinetic, latent, positional, voluntary or congenital nystagmus
6. Decreased vision
7. Problems with color vision
   a. Color vision defect
   b. Objects have yellow or green tinge
8. Visual hallucinations
9. Eyelids or conjunctiva
   a. Allergic reactions
   b. Conjunctivitis – non-specific
   c. Edema
   d. Photosensitivity
   e. Angioneurotic edema
   f. Urticaria
10. Decreased accommodation (primidone)
11. Keratoconjunctivitis sicca (primidone)
12. Abnormal ERG, VEP or critical flicker fusion
13. Cortical blindness (thiopental)

Possible
1. Optic nerve disorders (chronic use)
   a. Retrobulbar or optic neuritis
   b. Papilledema
   c. Optic atrophy
2. Visual fields
   a. Scotomas
   b. Constriction
3. Subconjunctival or retinal hemorrhages secondary to drug-induced anemia
4. Eyelids or conjunctiva
   a. Lupoid syndrome
   b. Erythema multiforme
   c. Stevens-Johnson syndrome
   d. Exfoliative dermatitis
   e. Lyell's syndrome

Ocular teratogenic effects (primidone)
Possible
1. Optic atrophy
2. Ptosis
3. Hypertelorism
4. Epicanthus
5. Strabismus

Clinical significance

New classes of drugs are generally replacing these short- and long-acting barbiturates. Numerous adverse ocular side effects have been attributed to barbiturate usage, yet nearly all significant ocular side effects are in acute barbiturate poisoning or habitual users. Few toxic ocular reactions are found due to barbiturate usage at therapeutic dosages or on short-term therapy. The most common ocular abnormalities are disturbances of ocular movement, such as decreased convergence, paresis of extraocular muscles or nystagmus. The pupillary response to barbiturate intake is quite variable, so this sign has questionable clinical value. Phenobarbital has the most frequently reported ocular side effects; however, all barbiturates may produce adverse ocular effects. Chronic barbiturate users have a 'tattle-tale' ptosis and blepharoclonus. Normally, a tap on the glabella area of the head produces a few eyelid blinks, but in the barbiturate addict the response will be a rapid fluttering of the eyelids (Hamburger 1965). Bilateral blindness or decreased vision after barbiturate-induced coma usually returns to normal vision. There are a few reports, however, of permanent blindness. Optic neuropathy with complete recovery in a 12-year-old boy from chronic phenobarbital medication is a unique case (Homma et al 1989). The barbiturates do not appear to have teratogenic effects, except possibly primidone. Primidone has been shown to be associated with acute attacks of porphyria. Acute onset of severe photophobia and/or lid reactions is an indicator of ocular porphyria.

REFERENCES AND FURTHER READING

Alpert JN. Downbeat nystagmus due to anticonvulsant toxicity. Ann Neurol 4: 471, 1978.

Amarenco P, Royer I, Guillevin L. Ophthalmoplegia externa in barbiturate poisoning. Presse Med 13: 2453, 1984.

Clarke RSJ, Fee JH, Dundee JW. Hypersensitivity reactions to intravenous anaesthetics. In: Adverse Response to Intravenous Drugs, Watkins J, Ward A (eds), Grune & Stratton, New York, pp 41–47, 1978.

Crosby SS, et al. Management of Stevens-Johnson syndrome. Clin Pharm 5: 682, 1986.

Hamburger E. Identification and treatment of barbiturate abusers. JAMA 193: 143–144, 1965.

Homma K, Wakakura M, Ishikawa S. A case of phenobarbital-induced optic neuropathy. Neuro-Ophthalmol 9(6): 357–359, 1989.

Martin E, Thiel T, Joeri P, et al. Effect of pentobarbital on visual processing in man. Hum Brain Mapp 10: 132–139, 2000.

Müller E, Huk W, Pauli E, et al. Maculo-papillary branch retinal artery occlusions following the Wada test. Graefe's Arch Clin Exp Ophthalmol 238: 715–718, 2000.

Murphy DF. Anesthesia and intraocular pressure. Anesth Analg 64: 520, 1985.

Nakame Y, et al. Multi-institutional study on the teratogenicity and fetal toxicity of antiepileptic drugs: a report of a collaborative study group in Japan. Epilepsia 21: 663, 1980.

Raitta C, et al. Changes in the electroretinogram and visual evoked potentials during general anesthesia. Graefe's Arch Clin Exp Ophthalmol 211: 139, 1979.

Tedeschi G, et al. Specific oculomotor deficits after amylobarbitone. Psychopharmacology 79: 187, 1983.

Tseng SCG, et al. Topical retinoid treatment for various dry-eye disorders. Ophthalmology 92: 717, 1985.

Wallar PH, Genstler DE, George CC. Multiple systemic and periocular malformations associated with the fetal hydantoin syndrome. Ann Ophthalmol 10: 1568, 1978.

Generic name: Chloral hydrate.

Proprietary name: Aquachloral.

Primary use

This non-barbiturate sedative-hypnotic is effective in the treatment of insomnia.

Ocular side effects

Systemic administration

Certain
1. Decreased vision
2. Pupils
   a. Mydriasis – toxic states
   b. Miosis
3. Visual hallucinations
4. Ptosis
5. Decreased convergence
6. Eyelids or conjunctiva
   a. Allergic reactions
   b. Hyperemia
   c. Edema
7. Lacrimation
8. Non-specific ocular irritation
9. Nystagmus
10. Extraocular muscles – toxic states
    a. Paralysis
    b. Jerky pursuit movements

Possible
1. Eyelids or conjunctiva
   a. Stevens-Johnson syndrome
   b. Erythema multiforme

Clinical significance

While the more serious ocular side effects due to chloral hydrate occur at excessive dosage levels, decreased convergence, miosis and occasionally ptosis are seen at recommended therapeutic dosages. The ptosis may be unilateral. Lilliputian hallucinations (in which objects appear smaller than their actual size) are said to be almost characteristic for chloral hydrate-induced delirium. Mydriasis only occurs in severely toxic states. Chloral hydrate not infrequently can cause lid edema with or without dermatitis. Ocular hyperemia and chemosis of the conjunctiva may also be seen.

REFERENCES AND FURTHER READING

Goldstein JH. Effects of drugs on cornea, conjunctiva, and lids. Int Ophthalmol Clin 11(2): 13, 1971.

Hermans G. Les psychotropes. Bull Soc Belge Ophtalmol 160: 15, 1972.

Lane RJM, Routledge PA. Drug-induced neurological disorders. Drugs 26: 124, 1983.

Levy DL, Lipton RB, Holzman PS. Smooth pursuit eye movements: effects of alcohol and chloral hydrate. J Psychiatr Res 16: 1, 1981.

Lubeck MJ. Effects of drugs on ocular muscles. Int Ophthalmol Clin 11(2): 35, 1971.

Margetts EL. Chloral delirium. Psychiatr Quart 24: 278–279, 1950.

Mowry JB, Wilson GA. Effect of exchange transfusion in chloral hydrate overdose. Vet Human Toxicol 25(Suppl. 1): 15, 1983.

Sweetman S. Martindale: The Complete Drug Reference, Pharmaceutical Press, London, Electronic Version, 2005.

Walsh FB, Hoyt WF. Clinical Neuro-Ophthalmology, 3rd edn, Vol. III, Williams & Wilkins, Baltimore, p 2619, 1969.

ANALGESICS, NARCOTIC ANTAGONISTS AND AGENTS USED TO TREAT ARTHRITIS

CLASS: AGENTS USED TO TREAT GOUT

Generic name: Allopurinol.

Proprietary names: Aloprim, Lopurin, Zyloprim.

Primary use

This potent xanthine oxidase inhibitor is primarily used in the treatment of chronic hyperuricemia.

Ocular side effects

Systemic administration

Certain
1. Decreased vision
2. Cataracts (Fig. 7.3a)
3. Eyelids or conjunctiva
   a. Allergic reactions
   b. Erythema
   c. Conjunctivitis – non-specific
   d. Edema
   e. Photosensitivity
   f. Ulceration
   g. Urticaria
   h. Purpura

Possible
1. Subconjunctival or retinal hemorrhages secondary to drug-induced anemia
2. Eyelids or conjunctiva
   a. Lupoid syndrome
   b. Erythema multiforme
   c. Stevens-Johnson syndrome
   d. Exfoliative dermatitis
   e. Lyell's syndrome
   f. Loss of eyelashes or eyebrows

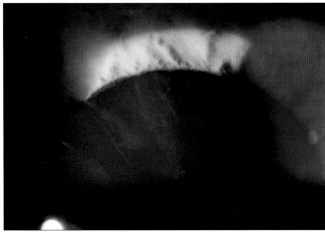

Fig. 7.3a Allopurinol-induced cataracts.

Clinical significance

The only side effects of major clinical importance are the lens changes associated with prolonged use of this agent. Lerman et al (1982) implicated the role of ultraviolet radiation as the instigator of this process. Garbe et al (1998) performed a large-scale population-based epidemiological study showing that patients taking a cumulative dose of more than 400 g of allopurinol for longer than 3 years were associated with a two-fold increased risk for cataract surgery. This type of study is rare for ophthalmology, but gives definitive proof of an association between allopurinol and cataract formation. Leske et al (1991) implicated the gout medications as second only to steroids as a major risk factor in cataractogenesis. The lens changes seen with allopurinol are anterior and posterior capsular changes with anterior subcapsular vacuoles. With time, wedge-shaped anterior and posterior cortical haze occurs. This may progress to dense posterior subcapsular opacities. While there are a few cases of macular changes reported in the literature and a number in the National Registry, to date there is no clear-cut association between allopurinol and macular changes. Almost 90% of allopurinol systemic drug side effects are skin related. Since the eyelids have some of the thinnest skin on the body, eyelid changes occur.

Recommendations

1. Patients taking allopurinol should wear ultraviolet blocking glasses. This is especially true in occupations, hobbies, etc. with increased sunlight exposure.
2. In keeping with the American Academy of Ophthalmology, patients probably should have an ophthalmic examination every 2 years.
3. Ultraviolet blocking lenses should decrease the incidence of lens changes and eyelid changes secondary to the photosensitivity effects of this drug. While there is no proof that the drug causes macular changes, the lens may protect the macula as well.

REFERENCES AND FURTHER READING

Dan M, et al. Allopurinol-induced toxic epidermal necrolysis. Int J Dermatol 23: 142, 1984.

Fraunfelder FT, Lerman S. Allopurinol and cataracts. Am J Ophthalmol 99: 215, 1985.

Fraunfelder FT, et al. Cataracts associated with allopurinol therapy. Am J Ophthalmol 94: 137, 1982.

Garbe E, Suissa S, LeLorier J. Exposure to allopurinol and the risk of cataract extraction in elderly patients. Arch Ophthalmol 116: 1652–1656, 1998.

Jick H, Brandt DE. Allopurinol and cataracts. Am J Ophthalmol 98: 355, 1984.

Laval J. Allopurinol and macular lesions. Arch Ophthalmol 80: 415, 1968.

Lerman S, Megaw JM, Gardner K. Allopurinol therapy and human cataractogenesis. Am J Ophthalmol 94: 141, 1982.

Leske MC, Chylack LT, Wu S. The lens opacities case-control study. Risk factors for cataract. Arch Ophthalmol 109: 244–251, 1991.

Pennell DJ, et al. Fatal Stevens-Johnson syndrome in a patient on captopril and allopurinol. Lancet 1: 463, 1984.

Pinnas G. Possible association between macular lesions and allopurinol. Arch Ophthalmol 79: 786, 1968.

Generic name: Colchicine.

Proprietary name: Multi-ingredient preparations only.

Primary use

This alkaloid is used in the prophylaxis and treatment of acute gout. It is also used for treating familial Mediterranean fever, Behçet's disease, rheumatoid arthritis and primary cholangitis.

Ocular side effects

Systemic administration
Certain
1. Reduction or inhibition of fibrosis
   a. Delays wound healing
   b. Enhances filtration surgery success

Probable
1. Inhibition of mitosis and migration of epithelial cells with delayed healing
   a. Dellen
   b. Corneal erosion
   c. Corneal ulcers
   d. Conjunctival wound, i.e. strabismus surgery

Possible
1. Subconjunctival or retinal hemorrhages secondary to drug-induced anemia
2. Papilledema – toxic states
3. Eyelids or conjunctiva
   a. Stevens-Johnson syndrome
   b. Toxic epidermal necroylsis

Inadvertent ocular exposure
Certain
1. Decreased vision
2. Conjunctival hyperemia
3. Corneal clouding

Clinical significance

Ocular side effects secondary to colchicine, while rare, have clinical importance. Alster et al (1997) and Biedner et al (1977) both warn that cessation of colchicine should be considered in patients who have corneal ulcers, dellen, corneal or conjuctional epithelial defects, or any ocular wounds that are refractory to conventional treatment. While these complications are probably colchicine side effects, most of the proof comes in part from animal data. Vignes et al (1998) described a case of colchicine-induced intracranial hypertension. Dickenson and Yates (2002) described a case of bilateral eyelid necrosis secondary to pseudomonal septicemia brought on by colchicine-induced neutropenia. Optic nerve changes have been found in animals, but to date no cases have been reported to the National Registry.

REFERENCES AND FURTHER READING

Alster Y, Varssano D, Loewenstein A, et al. Delay of corneal wound healing in patients treated with colchicine. Ophthalmology 104: 118–119, 1997.

Arroyo MP, Saunders S, Yee H, et al. Toxic epidermal necrolysis-like reaction secondary to colchicines overdose. Br J Dermatol 150: 581–588, 2004.

Biedner BZ, et al. Colchicine suppression of corneal healing after strabismus surgery. Br J Ophthalmol 61: 496, 1977.

Dickenson AJ, Yates J. Bilateral eyelid necrosis as a complication of pseudomonal septicaemia. Br J Oral Maxillofac Surg 40: 175–176, 2002.

Estable JJ. The ocular effect of several irritant drugs applied directly to the conjunctiva. Am J Ophthalmol 31: 837, 1948.

Heaney D, et al. Massive colchicine overdose: a report on the toxicity. Am J Med Sci 271: 233, 1976.

Naidus RM, Rodvien R, Mielke CH Jr. Colchicine toxicity. A multisystem disease. Arch Intern Med 137: 394, 1977.

Stapczynski JS, et al. Colchicine overdose: report of two cases and review of the literature. Ann Emerg Med 10: 364, 1981.

Vignes S, Vidailhet M, Dormont D, et al. Pseudotumorous presentation of neuro-Behçet: role of the withdrawal of colchicine. Revue de Medecine Interne 19(1): 55–59, 1998.

CLASS: ANTIRHEUMATIC AGENTS

Generic name: 1. Adalimumab; 2. etanercept; 3. infliximab.

Proprietary name: 1. Humira; 2. Enbrel; 3. Remicade.

Primary use

These agents block the activity of tumor necrosis factor (TNF). These drugs are primarily used in the management of various arthritic diseases and Crohn's disease.

Ocular side effects

Systemic administration
Certain
1. Optic or retrobulbar neuritis
2. Visual field defects
   a. Peripheral vision loss
   b. Various scotomas

Possible
1. Uveitis (etanercept)
2. Ocular sicca
3. Systemic lupus erythematous

Conditional/Unclassified
1. Orbit
   a. Cellulitis
   b. Myositis
2. Activation of toxoplasmosis (infliximab)
3. Retinal hemorrhage

Clinical significance

These relatively new agents have few clear-cut ocular side effects but there are areas of concern, with causation yet to be determined. Smith et al (2001) reported 60 cases of etanercept and optic neuritis. Symptoms develop within 1 to 14 months after starting therapy with a mean development time of 9.5 months. Nine patients had positive dechallenges and three had positive rechallenges. Tauber et al (2005) and Noguera-Pons et al (2005) also reported an association of this drug with optic neuritis. Fooroozan et al (2002), Mejico (2004), ten Tusscher et al (2003), Strong et al (2004), and Tran et al (2005) suggested an association of optic or retrobulbar neuritis with infliximab usage. Chung et al (2006) report two cases of optic neuritis associated with adalimumab use. There are five cases in the WHO database, making this whole class of drugs suspect as to an association with optic nerve disease. There are three cases in the National Registry showing uveitis. Some have suggested that these drugs cause or exacerbate systemic demylenating disease. This was postulated as the possible cause of a third nerve palsy with infliximab use (Farukhi et al 2006).

The question of whether or not these agents cause intraocular inflammation is confused by the fact that the diseases the drugs are used to treat may also cause uveitis. There are two cases in the literature (Reddy and Backhouse 2003) and a case in the National Registry showing uveitis occurring each time etanercept was started and clearing each time the drug was stopped. Taban et al (2006) reported a case of positive double rechallenge of etanercept exacerbating anterior uveitis. Hashkes and Shajrawi (2003) reported sarcoid related uveitis occurring during etanercept therapy. De Vos et al (1995) have shown exacerbation of uveitis with anti-tumor necrosis factor in animals. It is possible one may find a subset of patients for which etanercept may cause or aggravate uveitis. Infliximab seems to be free of causing uveitis.

While some suggest etanercept as a treatment for scleritis there are three cases in the National Registry where this drug is implicated as causing or exacerbating scleritis. Since the disease these drugs are used to treat can also cause scleriis, at this time a drug-induced effect is suspect. Since these drugs can cause a dry mouth, they may aggravate ocular sicca. Reports of these drugs causing systemic vasculitis and suppression of the hemopoetic systems possibly supports occasional reports of retinal vascular abnormalities and vitreous hemorrhage.

Single cases of possible retinal toxicity causing visual field changes with etanercept (Clifford and Rossiter 2004), orbital myositis (Caramaschi et al 2003) and orbital cellutitis (Roos and Ostor 2006) have been reported. We have no cases of either of these in the National Registry.

REFERENCES AND FURTHER READING

Bleumink BS, terBorg EJ, Ramselaar CG, et al. Etanercept-induced subacute cutaneous lupus erythematosus. Rheumatology 40: 1317–1319, 2001.

Caramaschi P, Carletto A, Biasi D, et al. Orbital myositis in rheumatoid arthritis patient during etanercept treatment. Clin Exp Rheumotol 21: 136–137, 2003.

Chung JH, Van Stavern GP, Frohman LP, et al. Adalimumab-associated optic neuritis. J Neurol Sci 244: 133–136, 2006.

Clifford LJ, Rossiter JD. Peripheral visual field loss following treatment with etanercept. Br J Ophthalmol 88: 842, 2004.

De Vos AF, Van Haren MAC, Verhagen C, et al. Systemic anti-tumor necrosis factor antibody treatment exacerbates endotoxin-induced uveitis in the rat. Exp Eye Res 61: 667–675, 1995.

Farukhi FI, Bollinger K, Ruggieri P, et al. Infliximab-associated third nerve palsy. Arch Ophthalmol 124: 1055–1057, 2006.

Foroozan R, Buono LM, Sergott RC, et al. Retrobulbar optic neuritis associated with infliximab. Arch Ophthalmol 120: 985–987, 2002.

Hashkes PJ, Shajrawi I. Sarcoid-related uveitis occurring during etanercept therapy. Clin Exp Rheumatol 21: 645–646, 2003.

Hernandez-Illas M, Tozman E, Fulcher AFA, et al. Recombinant human tumor necrosis factor receptor fc fusion protein (etanercept): experience as a therapy for sight-threatening scleritis and sterile corneal ulceration. Eye Contact Lens 30: 2–5, 2004.

Koizumi K, Poulaki V, Doehmen S, et al. Contribution of TNF-alpha to leukocyte adhesion, vascular leakage, and apoptotic cell death in endotoxin-induced uveitis in vivo. Invest Ophthalmol Vis Sci 44: 2184–2191, 2003.

Mejico LJ. Infliximab-associated retrobulbar optic neuritis. Arch Ophthalmol 122: 793–794, 2004.

Noguera-Pons R, Borrás-Blasco J, Romero-Crespo I, et al. Optic neuritis with concurrent etanercept and isoniazid therapy. Ann Pharmacother 39: 2131–2135, 2005.

Rajaraman RT, Kimura Y, Li S, et al. Retrospective case review of pediatric patients with uveitis treated with infliximab. Ophthalmology 113: 308–314, 2006.

Reddy AR, Backhouse OC. Does etanercept induce uveitis? Br J Ophthalmol 87: 925, 2003.

Reiff A, Takei S, Sadeghi S, et al. Etanercept therapy in children with treatment-resistant uveitis. Arthritis Rheum 44: 1411–1415, 2001.

Roos JCP, Ostor AJK. Orbital cellulitis in a patient receiving infliximab for ankylosing spondylitis. Am J Ophthalmol 141: 767–769, 2006.

Rosenbaum JT. Effect of etanercept on iritis in patients with ankylosing spondylitis. Arthritis Rheum 50: 3736–3737, 2004.

Scheinfeld N. A comprehensive review and evaluation of the side effects of the tumor necrosis factor alpha blockers etanercept, infliximab and adalimumab. J Dermatol Treat 15: 280–294, 2004.

Smith JR, Levinson RD, Holland GN, et al. Differential efficacy of tumor necrosis factor inhibition in the management of inflammatory eye disease and associated rheumatic disease. Arthritis Care Res 45: 252–257, 2001.

Strong BYC, Erny BC, Herzenberg H, et al. Retrobulbar optic neuritis associated with infliximab in a patient with Crohn disease. Ann Intern Med 140: 677–678, 2004.

Swale VJ, Perrett CM, Denton CP. Etanercept-induced systemic lupus erythematosus. Clin Exp Dermatol 28: 604–607, 2003.

Taban M, Dupps WJ, Mandell B, et al. Etanercept (enbrel)-associated inflammatory eye disease: case report and review of the literature. Ocul Immunol Inflamm 14: 145–150, 2006.

Tauber T, Daniel D, Barash J, et al. Optic neuritis associated with etanercept therapy in two patients with extended oligoarticular juvenile idiopathic arthritis. Rheumatology 44: 405, 2005.

Tiliakos AN, Tiliakos NA. Ocular inflammatory disease in patients with rheumatoid arthritis taking etanercept: is discontinuation of etanercept necessary? J Rheumatol 30: 2727, 2003.

ten Tusscher MPM, Jacobs PJC, Busch MJWM, et al. Bilateral anterior toxic neuropathy and the use of infliximab. BMJ 326: 579, 2003.

Tran TH, Milea D, Cassoux N, et al. Optic neuritis associated with infliximab. J Fr Ophtalmol 28: 201–204, 2005.

Young JD, McGwire BS. Infliximab and reactivation of cerebral toxoplasmosis. N Engl J Med 353: 1530–1531, 2005.

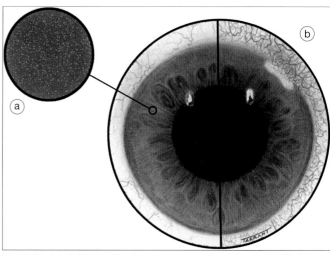

Fig. 7.3b Dust-like or glittering purple granules (a) and marginal keratitis (b) related to systemic auranofin use. Photo courtesy of Kanski JJ. Clinical Diagnosis in Ophthalmology, Mosby Elsevier, London, 2006.

Generic names: 1. Auranofin; 2. aurothioglucose; 3. sodium aurothiomalate (gold sodium thiomalate).

Proprietary names: 1. Ridaura; 2. Solganal; 3. Aurolate, Myocrysine.

Primary use

These heavy metals are used in the treatment of active rheumatoid arthritis and non-disseminated lupus erythematosus.

Ocular side effects

Systemic administration
Certain

1. Red, violet, purple or brown gold deposits (Fig. 7.3b)
   a. Eyelids
   b. Conjunctiva
   c. Cornea
   d. Surface of lens
2. Eyelids or conjunctiva
   a. Allergic reactions
   b. Hyperemia
   c. Erythema
   d. Blepharoconjunctivitis
   e. Edema
   f. Photosensitivity
   g. Symblepharon
   h. Angioneurotic edema
   i. Urticaria
   j. Purpura
3. Photophobia

4. Cornea
   a. Keratitis
   b. Ulceration
   c. Stromal melting
5. Iris and ciliary body
   a. Hyperemia
   b. Inflammation
   c. Cells and flare

Probable

1. May activate
   a. Herpes infections
   b. Guillain-Barre syndrome

Possible

1. Myasthenia gravis
   a. Diplopia
   b. Ptosis
   c. Paresis of extraocular muscles
2. Nystagmus
3. Subconjunctival or retinal hemorrhages secondary to drug-induced anemia
4. Eyelids or conjunctiva
   a. Lupoid syndrome
   b. Erythema multiforme
   c. Stevens-Johnson syndrome
   d. Exfoliative dermatitis
   e. Lyell's syndrome

Clinical significance

Patients taking any of the gold agent may show one of two patterns of ocular chrysiasis. The more common pattern is where gold salts are deposited in the conjunctiva, all layers of the cornea and in the crystalline lens. Gold deposition in the cornea may take a Hudson-Stähli line distribution or a vortex distribution, not unlike Fabry's disease. The gold deposits tend to be increased in areas of corneal scarring. Deep corneal deposition is usually in the posterior half of the cornea and denser inferiorly, while the superior cornea and perilimbal areas are more often spared. Lens deposits of gold are much less frequent than corneal deposits and are of little to no clinical importance. These deposits are reversible after stopping gold therapy but may take 3–12 months, and in some cases many years, to resolve. Visual acuity is unaffected, and deposition of gold in the cornea or lens is not an indication for cessation of therapy. In general, a total of over 1 g of gold deposited is needed before corneal changes are seen. In total dosages of 1.5 g 40–80% of patients will have gold deposition in the cornea. While lens deposits have previously been considered rare, 55% of patients on daily dosages over 1 g for 3 or more years have been reported to develop lens deposits. Corneal deposits may be seen as early as 1 month after starting therapy. It has been suggested that gold deposits in the cornea and lens are secondary to metal from the aqueous fluid or perilimbal blood vessels.

The second variant of ocular chrysiasis is much less common. This type presents as an inflammatory response secondary to gold, including corneal ulceration, subepithelial white perilimbal infiltrates, brush-like perilimbal stromal vascularization and interstitial keratitis (Arffa 1991; McCormick et al 1985). Corneal ulceration is more often marginal, crescent shaped and may be 2–3 mm in length. This response is felt to be an idiosyncratic allergic reaction, may be unilateral or bilateral, and is an indication in most patients to stop therapy. Zamir et al (2001) point out in patients presenting with marginal keratitis that this variant of chrysiasis should be considered. Stopping gold therapy along with looking for systemic toxicity is often warranted. Patients must be continuously followed since stromal inflammation may reoccur even after gold is stopped.

REFERENCES AND FURTHER READING

Arffa RC. Drugs and metals. In: Grayson's Diseases of the Cornea. 3rd edn, Arffa RC (ed), Mosby, St Louis, pp 617–631, 1991.
Bron A, McLendon B, Camp A. Epithelial deposition of gold in the cornea in patients receiving systemic therapy. Am J Ophthalmol 88: 354–360, 1979.
Dick D, Raman D. The Guillain-Barre syndrome following gold therapy. Scand J Rheumatol 11: 119, 1982.
Evanchick CC, Harrington TM. Transient monocular visual loss after aurothioglucose. J Rheumatol 12: 619, 1985.
Fam AG, Paton TW, Cowan DH. Herpes zoster during gold therapy. Ann Intern Med 94: 712, 1981.
Gottlieb NL, Major JC. Ocular chrysiasis correlated with gold concentrations in the crystalline lens during chrysotherapy. Arthritis Rheum 21: 704–708, 1978.
Kincaid MC, et al: Ocular chrysiasis. Arch Ophthalmol 100: 1791, 1982.
Lopez JD, Benitez del Castillo JM, Lopez CD, et al. Confocal microscopy in ocular chrysiasis. Cornea 22: 573–575, 2003.
McCormick SA, et al. Ocular chrysiasis. Ophthalmology 92: 1432, 1985.
Moore AP, et al. Penicillamine-induced myasthenia reactivated by gold. BMJ 288: 192, 1984.
Segawa K. Electron microscopy of the trabecular meshwork in open-angle glaucoma associated with gold therapy. Glaucoma 3: 257, 1981.
Weidle EG. Lenticular chrysiasis in oral chrysotherapy. Am J Ophthalmol 103: 240, 1987.
Zamir E, Read RW, Affeldt JC. Gold induced interstitial keratitis. Br J Ophthalmol 85: 1386–1387, 2001.

Generic names: 1. Celecoxib; 2. etolodac; 3. nimesulide; 4. rofecoxib; 5. valdecoxib.

Proprietary names: 1. Celebrex; 2. Lodine; 3. Ainex; 4. Vioxx; 5. Bextra.

Primary use

These non-steroidal anti-inflammatory drugs are selective inhibitors of cyclooxygenase-2 and are used in various forms in the treatment of arthritis, acute pain and dysmenorrhea.

Ocular side effects

Systemic administration
Certain
1. Blurred vision
2. Eyelids and conjunctiva – conjunctivitis

Possible
1. Retinal venous occlusions
2. Eyelids or conjunctiva
   a. Stevens-Johnson syndrome
   b. Toxic epidermal necrolysis

Conditional/Unclassified
1. Visual field defects
   a. Orange spots
   b. Central scotomas
2. Temporary blindness
3. Scintillating scotoma
4. Teichopsia

Clinical significance

The above-mentioned side effects are extremely rare. Fraunfelder et al (2006) reported blurred vision and conjunctivitis with multiple cases of positive rechallenge. The onset may occur within a few hours to days and if the drug is discontinued, resolves within 72 hours. Meyer et al (2006) made known a possible association of thrombotic events in selected patients. These findings include central retinal vein or other retinal venous occlusions. Meyer et al (2006) pointed out that the US FDA strongly associate the use of COX-2 inhibitors with Stevens-Johnson syndrome and toxic epidermal necrolysis. Coulter and Clark (2004) reported a case of temporary blindness and another with bilateral jellybean shaped loss of central vision. Lund and Neiman (2001) reported a case of orange spots in both visual fields. All signs and symptoms are fully reversible. The mechanism of action is postulated as inhibition of synthesis of prostaglandins that control blood flow. Also, most of these agents are sulfonamides with known drug-induced transient myopia.

REFERENCES AND FURTHER READING

Coulter DM, Clark DW. Disturbance of vision by cox-2 inhibitors. Expert Opin Drug Saf 3: 607–614, 2004.
Coulter D, Clark D. Visual disturbances with cox-2 inhibitors. Prescr Update 25: 8–9, 2004.
Coulter DM, Clark DWJ, Savage RL. Celecoxib, rofecoxib, and acute temporary visual impairment. BMJ 327: 1214–1215, 2003.
Cyclooxygenase-2 inhibitors: reports of visual disturbances. WHO Pharmaceuticals Newsletter. 3: 4, 2004.
Fraunfelder FW, Solomon J, Mehelas TJ. Ocular adverse effects associated with cyclooxygenase-2 inhibitors. Arch Ophthalmol 124: 277–278, 2006.
Lund BC, Neiman RF. Visual disturbance associated with celecoxib. Pharmacotherapy 21: 114–115, 2001.
Meyer CH, Mennel S, Schmidt JC, et al: Adverse effects of cyclooxygenase-2 inhibitors on ocular vision. Arch Ophthalmol 124: 1368, 2006.

Generic name: Fenoprofen calcium.

Proprietary name: Nalfon.

Primary use

This non-steroidal anti-inflammatory agent is used in the management of rheumatoid arthritis.

Ocular side effects

Systemic administration
Certain
1. Decreased vision
2. Diplopia
3. Eyelids or conjunctiva
   a. Erythema
   b. Conjunctivitis – non-specific
   c. Angioneurotic edema
   d. Urticaria

Possible
1. Optic neuritis
2. Visual field defects
   a. Scotomas – centrocecal or paracentral
   b. Enlarged blind spot
   c. Constriction
3. Subconjunctival or retinal hemorrhages secondary to drug-induced anemia
4. Eyelids or conjunctiva
   a. Erythema multiforme
   b. Stevens-Johnson syndrome
   c. Exfoliative dermatitis
   d. Toxic epidermal necrolysis

Clinical significance

Ocular side effects are seldom of clinical significance with fenoprofen. The most common adverse events are transient blurred vision and diplopia. Many of the adverse events associated with the other non-steroidal anti-inflammatories have been reported to the National Registry with fenoprofen, however, the numbers are small. Any skin lesion associated with the use of this drug requires stopping the drug and obtaining dermatologic consultation since a small number go on to severe systemic disease. Again, as with others in this group of drugs, there appears to be a rare idiosyncratic optic nerve response that may be associated with the use of this drug. There have been cases reported to the National Registry where there was a unilateral or bilateral decrease in visual acuity ranging from 20/80 to 20/200 after 6 months of therapy. Visual fields may show various types of scotoma. If the medication is stopped, the visual acuity usually returns to normal in 1 to 3 months. It has, however, taken over 8 months for color vision to return. It is not possible to state a positive cause-and-effect relationship between optic neuritis and this drug. It is prudent, however, to stop the medication if optic neuritis occurs. There are no reports in the literature or in the National Registry of this agent causing intracranial hypertension.

REFERENCES AND FURTHER READING

Bigby M, Stern R. Cutaneous reactions to nonsteroidal anti-inflammatory drugs. A review. J Am Acad Dermatol 12: 866, 1985.
McEvoy GK (ed). American Hospital Formulary Service Drug Information 87, American Society for Hospital Pharmacists, Bethesda, pp 914–917, 1987.
Sweetman SC (ed). Martindale: The Complete Drug Reference. 34th edn. Pharmaceutical Press, London, p 39, 2004.
Treusch PJ, et al. Agranulocytosis associated with fenoprofen. JAMA 241: 2700, 1979.

Generic name: Flurbiprofen.

Proprietary names: Ansaid, Ocufen.

Primary use

Systemic
This non-steroidal anti-inflammatory agent is used in the treatment of rheumatoid arthritis.

Ophthalmic
Flurbiprofen is used for the inhibition of intraoperative miosis.

Ocular side effects

Systemic administration
Possible
1. Decreased vision
2. Eyelids or conjunctiva
   a. Erythema
   b. Conjunctivitis – non-specific
   c. Urticaria
3. Diplopia
4. Subconjunctival or retinal hemorrhages secondary to drug-induced anemia

Local ophthalmic use or exposure
Certain
1. Irritation
   a. Hyperemia
   b. Burning sensation
2. Cornea
   a. Punctate keratitis
   b. Delayed wound healing

Probable
1. May aggravate herpes infections
2. Increased ocular or periocular bleeding

Clinical significance

Ocular side effects secondary to systemic administration are infrequent. While side effects reported with other non-steroidal anti-inflammatory agents must be looked for, to date no cases of optic neuritis or intracranial hypertension have been reported to the National Registry.

Generally, short-term therapy with ophthalmic flurbiprofen has been well tolerated; the most frequent adverse reactions have been mild transient stinging and burning on instillation. Flurbiprofen has been shown to inhibit corneal scleral wound healing, decrease leukocytes in tears and increase complications of herpetic keratitis. Flurbiprofen is one of the more potent non-steroidal anti-inflammatory drugs, which can interfere with thrombocyte aggregation. This may cause intraoperative bleeding as a rare event. This is more common if the patient is already on anticoagulants.

REFERENCES AND FURTHER READING

Bergamini MVW. Pharmacology of flurbiprofen, a nonsteroidal anti-inflammatory drug. Int Ophthalmol Rep 6: 2, 1981.

Feinstein NC. Toxicity of flurbiprofen sodium. Arch Ophthalmol 106: 311, 1988.

Flurbiprofen – an ophthalmic NSAID. Med Lett Drugs Ther 29: 58, 1987.

Gimbel HV. The effect of treatment with topical nonsteroidal anti-inflammatory drugs with and without intraoperative epinephrine on the maintenance of mydriasis during cataract surgery. Ophthalmology 96(5): 585–588, 1989.

Miller D, et al. Topical flurbiprofen or prednisolone. Effect on corneal wound healing in rabbits. Arch Ophthalmol 99: 681, 1981.

Romano A, Pietrantonio F. Delayed hypersensitivity to flurbiprofen. J Int Med 241(1): 81–83, 1997.

Samples JR. Sodium flurbiprofen for surgically induced miosis and the control of inflammation. J Toxico Cut Ocular Toxico 8(2): 163–166, 1989.

Trousdale MD, Dunkel EC, Nesburn AB. Effect of flurbiprofen on herpes simplex keratitis in rabbits. Invest Ophthalmol Vis Sci 19: 267, 1980.

Generic name: Ibuprofen.

Proprietary names: Advil, Ibu, Ibu-tab, Genpril, Motrin, Nuprin.

Primary use

This antipyretic analgesic is used in the treatment of rheumatoid arthritis and osteoarthritis.

Ocular side effects

Systemic administration
Certain
1. Decreased vision
2. Diplopia
3. Problems with color vision
   a. Color vision defect, red-green defect
   b. Colors appear faded
4. Abnormal visual sensations
   a. Moving mosaic of colored lights
   b. Shooting streaks
5. Abnormal ERG or VEP
6. Keratoconjunctivitis sicca
7. Photophobia
8. Visual hallucinations
9. Eyelids or conjunctiva
   a. Erythema
   b. Conjunctivitis – non-specific
   c. Edema
   d. Photosensitivity
   e. Angioneurotic edema
   f. Urticaria
   g. Purpura
10. Cornea – vortex keratopathy

Probable
1. Periorbital edema

Possible
1. Optic or retrobulbar neuritis
2. Myopia
3. Papilledema secondary to intracranial hypertension
4. Visual fields
   a. Scotomas – centrocecal or paracentral
   b. Constriction
   c. Hemianopsia
   d. Enlarged blind spot
5. Toxic amblyopia
6. Macular edema
7. Subconjunctival or retinal hemorrhages secondary to drug-induced anemia
8. Eyelids or conjunctiva
   a. Lupoid syndrome
   b. Erythema multiforme
   c. Stevens-Johnson syndrome
   d. Lyell's syndome
   e. Lupus erythematosus

Clinical significance

Ibuprofen is one of the largest selling antiarthritic agents in the world. The adverse ocular event most commonly associated with this drug is transient blurred vision. In those patients who have experienced a drug rechallenge, refractive error changes, diplopia, photophobia, dry eyes and decrease in color vision appear to be well documented. A typical vortex keratopathy with deposition limited to the corneal epthelium has been described. Once the drug was stopped, this resolved within 3 weeks. Other nonsteroidal inflammatories such as indometacin and naproxen can also cause corneal epithelial deposition. While sicca has been attributed to this drug, one suspects that this in part is secondary to the drug being in the tears and aggravating an already dry eye. Palungwachira et al (2005) described a case of periorbital edema due to ibuprofen and there is one case of this in the National Registry as well. Nicastro (1989) described three young females who were long-term ibuprofen users who possibly developed macular edema with vision in the 20/30 to 20/50 range. Once the drug was stopped, vision returned to 20/20. Reversible toxic ambyopia has been reported (Ravi et al 1986; Clements et al 1990).

This drug can cause other CNS changes, including aseptic meningitis with secondary effects on the visual system. If ibuprofen is not discontinued, permanent visual loss may result. For a drug so commonly used in combination with other agents, it is not possible to implicate specifically this agent. However, many of the cases are outside the usual multiple sclerosis age group and occur shortly after starting this medication. Patients on this drug should therefore be told to stop this medication if a sudden decrease in vision occurs. If there is an unexplained decrease in vision that occurs while on ibuprofen, tests to rule out optic nerve abnormalities should be considered. There may be a rare idiosyncratic optic nerve response associated with the use of this drug. The typical sequence is that after a few months of therapy, a unilateral or bilateral marked decrease in visual acuity occurs, with vision receding to the 20/80 to 20/200 range. Visual fields may show various types of scotomas. If the medication is stopped, visual acuity usually returns to normal in 1–3 months, but it may take up to 8 months for color vision to return to normal.

Ibuprofen, as well as other non-steroidal anti-inflammatories, may possibly cause intracranial hypertension. This is more common if used in combination with other antiarthritic agents, which can also induce this side effect.

REFERENCES AND FURTHER READING

Asherov J, et al. Diplopia following ibuprofen administration. JAMA 248: 649, 1982.

Bernstein HN. Some iatrogenic ocular diseases from systemically administered drugs. Int Ophthalmol Clin 10: 553–619, 1970.

Birch J, et al. Acquired color vision defects. In: Congenital and Acquired Color Vision Defects, Pokorny J et al (eds), Grune & Stratton, New York, 1979, p 243–350.

Clements D, et al. Colitis associated with ibuprofen. BMJ 301: 987, 1990.

Collum LMT, Bowen DI. Ocular side-effects of ibuprofen. Br J Ophthalmol 55: 472–477, 1971.

Court H, Streete P, Volans GN. Acute poisoning with ibuprofen. Human Toxicol 2: 381, 1983.

Dua HS, Forrester JV. The corneoscleral limbus in human corneal epithelial wound healing. Am J Ophthalmol 110: 646–656, 1990.

Fraunfelder FT. Interim report: National Registry of Possible Drug-Induced Ocular Side Effects. Ophthalmology 87: 87, 1980.

Hamburger HA, Beckman H, Thompson R. Visual evoked potentials and ibuprofen (Motrin) toxicity. Ann Ophthalmol 16: 328, 1984.

Melluish JW, et al. Ibuprofen and visual function. Arch Ophthalmol 93: 781, 1975.

Nicastro NJ. Visual disturbances associated with over-the-counter ibuprofen in three patients. Ann Ophthalmol 29: 447–450, 1989.

Palmer CAL. Toxic amblyopia from ibuprofen. BMJ 3: 765, 1972.

Palungwachira P, Palungwachira P, Ogawa H. Localized periorbital edema induced by ibuprofen. J Dermatol 32: 969–971, 2005.

Quinn JP, et al. Eosinophilic meningitis and ibuprofen therapy. Neurology 34: 108, 1984.

Ravi S, et al. Colitis caused by non-steroidal anti-inflammatory drugs. Postgrad Med J 62: 773–776, 1986.

Szmyd L, Perry HD. Keratopathy associated with the use of naproxen. Am J Ophthalmol 99: 598, 1985.

Tullio CJ. Ibuprofen-induced visual disturbance. Am J Hosp Pharm 38: 1362, 1981.

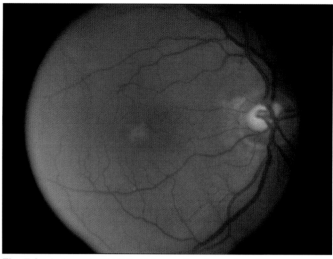

Fig. 7.3c Indomethacin induced macular pigment mottling.

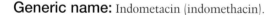

Generic name: Indometacin (indomethacin).

Proprietary names: Indocin, Indocin SR, Indo-lemmon, Indomethegan G.

Primary use

Systemic

This non-steroidal anti-inflammatory drug is a methylated indole derivative used as an antipyretic, analgesic or anti-inflammatory agent in the treatment of rheumatoid arthritis, rheumatoid spondylitis and degenerative joint disease.

Ophthalmic

Indometacin has been advocated for the treatment of cystoid macular edema or preoperatively to enhance mydriasis at cataract surgery. It has also been advocated in the management of symptoms due to corneal scars, edema, erosions or post refractory surgery pain.

Ocular side effects

Systemic administration
Certain
1. Blurred vision – transitory
2. Conjunctiva and cornea
   a. Irritation
   b. Keratitis
   c. Corneal deposits
   d. Corneal erosions

3. Abnormal ERG or EOG
4. Problems with color vision – color blue defect, yellow defect
5. Retina or macula
   a. Edema
   b. Degeneration
   c. Pigment mottling (Fig. 7.3c)
6. Visual fields
   a. Scotoma
   b. Constriction
   c. Enlarged blind spot

Possible
1. Intracranial hypertension
   a. Papilledema
   b. 6th nerve palsy
2. Optic neuritis
3. Induced anemia
   a. Conjunctival – hemorrhages
   b. Retinal – hemorrhages

Local ophthalmic use or exposure - topical ocular
Certain
1. Irritation
   a. Burning sensation
2. Superficial punctate keratitis
3. Eyelids
   a. Edema
   b. Erythema
   c. Contact dermatitis
4. Decreases miosis during intraocular surgery (weak)
5. Local anesthesia

Clinical significance

Indometacin has been used for over four decades with few ocular side effects unless the drug is used for prolonged periods in high doses. Its most serious side effect is retinal pigmentary retinopathy, with macular atrophy and a waxy disk (Burns 1968; Henkes et al 1972). This is associated with depressed ERG and constricted visual fields. While blurred vision may occur after starting this agent, seldom is it of clinical significance. The drug is probably secreted in the tears, thereby causing corneal deposits, irritation and occasionally a keratitis. Intracranial hypertension and optic neuritis have been reported with indometacin use.

Keratorefractive surgery has brought topical ocular indometacin back into clinical use in large part because it has fewer side effects than steroids. Its main use is as a local anesthetic, showing less damage to the corneal epithelium (Badalá et al 2004) in the immediate post-operative period. Sheehan and Kutzner (1989) reported a case of possible acute asthma due to topical ocular indometacin.

REFERENCES AND FURTHER READING

Badalá F, Fiorett M, Macrí A. Effect of topical 0.1% indomethacin solution versus 0.1% fluorometholon acetate on ocular surface and pain control following laser subepithelial keratomileusis (LASEK). Cornea 23: 550–553, 2004.

Birch J, et al. Acquired color vision defects. In: Congenital and Acquired Color Vision Defects, Pokorny J, et al. Grune & Stratton, New York, 1979, pp 243–350.

Burns CA. Indomethacin, reduced retinal sensitivity, and corneal deposits. Am J Ophthalmol 66: 825–835, 1968.

Carr RE, Siegel IM. Retinal function in patients treated with indomethacin. Am J Ophthalmol 75: 302–306, 1973.

Fraunfelder FT, Samples JR, Fraunfelder FW. Possible optic nerve side effects associated with nonsteroidal anti-inflammatory drugs. J Toxicol Cut Ocular Toxicol 13(4): 311–316, 1994.

Frucht-Pery J, Levinger S, Zauberman H. The effect of topical administration of indomethacin on symptoms in corneal scars and edema. Am J Ophthalmol 112(2): 186–190, 1991.

Frucht-Pery J, Siganos CS, Solomon A, et al. Topical indomethacin solution versus Dexamethasone solution for treatment of inflamed pterygium and pinguecula: a prospective randomized clinical study. Am J Ophthalmol 127: 148–152, 1999.

Gimbel HW. The effect of treatment with topical nonsteroidal anti-inflammatory drugs with and without intraoperative epinephrine on the maintenance of mydriasis during cataract surgery. Ophthalmology 96(5): 585–588, 1989.

Gomez A, Florido JF, Quiralte J, et al. Allergic contact dermatitis due to indomethacin and diclofenac. Contact Dermatitis 43: 59, 2000.

Graham CM, Blach RK. Indomethacin retinopathy: case report and review. Br J Ophthalmol 72: 434–438, 1988.

Henkes HE, van Lith GHM, Canta LR. Indomethacin retinopathy. Am J Ophthalmol 73: 846–856, 1972.

Katz IM. Indomethacin. Ophthalmology 88: 455, 1981.

Katzman B, Lu L, Tiwari RP, et al. Pseudotumor cerebri: an observation and review. Ann Ophthalmol 13: 887, 1981.

Palimeris G, Koliopoulos J, Velissaropoulos P. Ocular side effects of indomethacin. Ophthalmologica 164: 339–353, 1972.

Procianoy RS, Garcia-Prats JA, Hittner HM, et al. Use of indomethacin and its relationship to retinopathy of prematurity in very low birthweight infants. Arch Dis Child 55: 362–364, 1980.

Rich LF. Toxic drug effects on the cornea. J Toxicol Cut Ocular Toxicol I: 267, 1982–1983.

Sheehan GJ, Kutzner MR. Acute asthma attack due to ophthalmic indocin. Ann Int Med 111: 337–338, 1989.

Toler SM. Oxidative stress plays an important role in the pathogenesis of drug-induced retinopathy. Exp Biol Med 229: 607–615, 2004.

Yoshizumi MO, Schwartz S, Peterson M. Ocular toxicity of topical indomethacin eye drops. J Toxicol 10(3): 201–206, 1991.

Generic name: Ketoprofen.

Proprietary name: Oruvail.

Primary use

This non-steroidal anti-inflammatory drug with antipyretic and analgesic properties is used in the treatment of rheumatoid arthritis, osteoarthritis, ankylosing spondylitis and gout.

Ocular side effects

Systemic administration
Probable
1. Eyelids or conjunctiva
   a. Erythema
   b. Conjunctivitis – non-specific
   c. Edema
   d. Discoloration
   e. Photosensitivity
   f. Urticaria
   g. Purpura
   h. Contact dermatitis
   i. Angioneurotic edema
2. Non-specific ocular irritation
   a. Hyperemia
   b. Ocular pain
3. Visual hallucinations

Possible
1. Subconjunctival or retinal hemorrhages – secondary to systemic anemia
2. Decreased vision
3. Keratoconjunctivitis sicca
4. May aggravate the following disease
   a. Myasthenia gravis
   b. Herpes infections
5. Eyelids or conjunctiva
   a. Exfoliative dermatitis
   b. Eczema

Conditional/Unclassified
1. Paralysis of extraocular muscles

Clinical significance

Ketoprofen rarely causes ocular problems. There has only been one case each of intracranial hypertension or a possible optic neuritis reported to the National Registry, so a causative relationship is highly unlikely. Ketoprofen, however, has been associated with precipitating cholinergic crises. It has also been associated with herpes simplex activation systemically and ocularly. We are not convinced that this agent causes keratoconjunctivitis sicca. However, since the drug is secreted in the tears, it would have the potential to aggravate patients with borderline sicca or those with pre-existing sicca. This agent is a photosensitizing agent may cause ocular phototoxicity. There is only one report (McDowell and McConnell 1985) of precipitating a cholinergic crisis in a patient with myasthenia gravis.

REFERENCES AND FURTHER READING

Alomar A. Ketoprofen photodermatitis. Contact Dermatitis 12: 112, 1985.

Dukes MNG (ed). Meyler's Side Effects of Drugs, Vol. X. Excerpta Medica, Amsterdam, p 163, 1984.

Fraunfelder FT, Samples JR, Fraunfelder FW. Possible optic nerve side effects associated with nonsteroidal anti-inflammatory drugs. J Toxicol Cut Ocular Toxicol 13(4): 311–316, 1994.

Larizza D, et al. Ketoprofen causing pseudotumor cerebri in Bartter's syndrome. N Engl J Med 300: 796, 1979.
Le Coz CJ, Bottlaender A, Scrivener JN, Santinelli F. Photocontact dermatitis from ketoprofen and tiaprofenic acid: cross-reactivity study in 12 consecutive patients. Contact Dermatitis 38(5): 245–252, 1998.
McDowell IFW, McConnell JB. Cholinergic crisis in myasthenia gravis precipitated by ketoprofen. BMJ 291: 1094, 1985.
Umez-Eronini EM. Conjunctivitis due to ketoprofen. Lancet 2: 737, 1978.

Generic name: Naproxen.

Proprietary names: Aleve, Anaprox, Anaprox DS, Ec-naprosyn, Naprelan, Naprosyn.

Primary use

This antipyretic analgesic is used in the treatment of rheumatoid arthritis, osteoarthritis and ankylosing spondylitis.

Ocular side effects

Systemic administration
Certain
1. Decreased vision
2. Papilledema secondary to intracranial hypertension
3. Photophobia
4. Corneal opacities – verticillate pattern
5. Eyelids or conjunctiva
    a. Allergic reactions
    b. Erythema
    c. Conjunctivitis – non-specific
    d. Edema
    e. Photosensitivity
    f. Angioneurotic edema
    g. Urticaria
    h. Purpura
    i. Loss of eyelashes or eyebrows

Probable
1. Problems with color vision
    a. Color vision defect
    b. Objects have green or red tinge
2. Optic or retrobulbar neuritis
3. Visual field defects
    a. Scotomas – centrocecal or paracentral
    b. Constriction
    c. Hemianopia
    d. Enlarged blind spot

Possible
1. Subconjunctival or retinal hemorrhages secondary to drug-induced anemia
2. Eyelids or conjunctiva
    a. Erythema multiforme
    b. Stevens-Johnson syndrome
    c. Exfoliative dermatitis
    d. Lyell's syndrome

Conditional/Unclassified
1. Exacerbation of glaucoma
2. Cornea – peripheral ulcerations

Clinical significance

With increased use of this non-steroidal anti-inflammatory agent, more adverse ocular effects have been reported. Although some patients complain of decreased vision, this is seldom a significant finding and occurs in less than 5% of patients. In rare instances, it is possible that this agent can cause optic or retrobulbar neuritis. This, however, is not proven, although this group of drugs can cause numerous CNS side effects. Typically, these patients are on the drug for about a year before the optic neuritis, often unilateral, presents. There are cases in the National Registry of this occurring in only a few months of therapy. The drug should be discontinued until an etiology of the neuritis is established. This probable side effect seems to be more common in patients with renal disease, on multiple other drugs or with autoimmune disease. Intracranial hypertension seems to be well documented to occur with naproxen. Well-described aseptic meningitis is seen with this agent with secondary effects on the visual system. Whether or not this agent causes anterior or posterior cataracts is unknown; there are 20 such reports in the National Registry, but there is neither pattern nor proof to date of a cause-and-effect relationship. Whorl-like corneal opacities have been associated (Sznyd and Perry 1985) with the use of naproxen, and the National Registry has also received several reports of peripheral corneal ulcerations. This agent is one of the more potent photosensitizing non-steroidal anti-inflammatory agents. Ultraviolet light blocking lenses may be indicated in selected patients. Fincham (1989) reported a case of exacerbation of glaucoma, which may be secondary to naproxen.

REFERENCES AND FURTHER READING

Fincham JE. Exacerbation of glaucoma in an elderly female taking naproxen sodium: a case report. J Geriatr Drug Ther 3: 139–143, 1989.
Fraunfelder FT. Interim report: National Registry of Possible Drug-Induced Ocular Side Effects. Ophthalmology 86: 126, 1979.
Fraunfelder FT, Samples JR, Fraunfelder FW. Possible optic nerve side effects associated with nonsteroidal anti-inflammatory drugs. J Toxicol Cut Ocular Toxicol 13(4): 311–316, 1994.
Harry DJ, Hicks H. Naproxen hypersensitivity. Hosp Form 18: 648, 1983.
McEvoy GK. American Hospital Formulary Service Drug Information 87. American Society of Hospital Pharmacists, Bethesda, p 942–946, 1987.
Mordes JP, Johnson MW, Soter NA. Possible naproxen associated vasculitis. Arch Intern Med 140: 985, 1980.
Shelley WB, et al. Naproxen photosensitization demonstrated by challenge. Cutis 38: 169, 1986.
Svihovec J. Anti-inflammatory analgesics and drugs used in gout. In: Meyler's Side Effects of Drugs, Dukes MNG (ed), Excerpta Medica, Vol. IX, Amsterdam, p 152, 1980.
Szmyd L Jr., Perry HD. Keratopathy associated with the use of naproxen. Am J Ophthalmol 99: 598, 1985.

Generic name: Piroxicam.

Proprietary name: Feldene.

Primary use

This non-steroidal anti-inflammatory drug is used in the treatment of osteoarthritis and rheumatoid arthritis.

Ocular side effects

Systemic administration
Certain
1. Non-specific ocular irritation
   a. Lacrimation
   b. Hyperemia
   c. Edema
   d. Burning sensation

Probable
1. Decreased vision
2. Eyelids or conjunctiva
   a. Erythema
   b. Conjunctivitis – non-specific
   c. Photosensitivity
   d. Angioneurotic edema
3. Visual hallucinations

Possible
1. Optic neuritis
2. Alopecia
3. Eyelids or conjunctiva
   a. Urticaria
   b. Purpura
   c. Erythema multiforme
   d. Stevens-Johnson syndrome
   e. Exfoliative dermatitis
   f. Lyell's syndrome
   g. Pemphigoid lesion
   h. Eczema
   i. Loss of eyelashes or eyebrows

Clinical significance

Piroxicam is one of the most widely prescribed non-steroidal anti-inflammatory drugs and appears to have no serious ocular side effects except a questionable optic neuritis. This possible drug-related event is described by Fraunfelder et al (1994). Piroxicam is one of the few non-steroidal anti-inflammatory agents with which intracranial hypertension has not been reported. Ocular side effects are infrequent and usually transient. This agent is a strong photosensitizer, and ultraviolet light-blocking lenses may be indicated. Patients allergic to thimersol have a high prevalence of piroxicam photosensitivity (Varela et al 1998).

REFERENCES AND FURTHER READING

Duro JC, et al. Piroxicam-induced erythema multiforme. J Rheumatol 11: 554, 1984.
Fraunfelder FT, Samples JR, Fraunfelder FW. Possible optic nerve side effects associated with nonsteroidal anti-inflammatory drugs. J Toxicol Cut Ocular Toxicol 13(4): 311–316, 1994.
Halasz CLG. Photosensitivity to the nonsteroidal anti-inflammatory drug piroxicam. Cutis 39: 37, 1987.
Roujeau JC, et al. Sjogren-like syndrome after drug-induced toxic epidermal necrolysis. Lancet 1: 609, 1985.
Stern RS, Bigby M. An expanded profile of cutaneous reactions to nonsteroidal anti-inflammatory drugs. Reports to a specialty-based system for spontaneous reporting of adverse reactions to drugs. JAMA 252: 1433, 1984.
Varela P, Amorim I, et al. Photosensitivity induced by piroxicam. Acta Med Portuguesa 11(11): 997–1001, 1998.
Vasconcelos C, Magina S, et al. Cutaneous drug reactions to piroxicam. Contact Dermatitis 39(3): 145, 1998.

CLASS: MILD ANALGESICS

Generic names: Aspirin (acetylsalicylic acid).

Proprietary names: Bayer aspirin tablets, St Joseph Aspirin, Ecotrin enteric coated aspirin.

Primary use

This salicylate is used as an antipyretic analgesic in the management of gout, acute rheumatic fever, rheumatoid arthritis, subacute thyroiditis and renal calculi.

Ocular side effects

Systemic administration
Certain
1. Blurred vision
2. Myopia – transient
3. Drug secreted in tears
   a. Sicca – aggravate
   b. Superficial punctate keratitis
4. Eyelids or conjunctiva
   a. Allergic reactions
   b. Conjunctivitis – non-specific
   c. Edema
   d. Angioneurotic edema
   e. Urticaria
   f. Purpura

Possible
1. Retina – may increase retinal bleeding (Fig 7.3d)
2. Eyelids or conjunctiva
   a. Erythema multiforme
   b. Stevens-Johnson syndrome
   c. Lyell's syndrome
   d. Pemphigoid lesion

Conditional/Unclassified
1. Cataract – weak cataracogenesis

Toxic states
Certain
1. Problems with color vision
   a. Color vision defect – red-green defect
   b. Objects have yellow tinge
2. Paralysis of extraocular muscles
3. Diplopia
4. Visual hallucinations
5. Decreased intraocular pressure
6. Nystagmus
7. Pupils
   a. Mydriasis
   b. Decreased or absent reaction to light
8. Visual field defects
   a. Scotomas
   b. Constriction
   c. Hemianopsia
9. Scintillating scotomas
10. Papilledema
11. Retinal edema
12. Subconjunctival or retinal hemorrhages (Fig. 7.3d)
13. Toxic amblyopia
14. Optic atrophy

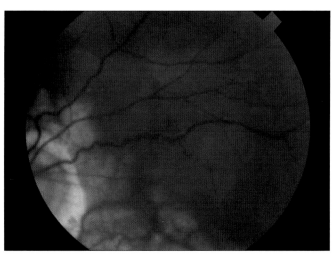

Fig. 7.3d Subretinal hemorrhage. Photo courtesy of Chak M, et al. Spontaneous suprochoroidal haemorrhage associated with high myopia and aspirin. Eye 17: 525-527, 2003.

Inadvertent ocular exposure or self-mutilation
Certain

1. Conjunctiva and cornea
   a. Edema
   b. Keratitis
   c. Ulceration
   d. Vascularization

Clinical significance

Acetylsalicylic acid (ASA) is one of the most commonly in-gested medications in the world. This drug rarely causes ocular problems at normal dosages; however, at higher dosages such problems may become clinically significant. This drug can be secreted in the tears, so transient blurred vision, aggravation of sicca and a keratitis can occur. In rare instances, transient myopia can take place. There are well-documented cases in the National Registry with multiple rechallenge data that acetylsali-cylic acid may cause blurred vision lasting 3 to 4 weeks even after one dosage. Christen et al (2001) suggested a small in-creased risk in cataracts with chronic aspirin use. Idiosyncratic or hypersensitivity reactions do occur. Those most susceptible to this are middle-aged females, and those with asthma, chronic urticaria, rhinitis, a history of atopy or a history of nasal pol-yps. These hypersensitivity reactions may involve many organ systems, but from the ocular viewpoint they mainly involve al-lergic ocular reactions, including erythema multiforme. It has been suggested that corneal donors on high doses of aspirin may have the potential for cytotoxic concentrations of the drug to the donor graft endothelium.

This agent increases bleeding time, decreases platelet adhe-siveness and can cause hypoprothrombinanemia. It can irrevers-ibly prevent platelet aggregation for the 10-day life span of the affected platelet. Conjunctival or retinal bleeds from a clinical perspective seem larger in patients on aspirin and clearly bleed-ing at ocular surgery is prolonged. Regardless of this, there is significant disagreement among ocular surgeons about whether or not aspirin should be stopped prior to ocular surgery (Assia et al 1998; Kokolakis et al 1999). However, most surgeons do not stop aspirin. Parkin and Manners (2000) pointed out that some oculoplastic surgeons, where appropriate, will limit ASA use pre and immediately post operatively. The use of aspirin in exuda-tive AMD is usually not contraindicated. Wilson et al (2004) found ASA protective for choroidal neovascularization in AMD

patients. When used in diabetes, Banerjee et al (2004) found no increase in the onset of first-time vitrious hemorrhages.

Toxicity can occur from increased dosages to control pain, cross-sensitivity, additive effects with other non-steroidal anti-inflammatory agents, suicide attempts and other drugs which allow aspirin to more easily pass through the blood-brain barrier. Oral acetazolamide is a classic example of a drug that causes the latter. ASA in toxic states affects the occipital visual cortex, causing transitory blindness lasting from 3 to 24 hours, dilated pupils (which react to light), narrow retinal vascular tree, color vision problems, nystagmus and optic nerve atrophy. Cases of scintillating scotoma, diplopia, papilledema, color vision defects, pupillary changes and visual field problems may rarely occur.

Sacca et al (1988) pointed out the safety of 1–3% aspirin collyrium on the eye for treatment of allergic conjunctivitis. However, as in self-mutilation, the 'crushed' tablets can cause mechanical abrasions, leading to ulceration, secondary infection and even loss of the eye. Aspirin needs to be considered in any self-mutilation ocular case.

REFERENCES AND FURTHER READING

Assia EI, Raskin T, Kaiserman I, et al. Effect of aspirin intake on bleeding during cataract surgery. J Cataract Refract Surg 24: 1243–1246, 1998.

Banerjee S, Denniston AKO, Gibson JM, et al. Does cardiovascular therapy affect the onset and recurrence of preretinal and vitreous haemorrhage in diabetic eye disease? Eye 18: 821–825, 2004.

Basu PK, et al. Should corneas from donors receiving a high dose of sali-cylate be used as grafts: an animal experimentation. Exp Eye Res 39: 393, 1984.

Benawra R, Mangurten HH, Duffell DR. Cyclopia and other anomalies following maternal ingestion of salicylates. Pediatrics 96: 1069, 1980.

Birch J, et al. Acquired color vision defects. In: Congenital and Acquired Color Vision Defects, Pokorny J, et al (eds), Grune & Stratton, New York, p 243–350, 1979.

Black RA, Bensinger RE. Bilateral subconjunctival hemorrhage after acetyl-salicylic acid overdose. Ann Ophthalmol 14: 1024, 1982.

Chak M, Williamson TH. Spontaneous suprachoroidal haemorrhage associ-ated with high myopia and aspirin. Eye 17: 525–527, 2003.

Cheng H. Aspirin and cataract (Editorial). Br J Ophthalmol 76: 257–258, 1992.

Chew EY, et al. Effects of aspirin on vitreous/preretinal hemorrhage in patients with diabetes mellitus. Arch Ophthalmol 113: 52–55, 1995.

Christen WG, Ajani UA, Schaumberg DA, et al. Aspirin use and risk of cataract in posttrial follow-up of physicians' health study I. Arch Ophthalmol 119: 405–412, 2001.

Cumming RG, Mitchell P. Medications and cataract. The Blue Mountains Eye Study. Ophthalmology 105: 1751–1757, 1999.

Early Treatment Diabetic Retinopathy Study Research Group. Effects of aspirin treatment on diabetic retinopathy. Ophthalmology 98: 757–765, 1991.

Ganley JP, et al. Aspirin and recurrent hyphema after blunt ocular trauma. Am J Ophthalmol 96: 797, 1983.

Kageler WV, Moake JL, Garcia CA. Spontaneous hyphema associated with ingestion of aspirin and alcohol. Am J Ophthalmol 82: 631–634, 1976.

Kokolakis S, Zafirakis P, Livir-Rallatos G, et al. Aspirin intake and bleeding during cataract surgery. J Cataract Refract Surg 25: 301–302, 1999.

Lumme P, Laatikainen LT. Risk factors for intraoperative and early postop-erative complications in extracapsular cataract surgery. Eur J Ophthal-mol 4: 151–158, 1994.

MakeIa A-L, Lang H, Korpela P. Toxic encephalopathy with hyperammo-naemia during high-dose salicylate therapy. Acta Neurol Scand 61: 146, 1980.

Ong-Tone L, Paluck EC, Hart-Mitchell RD. Perioperative use of warfarin and aspirin in cataract surgery by Canadian Society of Cataract and Refrac-tive Surgery members: survey. J Cataract Refract Surg 31: 991–996, 2005.

Paris GL, Waltuch GF. Salicylate-induced bleeding problem in ophthalmic plastic surgery. Ophthalmic Surg 13: 627, 1982.

Parkin B, Manners R. Aspirin and warfarin therapy in oculoplastic surgery. Br J Ophthalmol 84: 1426–1427, 2000.

Price KS, Thompson DM. Localized unilateral periorbital edema induced by aspirin. Comment in Ann Allergy Asthma Immunol 79: 420–422, 1997.

Ruocco V, Pisani M. Induced pemphigus. Arch Dermatol Res 274: 123, 1982.

Sacca SC, Cerqueti PM, et al. Topical use of aspirin in allergic conjunctivitis. Bull Ocul 67(Suppl 4): 193–196. 1988 (Italian).

Schachat AP. Can aspirin be used safely for patients with proliferative diabetic retinopathy? Arch Ophthalmol 110: 180, 1992.

Spaeth GL, Nelson LB, Beaudoin AR. Ocular teratology. In: Ocular Anatomy, Embryology and Teratology, Jakobiec FA (ed), JB Lippincott, Philadelphia, p 955–975, 1982.

Tilanus MA, Vaandrager W, Cuyper MH, et al. Relationship between anticoagulant medication and massive intraocular hemorrhage in age-related macular degeneration. Graefes Arch Clin Exp Ophthalmol 238: 482–485, 2000.

Valentic JP, Leopold IH, Dea FJ. Excretion of salicylic acid into tears following oral administration of aspirin. Ophthalmology 87: 815, 1980.

Wilson HL, Schwartz DM, Bhatt HRF, et al. Statin and aspirin therapy are associated with decreased rates of choroidal neovascularization among patients with age-related macular degeneration. Am J Ophthalmol 137: 615–624, 2004.

Generic names: 1. Codeine; 2. dextropropoxyphene.

Proprietary names: 1. Multi-ingredient preparations only; 2. Darvon.

Primary use

These mild analgesics are used for the relief of mild to moderate pain. Codeine is also used as an antitussive agent.

Ocular side effects

Systemic administration
Certain
1. Pupils
   a. Miosis – acute and toxic states
   b. Pinpoint pupils – initial
   c. Mydriasis – withdrawal
2. Eyelids or conjunctiva – angioneurotic edema (codeine)

Possible
1. Decreased vision
2. Myopia (codeine)
3. Visual hallucinations
4. Keratoconjunctivitis sicca (dextropropoxyphene)
5. Lacrimation – withdrawal states
6. Eyelids or conjunctiva
   a. Erythema multiforme (codeine)
   b. Exfoliative dermatitis (codeine)
   c. Urticaria (codeine)

Conditional/Unclassified
1. Optic atrophy – toxic states (dextropropoxyphene)

Clinical significance

Codeine and dextropropoxyphene seldom cause significant ocular side effects. While codeine may cause miosis, dextropropoxyphene does so only in overdose situations. Visual disturbances are usually insignificant. Cases have been reported to the National Registry of codeine causing transient myopia.

Bergmanson and Rios (1981) reported that darvocet-N, a compound containing dextropropoxyphene and acetaminophen, caused reduce tear secretion, which resulted in soft contact lens dehydration and corneal epithelial abrasion. Weiss (1982) reported bilateral optic atrophy possibly associated with an overdose of Darvon, a compound containing dextropropoxyphene, aspirin and caffeine. Other contributing factors in this patient may have been acidosis, hypokalemia or hypoxia. Cases of transient internuclear ophthalmoplegia (El-Mallakh 1986; Rizzo and Corbett 1983) have been reported, but it is difficult to prove a cause-and-effect relationship. Intravenous naloxone, however, caused the opthalmoplegia to return to normal.

REFERENCES AND FURTHER READING

Bergmanson JPG, Rios R. Adverse reaction to painkiller in Hydrogel lens wearer. Am Optom Assoc 52: 257, 1981.

El-Mallakh RS. Internuclear ophthalmoplegia with narcotic overdosage. Ann Neurol 20: 107, 1986.

Leslie PJ, Dyson EH, Proudfoot AT. Opiate toxicity after self poisoning with aspirin and codeine. BMJ 292: 96, 1986.

Ostler HB, Conant MA, Groundwater J. Lyell's disease, the Stevens-Johnson syndrome, and exfoliative dermatitis. Trans Am Ophthalmol Otolaryngol 74: 1254, 1970.

Ponte CD. A suspected case of codeine-induced erythema multiforme. Drug Intell Clin Pharm 17: 128, 1983.

Rizzo M, Corbett J. Bilateral internuclear ophthalmoplegia reversed by naloxone. Arch Neurol 40: 242–243, 1983.

Wall R, Linford SMJ, Akhter MI. Addiction to Distalgesic (dextropropoxyphene). BMJ 280: 1213, 1980.

Weiss IS. Optic atrophy after propoxyphene overdose. Report of a case. Ann Ophthalmol 14: 586, 1982.

Generic names: Paracetamol (acetaminophen).

Proprietary names: Acephen, Excedrin, Neopap, Tylenol.

Primary use

This para-aminophenol derivative is used in the control of fever and mild pain.

Ocular side effects

Systemic administration
Certain
1. Problems with color vision – objects have yellow tinge
2. Visual hallucinations
3. Green or chocolate discoloration of subconjunctival or retinal blood vessels
4. Pupils
   a. Mydriasis – toxic states
   b. Decreased reaction to light – toxic states

Probable
1. Eyelids or conjunctiva
   a. Allergic reactions
   b. Erythema
   c. Conjunctivitis – non-specific
   d. Edema
   e. Angioneurotic edema
   f. Urticaria
   g. Icterus

Possible
1. Subconjunctival or retinal hemorrhages secondary to drug-induced anemia
2. Decreased vision
3. Eyelids or conjunctiva
   a. Erythema multiforme
   b. Stevens-Johnson syndrome
   c. Lyell's syndrome

Clinical significance

Ocular side effects due to this analgesic are extremely rare except in toxic states. Data in the National Registry suggest that adverse reactions have occurred at quite low doses, implying a drug idiosyncrasy, a peculiar sensitivity or just a chance event not related to the drug. Toxic responses, mostly self-inflicted, have been reported due to paracetamol. In chronic therapy, this drug can produce sulfhemoglobinemia, which accounts for the greenish or chocolate color change in the subconjunctival or retinal blood vessels.

REFERENCES AND FURTHER READING

Gerard A, et al. Drug-induced Lyell's syndrome. Nine cases. Therapie 37: 475, 1982.

Johnson DAW. Drug-induced psychiatric disorders. Drugs 22: 57, 1981.

Kashihara M, et al. Bullous pemphigoid-like lesions induced by Phenacetin. Report of a case and an immunopathologic study. Arch Dermatol 120: 1196, 1984.

Kneezel LD, Kitchens CS. Phenacetin-induced sulfhemoglobinemia: Report of a case and review of the literature. Johns Hopkins Med J 139: 175, 1976.

Krenzelok EP, Best L, Manoguerra AS. Acetaminophen toxicity. Am Hosp Pharm 34: 391, 1977.

Malek-Ahmadi P, Ramsey M. Acute psychosis associated with codeine and acetaminophen: a case report. Neurobehav Toxicol Teratol 7: 193, 1985.

McEvoy GK (ed). American Hospital Formulary Service Drug Information 87, American Society of Hospital Pharmacists, Bethesda, p 998–1002, 1987.

Neetans A, et al. Possible iatrogenic action of phenacetin at the levels of the visual pathway. Bull Soc Belge Ophthalmol 178: 65, 1977.

CLASS: NARCOTIC ANTAGONISTS

Generic names: 1. Naloxone hydrochloride; 2. naltrexone.

Proprietary names: 1. Narcan; 2. Revia.

Primary use

These narcotic antagonists are used primarily in the management of narcotic-induced respiratory depression.

Ocular side effects

Systemic administration
Certain
1. Pupils
   a. Mydriasis – if a recent narcotic user
   b. Miosis
2. Visual hallucinations
3. Lacrimation – withdrawal states

Probable
1. Eyelids or conjunctiva
   a. Allergic reactions
   b. Erythema
   c. Photosensitivity (naltrexone)
   d. Urticaria
2. Non-specific ocular irritation (naltrexone)
   a. Photophobia
   b. Ocular pain
   c. Edema
   d. Burning sensation

Possible
1. Decreased vision
2. Pseudoptosis
3. Eyelids or conjunctiva
   a. Erythema multiforme (naloxone)
   b. Exfoliative dermatitis (naltrexone)

Local ophthalmic use or exposure (naloxone)
Certain
1. Pupils
   a. Mydriasis – if a recent narcotic user
   b. Miosis

Clinical significance

Although ocular side effects due to these narcotic antagonists are common, they have little clinical significance other than as a screening test to discover narcotic users. These narcotic antagonists produce either a miosis or no effect on the pupils when administered to non-addicts, but in addicts they cause mydriasis. Vivid visual hallucinations are seen both as an adverse ocular reaction and as a withdrawal symptom. Naloxone has only been reported to cause pupillary changes and erythema multiforme.

REFERENCES AND FURTHER READING

Bellini C, et al. Naloxone anisocoria: a non-invasive inexpensive test for opiate addiction. Int I Clin Pharm Res 11: 55, 1982.

Drago F, et al. Ocular instillation of naloxone increases intraocular pressure in morphine-addicted patients: a possible test for detecting misuse of morphine. Experimentia 41: 266, 1985.

Fanciullacci M, et al. The naloxone conjunctival test in morphine addiction. Eur J Pharmacol 61: 319, 1980.

Jasinski DR, Martin WR, Haertzen C. The human pharmacology and abuse potential of N-Allylnoroxymorphone. (Naloxone). I Pharmacol Exp Ther 157: 420, 1967.

Martin WR. Opioid antagonists. Pharmacol Rev 19: 463, 1967.

Nomof N, Elliott HW, Parker KD. The local effect of morphine, nalorphine, and codeine on the diameter of the pupil of the eye. Clin Pharmacol Ther 9: 358, 1968.

CLASS: STRONG ANALGESICS

Generic name: Diacetylmorphine (diamorphine, heroin).

Proprietary names: None.

Street names: Boy, brother, brown sugar, caballo, ca-ca, crap, h, harry, horse, junk, poison, scag, schmeck, shit, smack, stuff, tecata.

Primary use

This potent narcotic analgesic is administered pre- and post-operatively and in the terminal stage of cancer for the relief of severe pain.

Ocular side effects

Systemic administration
Certain
1. Pupils
   a. Miosis
   b. Pinpoint pupils – toxic states
   c. Absence of reaction to light
   d. Mydriasis – withdrawal states
   e. Anisocoria – withdrawal states
2. Decreased accommodation
3. Non-specific ocular irritation
   a. Lacrimation
   b. Photophobia
4. Eyelids or conjunctiva
   a. Hyperemia
   b. Erythema
   c. Edema
   d. Urticaria
   e. Decreased blink rate
5. Ocular motility
   a. Esotropia (on withdrawal)
   b. Exotropia

Probable
1. Intranuclear ophthalmoplegia (toxic)

Possible
1. Horner's syndrome
   a. Ptosis
   b. Increased sensitivity to sympathetic agents

Ocular teratogenic effects
Probable
1. Strabismus

Clinical significance

Heroin can cause pupillary changes, which are often used to identify probable users. Ocular irritation and conjunctival changes are common. However, recently Firth (2005), Kowal et al (2003) and Sutter and Landau (2003) have well documented that esotropia with double vision occurs with heroin withdrawal and its use can cause intermittent or persistent exotropia. Awareness of these ocular side effects is essential to avoid neurologic referrals. Heroin addiction has been associated with bacterial and fungal endophthalmitis, probably due to intravenous administration and impurities on an embolus basis. If undiagnosed and incompletely treated, these indirect drug-related entities can result in permanent loss of vision. Horner's syndrome has been reported in chronic addicts. Withdrawal of diacetylmorphine in the addict may cause excessive tearing, irregular pupils and decreased accommodation.

In opiate-dependent mothers, primarily on methadone, Gill et al (2003) estimated at least a 10-fold increase over the general population of ocular strabismus.

REFERENCES AND FURTHER READING

Alinlari A, Hashem B. Effect of opium addiction on intraocular pressure. Glaucoma 7: 69, 1985.
Caradoc-Davies TH. Opiate toxicity in elderly patients. BMJ 283: 905, 1981.
Cosgriff TM. Anisocoria in heroin withdrawal. Arch Neurol 29: 200, 1973.
Crandall DC, Leopold IH. The influence of systemic drugs on tear constituents. Ophthalmology 86: 115, 1979.
Dally S, Thomas G, Mellinger M. Loss of hair, blindness and skin rash in heroin addicts. Vet Human Toxicol 24(Suppl): 62, 1982.
Firth AY. Heroin and diplopia. Addiction 100: 46–50, 2005.
Gill AC, Oei J, Lewis NL, et al. Strabismus in infants of opiate-dependent mothers. Acta Paediatr 92: 379–385, 2003.
Gomezz Manzano C, et al. Internuclear ophthalmopathy associated with opiate overdose. Medicina Clinica 94: 637, 1990.
Hawkins KA, Bruckstein AH, Guthrie TC. Percutaneous heroin injection causing heroin syndrome. JAMA 237: 1963,1977.
Hogeweg M, De Jong PTVM. Candida endophthalmitis in heroin addicts. Doc Ophthalmol 55: 63, 1983.
Kowal L, et al. Acute esotropia in heroin withdrawal: a case series. Binocul Vis Strabismus Q 18: 163–166, 2003.
Rathod NH, De Alarcon R, Thomson IG. Signs of heroin usage detected by drug users and their parents. Lancet 2: 1411, 1967.
Salmon JF, Partridge BM, Spalton DJ. Candida endophthalmitis in a heroin addict: a case report. Br J Ophthalmol 67: 306, 1983.
Siepser SB, Magargal LE, Augsburger JJ. Acute bilateral retinal microembolization in a heroin addict. Ann Ophthalmol 13: 699, 1981.
Sutter FK, Landau K. Heroin and strabismus. Swiss Med Wkly 133: 293–294, 2003.
Tarr KH. Candida endophthalmitis and drug abuse. Aust J Ophthalmol 8: 303, 1980.
Vastine DW, et al. Endogenous candida endophthalmitis associated with heroin use. Arch Ophthalmol 94:1805, 1976.

Generic names: 1. Hydromorphone hydrochloride (dihydromorphinone); 2. oxymorphone hydrochloride.

Proprietary names: 1. Dilaudid, Dilaudid-HP; 2. Numorphan.

Primary use

These hydrogenated ketones of morphine are used for the relief of moderate to severe pain.

Ocular side effects

Systemic administration
Certain
1. Decreased vision
2. Decreased accommodation
3. Pupils
   a. Miosis
   b. Pinpoint pupils – toxic states
   c. Mydriasis – hypoxic states
4. Eyelids or conjunctiva
   a. Allergic reactions
   b. Urticaria
   c. Contact dermatitis

Probable
1. Extraocular muscles
   a. Nystagmus
   b. Diplopia

Clinical significance

Adverse ocular effects due to these drugs, although not uncommon, are rarely significant. All ocular side effects are reversible and transitory. Difficulty in focusing is probably the most frequent complaint.

REFERENCES AND FURTHER READING

Acute drug abuse reactions. Med Lett Drugs Ther 27: 77, 1985.
De Cuyper C, Goeteyn M. Systemic contact dermatitis from subcutaneous hydromorphone. Contact Dermatitis 27(4): 220–223, 1992.
Drug Evaluations, 6th edn, American Medical Association, Chicago, p 59, 1986.
Gilman AG, Goodman LS, Gilman A (eds). The Pharmacological Basis of Therapeutics. 6th edn. Macmillan, New York, pp 495–511, 1980.
Katcher J, Walsh D. Opioid-induced itching: morphine sulfate and hydromorphone hydrochloride. J Pain Symptom Manage 17(1): 70–72, 1999.
Sweetman SC (ed). Martindale: The Complete Drug Reference. 34th edn. Pharmaceutical Press, London, pp 45–76, 2004.

Generic name: Methadone hydrochloride.

Proprietary names: Dolophine hydrochloride, Methadose.

Street names: Dolly, doses, juice, meth.

Primary use

This synthetic analgesic is useful in the treatment of chronic painful conditions and in the detoxification treatment of patients dependent on heroin or other morphine-like agents.

Ocular side effects

Systemic administration
Certain
1. Pupils
   a. Miosis – toxic states
   b. Pinpoint pupils – toxic states
   c. Mydriasis – withdrawal states
2. Talc retinopathy (intravenous)
3. Decreased vision
4. Decreased spontaneous eye movements

Probable
1. Eyelids – urticaria

Ocular teratogenic effects
Certain
1. Increased incidences of strabismus

Clinical significance

Methadone seldom causes significant ocular side effects. Miosis is uncommon but may occur at therapeutic dosages. In severe toxic states, there may be 'pinpoint' pupils. Talc emboli, appearing as small white glistening dots in the macular area, have been reported in addicts who intravenously inject oral medications that contain talc as a filler. A case of cortical blindness, apparently secondary to anoxia, has been reported in a child who experienced severe respiratory depression. Nelson et al (1987) and Gill et al (2003) reported the incidence of strabismus in infants of methadone-dependent mothers to be at least 10 times greater then that seen in the general population.

REFERENCES AND FURTHER READING

Gill AC, Oei J, Lewis NL, et al. Strabismus in infants of opiate-dependent mothers. Acta Paediatr 92: 379-385, 2003.
Linzmayer L, Fischer G, Grunberger J. Pupillary diameter and pupillary reactions in heroin dependent patients and in patients participating in a methadone and morphine replacement program. Weiner Medizinische Wochenschrift 147(3): 67-69, 1997.
Murphy SB, Jackson WB, Pare JAP. Talc retinopathy. Can J Ophthalmol 13: 152, 1978.
Nelson LB, et al. Occurrence of strabismus in infants born to drug-dependent women. Am J Dis Child 141: 175-178, 1987.
Ratcliffe SC. Methadone poisoning in a child. BMJ 1: 1056-1070, 1963.
Rothenberg S, et al. Methadone depression of visual signal detection performance. Pharmacol Biochem Behav 11: 521, 1979.
Rothenberg S, et al. Specific oculomotor deficit after acute methadone. I. Saccadic eye movements. Psychopharmacology 67: 221, 1980.
Rothenberg S, et al. Specific oculomotor deficit after acute methadone. II. Smooth pursuit eye movements. Psychopharmacology 67: 229, 1980.
Sweetmand SC (ed). Martindale: The Complete Drug Reference. 34th edn. Pharmaceutical Press, London, pp 57-59, 2004.

Generic names: 1. Morphine; 2. opium.

Proprietary names: 1. Astramorph PF, Avinza, DepoDur, Duramorph PF, Infumorph, Kadian, MS Contin, Oramorph SR.

Street names: 1. M, morf, white stuff; 2. joy plant, pen yan, skee.

Primary use

These opioids are used for the relief of severe pain. Morphine is the alkaloid that gives opium its analgesic action.

Ocular side effects

Systemic administration
Certain
1. Pupils
   a. Miosis
   b. Pinpoint pupils – toxic states
   c. Mydriasis – withdrawal or extreme toxic states
   d. Irregularity – withdrawal states
2. Decreased vision
3. Decreased accommodation
4. Decreased convergence
5. Decreased intraocular pressure
6. Visual hallucinations
7. Lacrimation
   a. Increased – withdrawal states
   b. Decreased
8. Eyelids or conjunctiva
   a. Allergic reactions
   b. Conjunctivitis – non-specific

c. Urticaria
d. Pruritis
9. Ptosis (opium)

Probable
1. Accommodative spasm
2. Diplopia

Possible
1. Myopia
2. Keratoconjunctivitis

Local ophthalmic use or exposure – morphine
Certain
1. Miosis
2. Increased intraocular pressure

Epidural or intravenous exposure
Certain
1. Vertical nystagmus

Ocular teratogenic effects
Probable
1. Increased incidence of strabismus

Clinical significance

These narcotics seldom cause significant ocular side effects, and all proven drug-induced toxic effects are transitory. Miosis is the most frequent ocular side effect and is commonly seen at therapeutic dosage levels. Ocular side effects reported in long-term addicts may include color vision or visual field changes, which are probably due to vitamin deficiency rather than to the drug itself. Withdrawal of morphine or opium in the addict may cause excessive tearing, irregular pupils, decreased accommodation and diplopia. Epidural (Fish and Rosen 1990) and intravenous opioids (Henderson and Wijdicks 2000) have been reported to cause vertical nystagmus. Castano and Lyons (1999) recently reported that intravenous morphine could cause eyelid pruritus.

Gill et al (2003) reported that the incidence of strabismus in infants of opiate-dependent mothers is at least 10 times greater then that seen in the general population.

REFERENCES AND FURTHER READING

Aminlari A, Hashem B. Effect of opium addiction on intraocular pressure. Glaucoma 7: 69, 1965.
Andersen PT. Alopecia areata after epidural morphine. Anesth Analg 63: 1142, 1984.
Castano G, Lyons CJ. Eyelid pruritus with intravenous morphine. J Am Assoc Pediatr Ophthalmol Strabismus 3(1): 60, 1999.
Crandall DC, Leopold IH. The influence of systemic drugs on tear constituents. Ophthalmology 86: 115, 1979.
Fish DJ, Rosen SM. Epidural opioids as a cause of vertical nystagmus. Anesthesiology 73: 785-786, 1990.
Gill AC, Oei J, Lewis NL, et al: Strabismus in infants of opiate-dependent mothers. Acta Paediatr 92: 379-385, 2003.
Henderson RD, Wijdicks EFM. Downbeat nystagmus associated with intravenous patient-controlled administration of morphine. Anesth Analg 91: 691-692, 2000.
Murphy DF. Anesthesia and intraocular pressure. Anesth Analg 64: 520, 1985.
Shelly MP, Park GR. Morphine toxicity with dilated pupils. BMJ 289: 1071, 1984.
Stevens RA, Sharrock NE. Nystagmus following epidural morphine. Anesthesiology 74: 390-391, 1991.

Ueyama H, Nishimura M, Tashiro C. Naloxone reversal of nystagmus associated with intrathecal morphine [letter]. Anesthesiology 76: 153, 1992.

Generic name: Pethidine hydrochloride (meperidine).

Proprietary name: Demerol.

Primary use

This phenylpiperidine narcotic analgesic is used for the relief of pain, as a preoperative medication and to supplement surgical anesthesia.

Ocular side effects

Systemic administration
Probable
1. Pupils
   a. Mydriasis
   b. Miosis
   c. Decreased reaction to light (overdose)
2. Decreased intraocular pressure
3. Decreased vision
4. Eyelids or conjunctiva
   a. Allergic reactions
   b. Erythema
   c. Urticaria
5. Visual hallucinations

Possible
1. Nystagmus
2. Ocular signs of drug-induced Parkinson's disease
   a. Paralysis of extraocular muscles
   b. Ptosis
   c. Diplopia

Inadvertent ocular exposure
Certain
1. Blepharitis
2. Conjunctivitis – non-specific

Clinical significance

None of the ocular side effects due to pethidine are of major clinical importance and all are transitory. Miosis is uncommon at therapeutic dosages and seldom significant. Mydriasis and decreased pupillary light reflexes are only seen in acute toxicity or in long-term addicts. Decrease in intraocular pressure is minimal. Ocular side effects, such as blepharitis or conjunctivitis, have been seen secondary to pethidine dust.

REFERENCES AND FURTHER READING

Bron AJ. Vortex patterns of the corneal epithelium. Trans Ophthalmol Soc UK 93: 455, 1973.
Carlson VR. Individual pupillary reactions to certain centrally acting drugs in man. J Pharmacol Exp Ther 121: 501–506, 1957.
Goetting MG, Thirman MJ. Neurotoxicity of meperidine. Ann Emerg Med 14: 1007, 1985.
Hovland KH. Effects of drugs on aqueous humor dynamics. Int Ophthalmol Clin 11(2): 99, 1971.
Johnson DAW. Drug-induced psychiatric disorders. Drugs 22: 57, 1981.

Lubeck MJ. Effects of drugs on ocular muscles. Int Ophthalmol Clin 11(2): 35, 1971.

Waisbren BA, Smith MB. Hypersensitivity to meperidine. JAMA 239: 1395, 1978.

Generic name: Pentazocine.

Proprietary name: Talwin.

Primary use

This benzomorphan narcotic analgesic is used for the relief of pain, as a preoperative medication and to supplement surgical anesthesia.

Ocular side effects

Systemic administration
Certain
1. Miosis
2. Decreased vision
3. Visual hallucinations

Probable
1. Nystagmus
2. Diplopia
3. Lacrimation – abrupt withdrawal states
4. Decreased accommodation
5. Eyelids or conjunctiva
   a. Erythema
   b. Conjunctivitis – non-specific
   c. Edema
   d. Urticaria
6. Decreased spontaneous eye movements

Possible
1. Oculogyric crisis

Clinical significance

Ocular side effects due to pentazocine are usually insignificant and reversible. Miosis is the most frequent and is seen routinely even at suggested dosage levels. Although visual complaints are seldom of major consequence, diplopia may be incapacitating. Vivid visual hallucinations, some of which are threatening, have been reported with this drug. Once pentazocine is discontinued, the hallucinations cease. Burstein and Fullerton (1993) reported oculogyric crisis possibly related to this drug.

REFERENCES AND FURTHER READING

Belleville JP, Dorey F, Bellville JW. Effects of nefopam on visual tracking. Clin Pharmacol Ther 26: 457, 1979.

Burstein AH, Fullerton T. Oculogyric crisis possibly related to pentazocine. Ann Pharm 27(7–8): 874–876, 1993.

Davidson SI. Reports of ocular adverse reactions. Trans Ophthalmol Soc UK 93: 495-510, 1973.

Gould WM. Central nervous disturbance with pentazocine. BMJ 1: 313–314, 1972.

Jones KD. A novel side-effect of pentazocine. Br J Clin Pract 29: 218, 1975.

Martin WR. Opioid antagonists. Pharmacol Rev 19: 463, 1967.

SECTION 4
AGENTS USED IN ANESTHESIA

CLASS: ADJUNCTS TO ANESTHESIA

Generic name: Hyaluronidase.

Proprietary names: Amphadase, Hydase, Vitrase.

Primary use

This enzyme is added to local anesthetic solutions to enhance the effect of infiltrative anesthesia. It has also been used in paraphimosis, lepromatous nerve reactions and in the management of carpal tunnel syndrome.

Ocular side effects

Subconjunctival or retrobulbar injection
Certain
1. Eyelids or conjunctiva
   a. Allergic reactions
   b. Conjunctivitis – follicular
   c. Angioneurotic edema
2. Irritation
3. Myopia
4. Astigmatism
5. Decreases the length of action of local anesthetics
6. Increases the frequency of local anesthetic reactions

Probable
1. Allergic reaction simulated expulsive choroidal or retrobulbar hemorrhage
2. May spread infection

Possible
1. May spread tumor
2. Decrease local anesthetic toxicity to adjacent extra ocular muscles and nerves

Conditional/Unclassified
1. Cystoid macular edema

Clinical significance

Adverse ocular reactions due to periocular injection of hyaluronidase are either quite rare or masked by postoperative surgical reactions. Subconjunctival injection of this drug causes myopia and astigmatism secondary to changes in the corneal curvature. This is a transitory phenomenon with recovery occurring within 2–6 weeks. Irritative or allergic reactions are often stated to be due to impurities in the preparation since pure hyaluronidase is felt to be non-toxic. Minning (1994) reported allergic reactions secondary to retrobulbar hyaluronidase. This occurred as an acute process simulating an expulsive choroidal or retrobulbar hemorrhage. Massive retrobulbar, peribulbar and intraorbital swelling may occur. Cases similar to this have been reported to the National Registry. Hyaluronidase decreases the duration of action of local anesthetic drugs by allowing them to diffuse out of the tissue more rapidly. Brown et al (1999) and Jehan et al (2001) pointed out that hyaluronidase may be important in decreasing or preventing damage from local anesthetics on adjacent extraocular muscles and nerves. This may occur, in part, by diffusion of the anesthetic, thereby decreasing the anesthetic concentration adjacent to muscle tissue. Miller (2000) has not found this to be true since he has not seen restrictive diplopia in over 7000 ocular procedures without using hyaluronidase.

Some side effects of the local anesthetic are probably more frequent when it is used with hyaluronidase, since its absorption rate is increased. Infection or tumor cells may be allowed to spread as well, based on the same mechanism. A prospective double-blind study that suggests cystoid macular edema is possibly caused by the use of hyaluronidase is of clinical importance. To date, these data are not completely accepted (Kraff et al 1983) and some of these cases may be secondary to inadvertent intraocular injection. If the patient is on heparin or if there is associated bleeding in the area of injection, the effect of hyaluronidase may be decreased since both human serum and heparin inhibit this agent.

REFERENCES AND FURTHER READING

Ahluwalia HS, Lukaris A, Lane CM. Delayed allergic reaction to hyaluronidase: A rare sequel to cataract surgery. Eye 17: 263–266, 2003.

Barton D. Side reactions to drugs in anesthesia. Int Ophthalmol Clin 11(2): 185, 1971.

Brown SM, Brooks SE, Mazow ML, et al. Cluster diplopia cases after periocular anesthesia without hyaluronidase. J Cataract Refract Surg 25: 1245–1249, 1999.

Brown SM, Coats DK, Collins MLZ, et al. Second cluster of strabismus cases after periocular anesthesia without hyaluronidase. J Cataract and Refract Surg 27: 1872–1875, 2001.

Eberhart AH, Weiler CR, Erie JC. Angioedema related to the use of hyaluronidase in cataract surgery. Am J Ophthalmol 138: 142–143, 2004.

Hagan JC III, Whittaker TJ, Byars SR. Diplopia cases after periocular anesthesia without hyaluronidase. J Cataract Refract Surg 25: 1560–1561, 1999.

Jehan FS, Hagan JC III, Whittaker TJ, et al. Diplopia and ptosis following injection of local anesthesia without hyaluronidase. J Cataract Refract Surg 27: 1876–1879, 2001.

Kraff MC, Sanders DR, Jampol LM, et al. Effect of retrobulbar hyaluronidase on pseudophakic cystoid macular edema. Am Intra-Ocular Implant Soc J 9: 184–185, 1983.

Miller RD. Hyaluronidase and diplopia. J Cataract Refract Surg 26: 478–480, 2000.

Minning CA. Hyaluronidase allergy simulating expulsive choroidal hemorrhage. Case reports. Arch Ophthal 112: 585, 1994.

Roper DL, Nisbet RM. Effect of hyaluronidase on the incidence of cystoid macular edema. Ann Ophthalmol 10: 1673, 1978.

Salkie ML. Inhibition of wydase by human serum. Can Med Assoc J 121: 845, 1979.

Singh D. Subconjunctival hyaluronidase injection producing temporary myopia. J Cataract Refract Surg 21(4): 477–478, 1995.

Taylor IS, Pollowitz JA. Little known phenomenon. Ophthalmology 91: 1003, 1984.

Treister G, Romano A, Stein R. The effect of subconjunctivally injected hyaluronidase on corneal refraction. Arch Ophthalmol 81: 645, 1969.

Generic names: 1. Hyoscine (scopolamine); 2. hyoscine methobromide (methscopolamine).

Proprietary names: 1. Transderm scop; 2. Pamine.

Primary use

Systemic
These quaternary ammonium derivatives are used as preanesthetic medications to decrease bronchial secretions, as sedatives and antispasmodics, and in the prophylaxis of motion sickness.

Topical
Hyoscine is used in the prevention of nausea and vomiting associated with motion sickness.

Ocular side effects

Systemic administration
Certain
1. Mydriasis – may precipitate angle-closure glaucoma
2. Decrease or paralysis of accommodation
3. Decreased vision
4. Decreased lacrimation
5. Visual hallucinations
6. Decreased tear lysozymes
7. Impairment of saccadic eye movements (IM injection)

Local ophthalmic use or exposure
Certain
1. Decreased vision
2. Mydriasis – may precipitate angle-closure glaucoma
3. Decrease or paralysis of accommodation
4. Eyelids or conjunctiva
   a. Allergic reactions
   b. Conjunctivitis – follicular
   c. Eczema
5. Irritation
   a. Hyperemia
   b. Photophobia
   c. Edema
6. Increased intraocular pressure
7. Decreased lacrimation
8. Visual hallucinations

Systemic absorption or finger to eye cross-contamination from topical application to the skin
Certain
1. Pupils
   a. Mydriasis – may precipitate narrow-angle glaucoma
   b. Anisocoria
   c. Absent reaction to light – toxic states
2. Decrease or paralysis of accommodation
3. Decreased vision
4. Decreased lacrimation
5. Visual hallucinations
6. Nystagmus

Systemic side effects

Local ophthalmic use or exposure
Certain
1. Psychosis
2. Agitation
3. Confusion
4. Hallucinations
5. Hostility
6. Amnesia
7. Ataxia
8. Vomiting
9. Urinary incontinence
10. Somnolence
11. Fever
12. Vasodilation

Clinical significance
Although ocular side effects from systemic administration of these drugs are common, they are reversible and seldom serious. Occasionally, patients on scopolamine have aggravated keratoconjunctivitis sicca problems due to decreased tear

production. This is the only autonomic drug that has been reported to cause decreased tear lysozymes. Mydriasis and paralysis of accommodation are intended ocular effects resulting from topical ophthalmic application of hyoscine but may also occur from oral administration. This drug may elevate the intraocular pressure in open-angle glaucoma and can precipitate angle-closure glaucoma. Allergic reactions are not uncommon after topical ocular application. Transient impairment of ocular accommodation, including blurred vision and mydriasis, has also been reported following the application of transdermal hyoscine patches. Several case reports of unilateral dilated pupils with associated blurred vision and angle-closure glaucoma have been published, and inadvertent finger-to-eye contamination has been shown to be the cause.

Systemic side effects from topical ophthalmic use of hyoscine have been reported infrequently and are similar to those seen secondary to topical ophthalmic atropine. Toxic psychosis, however, especially in the elderly or visually impaired, has been reported in the literature and to the National Registry.

REFERENCES AND FURTHER READING

Firth AY. Visual side-effects from transdermal scopolamine (hyoscine). Dev Med Child Neurol 48: 137–138, 2006.

Fraunfelder FT. Transdermal scopolamine precipitating narrow-angle glaucoma. N Engl J Med 307: 1079, 1982.

Gleiter CN, et al. Transdermal scopolamine and basal acid secretion. N Engl J Med 311: 1378, 1984.

Goldfrank L, et al. Anticholinergic poisoning. J Toxicol Clin Toxicol 19: 17, 1982.

Kortabarria RP, Duran JA, Chaco JR. Toxic psychosis following cycloplegic eyedrops. DICP. Ann Pharmacother 24: 708–709, 1990.

Lin YC. Anisocoria from trandermal scopolamine. Paediatr Anaesth 11: 626–627, 2001.

MacEwan GW, et al. Psychosis due to transdermally administered scopolamine. Can Med Assoc J 133: 431, 1985.

McBride WG, Vardy PN, French J. Effects of scopolamine hydrobromide on the development of the chick and rabbit embryo. Aust I Biol Sci 35: 173, 1982.

Namborg-Petersen B, Nielsen MM, Thordal C. Toxic effect of scopolamine eye drops in children. Acta Ophthalmol 62: 485, 1984.

Namill MB, Suelflow JA, Smith JA. Transdermal scopolamine delivery system (Transderm-V) and acute angle-closure glaucoma. Ann Ophthalmol 15: 1011, 1983.

Oliva GA, Bucci MP, Fioravanti R. Impairment of saccadic eye movements by scopolamine treatment. Percept Motor Skills 76(1): 159–167, 1993.

Price BH. Anisocoria from scopolamine patches. JAMA 253: 1561, 1985.

Rengstorff RN, Doughty CB. Mydriatic and cycloplegic drugs: A review of ocular and systemic complications. Am J Optom Physiol Optics 59: 162, 1982.

Rubner O, Kummerhoff PW, Haase H. An unusual case of psychosis caused by long-term administration of a scopolamine membrane patch. Paranoid hallucinogenic and delusional symptoms. Nervenarzt 68(1): 77–79, 1997.

Seenhauser FN, Schwarz NP. Toxic psychosis from transdermal scopolamine in a child. Lancet 2: 1033, 1986.

Generic name: Suxamethonium chloride (succinylcholine).

Proprietary names: Anectine, Quelicin.

Primary use

This neuromuscular blocking agent is used as an adjunct to general anesthesia to obtain relaxation of skeletal muscles.

Ocular side effects

Systemic administration
Certain
1. Extraocular muscles
   a. Eyelid retraction (initial – lasting up to 5 minutes)
   b. Endophthalmos (initial – lasting up to 5 minutes)
   c. Globe rotates inferiorly
   d. Paralysis (initial – lasting up to 5 minutes)
   e. Adduction of abducted eyes (initial – lasting up to 5 minutes)
   f. Alters forced duction tests (initial – lasting up to 20 minutes)
2. Intraocular pressure
   a. Increased (lasting 20–30 seconds)
   b. Decreased (late)
3. Ptosis
4. Diplopia
5. Eyelids or conjunctiva
   a. Allergic reactions
   b. Erythema
   c. Edema
   d. Urticaria

Conditional/Unclassified
1. Precipitates angle-closure glaucoma

Clinical significance

All ocular side effects due to suxamethonium chloride are transitory. The importance of the possible side effects of this drug effect on the 'open' eye is an ongoing debate. Some feel a transient contraction of extraocular muscles may cause 5–15 mmHg of intraocular pressure elevations within 20–30 seconds or increased choroidal blood flow (Robinson et al 1991) after suxamethonium is given, lasting from 1 to 4 minutes. While this short-term elevation of intraocular pressure has little or no effect in the normal or glaucomatous eye, it has the potential to cause expulsion of the intraocular contents in a surgically opened or perforated globe. McGoldrick (1993) considers the drug safe in human 'open' eyes with the benefits far outweighing the 'unproven' risks. There are at least 20 publications taking either side of this argument, with most recommending avoiding this agent in an 'open' eye. This may require anesthesiologists to use an agent they are not as familiar with, and the overall risk of this may be greater than that of using suxamethonium. Chidiac (2004) has suggested an algorithm that asks two questions with a total of three answers to help with the decision on whether or not to use this drug (see Recommendations). Brinkley and Henrick (2004) concur with this methodology. Eldor and Admoni (1989) report two cases of this agent, inducing acute glaucoma.

Extraocular muscle contraction induced by suxamethonium may cause lid retraction or an enophthalmos. This may cause the surgeon to misjudge the amount of resection needed in ptosis procedures. Eyelid retraction may be due to a direct action on Muller's muscle. Both eyelid retraction and enophthalmos seldom last for over 5 minutes after drug administration. Suxamethonium may cause abnormal forced duction tests up to 20 minutes after the drug is administered.

Prolonged respiratory paralysis may follow administration of suxamethonium during general anesthesia in patients with recent exposure to topical ocular echothiophate, anticholinesterase insecticides or in those with cholinesterase deficiency. Oral clonidine (Polarz et al 1992), thiopentone (Polarz et al 1993) and mivacurium (Chiu et al 1998) have been suggested to minimize suxamethonium ocular pressure effects on the eye.

Recommendations for use in open globe (after Chidiac 2004)

1. If intubation is easy, avoid using suxamethonium chloride.
2. If intubation is difficult, ask if eye is viable or not:
   a. If eye is viable then use suxamethonium
   b. If eye not viable then use fiber optic laryngoscopy.

REFERENCES AND FURTHER READING

Brinkley JR, Henrick A. Role of extraocular pressure in open globe injury. Anesthesiology 100: 1036, 2004.
Chidiac EJ. Succinylcholine and the open globe: Question unanswered. Anesthesiology 100: 1035–1036, 2004.
Chiu CL, Lang CC, Wong PK, et al. The effect of mivacurium pretreatment on intraocular pressure changes induced by suxamethonium. Anaesthesia 53(5): 501–505, 1998.
Cook JH. The effect of suxamethonium on intraocular pressure. Anaesthesia 36: 359, 1981.
Eldor J, Admoni M. Acute glaucoma following nonophthalmic surgery. Isr J Med Sci 25: 293–294, 1989.
France NK, et al. Succinylcholine alteration of the forced duction test. Ophthalmology 87: 1282, 1980.
Goldstein JH, Gupta MK, Shah MD. Comparison of intramuscular and intravenous succinylcholine on intraocular pressure. Ann Ophthalmol 13: 173, 1981.
Indu B, et al. Nifedipine attenuates the intraocular pressure response to intubation following succinylcholine. Can J Anesthesiol 36: 269–272, 1989.
Kelly RE, et al. Succinylcholine increases intraocular pressure in the human eye with the extraocular muscles detached. Anesthesiology 79: 948, 1993.
Lingua RW, Feuer W. Intraoperative succinylcholine and the postoperative eye alignment. J Pediatr Ophthalmol Strabismus 29(3): 167–170, 1992.
McGoldrick KE. The open globe: is an alternative to succinylcholine necessary? J Clin Anesthesia 5(1): 1–4, 1993.
Metz HS, Venkatesh B. Succinylcholine and intraocular pressure. J Pediatr Ophthalmol Strabismus 18: 12, 1981.
Meyers EF, Singer P, Otto A. A controlled study of the effect of succinylcholine self-taming on intraocular pressure. Anesthesiology 53: 72, 1980.
Mindel JS, et al. Succinylcholine-induced return of the eyes to the basic deviation. Ophthalmology 87: 1288, 1980.
Moreno RJ, et al. Effect of succinylcholine on the intraocular contents of open globes. Ophthalmology 98: 636–638, 1991.
Nelson LB, Wagner RS, Harley RD. Prolonged apnea caused by inherited cholinesterase deficiency after strabismus surgery. Am J Ophthalmol 96: 392, 1983.
Polarz H, Bohrer H, Fleischer F, et al. Effects of thiopentone/suxamethonium on intraocular pressure after pretreatment with alfentanil. Eur J Clin Pharmacol 43(3): 311–313, 1992.
Polarz H, Bohrer H, Martin E, et al. Oral clonidine premedication prevents the rise in intraocular pressure following succinylcholine administration. Germ J Ophthalmol 2(2): 97–99, 1993.
Robinson R, White M, et al. Effect of anaesthesia on intraocular blood flow. Br J Ophthalmol 75: 92–93, 1991.
Vachon CA, Warner DO, Bacon DR. Succinylcholine and the open globe. Anesthesiology 99: 220–223, 2003.

CLASS: GENERAL ANESTHESIA

Generic name: Ether (anesthetic ether).

Proprietary names: None.

Primary use

This potent inhalation anesthetic, analgesic and muscle relaxant is used during induction of general anesthesia.

Ocular side effects

Systemic administration
Certain

1. Pupils – dependent on plane of anesthesia
   a. Mydriasis – reactive to light (initial)
   b. Miosis – reactive to light (deep level of anesthesia)
   c. Mydriasis – non-reactive to light (coma)
2. Extraocular muscles – dependent on plane of anesthesia
   a. Slow oscillations (initial)
   b. Eccentric placement of globes (initial)
   c. Concentric placement of globes (coma)
3. Non-specific ocular irritation
4. Conjunctival hyperemia
5. Lacrimal secretion – dependent on plane of anesthesia
   a. Increased (initial)
   b. Decreased (coma)
   c. Abolished (coma)
6. Decreased intraocular pressure
7. Decreased vision
8. Cortical blindness

Inadvertent ocular exposure
Certain

1. Irritation
   a. Hyperemia
   b. Edema
2. Punctate keratitis
3. Corneal opacities

Clinical significance

Adverse ocular reactions due to ether are common, reversible and seldom of clinical importance other than in the determination of the plane of anesthesia. Ether decreases intraocular pressure, probably on the basis of increasing outflow facility. Ether vapor is an irritant to all mucous membranes, including the conjunctiva. In addition, either vapor has a vasodilator property. Permanent corneal opacities have been reported due to direct contact of liquid ether with the cornea. Blindness after induction of general anesthesia is probably due to asphyxic cerebral cortical damage.

REFERENCES AND FURTHER READING

Gilman AG, Goodman LS, Gilman A (eds). The Pharmacological Basis of Therapeutics, 6th edn, Macmillan, New York, p 291, 1980.
Murphy DF. Anesthesia and intraocular pressure. Anesth Analg 64: 520, 1985.
Smith MB. Handbook of Ocular Toxicology, Publishing Sciences Group, Acton, pp 356–357, 1976.
Sweetman SC (ed). Martindale: The Complete Drug Reference, 34th edn, Pharmaceutical Press, London, pp 1298–1299, 2004.
Tripathi RC, Tripathi BC. The Eye. Riddell RH (ed), Pathology of Drug-Induced and Toxic Diseases, Churchill Livingstone, New York, pp 377–450, 1982.

Generic name: Ketamine hydrochloride.

Proprietary name: Ketalar.

Primary use

This intravenous non-barbiturate anesthetic is used for short-term diagnostic or surgical procedures. It may also be used as an adjunct to anesthesia.

Ocular side effects

Systemic administration
Certain
1. Decreased vision
2. Diplopia
3. Horizontal nystagmus
4. Postsurgical visually induced 'emergence reactions'
5. Extraocular muscles
   a. Abnormal conjugate deviations
   b. Random ocular movements
6. Lacrimation
7. Visual hallucinations
8. Distortion of visual perception

Probable
1. Increased intraocular pressure – minimal (deep level of anesthesia)

Conditional
1. Optic neuritis
2. Blindness – transient

Clinical significance

All ocular side effects due to ketamine are transient and reversible. After ketamine anesthesia, diplopia may persist for up to 30 minutes during the recovery phase and may be particularly bothersome to some patients. 'Emergence reactions' occur in 12% of patients and may consist of various psychological manifestations from pleasant dream-like states to irrational behavior. The incidence of these reactions is increased by visual stimulation as the drug is wearing off. El'kin et al (2000) showed inadequate evaluation of size, shape and velocity in visual perception for the first 24 hours post anesthesia. Fine et al (1974) report three cases of transient blindness following ketamine anesthesia lasting about half an hour with complete restoration of sight and no apparent sequelae. This is thought to be a toxic cerebral-induced phenomenon or an anoxic insult. The effect of ketamine on intraocular pressure is somewhat confusing, with various authors obtaining different results. Intraocular pressure is probably not elevated in the first 8–10 minutes after the drug is administered; however, after this there may be increased muscle tone with a resultant increase in intraocular pressure. Fantinati et al (1988) reported a case of bilateral optic neuritis after a general anesthesia induced by ketamine. Ketamine is also used as a recreational drug for its psychedelic effect, and abusers may develop visual hallucinations, coarse horizontal nystagmus, abnormal conjugate eye deviations and diplopia.

REFERENCES AND FURTHER READING

Ausinsch B, et al. Ketamine and intraocular pressure in children. Anesth Analg 55: 773, 1976.

Crandall DC, Leopold IH. The influence of systemic drugs on tear constituents. Ophthalmology 86(1): 115–125, 1979.

Drugs that cause psychiatric symptoms. Med Lett Drugs Ther 28: 81, 1986.

El'kin IO, Verbuk AM, Egorov VM. Comparative characterization of changes in visual perception after ketamine and brietal anesthesia in children. Anesteziol Reanimatol 1: 17–19, 2000.

Fantinati S, Casarotto R, et al. Bilateral retrobulbar neuritis after general anesthesia. Ann Ophthalmol 114: 649, 1988.

Fine J, Weissman J, Finestone SC. Side effects after ketamine anesthesia: Transient blindness. Anesth Analg 53: 72, 1974.

MacLennan FM. Ketamine tolerance and hallucinations in children. Anaesthesia 37: 1214, 1982.

Meyers EF, Charles P. Prolonged adverse reactions to ketamine in children. Anesthesiology 49: 39, 1979.

Shaw IH, Moffett SP. Ketamine and video nasties. Anaesthesia 45: 422, 1990.

Whitwam JG. Adverse reactions to intravenous agents: side effects, Thorton JA (ed), Adverse Reactions to Anaesthetic Drugs, Elsevier, New York, pp 47–57, 1981.

Generic name: Methoxyflurane.

Proprietary name: Penthrane.

Primary use

This methyl ether is used as an inhalation anesthetic with good analgesic and muscle relaxant properties.

Ocular side effects

Systemic administration
Certain
1. 'Flecked retinal syndrome'
2. Fluorescein angiography – window defects

Probable
1. Decreased intraocular pressure
2. Myasthenia gravis
   a. Diplopia
   b. Ptosis
   c. Paresis of extraocular muscles

Clinical significance

Ocular side effects due to methoxyflurane are rare, but a unique adverse ocular reaction has been reported. Oxalosis occurs for unknown reasons, with calcium oxalate crystal deposits throughout the body. These deposits have a predilection for the retinal pigment epithelium and around retinal arteries and arterioles. They may be found in any ocular tissue, but mainly in vascularized tissue. Seldom does this interfere with vision. The deposition of these crystals in the retina gives the clinical picture of an apparent 'flecked retinal syndrome'. With time the crystals become less prominent, but may remain visible for many years. There is no known effective treatment. This drug can also aggravate or unmask myasthenia gravis.

REFERENCES AND FURTHER READING

Albert DM, et al. Flecked retina secondary to oxalate crystals from methoxyflurane anesthesia: Clinical and experimental studies. Trans Am Acad Ophthalmol Otolaryngol 79: 817, 1975.

Argov Z, Mastaglia FL. Disorders of neuromuscular transmission caused by drugs. N Engl J Med 301: 409, 1979.

Bullock JD, Albert DM. Flecked retina. Arch Ophthalmol 93: 26, 1975.

Kaeser NE. Drug-induced myasthenic syndromes. Acta Neurol Scand 70(Suppl. 100): 39, 1984.

Novak MA, Roth AS, Levine MR. Calcium oxalate retinopathy associated with methoxyflurane abuse. Retina 8: 230–236, 1988.

Schettini A, Owre ES, Fink AI. Effect of methoxyflurane anesthesia on intraocular pressure. Can Anaesth Soc J 15: 172, 1968.

Sweetman SC (ed). Martindale: The Complete Drug Reference, 34th edn, Pharmaceutical Press, London, p 1304, 2004.

Tammisto O, Hamalainen L, Tarkkanen L. Halothane and methoxyflurane in ophthalmic anesthesia. Acta Anaesth Scand 9: 173–177, 1965.

Generic name: Nitrous oxide.

Proprietary name: None.

Primary use
This inhalation anesthetic and analgesic is used in dentistry, in the second stage of labor in pregnancy and during induction of general anesthesia.

Ocular side effects.

Systemic administration
Certain
1. Pupils – dependent on plane of anesthesia
   a. Mydriasis – reactive to light (initial)
   b Miosis – reactive to light (deep level of anesthesia)
   c. Mydriasis – non-reactive to light (coma)
2. Intraocular pressure
   a. Increased during anesthesia
   b. Decreased immediately post anesthesia
3. Decreased vision
4. Decreased lacrimation
5. Abnormal ERG or VEP
6. Cortical blindness

Intravitreal injection of gas during vitrectomy
Certain
1. Nitrous oxide gas increases in volume up to 42 days (Fig. 7.4a)
2. Acute glaucoma
3. Central retinal artery occlusion
4. Optic atrophy
5. Pupillary block

Clinical significance
Pupillary changes due to nitrous oxide are common; however, other than aiding in determination of the anesthetic plane, they are seldom of importance. Nitrous oxide, as well as other anesthetics, produces the transitory effect of decreased basal tear production during general anesthesia. Although decreased vision or blindness after induction of general anesthesia is quite rare, this phenomenon is more frequent with nitrous oxide than with most other general anesthetics. Visual loss is probably secondary to asphyxic cerebral cortical damage.

Nitrogen from the bloodstream can enter an intraocular gas bubble from retinal surgery, causing it to expand. Nitrous oxide's solubility is 34 times that of nitrogen, therefore long-lasting insoluble gases for retinal tamponades have expanded to cause central artery occlusion, pupillary block and acute glaucoma in a closed globe (Fig. 7.4a). While most gases will absorb within 10 days, Lee reports the onset of this complication at 3–7 days and Seaberg et al at 42 days post anesthesia. If these gases are used, therefore, nitrous oxide anesthesia is contraindicated and patients should be instructed to wear identifying bracelets (Fig. 7.4b) until the gas bubble is absorbed.

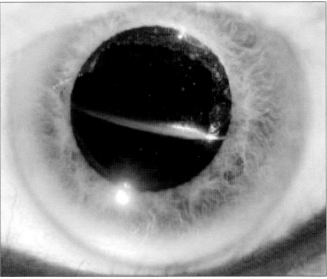

Fig. 7.4a Vitreous cavity about 50% full of gas. Photo courtesy of Yang YF, et al. Nitrous oxide anaesthesia in the presence of intraocular gas can cause irreversible blindness. BMJ 325: 532–533, 2002.

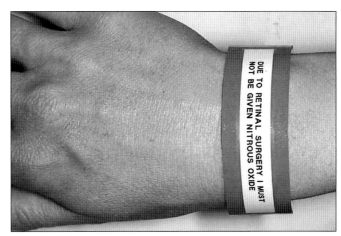

Fig. 7.4b Wristband worn by patient after retinal surgery using intraocular gas. Photo courtesy of Hart RH, et al. Loss of vision caused by expansion of intraocular perflurorpropan gas during nitrous oxide anesthesia. Am J Ophthalmol 134:761–763, 2002.

REFERENCES AND FURTHER READING
Boucher MC, Meyers E. Effects of nitrous oxide anesthesia on intraocular air volume. Can J Ophthalmol 18: 246, 1983.

Crandall DC, Leopold IN. The influence of systemic drugs on tear constituents. Ophthalmology 86: 115, 1979.

Fenwick PBC, et al. Changes in the pattern reversal visual evoked potential as a function of inspired nitrous oxide concentration. Electroencephalogr Clin Neurophysiol 57: 178, 1984.

Fu AR, McDonald HR, Eliott D, et al. Complications of general anesthesia using nitrous oxide in eyes with preexisting gas bubbles. Retina 22: 569–574, 2002.

Hart RH, Vote BJ, Borthwick JH, et al. Loss of vision caused by expansion of intraocular perfluoropropane (C_3F_8) gas during nitrous oxide anesthesia. Am J Ophthalmol 134: 761–763, 2002.

Lane GA, et al. Anesthetics as teratogens: Nitrous oxide is fetotoxic, xenon is not. Science 210: 899, 1980.

Lee EJK. Use of nitrous oxide causing severe visual loss 37 days after retinal surgery. Br J Anaesth 93: 464–466, 2004.

Mostafa SM, Wong SH, Snowdown SL, et al. Nitrous oxide and internal tamponade during vitrectomy. Br J Ophthalmol 75(12): 726–728, 1991.

Ratta C, et al. Changes in the electroretinogram and visual evoked potentials during general anaesthesia. Graefes Arch Clin Exp Ophthalmol 211: 139, 1979.

Seaberg RR, Freeman WR, Goldbaum MH, et al. Permanent postoperative
vision loss associated with expansion of intraocular gas in the presence of
nitrous oxide-containing anesthetic. Anesthesiology 97: 1309–1310, 2002.
Sebel PS, Flynn PJ, Ingram DA. Effect of nitrous oxide on visual, auditory
and somatosensory evoked potentials. Br J Anaesth 56: 1403, 1984.
Vote BJ, Hart RH, Worsley DR, et al. Visual loss after use of nitrous oxide gas
with general anesthetic in patients with intraocular gas still persistent
up to 30 days after vitrectomy. Anesthesiology 97: 1305–1308, 2002.
Wolf GE, Capuano C, Hartung J. Effect of nitrous oxide on gas bubble volume in the anterior chamber. Arch Ophthalmol 103: 418–419, 1985.
Yang YF, Herber L, Rüschen RJ, Colling RJ. Nitrous oxide anaesthesia in the
presence of intraocular gas can cause irreversible blindness. BMJ 325:
532–533, 2002.

Generic name: Propofol.

Proprietary name: Diprivan.

Primary use

An intravenous sedative-hypnotic used in the induction and maintenance of anesthesia or sedation.

Ocular side effects

Intravenous administration
Certain
1. Extraocular muscles
   a. Diplopia
   b. Palsy
   c. Paresis
   d. External ophthalmoplegia
2. Inability to open eyes
3. Eyelids
   a. Rash
   b. Edema

Probable
1. Blurred vision
2. Nystagmus

Accidental ocular exposure
Certain
1. Intense ocular burning
2. Temporary blindness
3. Keratitis

Clinical significance

Propofol is an intravenous medication that can cause transitory visual complications. To date, none of the reported events in the literature or in the National Registry have been permanent. One of the more unusual side effects is that after patients have recovered from anesthesia (i.e. respond to verbal commands and have a return of muscular power) they are unable to open their eyes either spontaneously or in response to a command for 3–20 minutes. This may include the transitory loss of all ocular or periocular muscle movements, including the lids and rectus muscles. Blurred vision can occur, but it is usually inconsequential. Associated exposure keratitis occurs due to lack of eyelid control and restriction of Bell's phenomena. While nystagmus has been reported to the National Registry, it is difficult to prove a cause-and-effect relationship. Neel et al (1995) reported that

with a single low-dose bolus intravenous sedation before cataract surgery there was a moderate reduction in intraocular pressure.

Reddy (2002) reported that as an anesthetist he inadvertently got this liquid drug on his eyes and experienced intense burning for several minutes until his eye could be irrigated. He could not continue giving the anesthetic as he was experiencing a complete loss of vision. Ameen (2001) had a similar experience but could continue and eventually developed a keratitis, which resolved without sequelae.

REFERENCES AND FURTHER READING

Ameen H. Can propofol cause keratitis? Anaesthesia 56: 1017–1018, 2001.
Kumar CM, McNeela BJ. Ocular manifestation of propofol allergy. Anaesthesia 44: 266, 1989.
Lenart SB, Garrity JA. Eye care for patients receiving neuromuscular block-
ing agents or propofol during mechanical ventilation. Am J Crit Care 9:
188–191, 2000.
Marsch SC, Schaefer HG. External ophthalmoplegia after total intravenous
anaesthesia. Anaesthesia 49(6): 525–527, 1994.
Marsch SCU, Schaefer HG. Problems with eye opening after propofol
anesthesia. Anesth Analg 70: 127–128, 1990.
Neel S, Deitch R, Moorthy SS, et al. Changes in intraocular pressure during
low dose intravenous sedation with propofol before cataract surgery.
Br J Ophthalmol 79: 1093–1097, 1995.
Reddy MB. Can propofol cause keratitis? Anaesthesia 57: 183–208, 2002.

CLASS: LOCAL ANESTHETICS

Generic names: 1. Bupivacaine hydrochloride; 2. chloro-procaine hydrochloride; 3. lidocaine; 4. mepivacaine hydrochloride; 5. prilocaine; 6. procaine hydrochloride.

Proprietary names: 1. Sensorcaine, Marcaine Hydrochloride; 2. Nescaine, Nescaine-MPF; 3. Anestacon, Laryng-o-jet kit, Lidoderm, Lidopen, LTA II Kit, Xylocaine, Xylocaine Viscous; 4. Carbocaine, Isocaine Hydrochloride, Polocaine, Polocaine-MPF, Scandonest Plain; 5. Citanest Plain; 6. Novocain.

Primary use

These amides or esters of para-aminobenzoic acid are used in infiltrative, epidural block and peripheral or sympathetic nerve block anesthesia or analgesia.

Ocular side effects

Systemic administration – spiral, caudal, epidural, extradural injections
Certain
1. Extraocular muscles
   a. Paresis or paralysis (Fig. 7.4c)
   b. Diplopia
   c. Nystagmus
   d. Jerky pursuit movements – toxic states
   e. Abnormal doll's head movements – toxic states
2. Decreased vision
3. Horner's syndrome
   a. Miosis
   b. Ptosis
4. Pupils
   a. Mydriasis – toxic states
   b. Anisocoria – toxic states
5. Problems with color vision – color vision defect (lidocaine)
6. Visual hallucinations (lidocaine)

Probable
1. Retinal hemorrhages (caudal block)
2. Macular edema
3. Photosensitivity

Local ophthalmic use or exposure – retrobulbar parabulbar injection (bupivacaine, lidocaine, mepivacaine, procaine)
Certain
1. Decreased or loss of vision – temporary
2. Paresis or paralysis of extraocular muscles, including contralateral 6th nerve (Fig. 7.4c)
3. Decreased intraocular pressure
4. Eyelids or conjunctiva
   a. Allergic reactions
   b. Hyperemia
   c. Blepharoconjunctivitis
   d. Edema
   e. Urticaria
   f. Blepharoclonus
5. Pain – dependent in part on temperature of solution

Possible
1. Eyelids or conjunctiva – exfoliative dermatitis

Conditional/Unclassified
1. Orbital inflammation

Inadvertent topical intraocular injection - anterior or posterior segment
Certain
1. Vision loss
2. Corneal edema
3. Endothelial cell loss
4. Increased intraocular pressure (transitory)

5. Uveitis
6. Hypotony
7. Decreased pupillary function
8. Pigment dispersion syndrome
9. Cataracts
10. Chronic Descemet's membrane wrinkling

Inadvertent ocular exposure (lidocaine)
Certain
1. Pupils
   a. Mydriasis
   b. Absence of reaction to light
2. Decreased vision
3. Superficial punctate keratitis

Systemic side effects

Local ophthalmic use or exposure retrobulbar injection
Certain
1. Convulsion
2. Apnea
3. Cardiac arrest
4. Methaemoglobin (prilocaine)

Clinical significance

Spinal, caudal, epidural and extradural injections of local anesthetics rarely cause ocular side effects. The most common ocular adverse event is an extraocular nerve palsy or paralysis. This may start with or without a headache followed by a weakness of the 6th nerve, although the 3rd and 4th nerves may also be involved. This may occur as soon as 2 hours after the spinal injection or up to 3 weeks later. Recovery usually occurs in 3 days to 3 weeks but has required up to 18 months. Acute bilateral central scotomas, possible due to hypotension or macular ischemia,

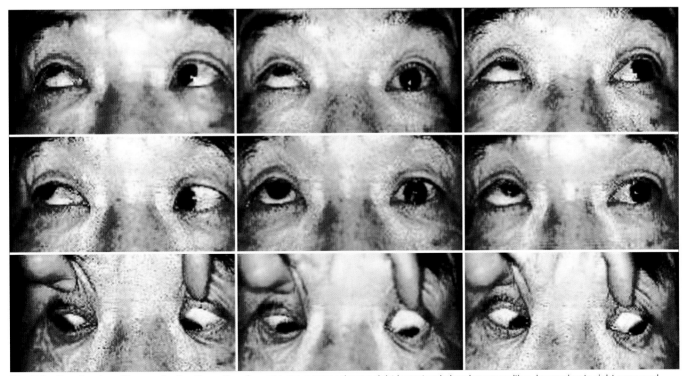

Fig. 7.4c Results of motility examination 6 months after cataract surgery show a right hypertropia in primary position, increasing to right gaze and decreasing to left gaze. Photo courtesy of Han SK, et al. Persistent diplopia after retrobulbar anesthesia. J Cataract Refract Surg. 30: 1248–1253, 2004.

have been reported. These side effects were more common decades ago when the purity of some products was in doubt or before the detergents used to clean equipment were found to be toxic.

Regional anesthesia has caused ocular adverse events but it is difficult to rule out mechanical (speed of injection, bolus effect, increased local pressure) emboli from a toxic effect. Case reports include diplopia after a dental procedure (Walker et al 2004), bilateral transient blindness during hand surgery (Sawyer et al 2002) and permanent uniocular blindness after a dental extraction (Rishiraj et al 2005).

Adverse events secondary to retrobulbar or peribulbar injections of anesthetics are seldom of clinical importance. However, problems may arise secondary to injections into the optic nerve sheath or nerve itself. Irreversible ischemic changes secondary to pressure effects that impede ocular blood flow, direct toxicity to muscle or needle-induced trauma may occur. Myotoxic effects of local anesthetics, which could cause degeneration and subsequent regeneration of extraocular muscles, could explain some cases of postoperative diplopia and ptosis. Han et al (2004) state that persistent diplopia post-retrobulbar anesthesia is due to drug myotoxicity or from direct trauma. Transient loss of vision is practically routine from retrobulbar injections of lidocaine or procaine. There have been occasional reports of cardiopulmonary arrest or grand mal seizures following the retrobulbar administration of bupivacaine, lidocaine, mepivacaine or procaine. Warming the anesthetic prior to injection was found by Ursell and Spalton (1996) to decrease the iatrogenic pain of the injection.

Inadvertent intraocular injection of a local anesthetic into the anterior chamber is a rare but potentially devastating event. Instances of toxicity to the corneal endothelial cell secondary to local anesthesia have recently increased due to the use of intracameral anesthesia. Judge et al (1997) has reviewed this in animals. Shah et al (2004), along with others, point out that if one uses preservative-free 1% xylocaine (lidocaine), the endothelium is not adversely affected during phacoemulsification. Eggeling et al (2000) concur that lidocaine at 1% appears safe. Dance et al (2005) point out that some patients allergic to 'caines' do not react adversely to preservative-free lidocaine. Lee et al (2003) confirm that intracameral 1% lidocaine causes pupillary dilation in the eyes, which are difficult to dilate. Higher concentrations of local anesthetics are toxic to the lens and cornea epithelium.

Inadvertent intraocular injection of lidocaine has been reported to cause cataracts. Pigment dispersion is common, and much of this may be mechanical due to the fire hose effect of a fluid under pressure being forced out through a small gauge needle. The resultant stream has a shearing effect on the tissue it comes into contact with. Pupillary function is often decreased and even absent, partially due to acute secondary glaucoma, synechiae or a direct drug effect. The spectrum of injury is broad; however, if the posterior segment is not involved and chronic glaucoma is avoided, the prognosis may be good with corneal surgery. The outcome of inadvertent local anesthetic injected in the posterior segment is often dependent on the direct effect of the penetration trauma. Although a double perforation may have a better prognosis than a single perforation, an injection through the pars plana may be devoid of significant effects other than the acute rise in intraocular pressure. The immediate effect of the injection is a marked increase in intraocular pressure, with or without pupillary dilation, corneal edema or loss of vision. All of the above are transitory since there appear to be no significant long-term toxic effects of the local anesthetic on the retina or optic nerve. The chief concern is control of the acute rise in pressure, which may be severe enough to cause central retinal

venous or arterial occlusion. Next are the problems from retinal perforation, vitreous adhesion or retinal detachment. Lemagne et al (1990) reported a case of Purtscher-like retinopathy with a retrobulbar injection of a local anesthetic. The exudates and hemorrhages disappeared while a localized paracentral scotoma and afferent pupillary defect were permanent.

Numerous systemic reactions from topical ocular applications of local anesthetics have been reported. Many of these occur in part from the fear of the impending procedure or possibly an oculocardiac reflex. Side effects reported include syncope, convulsions and anaphylactic shock.

Local anesthetics applied to the eye are seldom of importance except with multiple repeat exposures.

REFERENCES AND FURTHER READING

Anderson NJ, Woods WD, Terry K, et al. Intracameral anesthesia. Arch Ophthalmol 117: 225–232, 1999.

Antoszyk AN, Buckley EG. Contralateral decreased visual acuity and extraocular palsies following retrobulbar anesthesia. Ophthalmology 93: 462, 1986.

Breslin CW, Nershenfeld S, Motolko M. Effect of retrobulbar anesthesia on ocular tension. Can J Ophthalmol 18: 223, 1983.

Carruthers JDA, Sanmugasunderan S, Mills K, et al. The efficacy of topical corneal anesthesia with 0.5% bupivacaine eyedrops. Can J Ophthalmol 30(5): 264–266, 1995.

Cohen RG, Hartstein M, Ladav M, et al. Ocular toxicity following topical application of anesthetic cream to the eyelid skin. Ophthalmic Surg Lasers 27: 374–377, 1996.

Dance D, Basti S, Koch DD. Use of preservative-free lidocaine for cataract surgery in a patient allergic to 'caines'. J Cataract Refract Surg 31: 848–850, 2005.

Duker JS, et al. Inadvertent globe perforation during retrobulbar and peribulbar anesthesia. Patient characteristics, surgical management, and visual outcome. Ophthalmology 98(4): 519–526, 1991.

Eggeling P, Pleyer U, Hartmann C, et al. Corneal endothelial toxicity of different lidocaine concentrations. J Cataract Refract Surg 6: 1403–1408, 2000.

Eltzschig H, Rohrbach M, Hans Schroeder T. Methaemoglobinaemia after peribulbar blockade: An unusual complication in ophthalmic surgery. Br J Ophthalmol 84: 439, 2000.

Gild WM, et al. Eye injuries associated with anesthesia. A closed claims analysis. Anesthesiology 76: 204–208, 1992.

Gills JP. Effect of lidocaine on lens epithelial cells. J Cataract Refract Surg 30: 1152–1153, 2004.

Haddad R. Fibrinous iritis due to oxybuprocaine. Br J Ophthalmol 73: 76–77, 1989.

Han SK, Kim JH, Hwang J-M. Persistent diplopia after retrobulbar anesthesia. J Cataract Refract Surg 30: 1248–1253, 2004.

Judge AJ, Najafi K, Lee DA, et al. Corneal endothelial toxicity of topical anesthesia. Ophthalmology 104: 1373–1379, 1997.

Kim T, Holley GP, Lee JH, et al. The effects of intraocular lidocaine on the corneal endothelium. Ophthalmology 105(1): 125–130, 1998.

Lee JJ, Moster MR, Henderer JD, et al. Pupil dilation with intracameral 1% lidocaine during glaucoma filtering surgery. Am J Ophthalmol 136: 201–203, 2003.

Lemagne JM, et al. Purtscher-like retinopathy after retrobulbar anesthesia. Ophthalmology 97(7): 859–861, 1990.

Lincoff N, et al. Intraocular injection of lidocaine. Ophthalmology 92: 1587, 1985.

Meyer D, Hamilton RC, Gimbel HV. Myasthenia gravis-like syndrome induced by topical ophthalmic preparations. A case report. J Clin Neuro-ophthalmol 12(3): 210–212, 1992.

Mukherji S, Esakowitz L. Orbital inflammation after sub-tenon's anesthesia. J Cataract Refract Surg 31: 2221–2223, 2005.

Rishiraj B, Epstein JB, Fine D, et al. Permanent vision loss in one eye following administration of local anesthesia for a dental extraction. Int J Oral Maxillofac Surg 34: 220–223, 2005.

Salama H, Farr AK, Guyton DL. Anesthetic myotoxicity as a cause of restrictive strabismus after scleral buckling surgery. Retina 20: 478–482, 2000.

Sawyer RJ, von Schroeder H. Temporary bilateral blindness after acute lidocaine toxicity. Anesth Analg 95: 224–226, 2002.

Shah AR, Diwan RP, Vasavada AR, et al. Corneal endothelial safety of intracameral preservative-free 1% xylocaine. Indian J Ophthalmol 52: 133–138, 2004.

Sprung J, Haddox JD, Maitra-D'Cruze AM. Horner's syndrome and trigeminal nerve palsy following epidural anaesthesia for obstetrics. Can J Anaesthesia 38(6): 767–771, 1991.

Sullivan KL, et al. Retrobulbar anesthesia and retinal vascular obstruction. Ophthalmology 90: 373, 1983.

Ursell PG, Spalton DJ. The effect of solution temperature on the pain of peribulbar anesthesia. Ophthalmology 103(5): 839–841, 1996.

Walker M, Drangsholt M, Czartoski TJ, et al. Dental diplopia with transient abducens palsy. Neurology 63: 2449–2450, 2004.

Wittpenn JR, et al. Respiratory arrest following retrobulbar anesthesia. Ophthalmology 93: 867, 1986.

CLASS: THERAPEUTIC GASES

Generic name: Carbon dioxide.

Proprietary name: None.

Primary use

This odorless, colorless gas is used as a respiratory stimulant to increase cerebral blood flow and in the maintenance of acid-base balance.

Ocular side effects

Systemic administration – extreme concentrations
Certain
1. Decreased vision
2. Decreased convergence
3. Paralysis of accommodation
4. Decreased dark adaptation
5. Photophobia
6. Visual fields
   a. Constriction
   b. Enlarged blind spot
7. Problems with color vision
   a. Color vision defect
   b. Objects have yellow tinge
8. Retinal vascular engorgement
9. Pupils
   a. Mydriasis
   b. Absence of reaction to light
10. Visual hallucinations
11. Diplopia
12. Abnormal conjugate deviations
13. Papilledema
14. Increased intraocular pressure
15. Ptosis
16. Decreased corneal reflex
17. Proptosis
18. Decreased ability to detect coherent motion

Clinical significance

Although ocular side effects due to carbon dioxide are numerous, they are rare and nearly all significant findings are in toxic states. Transient elevation of intraocular pressure has been reported in the inhalation of 10% carbon dioxide. It is of interest in evaluating 'sick building syndrome' (Hempel-Jorgensen et al 1997; Kjaergaard et al 1992) that the percentage of CO_2 in the air may be correlated with ocular stinging and discomfort. Yang (1997) reported that a 2.5% rise in CO_2 in the air may cause temporary impairment of the ability to detect coherent motion.

REFERENCES AND FURTHER READING

Duke-Elder S. Systems of Ophthalmology, Vol. XIV, Part 2, Mosby, St Louis, pp 1350–1351, 1972.

Dumont L, Mardirosoff C, Dumont C, et al. Bilateral mydriasis during laparoscopic surgery. Acta Anaesthesiologica Belgica 49(1): 33–37, 1998.

Freedman A, Sevel D. The cerebro-ocular effects of carbon dioxide poisoning. Arch Ophthalmol 76: 59, 1966.

Hempel-Jorgensen A, Kjaergaard SK, Molhave L. Integration in human eye irritation. Int Arch Occup Environ Health 69(4): 289–294, 1997.

Kjaergaard S, Pedersen OF, Molhave L. Sensitivity of the eyes to airborne irritant stimuli: Influence of individual characteristics. Int Arch Occup Environ Health 47(1): 45–50, 1992.

Lincoff A, et al. Selection of xenon gas for rapidly disappearing retinal tamponade. Arch Ophthalmol 100: 996–997, 1982.

Podlekareva D, Pan Z, Kjaergaard S, et al. Irritation of the human eye mucous membrane caused by airborne pollutants. Int Arch Occup Environ Health 75: 359–364, 2002.

Sevel D, Freedman A. Cerebro-retinal degeneration due to carbon dioxide poisoning. Br J Ophthalmol 51: 475, 1967.

Sieker NO, Nickam JB. Carbon dioxide intoxication: The clinical syndrome, its etiology and management, with particular reference to the use of mechanical respirators. Medicine 35: 389, 1956.

Walsh FB, Noyt WF. Clinical Neuro-Ophthalmology 3rd edn, Vol. III, Williams & Wilkins, Baltimore, pp 2601–2602, 1969.

Wolbarsht ML, et al. Speculation on carbon dioxide and retrolental fibroplasia. Pediatrics 71: 859, 1983.

Yang Y, Sun C, Sun M. The effect of moderately increased CO_2 concentration on perception of coherent motion. Aviation Space Environ Med 68(3): 187–191, 1997.

Generic names: Oxygen, oxygen-ozone.

Proprietary names: None.

Primary use

This colorless, odorless, tasteless gas is used in inhalation anesthesia and in hypoxia. Oxygen-ozone (O_2O_3) is used as intradiscal injections for the treatment of lumbar sciatic pain peridurally and lumbar disc herniation.

Ocular side effects

Systemic administration
Certain
1. Retinal vascular changes
   a. Constriction
   b. Spasms
   c. Hemorrhages (Fig. 7.4d)
2. Decreased vision
3. Visual fields
   a. Constriction
4. Retrolental fibroplasia – in newborns or young infants
5. Heightened color perception
6. Retinal detachment
7. Abnormal ERG
8. Decreased dark adaptation
9. Myopia
10. Cataracts – nuclear

Possible
1. Retinal hemorrhage (oxygen-ozone) (Fig. 7.4d)

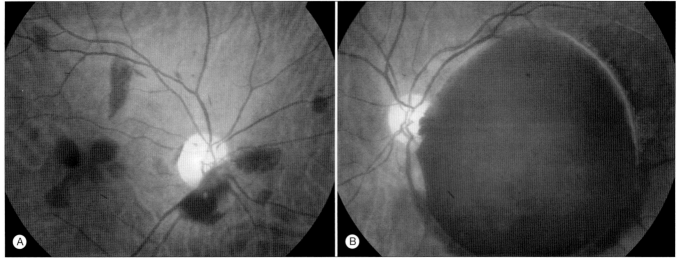

Fig. 7.4d A: Right eye with multiple retinal, intraretinal and preretinal hemorrhages surrounding the optic nerve head and the posterior pole. B: An extensive premacular subhyaloid hemorrhage involving the left macular region due to oxygen-ozone therapy. Photo courtesy of Giudice GL, et al: Acute bilateral vitreo-retinal hemorrhages following oxygen-ozone therapy for lumbar disk herniation. Am J Ophthalmol 138: 175-177, 2004.

Clinical significance

Toxic ocular effects due to oxygen are more prominent in premature infants but may be found in any age group under hyperbaric oxygen therapy. Otherwise, ocular side effects secondary to oxygen therapy are rare. While ocular changes due to retrolental fibroplasia are irreversible, most other side effects are transient after use of oxygen is discontinued. Permanent bilateral blindness probably due to 80% oxygen during general anesthesia has been reported. It has been suggested that in susceptible people, severe retinal vasoconstriction or even direct retinal toxicity may occur from oxygen therapy. Bilateral retinal hemorrhages with permanent partial visual loss have been reported secondary to a sudden increase in cerebral spinal fluid pressure after an excessive volume of oxygen was used in a myelogram contrast study. A slow increase in myopia following prolonged hyperbaric oxygen has been seen in premature infants and adults. In addition, oxidative damage to the lens proteins has been postulated as a cause of nuclear cataracts in patients exposed to hyperbaric oxygen treatments.

In a single case report, Giudice et al (2004) described O_2O_3 injected spinal disc infiltration causing bilateral retinal hemorrhage.

REFERENCES AND FURTHER READING

Anderson B Jr, Farmer JC Jr. Hyperoxic myopia. Trans Am Ophthalmol Soc 76: 116, 1978.

Ashton N. Oxygen and the retinal vessels. Trans Ophthalmol Soc UK 100: 359, 1980.

Campbell PB, et al. Incidence of retinopathy of prematurity in a tertiary newborn intensive care unit. Arch Ophthalmol 101: 1686, 1983.

Fisher AB. Oxygen therapy. Side effects and toxicity. Am Rev Respir Dis 122: 61, 1980.

Gallin-Cohen PF, Podos SM, Yablonski ME. Oxygen lowers intraocular pressure. Invest Ophthalmol Vis Sci 19: 43, 1980.

Giudice GL, Valdi F, Gismondi M, et al. Acute bilateral vitreo-retinal hemorrhages following oxygen-ozone therapy for lumbar disk herniation. Am J Ophthalmol 138: 175–177, 2004.

Handelman IL, et al. Retinal toxicity of therapeutic agents. J Toxicol Cut Ocular Toxicol 2: 131, 1983.

Kalina RE, Karr DJ. Retrolental fibroplasia. Ophthalmology 89: 91, 1982.

Lyne AJ. Ocular effects of hyperbaric oxygen. Trans Ophthalmol Soc UK 98: 66, 1978.

Nissenkorn I, et al. Myopia in premature babies with and without retinopathy of prematurity. Br J Ophthalmol 67: 170, 1983.

Oberman J, Cohn N, Grand MG. Retinal complications of gas myelography. Arch Ophthalmol 97: 1905, 1979.

Palmquist BM, Philipson B, Barr PO. Nuclear cataract and myopia during hyperbaric oxygen therapy. Br J Ophthalmol 68: 113, 1984.

SECTION 5
GASTROINTESTINAL AGENTS

CLASS: AGENTS USED TO TREAT ACID PEPTIC DISORDERS

Generic names: 1. Cimetidine; 2. famotidine; 3. nizatidine; 4. ranitidine.

Proprietary names: 1. Tagamet; 2. Pepcid; 3. Axid; 4. Zantac.

Primary use

These histamine H_2 receptor antagonists are used in the treatment of duodenal ulcers.

Ocular side effects

Systemic administration
Certain
1. Visual hallucinations
2. Photophobia
3. Eyelids or conjunctiva
   a. Hyperemia
   b. Erythema
   c. Conjunctivitis – non-specific
   d. Urticaria
   e. Purpura
   f. Photosensitivity reactions

Probable

1. Decreased vision
2. Pupils – toxic states
   a. Mydriasis – may precipitate angle-closure glaucoma
   b. Decreased reaction to light

Possible

1. Decreased color vision
2. Myopia
3. Immune modulation (cimetidine) (Fig. 7.5a)
4. Eyelids or conjunctiva
   a. Stevens-Johnson syndrome
   b. Exfoliative dermatitis
5. Subconjunctival or retinal hemorrhages secondary to drug-induced anemia

Conditional/Unclassified

1. Retinopathy (famotidine)

Clinical significance

Adverse ocular effects secondary to these agents are uncommon. While the National Registry has hundreds of possible adverse ocular reactions with these agents, there are few patterns, and most are probably just background noise. However, transient myopia, yellow or pink tinge to objects, and sicca-like symptoms are all possibly drug related. Visual hallucinations have occurred, particularly with high doses in elderly patients with renal impairment. All adverse ocular reactions are transient and disappear with withdrawal of drug therapy. There is debate on whether or not these agents cause changes in intraocular pressure. The case by Dobrilla et al (1982) along with the National Registry suggests that in rare instances this class of drugs may be associated with changes in intraocular pressure. However, data by Feldman and Cohen (1982), as well as Garcia-Rodríguez et al (1996) do not support this. If these drugs do cause pressure elevation, it is in all likelihood in predisposed eyes and is a rare event. Gardner et al (1995) showed that a combination of astemizole and ranitidine caused increased blood-retinal barrier permeability in patients with diabetic retinopathy. Lee and Wang (2006) reported a single case of bilateral irreversible decrease in vision after two dosages of famotidine. Shields et al (1991) reported improvement of diffuse conjunctival papillomatosis in an 11-year-old after starting cimetidine (Fig. 7.5b).

REFERENCES AND FURTHER READING

Agarwal SK. Cimetidine and visual hallucinations. JAMA 240: 214, 1978.

De Giacomo C, Maggiore G, Scotta MS. Ranitidine and loss of colour vision in a child. Lancet 2: 47, 1984.

Dobrilla G, et al. Exacerbation of glaucoma associated with both cimetidine and ranitidine. Lancet 1: 1078, 1982.

Feldman F, Cohen MM. Effect of histamine-2 receptor blockade by cimetidine on intraocular pressure in humans. Am J Ophthalmol 93: 351, 1982.

García-Rodríguez LA, et al. A cohort study of the ocular safety of anti-ulcer drugs. Br J Clin Pharmacol 42: 213–216, 1996.

Gardner TW, Eller AW, Fribert TR, et al. Antihistamines reduce blood-retinal barrier permeability in Type I (Insulin-dependent) diabetic patients with nonproliferative retinopathy. Retina 15(2): 134–140, 1995.

Horiuchi Y, Ikezawa K. Famotidine-induced erythema multiforme: Cross sensitivity with cimetidine. Ann Intern Med 131: 795, 1999.

Hoskyns BL. Cimetidine withdrawal. Lancet 1: 254, 1977.

Lee Y-C, Wang C-C. Famotidine-induced retinopathy. Eye 20: 260–263, 2006.

Shields CL, Lally MR, Singh AD, et al. Oral cimetidine (tagamet) for recalcitrant, diffuse conjunctival papillomatosis. Am J Ophthalmol 128: 362–364, 1999.

CLASS: ANTACIDS

Generic names: 1. Bismuth aluminate; 2. bismuth citrate; 3. bismuth oxide; 4. bismuth salicylate; 5. bismuth subcarbonate; 6. bismuth subgallate; 7. bismuth subnitrate.

Proprietary names: (1-7) Bismantrol, Children's Kaopectate, Devrom, Kaopectate, Maalox, Peptic Relief, Pepto-Bismol.

Primary use

Bismuth salts are primarily used as antacids and in the treatment of syphilis and yaws.

Ocular side effects

Systemic administration
Probable

1. Eyelids or conjunctiva – blue discoloration
2. Corneal deposits
3. Visual hallucinations – toxic states

Possible

1. Eyelids or conjunctiva
   a. Exfoliative dermatitis
   b. Lyell's syndrome

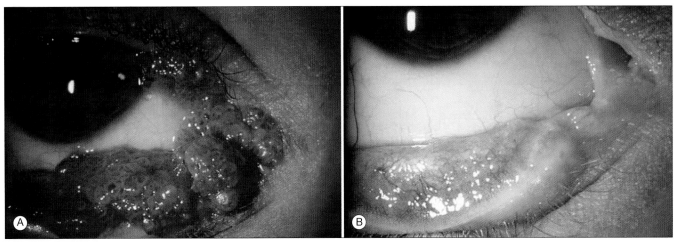

Fig. 7.5a A: Patient with recurrent conjunctival papillomatosis non-responsive to biopsy, cryotherapy or mitomycin C treatment. B: Resolution of papillomas after systemic cimetidine administration.

Local ophthalmic use or exposure
Probable
1. Eyelids or conjunctiva – contact dermatitis

Clinical significance

Adverse ocular reactions to bismuth preparations are quite rare and seldom of clinical significance except in toxic states. Bismuth-containing corneal deposits have been documented. Only one case of decreased vision has been reported after an overdose of bismuth.

Bismuth is used for its bacteriostasis on skin lesions. It is used in some eye ointment and can rarely cause allergic reactions.

REFERENCES AND FURTHER READING

Cohen EL. Conjunctival hemorrhage after bismuth injection. Lancet 1: 627, 1945.
Fischer FP. Bismuthiase secondaire de la cornee. Ann Oculist (Paris) 183: 615, 1950.
Goas JY, et al. Encephalopathie myoclinique par le sous-nitrate de Bismuth. Une observation recente. Nouv Presse Med 10: 3855, 1981.
Supino-Viterbo V, et al. Toxic encephalopathy due to ingestion of bismuth salts: Clinical and ERG studies of 45 patients. J Neurol Neurosurg Psychiatry 40: 748, 1977.
Wictorin A, Hansson C. Allergic contact dermatitis from a bismuth compound in an eye ointment. Contact Derm 24: 318, 2001.
Zurcher K, Krebs A. Cutaneous Side Effects of Systemic Drugs, S. Karger, Basel, p 302, 1980.

CLASS: ANTIEMETICS

Generic name: Metoclopramide.

Proprietary name: Reglan.

Primary use

This orthopramide is used as adjunctive therapy in roentgen-ray examination of the stomach and duodenum, for the prevention and treatment of irradiation sickness, and as an antiemetic.

Ocular side effects

Systemic administration
Certain
1. Extraocular muscles
   a. Oculogyric crises
   b. Diplopia
   c. Paralysis
   d. Nystagmus
   e. Strabismus
2. Eyelids or conjunctiva
   a. Edema
   b. Angioneurotic edema
   c. Urticaria

Probable
1. Decreased vision
2. Problems with color vision-color vision defect

Possible
1. Mydriasis – may precipitate narrow-angle glaucoma
2. Photophobia

Clinical significance

Ocular side effects secondary to metoclopramide are rare, but the drug can produce acute dystonic reactions, particularly in children. This includes transitory oculogyric crises, inability to close the eyes, nystagmus, and various extraocular muscle abnormalities. These dystonic reactions usually occur within 36 hours of starting treatment and subside within 24 hours of stopping the drug.

REFERENCES AND FURTHER READING

Berkman N, Frossard C, Moury F. Oculogyric crises and metoclopramide. Bull Soc Ophthalmol Fr 81: 153, 1981.
Bui NB, Marit G, Noerni B. High-dose metoclopramide in cancer chemotherapy-induced nausea and vomiting. Cancer Treat Rep 66: 2107, 1982.
Hyser CL, Drake ME, Jr. Myoclonus induced by metoclopramide therapy. Arch Intern Med 143: 2201, 1983.
Kofoed P-E, Kamper J. Extrapyramidal reactions caused by antiemetics during cancer chemotherapy. J Pediatr 105: 852, 1984.
Laroche J, Laroche C. Etude de l'action d'un 4e groupe de medicaments sur la discrimination des couleurs et recapitulation des resultats acquis. Ann Pharm Fr 38: 323, 1980.
Terrin BN, McWilliams NB, Maurer HM. Side effects of metoclopramide as an antiemetic in childhood cancer chemotherapy. J Pediatr 104: 138, 1984.

CLASS: ANTILIPIDEMIC AGENTS

Generic names: 1. Atorvastatin calcium; 2. fluvastatin sodium; 3. lovastatin; 4. pravastatin sodium; 5. rosuvastatin calcium; 6. simvastatin.

Proprietary names: 1. Lipitor; 2. Lescol; 3. Altoprev, Mevacor; 4. Pracachol; 5. Crestor; 6. Zocor.

Primary use

These inhibitors of 3-hydroxy-3-methylglutaryl-coenxyme A (HMG-CoA) reductase are used to treat patients with hypercholesterolemia by lowering total cholesterol and LDL cholesterol, and increasing HDL cholesterol. Fluvastatin and lovastatin are also indicated for preventing coronary atherosclerosis.

Ocular side effects

Systemic administration
Probable
1. Decreased rate of choroidal neovascularization
2. Type II diabetes retinopathy
   a. Reduces severity of hard exudates
   b. Reduces subfoveal lipid migration
   c. Reduces clinically significant macula edema
3. Retina
   a. Increases blood velocity and blood flow in arteries and veins
   b. Increases plasma in veins
4. Intraocular pressure
   a. Decreases
   b. Reduced risk of open-angle glaucoma
5. Diplopia

Possible
1. Myasthenia gravis
   a. Diplopia
   b. Ptosis
   c. Paresis of extraocular muscles
2. Blurred vision
3. Eyelids or conjunctiva
   a. Steven-Johnson syndrome
   b. Toxic epidermal necrolysis
   c. Erythema multiforme
   d. Xanthelasma decreases

4. External ophthalmoplegia (reversible)
5. Ptosis

Conditional/Unclassified
1. Lens opacities
   a. Improves
   b. Worsens
   c. Increase risk if taken with erythromycin
2. Keratitis sicca
3. Macular degeneration
   a. Impedes
   b. Increase

Clinical significance

This group of medications, commonly called the statins, is one of the largest groups of prescription drugs in the world. While there are millions of patients on long-term therapy with these agents and multiple peer review articles on their effects on the eye, little concrete data are available. There are no CERTAIN visual side effects, although some patients may complain of a decrease in vision from an unknown cause. This is not statistically significant compared to a placebo in phase III trials (Physicians' Desk Reference 2006). The side effects more likely, although still only POSSIBLE, are ptosis, diplopia and muscle paralysis. Fraunfelder and Fraunfelder (1999) described 71 cases of possible diplopia associated with the use of HMG-CoA reductase inhibitors, with 31 having positive dechallenge tests and two positive rechallenge. The National Registry has 60 additional cases of diplopia and eight of ptosis. Ertas et al (2006) described a case of unilateral ptosis possibly due to atorvastatin. The above may be related to the statins effect on muscle tissue by yet another mechanism. Purvin et al (2006) and Cartwright et al (2004) showed that statins can also exacerbate myasthenia gravis. Cases in the National Registry describe the statins associated with reversible external ophthalmoloplegia with a mechanism unknown.

There are numerous peer review papers on both sides on whether or not these drugs are cataractogenic. It has been suggested that they are possibly weakly cataractogenic, but Cumming and Mitchell (1998), along with others, have shown no clear association of a cataractogenic effect. Klein et al have reported that these drugs decrease the incidence of nucular sclerosis of aging. Another debate is if these drugs impede the development of age-related maculopathy. Several authors feel there is a plausible explanation to support a potential role of anticholesterol drugs, especially the statins, to protect against age-related maculopathy. A recent study by McGwin et al feels statins may increase the risk of age-related maculopathy. Wilson et al (2004) have shown a decreased rate of chorodial neovascularization in age-related maculopathy when patients are on statins. Klein and Klein pooled these findings in a perspective editorial. Nagaoka et al (2006) have shown an increase in blood velocity and blood flow in retinal arteries and veins, an increase in plasma nitrites/nitrates, and a decrease in intraocular pressure probably due to an increase in nitric oxide. Gupta et al (2004) have reported in patients on atorvastatin with type II diabetes and dyslipidema that statins reduced the severity of hard exudates and subfoveal lipid migration in clinically significant macular edema. McGwin et al suggest that long-term use of statins may be associated with a reduced risk of open-angle glaucoma, especially in patients with cardiovascular disease and lipid disease. The questions of the effect of statins on cataracts, age-related maculopathy, type II diabetes retinopathy, and glaucoma need additional confirmation to determine causation.

REFERENCES AND FURTHER READING

Cartwright MS, Jeffery DR, Nuss GR, et al. Statin-associated exacerbation of myasthenia gravis. Neurology 63: 2188, 2004.
Cumming RG, Mitchell P. Medications and cataract: The blue mountains eye study. Ophthalmology 105: 1751–1758, 1998.
Ertas FS, Ertas NM, Gulec S, et al. Unrecognized side effect of statin treatment: Unilateral blepharoptosis. Ophthal Plast Reconstr Surg 22: 222–224, 2006.
Fraunfelder FW, Fraunfelder FT, Edwards R. Diplopia and HMG-CoA reductase inhibitors. J Toxicol Cut Ocular Toxicol 18: 319–321, 1999.
Gupta A, Gupta V, Thapar S, et al. Lipid-lowering drug atorvastatin as an adjunct in the management of diabetic macular edema. Am J Ophthalmol 137: 675–682, 2004.
Hall NF, Gale CR, Syddall H, et al. Risk of macular degeneration in users of statins: Cross sectional study. BMJ 323: 375–376, 2001.
Klein R, Klein BEK. Do statins prevent age-related macular degeneration? Am J Ophthalmol 137: 747–749, 2004.
Klein R, Klein BEK, Tomany SC, et al. Relation of statin use to the 5-year incidence and progression of age-related maculopathy. Arch Ophthalmol 121: 1151–1155, 2003.
Klein BEK, Klein R, Lee KE, et al. Statin use and incident nuclear cataract. JAMA 295: 2752–2758, 2006.
McCarty CA, Mukesh BN, Guymer RH, et al. Cholesterol-lowering medication reduces the risk of age-related maculopathy progression. Let Med J Aust 175: 340, 2001.
McGwin G, Jr, Owsley C, Curcio CA, et al. The association between statin use and age related maculopathy. Br J Ophthalmol 87: 1121–1125, 2003.
McGwin G, Jr, McNeal S, Owsley C, et al. Statins and other cholesterol-lowering medication and the presence of glaucoma. Arch Ophthalmol 122: 822–826, 2004.
McGwin G, Jr, Modjarrad K, Hall TA, et al. 3-Hydroxy-3-methylglutaryl coenzyme a reductase inhibitors and the presence of age-related macular degeneration in the cardiovascular health study. Arch Ophthalmol 124: 33–37, 2006.
Nagaoka T, Takahashi A, Sato E, et al. Effect of systemic administration of simvastatin on retinal circulation. Arch Ophthalmol 124: 665–670, 2006.
Physicians' Desk Reference, 60th edn, Thomson PDR, Montevale NJ, pp 943–948, 2006.
Purvin V, Kawasaki A, Smith KH, et al. Statin-associated myasthenia gravis: Report of 4 cases and review of the literature. Medicine 85: 82–85, 2006.
van Leeuwen R, Vingerling JR, Hofman A, et al. Cholesterol lowering drugs and risk of age related maculopathy: Prospective cohort study with cumulative exposure measurement. BMJ 363: 255–256, 2003.
Wilson HL, Schwartz DM, Bhatt HRF, et al. Statin and aspirin therapy are associated with decreased rates of choroidal neovascularization amoung patients with age-related macular degeneration. Am J Ophthalmol 137: 615–624, 2004.

Generic name: Clofibrate.

Proprietary names: Generic only.

Ocular side effects

Systemic administration
Certain
1. Decreased vision
2. Eyelids or conjunctiva
   a. Erythema
   b. Conjunctivitis – non-specific
   c. Edema
   d. Urticaria
   e. Purpura
   f. Blepharoclonus
   g. Loss of eyelashes or eyebrows
   h. Pruritis

Possible
1. Subconjunctival or retinal hemorrhages secondary to drug-induced anemia

2. Hypermetropia
3. Decreased intraocular pressure
4. Myokymia
5. Eyelids or conjunctiva
   a. Lupoid syndrome
   b. Erythema multiforme

Clinical significance

Ocular side effects due to clofibrate are quite rare and seldom of major clinical significance. All reactions seem to clear on cessation of the drug. There are two reports that suggest this agent, by decreasing blood viscosity, has made glaucoma more easily managed. However, this has not been proven. Regression of xanthomas and diabetic retinopathy has been claimed as well. The drug can make hair more brittle, and alopecia may occur. One case in the National Registry documents a +2.50 refractive change, lasting for 6 weeks after cessation of the drug. Clements et al (1968) did a clinical study using this drug to treat retinal vein occlusions, but the drug was unsuccessful. Teravainen and Makitie (1976) described myokymia as a side effect of clofibrate.

REFERENCES AND FURTHER READING

Arif MA, Vahrman J. Skin eruption due to clofibrate. Lancet 2: 1202, 1975.
Clements DB, Elsby JM, Smith WD. Retinal vein occlusion. A comparative study of factors affecting the prognosis, including a therapeutic trial of Atromid S in this condition. Br J Ophthalmol 52: 111, 1968.
Cullen JF. Clofibrate in glaucoma. Lancet 2: 892, 1967.
Orban T. Clofibrate in glaucoma. Lancet 1: 47, 1968.
Teravainen H, Makitie J. Myokymia, unusual side-effect of clofibrate. Lancet 2: 1298, 1976.

CLASS: ANTISPASMODICS

Generic names: 1. Atropine; 2. homatropine.

Proprietary names: 1. Atropen, Atropine sulfate ansyr plastic syringe; 2. topical ocular multi-ingredient preparations only.

Primary use

Systemic

These anticholinergic agents are used in the management of gastrointestinal tract spasticity, peptic ulcers, hyperactive carotid sinus reflex, Parkinson's disease, in the treatment of dysmenorrhea and to decrease secretions of the respiratory tract.

Ophthalmic

These topical anticholinergic mydriatic and cycloplegic agents are used in refractions, semiocclusive therapy, accommodative spasms and uveitis.

Ocular side effects

Systemic administration
Certain
1. Decreased vision
2. Mydriasis – may precipitate angle-closure glaucoma
3. Decrease or paralysis of accommodation
4. Photophobia
5. Micropsia
6. Decreased lacrimation
7. Visual hallucinations
8. Problems with color vision
   a. Color vision defect
   b. Objects have red tinge

Local ophthalmic use or exposure – topical ocular application
Certain
1. Decreased vision
2. Decrease or paralysis of accommodation
3. Irritation
   a. Hyperemia
   b. Photophobia
   c. Ocular pain
   d. Edema
4. Mydriasis
   a. May precipitate angle-closure glaucoma
   b. May elevate intraocular pressure
5. Eyelids or conjunctiva
   a. Allergic reactions
   b. Blepharoconjunctivitis – follicular and/or papillary
6. Micropsia
7. Decreased lacrimation
8. Visual hallucinations

Local ophthalmic use or exposure – subconjunctival injection
Probable
1. Brawny scleritis
2. Conjunctival and/or necrosis (Fig. 7.5b)

Systemic side effects

Local ophthalmic use or exposure – topical application
Certain
1. Agitation
2. Confusion
3. Psychosis
4. Delirium
5. Hallucinations
6. Ataxia
7. Hostility
8. Fever
9. Dry mouth
10. Vasodilation
11. Dysarthria
12. Tachycardia
13. Convulsion
14. Cardiac dysrhythmias

Clinical significance

Atropine and homatropine have essentially the same ocular side effects whether they are administered systemically, via aerosols, or by topical ocular application. Systemic administration causes fewer and less severe ocular side effects because significantly smaller amounts of the drug reach the eye. Mydriasis is of greatest ocular concern from systemic anticholinergics. Data in the National Registry support the fact that acute glaucoma occurs much more commonly unilaterally and only very rarely is it precipitated bilaterally.

Topical ocular atropine and homatropine have the same ocular effects. The action of homatropine's cycloplegic and mydriatic actions are more rapid and of shorter duration than those of atropine. Irritation or allergic reactions of the eyelids or conjunctiva are the most frequent occurrences, followed by increased light sensitivity. Conjunctival papillary hypertrophy usually suggests

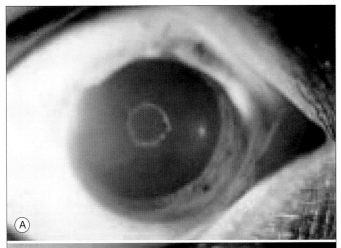

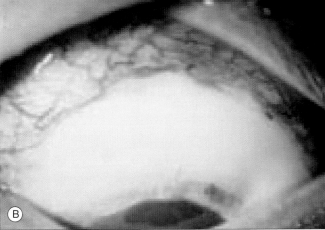

Fig. 7.5b A: Limbus necrosis. B: Conjunctival necrosis from subconjunctival injection of atropine.

a hypersensitivity reaction, while a follicular response suggests a toxic or irritative reaction to these agents. However, as with systemic exposure, the effect on the pupil and cillary body with resultant elevation in intraocular pressure with or without the precipitation of angle-closure glaucoma is of greatest concern.

Atropine, but not homatropine, is said to produce a greater pupillary response in patients with Down's syndrome. Permanent, fixed, dilated pupils may result from chronic atropinization, or large doses of atropine used in resuscitation. Geyer et al (1991) discuss the disagreement of whether or not long-term atropinization post keratoplasty can cause irreversible mydriasis. Unilateral atropinization during visual immaturity may cause amblyopia if used inappropriately (Morrison et al 2005). Seo et al (2002) and cases in the National Registry support the fact that subconjunctival atropine injection may cause necrosis of the sclera and conjunctiva.

Systemic reactions may occur after ocular instillation of these anticholinergic drugs, particularly in children or elderly patients. Symptoms of systemic toxicity include dryness of the mouth and skin, flushing, fever, rash, thirst, tachycardia, irritability, hyperactivity, ataxia, confusion, somnolence, hallucinations and delirium. These reactions have been observed most frequently after the use of atropine. Rarely, convulsions, coma and death have occurred after ocular instillation of atropine in infants and children, primarily if the solution form was used.

Mydriasis due to atropine can be distinguished by applying topical ocular 1.0% pilocarpine, which will not constrict the pupil if atropine is present.

REFERENCES AND FURTHER READING

Arnold RW, Goinet E, Hickel J, et al. Duration and effect of single-dose atropine: Paralysis of accommodation in penalization treatment of functional amblyopia. Binocular Vision Strabismus Quarterly 19: 81–86, 2004.

Chhabra A, Mishra S, Kumar A, et al. Atropine-induced lens extrusion in an open eye surgery. Pediatr Anaesth 16: 59–62, 2006.

Decraene T, Goossens A. Contact allergy to atropine and other mydriatic agents in eye drops. Contact Derm 45: 309–310, 2001.

Geyer O, Rothkoff L, Lazar M. Atropine in keratoplasty for keratoconus. Cornea 10(5): 372–373, 1991.

Gooding JM, Nolcomb MC. Transient blindness following intravenous administration of atropine. Anesth Analg 56: 872, 1977.

Merli GJ, et al. Cardiac dysrhythmias associated with ophthalmic atropine. Arch Intern Med 116: 45, 1986.

Morrison DG, Palmer NJ, Sinatra RB, et al. Severe amblyopia of the sound eye resulting from atropine therapy combined with optical penalization. J Pediatr Ophthalmol Strabismus 42: 52–53, 2005.

O'Brien D, Haake MW, Braid B. Atropine sensitivity and serotonin in mongolism. J Dis Child 100: 873–874, 1960.

Sanitato JJ, Burke MJ. Atropine toxicity in identical twins. Ann Ophthalmol 15: 380, 1983.

Seo KY, Kim CY, Lee JH, et al. Amniotic membrane transplantation for necrotizing conjunctival atropine injection. Br J Ophthalmol 86: 1316–1317, 2002.

The Pediatric Eye Disease Investigator Group. A randomized trial of atropine vs patching for treatment of moderate amblyopia in children. Arch Ophthalmol 120: 268–278, 2002.

The Pediatric Eye Disease Investigator Group. A randomized trial of atropine regimens for treatment of moderate amblyopia in children. Ophthalmology 111: 2076–2085, 2004.

Verma NP. Drugs as a cause of fixed, dilated pupils after resuscitation. JAMA 255: 3251, 1986.

von Noorden GK. Amblyopia caused by unilateral atropinization. Ophthalmology 88: 131, 1981.

Wark NJ, Overton JH, Marian P. The safety of atropine premedication in children with Down's syndrome. Anaesthesia 38: 871, 1983.

Wilhelm H, Wilhelm B, Schiefer U. Mydriasis caused by plant content. Fortschritte der Ophthalmologie 88(5): 588–591, 1991.

Wilson FM, II. Adverse external ocular effects of topical ophthalmic medications. Surv Ophthalmol 24: 57, 1979.

Wright BD. Exacerbation of a kinetic seizure by atropine eye drops. Br J Ophthalmol 76(3): 179–180, 1992.

Yung M, Herrema I. Persistent mydriasis following intravenous atropine in a neonate. Paediatr Anaesth 10: 438–440, 2000.

Generic names: 1. Dicycloverine hydrochloride (dicyclomine); 2. glycopyrronium bromide (glycopyrrolate); 3. mepenzolate bromide; 4. propantheline bromide; 5. tolterodine tartrate.

Proprietary names: 1. Antispas, Bentyl; 2. Robinul, Robinul Forte; 3. Cantil; 4. Pro-banthine; 5. Detrol, Unidet.

Primary use

Systemic
These anticholinergic agents are effective in the management of gastrointestinal tract spasticity and peptic ulcers.

Ophthalmic
These topical anticholinergic mydriatic and cycloplegic agents are used in refractions and fundus examinations.

Ocular side effects

Systemic administration
Certain
1. Decreased vision
2. Mydriasis – may precipitate angle-closure glaucoma

3. Paralysis of accommodation
4. Photophobia
5. Diplopia
6. Problems with color vision
   a. Color vision defect
   b. Colored flashing lights (propantheline)
7. Flashing lights
8. Eyelids or conjunctiva – allergic reactions
9. Visual hallucinations
10. Keratitis sicca (tolterodine)

Possible
1. Eyelids or conjunctiva
   a. Exfoliative dermatitis
   b. Contact dermatitis

Local ophthalmic use or exposure
Certain
1. Mydriasis may precipitate angle-closure glaucoma
2. Photophobia
3. Paralysis of accommodation
4. Eyelids or conjunctiva
   a. Allergic reactions
   b. Conjunctivitis – non-specific
   c. Contact dermatitis

Possible
5. Increased intraocular pressure

Inadvertent ocular exposure
Certain
1. Pupils (propantheline)
   a. Mydriasis
   b. Absence of reaction to light

Possible
1. Paralysis of accommodation

Clinical significance

Ocular side effects due to these anticholinergic agents vary depending on the drug. Adverse ocular reactions are seldom significant and are reversible. None of the preceding drugs has more than 10–15% of the anticholinergic activity of atropine. The most frequent ocular side effects are decreased vision, mydriasis, decreased accommodation and photophobia. While these effects are not uncommon with some of these agents, rarely are they severe enough to modify the use of the drug. The weak anticholinergic effect of these agents seldom aggravates open-angle glaucoma; however, it has the potential to precipitate narrow-angle glaucoma attacks. Varssano et al (1996) showed that topical ocular glycopyrronium may be faster, stronger and have a more persistent mydriatic effect than atropine. Some of these agents, especially tolterodine, may increase tear film breakup time and aggravate or cause keratitis sicca. Two cases of unilateral pupillary dilatation were seen in patients who inadvertently got antiperspirants containing propantheline on their fingers and transferred it to their eyes.

REFERENCES AND FURTHER READING

Altan-Yaycioglu R, Yaycioglu O, Aydin-Akova Y, et al. Ocular side-effects of tolterodine and oxybutynin, a single-blinded prospective randomized trial. Br J Clin Pharmacol 59: 588–592, 2005.

Brown DW, Gilbert GD. Acute glaucoma in patient with peptic ulcer. Am J Ophthalmol 36: 1735–1736, 1953.

Cholst M, Goodstein S, Bernes C. Glaucoma in medical practice, danger of use of systemic antispasmodic drugs in patients predisposed to or having glaucoma. JAMA 166: 1276–1280, 1958.

Grant WM. Toxicology of the Eye, 1st edn, Charles C Thomas, Springfield, p 160, 1962.

Henry DA, Langman MJS. Adverse effects of anti-ulcer drugs. Drugs 21: 444, 1981.

Hufford AR. Bentyl hydrochloride: Successful administration of a parasympatholytic antispasmodic in glaucoma patients. Am J Dig Dis 19: 257–258, 1952.

Leung DL, Kwong YY, Lam DS. Ocular side-effects of tolterodine and oxybutynin, a single-blind prospective randomized trial. Br J Clin Pharmacol 60: 668, 2005.

McHardy G, Brown DC. Clinical appraisal of gastrointestinal antispasmodics. South Med J 45: 1139–1144, 1952.

Mody MV, Keeney AH. Propantheline (Pro-Banthine) bromide in relation to normal and glaucomatous eyes: Effects on intraocular tension and pupillary size. JAMA 159: 113–114, 1955.

Nissen SN, Nielsen PG. Unilateral mydriasis after use of propantheline bromide in an antiperspirant. Lancet 2: 1134, 1977.

Schwartz N, Apt L. Mydriatic effect of anticholinergic drugs used during reversal of nondepolarizing muscle relaxants. Am J Ophthalmol 88: 609, 1979.

Varssano D, Rothman S, Haas K, Lazar M. The mydriatic effect of topical glycopyrrolate. Graefes Arch Clin Exp Ophthalmol 234(3): 205–207, 1996.

CLASS: GASTROINTESTINAL AND URINARY TRACT STIMULANTS

Generic name: Bethanechol chloride.

Proprietary names: Duvoid, Urecholine.

Primary use

This quaternary ammonium parasympathomimetic agent is effective in the management of postoperative abdominal distention and non-obstructive urinary retention.

Ocular side effects

Systemic administration
Certain
1. Non-specific ocular irritation
   a. Lacrimation
   b. Hyperemia
   c. Burning sensation
   d. Pruritus
2. Decreased accommodation
3. Miosis

Clinical significance

Adverse ocular reactions due to bethanechol are unusual, but they may continue long after use of the drug is discontinued. Some advocate use of this agent in the treatment of Riley Day syndrome and ocular pemphigoid because the drug is associated with an increase in lacrimal secretion.

REFERENCES AND FURTHER READING

Crandall DC, Leopold IH. The influence of systemic drugs on tear constituents. Ophthalmology 86: 115, 1979.

McEvoy GK (ed). American Hospital Formulary Service Drug information 87, American Society of Hospital Pharmacists, Bethesda, p 521–523, 1987.

Perritt RA. Eye complications resulting from systemic medications. Ill Med J 117: 423, 1960.

Physicians' Desk Reference, 60th edn, Thomson PDR, Montvale NJ, pp 2349–2350, 2006.

Generic name: Carbachol.

Proprietary names: Carbostat, Miostat.

Primary use

Systemic
This quaternary ammonium parasympathomimetic agent is effective in the management of postoperative intestinal atony and urinary retention.

Ophthalmic
This topical or intraocular agent is used for open-angle glaucoma.

Ocular side effects

Systemic administration
Certain
1. Decreased accommodation

Local ophthalmic use or exposure – topical application
Certain
1. Miosis
2. Decreased vision
3. Decreased intraocular pressure
4. Accommodative spasm
5. Eyelids or conjunctiva
   a. Allergic reactions
   b. Hyperemia
   c. Cojunctivitis – follicular
   d. Pemphigoid-like lesion with symblepharon and shortening of the fornices
6. Irritation
   a. Lacrimation
   b. Ocular pain
7. Blepharoclonus
8. Myopia
9. Retinal detachment
10. Problems with color vision – objects have yellow tinge
11. Cataract formation
12. Myokymia

Local ophthalmic use or exposure – intracameral injection
Certain
1. Miosis
2. Corneal edema
3. Decreased vision
4. Anterior chamber – cells and flare (increased after cataract surgery)

Systemic side effects

Local ophthalmic use or exposure – topical application

Certain
1. Headaches – frontal
2. Ocular or periocular pain
3. Dizziness
4. Vomiting
5. Diarrhea
6. Stomach pain
7. Intestinal cramps
8. Bradycardia
9. Arrhythmia
10. Hypotension
11. Syncope
12. Asthma – may aggravate
13. Salivation increase
14. Perspiration increase
15. Bronchospasm
16. Generalized muscle weakness

Clinical significance
Probably the most frequent ocular side effect due to carbachol is a decrease in vision secondary to miosis or accommodative spasms. In the younger age groups, transient drug-induced myopia also may occur. Follicular conjunctivitis often occurs after long-term therapy, but this in general is of limited clinical significance. Some of the topical ocular side effects may be aggravated or caused by the benzalkonium chloride preservative. Enhancement of cataract formation is probably common to all miotics after many years of exposure. Miotics can induce retinal detachments but probably only in eyes with pre-existing retinal pathology (Beasley and Fraunfelder 1979). This topical ocular medication may be one of the more toxic agents on the corneal epithelium. Roberts (1993) showed increased cells and flare post-cataract surgery due to carbachol by delaying the re-establishment of the blood aqueous barrier after surgery, causing a more prolonged inflammatory process. Phillips et al (1997) suggested that intraocular carbachol post surgery did not play a role in increasing postcapsular opacification.

If there are abrasions of the conjunctiva or corneal epithelium, care must be taken not to apply topical ocular carbachol since this enhances absorption and increases the incidences of systemic side effects. In general, systemic reactions to carbachol are rare, usually occurring only after excessive use of the medication.

REFERENCES AND FURTHER READING

Beasley H, Fraunfelder FT. Retinal detachments and topical ocular miotics. Ophthalmology 86: 95, 1979.

Beasley H, et al. Carbachol in cataract surgery. Arch Ophthalmol 80: 39, 1968.

Crandall DC, Leopold IH. The influence of systemic drugs on tear constituents. Ophthalmology 86: 115, 1979.

Fraunfelder FT. Corneal edema after use of carbachol. Arch Ophthalmol 97: 975, 1979.

Hesse RJ, et al. The effect of carbachol combined with intraoperative viscoelastic substances on postoperative IOP response. Ophthalmic Surg 19: 224, 1988.

Hung PT, Hsieh JW, Chiou GCY. Ocular hypotensive effects of N-demethylated carbachol on open angle glaucoma. Arch Ophthalmol 100: 262, 1982.

Krejci L, Harrison R. Antiglaucoma drug effects on corneal epithelium. A comparative study in tissue culture. Arch Ophthalmol 81: 766, 1970.

Monig H, et al. Kreislaufkollaps durch carbachol-haltige augentropgen. Dtsch Med Wochenschr 114(47): 1860, 1989.

Olson RJ, et al. Commonly used intraocular medications and the corneal endothelium. Arch Ophthalmol 98: 2224–2226, 1980.

Pape LG, Forbes M. Retinal detachment and miotic therapy. Am J Ophthalmol 85: 558, 1978.

Phillips B, Crandall AS, Mamalis N, Olson RJ. Intraoperative miotics and posterior capsular opacification following phacoemulsification with intraocular lens insertion. Ophthalmic Surg Lasers 28(11): 911–914, 1997.

Roberts CW. Intraocular miotics and postoperative inflammation. J Cat Refractive Surg 19(6): 731–734, 1993.

Vaughn ED, Hull DS, Green K. Effect of intraocular miotics on corneal endothelium. Arch Ophthalmol 96: 1897, 1978.

CLASS: AGENTS USED TO TREAT MIGRAINE

Generic names: 1. Ergometrine maleate (ergonovine); 2. ergotamine tartrate; 3. methylergometrine maleate (methylergonovine).

Proprietary names: 1. Ergotrate; 2. Ergomar; 3. Methergine.

Primary use
These ergot alkaloids and derivatives are effective in the management of orthostatic hypertension migraine or other vascular types of headaches and as oxytocic agents.

Ocular side effects

Systemic administration
Certain
1. Decreased vision
2. Miosis (ergotamine)
3. Eyelids or conjunctiva
   a. Allergic reactions
   b. Erythema
   c. Edema

Probable
1. Retinal vascular disorders
   a. Spasms
   b. Constriction
   c. Stasis
   d. Thrombosis
   e. Occlusion
2. Visual fields
   a. Scotomas
   b. Hemianopsia
3. Problems with color vision
   a. Color vision defect, red-green defect
   b. Objects have red tinge
4. Visual hallucinations
5. Decreased dark adaptation

Possible
1. Decreased intraocular pressure – minimal
2. Decreased accommodation
3. Eyelids or conjunctiva – lupoid syndrome

Clinical significance
Ocular side effects due to these ergot alkaloids are rare, but patients on standard therapeutic dosages can develop significant adverse ocular effects. This is probably due to an unusual susceptibility, sensitivity or a pre-existing disease which is exacerbated by the ergot preparations. Increased ocular vascular complications have been seen in patients with a pre-existing occlusive peripheral vascular disease, especially in dosages higher than normal. Crews (1963) reported a healthy 19-year-old in whom a standard therapeutic injection of ergotamine apparently precipitated a central retinal artery occlusion. Gupta and Strobos (1972) reported a bilateral ischemic optic neuritis that may have been due to ergotamine. Merhoff and Porter (1974) reported a case with possible drug-induced central scotoma, retinal vasospasms and retinal pallor. Heider et al (1986) reported the case of a long-term ergot user who developed reversible decreased vision with decreased sensitivity in the central 30° in his visual field. Sommer et al (1998) described a 31-year-old male who developed bilateral ischemic optic neuropathy after administration of ergotamine tartrate and macrolides. Mieler (1997) reported a 19-year-old female who received ergot alkaloids to control postpartum hemorrhage and had a toxic retinal reaction, including bilateral cystoid macular edema, central retinal vein occlusion papilitis and optic disc pallor. Ahmad (1991) described a case of ergometrine given intravenously that unmasked a previously 'cured' myasthenia gravis. According to Creze et al (1976) methylergometrine-induced cerebral vasospasm may have caused transitory cortical blindness. There are sporadic reports of cataracts in the literature, but these are rare and it is difficult to prove a cause-and-effect relationship.

REFERENCES AND FURTHER READING

Ahmad S. Ergonovine: unmasking of myasthenia gravis. Am Heart J 121: 1851, 1991.

Birch J, et al. Acquired color vision defects. In: Congenital and Acquired Color Vision Defects, Pokorny J, et al: (eds), Grune & Stratton, New York, pp 243–350, 1979.

Crews SJ. Toxic effects on the eye and visual apparatus resulting from systemic absorption of recently introduced chemical agents. Trans Ophthalmol Soc UK 82: 387–406, 1963.

Creze B, et al. Transitory cortical blindness after delivery using Methergin. Rev Fr Gynecol Obstet 71: 353, 1976.

Gupta DR, Strobos RJ. Bilateral papillitis associated with Cafergot therapy. Neurology 22: 793, 1972.

Heider W, Berninger T, Brunk G. Electroophthalmological and clinical findings in a case of chronic abuse of ergotamine. Fortschr Ophthalmol 83: 539–541, 1986.

Merhoff GC, Porter JM. Ergot intoxication. Ann Surg 180: 773, 1974.

Mieler WF. Systemic therapeutic agents and retinal toxicity. Am Academy Ophthalmol XV(12): 5, 1997.

Mindel JS, Rubenstein AE, Franklin B. Ocular ergotamine tartrate toxicity during treatment of Vacor-induced orthostatic hypotension. Am J Ophthalmol 92: 492, 1981.

Sommer S, Delemazure B, Wagner M. Bilateral ischemic optic neuropathy secondary to acute ergotism. J Fr Ophthalmol 21(2): 123–125, 1998.

Wollensak J, Grajewski O. Bilateral vascular papillitis following ergotamine medication. Klin Monatsbl Augenheilkd 173: 731, 1978.

CLASS: ANTIANGINAL AGENTS

Generic name: 1. Amyl nitrite; 2. butyl nitrite.

Proprietary names: None.

Street names: Ames, aroma of men, liquid gold, poppers, ram and thrust, rush.

Primary use
1. This short-acting nitrite anti-anginal agent is effective in the treatment of acute attacks of angina pectoris.
2. Smooth muscle relaxant and vasodilator used to enhance orgasms.

Ocular side effects

Inhalation administration
Certain
1. Mydriasis – transitory
2. Decreased vision – transitory

3. Problems with color vision
   a. Objects have yellow tinge
   b. Colored haloes around objects – mainly blue or yellow
4. Intraocular pressure
   a. Initially increased – momentarily
   b. Decreased – transient
5. Color hallucinations
6. Eyelids or conjunctiva – allergic reactions
7. Retinal vasodilatation – transitory

Conditional/Unclassified
1. Optic neuritis

Topical ocular application – inadvertent contact with liquid
Certain
1. Eyelids – erythema
2. Irritation – stinging pain
3. Cornea and conjunctiva
   a. Sloughing of epithelial
   b. Limbal ischemia
   c. Edema

Clinical significance
Ocular side effects due to amyl nitrite are transient, reversible, uncommon and seldom of clinical significance. There is no evidence that these drugs have precipitated angle-closure glaucoma. Becker (1955) attempted to use amyl nitrite as a provocative test for angle-closure glaucoma, but was unsuccessful. Amyl nitrite ordinarily causes a slight rise of <3 mm of mercury for several seconds followed by a fall in intraocular pressure for only 10–20 minutes. This decrease in pressure is felt to be secondary to a fall in blood pressure. Fledelius (1999) reported a case of optic neuritis with irreversible loss of vision after amyl nitrite inhalation. Pece et al (2004) reported possible bilateral decreased vision and small yellowish-white foveal spots with improvement in time after isobutyl nitrite abuse.

These agents are used as recreational drugs and can come into contact with the eye in a liquid form. Mearza et al (2001) showed that anterior injury can be extensive, but heals without complication in time.

REFERENCES AND FURTHER READING

Becker B. In: Symposium on Glaucoma. Transactions of the first conference, Newell FW (ed), Josiah Macy Jr. Foundation, New York, p 32, 1955.
Cristini G, Pagliarani N. Amyl nitrite test in primary glaucoma. Br J Ophthalmol 37: 741, 1953.
Cristini G, Pagliarani N. Slitlamp study of the aqueous veins in simple glaucoma during the amyl nitrite test. Br J Ophthalmol 39: 685, 1955.
Fledelius HC. Irreversible blindness after amyl nitrite inhalation. Acta Ophthalmol Scand 77: 719–721, 1999.
Grant WM. Physiological and pharmacological influences upon intraocular pressure. Pharmacol Rev 7: 143, 1955.
Mearza AA, Asaria RHY, Little B. Corneal burn secondary to amyl nitrite. Eye 15: 333–334, 2001.
Pece A, Patelli F, Milani P, et al. Transient visual loss after amyl isobutyl nitrite abuse. Semin Ophthalmol 19: 105–106, 2004.
Robertson D, Stevens RM. Nitrates and glaucoma. JAMA 237: 117, 1977.

Generic names: 1. Diltiazem hydrochloride; 2. nifedipine; 3. verapamil hydrochloride.

Proprietary names: 1. Cardizem, Cardizem, LA, Cardizem XT, Cartia XT, Dilacor XR, Dilt-CD, Diltzac, Taztia XT, Teczem, Tiazac; 2. Adalat CC, Afeditab CR, Procardia, Procardia XL; 3. Calan, Cover-HS, Isoptin, Isoptin SR, Verelan, Verelan pm.

Primary use
These calcium channel blockers are used in the treatment of vasospastic angina and chronic stable angina.

Ocular side effects

Systemic administration
Certain
1. Decreased vision
2. Eyelids or conjunctiva
   a. Chemosis
   b. Erythema
   c. Conjunctivitis – non-specific
   d. Photosensitivity
   e. Angioneurotic edema
   f. Urticaria
   g. Purpura
   h. Hyperpigmentation
3. Nystagmus – rotary (nifedipine, verapamil)

Probable
1. Periorbital edema
2. Visual hallucinations
3. Eyelids or conjunctiva – lupus erythematosus

Possible
1. Non-specific ocular irritation
   a. Lacrimation
   b. Photophobia (nifedipine)
   c. Ocular pain (nifedipine)
2. Eyelids or conjunctiva
   a. Stevens-Johnson syndrome
   b. Toxic epidermal necrolysis
   c. Erythema multiforme
3. Subconjunctival or retinal hemorrhages secondary to drug-induced anemia

Conditional/Unclassified
1. Blepharospasm
2. Retinal ischemia – transient (nifedipine)

Clinical significance
Ocular side effects are uncommon, reversible and seldom of enough clinical importance to stop the drug. The area of clinical interest is in the management of glaucoma. Intraocular pressure does not appear to be affected by calcium channel blockers, although there are questionable data that glaucoma patients may be more difficult to control on these agents. Nifedipine attenuates the intraocular pressure response to intubation following suxamethonium. Verapamil eyedrops have been shown to decrease episcleral venous pressure and intraocular pressure (Abreu et al 1998). There is increasing evidence that topical ocular beta blockers given to patients who are on calcium channel blockers may, in exceedingly rare cases, result in an arrythmia. This has been suggested in four separate reports by Pringle (1987), Sinclair and Benzie (1983), Staffurth and Emery (1981), Ansatassiades (1980), and in five cases within the National Registry. The proposed mechanism is that each agent acts in a different way to decrease the heart rate so the effects may be additive, causing an arrhythmia. Verapamil has been implicated in worsening myasthenia gravis (Swash and Ingram 1992) because of the drug's inhibition of potassium outflow from cells at the motor end

plate. A reversible reticulated slate-gray hyperpigmentation on sun-exposed skin areas can occur. Pitlik et al (1983) described a case of transient retinal ischemia felt to be associated with nifedipine.

REFERENCES AND FURTHER READING

Abreu MM, Kim YY, Shin DH, Netland PA. Topical verapamil and episcleral venous pressure. Ophthalmology 105(12): 2251–2255, 1998.

Ahmad S. Nifedipine interaction: CNS toxicity due to altered disposition of phenytoin. J Am College Card 3: 1582, 1984.

Anastassiades CJ. Nifedipine and beta blocker drugs. BMJ 281: 1251–1252, 1980.

Beatty JF, et al. Elevation of intraocular pressure by calcium channel blockers. Arch Ophthalmol 102: 1072, 1984.

Coulter DM. Eye pain with nifedipine and taste disturbance with captopril, a mutually controlled study demonstrating a method of post marketing surveillance. BMJ 296: 1086–1088, 1988.

Friedland S, Kaplan S, Lahav M, et al. Proptosis and periorbital edema due to diltiazem treatment. Arch Ophthalmol 111: 1027–1028, 1993.

Gubinelli E, Cocuroccia B, Girolomoni G. Subacute cutaneous lupus erythematosus induced by nifedipine. J Cutan Med Surg 7: 243–246, 2003.

Harris A, Evans DW, Cantor LB, Martin B. Hemodynamic and visual function effects of oral nifedipine in patients with normal-tension glaucoma. Am J Ophthalmol 124(3): 296–302, 1997.

Hockwin O, et al. Evaluation of the ocular safety of verapamil. Scheimpflug photography with densitometric image analysis of lens transparency in patients with hypertrophic cardiomyopathy subjected to long-term therapy with high doses of verapamil. Ophthalmic Res 16: 264, 1984.

Indu B, Batra YK, Puri GD, Singh H. Nifedipine attenuates the intraocular pressure response to intubation following succinylcholine. Can J Anesthes 36: 269–272, 1989.

Kelly SP, Walley TJ. Eye pain with nifedipine. BMJ 296: 1401, 1988.

Kuykendall-Ivy T, Collier SL, Johnson SM. Diltiazem-induced hyperpigmentation. Cutis 73: 239–240, 2004.

Manga P, Vythilingum S. Nifedipine: unstable angina. S Afr Med J 66: 144, 1984.

Opie LH, White DA. Adverse interaction between nifedipine and beta-blockade. BMJ 281: 1462, 1980.

Pitlik S, et al. Transient retinal ischaemia induced by nifedipine. BMJ 287: 1845, 1983.

Pringle SD, MacEwen CJ. Severe bradycardia due to interaction of timolol eye drops and verapamil. BMJ 294: 155–156, 1987.

Rainer G, Kiss B, Dallinger S, et al. A double masked placebo controlled study on the effect of nifedipine on optic nerve blood flow and visual field function in patients with open angle glaucoma. Br J Clin Pharmacol 52: 210–212, 2001.

Scherschun L, Lee MW, Lim HW. Diltiazem-associated photodistributed hyperpigmentation: a review of 4 cases. Arch Dermatol 137: 179–182, 2001.

Silverstone PH. Periorbital edema caused by nifedipine. BMJ 288: 1654, 1984.

Sinclair NI, Benzie JL. Timolol eye drops and verapamil – a dangerous combination. Med J Aust 1: 549, 1983.

Staffurth JS, Emery P. Adverse interaction between nifedipine and beta-blockade. BMJ 282: 225, 1981.

Swash M, Ingram DA. Adverse effect of verampil in myasthenia gravis. Muscle Nerve 15: 396–398, 1992.

Tordjman K, Itosenthal T, Bursztyn M. Nifedipine-induced periorbital edema. Am J Cardiol 55: 1445, 1985.

Generic names: 1. Flecainide acetate; 2. procainamide.

Proprietary names: 1. Tambocor; 2. Procanbid, Pronestyl, Pronestyl SR.

Primary use

These primary amine analogs of lidocaine are used in the treatment of resistant ventricular arrhythmia.

Ocular side effects

Systemic administration
Certain
1. Decreased vision (flecainide)

2. Various visual sensations (flecainide)
   a. 'Spots before eyes'
   b. Peripheral bright or flashing lights
   c. Photophobia
   d. Ocular pain
3. Rectus muscle (flecainide)
   a. Spasms
   b. Pain
   c. Diplopia
4. Corneal deposits (flecainide)
5. Nystagmus (flecainide)
6. Visual hallucinations (flecainide)
7. Eyelids or conjunctiva
   a. Erythema
   b. Angioneurotic edema
   c. Urticaria (flecainide)
   d. Loss of eyelashes or eyebrows
   e. Irritation
   f. Photosensitivity (procainamide)

Possible
1. Subconjunctival or retinal hemorrhages secondary to drug-induced anemia
2. Myasthenia gravis (procainamide)
   a. Diplopia
   b. Ptosis
   c. Paresis of extraocular muscles
3. Eyelids or conjunctiva
   a. Lupoid syndrome
   b. Exfoliative dermatitis (flecainide)
   c. Stevens-Johnson syndrome
   d. Lupus erythematosus

Conditional/Unclassified
1. Scleritis

Clinical significance

There is little data on ocular side effects from this class of drugs other than with flecainide. Gentzkow and Sullivan (1984) as well as others have stated that the most common side effects of flecainide are visual disturbances, with blurred vision occurring in about 30% of patients. Ikäheimo et al (2001) found that blurred vision occurred in 10.5% of patients in their series. This was only in lateral gaze, and lasted only for a few seconds. Decreased accommodation with non-specific visual symptoms such as 'spots before eye', peripheral bright lights and photophobia also occur. Well-documented cases of intermittent diplopia, rectus muscle spasms, decreased depth perception and nystagmus are in the literature and the National Registry. These can be dose dependent and resolve at lower dosages. Skander and Issacs (1985) reported painful lateral rectus muscle spasms. Moller et al (1991) reported two patients on flecainide who developed superficial gray whorl corneal deposits. Ikäheimo et al (2001) found brownish epithelial deposits in a thin horizontal linear pattern in the inferior cornea. This occurred in 14.5% of their patients, but did not appear to be dose or time related. High-pressure liquid chromatography suggested these are due to flecainide and peptide corneal depostion. Stopping the drug resulted in corneal clearing over a 3-month period. All ocular signs and symptoms are reversible either at decreased dosages or when the drug is discontinued.

Turgeon and Slamovits (1989) described a case of procainamide-induced lupus, which presented first with scleritis.

REFERENCES AND FURTHER READING

Cetnarowski AB, Rihn TL. Adverse reactions to tocainide and mexiletine. Cardiovasc Rev Reports 6: 1335, 1985.

Clarke CWF, el-Mahdi EO. Confusion and paranoia associated with oral tocainide. Postgrad Med J 61: 79, 1985.

Gentzkow GD, Sullivan JY. Extracardiac adverse effects of flecainide. Am J Cardiol 53: 101B, 1984.

Hopson JR, Buxton AE, Rinkenberger RL, et al. Safety and utility of flecainide acetate in the routine care of patients with supraventricular tachyarrhythmias: results of a multicenter trial. The Flecainide Supraventricular Tachycardia Study Group. Am J Card 77(3): 72A–82A, 1996.

Ikäheimo K, Kettunen R, Mäntyjärvi M. Adverse ocular effects of flecainide. Acta Ophthalmol Scand 79: 175–156, 2001.

Kaeser HE. Drug-induced myasthenic syndromes. Acta Neurol Scand 70: 39–47, 1984.

Keefe DLD, Kates RE, Harrison DC. New antiarrhythmic drugs: their place in therapy. Drugs 22: 363, 1981.

Moller HU, Thygesen K, Kruit PJ. Corneal deposits associated with flecainide. BMJ 302: 506–507, 1991.

Ramhamadany E, et al. Dysarthria and visual hallucinations due to flecainide toxicity. Postgrad Med J 62: 61, 1986.

Skander M, Issacs PET. Flecainide, ocular myopathy, and antinuclear factor. BMJ 291: 450, 1985.

Smith AG. Drug-induced photosensitivity. Adverse Drug React Bull 136: 508–511, 1989.

Turgeon PW, Slamovits TL. Scleritis as the presenting manifestation of procainamide-induced lupus. Ophthalmology 96: 68–71, 1989.

Vincent FM, Vincent T. Tocainide encephalopathy. Neurology 35: 1804, 1985.

with transient visual loss followed by a severe headache. Visual hallucinations have also been reported. This drug has been implicated in cases of intracranial hypertension. Inadvertent ocular exposure to nitroglycerin-containing pastes has caused conjunctival injection, pupil dilatation and eyelid reactions.

REFERENCES AND FURTHER READING

Afridi S, Kaube H, Goadsby PJ. Occipital activation in glyceryl trinitrate induced migraine with visual aura. J Neurol Neurosurg Psychiatry 76: 1158–1160, 2005.

Bánk J. Migraine with aura after administration of sublingual nitroglycerin tablets. Headache 41: 84–87, 2001.

McKenna KE. Allergic contact dermatitis from glyceryl trinitrate ointment. Contact Derm 42: 246, 2000.

Ohar JM, et al. Intravenous nitroglycerin-induced intracranial hypertension. Crit Care Med 13: 867, 1985.

Physicians' Desk Reference, 60th edn, Thomson PDR, Montvale NJ, pp 1161-1162, 1824, 3060–3062, 2006.

Purvin V, Dunn D. Nitrate-induced transient ischemic attacks. South Med J 74: 1130, 1981.

Robertson D, Stevens RM. Nitrates and glaucoma. JAMA 237: 117, 1977.

Shorey J, Bhardwaj N, Loscalzo J. Acute Wernicke's encephalopathy after intravenous infusion of high-dose nitroglycerin. Ann Intern Med 101: 500, 1984.

Sveska K. Nitrates may not be contraindicated in patients with glaucoma. Drug Intell Clin Pharm 19: 361, 1985.

Wizemann AJS, Wizemann V. Organic nitrate therapy in glaucoma. Am J Ophthalmol 90: 106, 1980.

Generic name: Nitroglycerin.

Proprietary names: Minitran, Nitro-dur, Nitrolingual, Nitropress, Nitrostat.

Primary use

This short-acting trinitrate vasodilator is effective in the treatment of acute attacks of angina pectoris.

Ocular side effects

Systemic administration
Certain
1. Vasodilatation – transitory
   a. Conjunctiva
   b. Retina
2. Visual hallucinations

Probable
1. Decreased vision – transitory
2. Problems with color vision – colored haloes around lights, mainly yellow or blue
3. Eyelids – allergic reactions
4. Papilledema secondary to intracranial hypertension
5. Precipitated visual auras

Possible
1. Eyelids – exfoliative dermatitis

Clinical significance

Oral nitroglycerin appears to have few to no significant ocular side effects. The Physicians' Desk Reference states that on rare occasions sublinguinal nitroglycerin can cause transient blurring of vision. Bánk (2001) and Afridi et al (2005) described cases where nitroglycerin-induced migraines start with a visual aura. Employees manufacturing this agent have reported acute intoxication

CLASS: ANTIARRYTHMIC AGENTS

Generic name: Amiodarone.

Proprietary names: Cordarone, Pacerone.

Primary use

This benzofuran derivative is effective in the treatment of various arrhythmias.

Ocular side effects

Systemic administration
Certain
1. Visual changes
   a. Photophobia
   b. Blurred vision
   c. Glare
   d. Halos around light – most prominent at night
2. Cornea
   a. Golden-brown superficial punctate deposits (Fig. 7.6a)
   b. Epithelial erosion
   c. Decreased sensation
3. Eyelids or conjunctiva
   a. Yellow-brown or gray deposits
   b. Blepharoconjunctivitis
   c. Photosensitivity reactions
   d. Keratoconjunctivitis
4. Keratitis
5. Lens
   a. Anterior subcapsular small yellow-white punctuate opacities
   b. Cortical changes
   c. Intraocular lenses – brown discoloration
6. Drug found in the tears

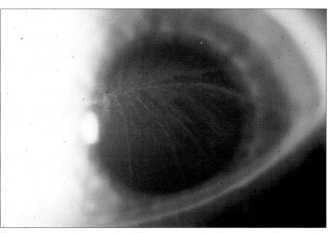

Fig. 7.6a Amiodarone whorl-like pattern of golden brown deposits in the anterior cornea.

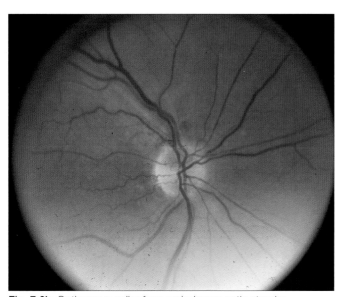

Fig. 7.6b Optic nerve pallor from amiodarone optic atrophy.

Probable

1. Loss of eyelashes or eyebrows
2. Thyroid eye disease
   a. Hypothyroid ocular signs
   b. Hyperthyroid ocular signs
3. Papilledema secondary to intracranial hypertension
4. Autoimmune reaction
   a. Dry mouth
   b. Dry eyes
   c. Peripheral neuropathy
   d. Pneumonitis

Possible

1. Optic neuropathy
   a. Visual loss
   b. Disc edema
   c. Disc hemorrhage
   d. Optic nerve pallor (Fig. 7.6b)
   e. Visual field defects

Clinical significance

Amiodarone was first introduced in the 1960s and its most frequent drug-induced side effects are ocular. These side effects, especially in the anterior segment, are dose and time dependent.

Corneal microdeposits due to aminodarone occur in all patients who are using the drug long term. The corneal epithelial whirl-like drug-related deposition is indistinguishable from that due to quinacrine, indomethacin, chlorpromazine, etc. The keratopathy may reach a steady state with no progression even with continued drug use. The usual pattern for corneal deposition (Klingele et al 1984) initially, in stage 1, is a horizontal, irregular, branching line near the junction of the mid and outer one-third of the cornea. In stage 2, this increases so that there are 6 to 10 branches, with an increase in length and curve superiorly. Any increase in the number of branches constitutes stage 3. Stage 4 is the whirl-like pattern with clumping deposits. The deposits may be seen as early as 2 weeks after starting the drug, but in general the visible keratopathy develops in most patients within 6 weeks after initiation of amiodarone therapy and reaches its peak within 3–6 months. Patients taking 100–200 mg/day have only minimal or even no visible corneal deposits. At dosages of 400 mg or more almost all patients will show corneal deposits. Once the drug is stopped most deposits completely regress in 3–7 months, but this may take up to 2 years. In patients using soft contact lenses, the keratopathy is significantly less. Visual changes due to these deposits are uncommon, but on occasion are severe enough to stop the drug. Patient complaints consist of photophobia, hazy vision or colored haloes around lights. Occasionally, a patient may complain that bright lights, especially headlights at night, will cause a significant glare problem. Keratitis sicca has been reported since the drug is secreted in tears, which may aggravate borderline sicca cases or enhance the evaporative form of sicca. A probable autoimmune reaction can occur, which is associated with dry mouth, dry eyes, peripheral neuropathy and pneumonitis. Slate-gray periocular skin pigmentation or blue skin discoloration has been seen secondary to photosensitivity reactions. Corneal ulcerations can rarely occur during treatment with amiodarone. Flach and Dolan (1990) first described subtle anterior subcapsular lens opacities in patients taking amiodarone long term. These changes primarily occur in the pupillary area and are yellow-white, loosely packed deposits that rarely interfere with vision. The location of the deposits suggests a photosensitizing effect of amiodarone on the lens. Cumming and Mitchell (1998) reported increased cortical cataracts.

Does amiodarone cause optic neuropathy? It is not known if this is simply a variant of non-arteritic ischemic optic neuropathy (NAION), in which swelling of the disc is prolonged, or if amiodarone is an independent risk factor of NAION. Regardless, from a practical point of view one may need to practice defensive medicine since the legal system has determined a relationship between amiodarone and NAION in a number of cases. Scientific data (along the guidelines of Murphy and Murphy 2005) are necessary to determine if a relationship exists or not. However, some feel amiodarone optic neuropathy is possibly characterized by an insidious onset, slower progression, which often has bilateral visual loss and protracted disc swelling. NAION may be characterized as an acute, unilateral visual loss that is usually complete at onset with resolution of disc edema over several weeks. Optic nerve swelling and peripapillary nerve fiber layer hemorrhages tend to persist for several months in amiodarone-induced optic neuropathy, while in NAION these usually resolve more quickly. After discontinuation of amiodarone, visual acuity and visual field defects tend to stabilize. Purvin et al (2006) have recently recommended (Table 7-6a) a systemic approach with well-defined diagnostic criteria to help the clinician manage these patients. Fraunfelder and Fraunfelder (2007) predict that, in time, the association of this drug causing a neuropathy will be 'probable'. Although the mechanism of amiodarone optic neuropathy, or even if it occurs,

Table 7-6a – Management of patients taking amiodarone (Purvin et al).

	Disc Edema	Management
Group I	Simultaneous and bilateral Further tests to rule out increased intracranial pressure giant cell arteritis	If other tests are negative, strongly consider discontinuation of amiodarone
Group II	Unilateral atypical NAION Insidious onset of symptoms, relatively mild optic nerve dysfunction, generous cup to disc ratio in fellow eye, prolonged disc edema	Strongly consider discontinuation of amiodarone
Group III	Unilateral typical NAION Immediate onset of disc edema, crowded contralateral disc, moderate to substantial defects of optic nerve dysfunction, no systemic symptoms of amiodarone	Continuation of amiodarone may be appropriate

is unknown, ultrastructural changes in the human optic nerve illustrate a primary lipidosis. Selective accumulation of intracytoplasmic lamellar inclusions in large optic nerve axons may mechanically or biochemically decrease axoplasmic flows. Resultant optic nerve head edema may persist as long as transport is inhibited (perhaps as long as several months following discontinuation of amiodarone, which has a half-life of up to100 days).

There is no documented evidence that this drug causes human retinal damage, although intracytoplasmic granulations have been found in the retinal pigment epithelium and choroid as well as the ciliary body, iris, cornea, conjunctiva and lens. This drug is a photosensitizing agent and in selected cases sunglasses that block UV rays from the sunlight to 400 nm may be considered for eyelid and lens changes.

Recommendations

1. Baseline ophthalmic examination before or shortly after starting amiodarone.
2. If any visual disturbances occur while on the drug, the patient should see an ophthalmologist.
3. If there is any suggestion of an optic neuropathy, discuss with the patient and their physician of the possibility of using alternative medication or obtain an informed consent as to the possible ocular side effects if amiodarone therapy is continued.
4. Carry out ophthalmic examinations on an annual basis.
5. In patients having photosensitizing side effects, consider UV-blocking lenses.
6. In children it is especially important to get informed consent and stress to the parent the difficulty in getting accurate vision and visual fields, which may delay diagnosis and limit the ability to follow progression accurately. In young children the inability to do these tests may require regular 3-month optic disc examinations.

REFERENCES AND FURTHER READING

Banerjee S, James CB. Amiodarone and dysthyroid eye disease (letter). Br J Ophthalmol 80: 851–852, 1996.

Cumming RG, Mitchell P. Medications and cataract – the Blue Mountain Eye Study. Ophthalmology 105: 1751–1757, 1998.

Dickerson EJ, Wolman RL. Sicca syndrome associated with amiodarone therapy. BMJ 293: 510, 1986.

Farwell AP, Abend SL, Huang SKS, et al. Thyroidectomy for amiodarone induced thyrotoxicosis. JAMA 263: 1526–1528, 1990.

Fikkers BG, et al. Pseudotumor cerebri with amiodarone. J Neurol Neurosurg Psychiatry 49: 606, 1986.

Flach AJ, Dolan BJ. Amiodarone-induced lens opacities: an 8-year follow-up study. Arch Ophthalmol 108: 1668–1669, 1990.

Fraunfelder FW, Fraunfelder FT. Scientific challenges in postmarketing surveillance of ocular adverse drug reactions. Am J Ophthalmol 143: 145–149, 2007.

Hawthorne GC, Campbell NPS, Geddes JS, et al. Amiodarone-induced hypothyroidism. A common complication of prolonged therapy: a report of eight cases. Arch Intern Med 145: 1016–1019, 1985.

Kaplan LJ, Cappaert WE. Amiodarone keratopathy. Correlation to dosage and duration. Arch Ophthalmol 100: 601, 1982.

Katai N, Yokoyama R, Yoshimura N. Progressive brown discoloration of silicone intraocular lenses after vitrectomy in a patient on amiodarone. J Cat Refract Surg 25: 451–452, 1999.

Klingele TG, Alves LE, Rose EP. Amiodarone keratopathy. Ann Ophthalmol 16: 1172–1176, 1984.

Lopez AC, et al. Acute intracranial hypertension during amiodarone infusion. Crit Care Med 13: 688, 1985.

Macaluso DC, Shults WT, Fraunfelder FT. Features of amiodarone optic neuropathy. Am J Ophthalmol 127: 610–613, 1999.

Mantyjarvi M, Tuppurainen K, Ikaheimo K. Ocular side effects of amiodarone. Surv Ophthalmol 42: 360–366, 1998.

Mindel JM. Amiodarone and optic neuropathy – a medicolegal issue (editorial). Surv Ophthalmol 42: 358–359, 1998.

Murphy MA, Murphy JF. Amiodarone and optic neuropathy: the heart of the matter. J Neuroophthalmol 25(3): 232–236, 2005.

Nagra PK, Forozoan R, Savino PJ, Castillo I, Sergott RC. Amiodarone induced optic neuropathy. Br J Ophthalmol 87: 420–422, 2003.

Orlando RG, Dangel ME, Schaal SF. Clinical experience and grading of amiodarone keratopathy. Ophthalmology 91: 1184, 1984.

Purvin V, Kawasaki A, Borruat F-X. Optic neuropathy in patients using amiodarone. Arch Ophthalmol 124: 696–701, 2006.

Roberts JE, Reme CE, Dillon J, Terman M. Exposure to bright light and the concurrent use of photosensitizing drugs. New Engl J Med 326(22): 1500–1502, 1992.

Ya mur M, Okan O, Ersöz, et al. Confocal microscopic features of amiodarone keratopathy. J Toxicol Cut Ocul Toxicol 22: 243–253, 2003.

Generic name: Disopyramide.

Proprietary names: Norpace, Norpace CR.

Primary use

This anticholinergic agent is indicated for suppression and prevention of recurrence of cardiac arrhythmias.

Ocular side effects

Systemic administration
Certain

1. Decreased vision

2. Eyelids or conjunctiva
   a. Erythema
   b. Conjunctivitis – non-specific
   c. Photosensitivity
3. Mydriasis – may precipitate angle-closure glaucoma
4. Decreased accommodation

Probable
1. Decreased lacrimation
2. Visual hallucinations

Conditional/Unclassified
1. Diplopia
2. Blepharospasm

Clinical significance

The anticholinergic effects of disopyramide can cause blurred vision and fluctuation of visual acuity, by up to 28% in one series. Since this drug can cause mydriasis there are cases in the literature and the National Registry of narrow-angle glaucoma occurring shortly after or up to 3 weeks after the patient started taking the medication. Nine cases of diplopia, two cases of paralysis of extraocular muscles and two cases of blepharospasms have also been reported to the National Registry. Some of these patients were also on other cardiac drugs, and some had other illnesses, which clouded a cause-and-effect relationship.

REFERENCES AND FURTHER READING

Ahmad S. Disopyramide: pulmonary complications and glaucoma. Mayo Clin Proc 65: 1030–1031, 1990.
Frucht J, Freimann I, Merin S. Ocular side effects of disopyramide. Br J Ophthalmol 68: 890, 1984.
Keefe DLD, Kates RE, Harrison DC. New antiarrhythmic drugs: their place in therapy. Drugs 22: 363, 1981.
Schwartz JB, Keefe D, Harrison DC. Adverse effects of antiarrhythmic drugs. Drugs 21: 23, 1981.
Trope GE, Hind VMD. Closed-angle glaucoma in patients on disopyramide. Lancet 1: 329, 1978.
Wayne K, Manolas E, Sloman G. Fatal overdose with disopyramide. Med J Aust 1: 231, 1980.

Generic name: Methacholine chloride.

Proprietary name: Provocholine.

Primary use

Systemic

This quaternary ammonium parasympathomimetic agent is primarily used in the management of paroxysmal tachycardia, Raynaud's syndrome and scleroderma.

Ophthalmic

This topical agent is used in the management of angle-closure glaucoma and in the diagnosis of Adie's pupil.

Ocular side effects

Systemic administration
Certain
1. Decreased accommodation
2. Lacrimation

Local ophthalmic use or exposure
Certain
1. Pupils
   a. No effect – normal pupil
   b. Miosis – Adie's pupil
2. Decreased intraocular pressure
3. Eyelids or conjunctiva
   a. Allergic reactions
   b. Hyperemia
4. Myopia
5. Blepharoclonus
6. Lacrimation

Systemic side effects

Local ophthalmic use or exposure – retrobulbar injection
Certain
1. Nausea
2. Vomiting
3. Heart block
4. Incontinence
5. Cardiac arrest

Clinical significance

Topical ocular application of methacholine causes a number of ocular side effects, but all are reversible and have minimal clinical importance. While miosis normally occurs with topical ocular 10% methacholine solutions, no effect is seen with 2.5% solutions, except in patients with Adie's pupil or familial dysautonomia.

REFERENCES AND FURTHER READING

Crandall DC, Leopold IH. The influence of systemic drugs on tear constituents. Ophthalmology 86: 115, 1979.
Ellis PP. Ocular Therapeutics and Pharmacology, 6th edn, Mosby, St Louis, p 57, 1981.
Gilman AG, Goodman LS, Gilman A (eds). The Pharmacological Basis of Therapeutics, 6th edn, Macmillan, New York, pp 91–96, 1980.
Havener WH. Ocular Pharmacology, 5th edn, Mosby, St Louis, 316–317, 1983.
Leopold IH. The use and side effects of cholinergic agents in the management of intraocular pressure. In: Glaucoma: Applied Pharmacology in Medical Treatment. Drance SM, Neufeld AH (eds), Grune & Stratton, New York, p 357–393, 1984.
Spaeth GL. The effect of autonomic agents on the pupil and the intraocular pressure of eyes treated with dexamethasone. Br J Ophthalmol 64: 426, 1980.
Sweetman SC (ed). Martindale: The Complete Drug Reference. 34th edn, Pharmaceutical Press, London, p 1492–1494, 2004.

Generic name: 1. Oxprenolol hydrochloride; 2. propranolol hydrochloride.

Proprietary names: 1. Kerpin; 2. Innopran XL, Inderal, Inderal LA.

Primary use

These beta-adrenergic blocking agents are effective in the management of angina pectoris, certain arrhythmias, hypertrophic subaortic stenosis, pheochromocytoma and certain hypertensive states.

Ocular side effects

Systemic administration
Certain
1. Decreased vision
2. Diplopia – transient

3. Visual hallucinations
4. Eyelids or conjunctivitis
    a. Allergic reactions
    b. Erythema
    c. Conjunctivitis – non-specific
    d. Urticaria
    e. Purpura
    f. Pemphigoid lesion
    g. Keratoconjunctivitis sicca
5. Non-specific ocular irritation
    a. Lacrimation
    b. Photophobia
    c. Ocular pain

Probable
1. Decreased intraocular pressure
2. Decreased lacrimation
3. Myasthenia gravis
    a. Diplopia
    b. Ptosis
    c. Paresis of extraocular muscles

Possible
1. Decreased accommodation
2. Exophthalmos – withdrawal states
3. Eyelids or conjunctiva
    a. Lupoid syndrome
    b. Erythema multiforme
    c. Stevens-Johnson syndrome
    d. Exfoliative dermatitis

Conditional/Unclassified
1. Intracranial hypertension

Local ophthalmic use or exposure
Certain
1. Local anesthetic effect (propranolol)
2. Irritation
    a. Hyperemia
    b. Ocular pain
    c. Burning sensation
3. Decreased intraocular pressure
4. Miosis

Clinical significance

Adverse ocular side effects due to these agents are usually insignificant and transient. Dennis et al (1991) reviewed a series of patients with side effects from oral beta blockers. The visual side effect 'changes in vision' was the fifth most common of all systemic complaints. As with all beta-adrenergic blocking agents, one needs to be aware of the possibility of sicca-like syndrome. There are many cases in the literature and in the National Registry to implicate these drugs in causing a keratoconjunctivitis sicca-like syndrome, probably on the basis of decreased lacrimation. This often appears as a sudden onset of ocular sicca with conjunctival hyperemia shortly after starting the drug. In the National Registry's experience, one of the most bothersome side effects is transient diplopia with an unknown cause. This may resolve even if these drugs are continued. Yeomans et al (1983) described a case where propanolol may have caused an inflammatory lymphoid process of the iris and ciliary body, which resolved without treatment when propranolol was discontinued. While propranol is structurally similar to practolol, to date there has been no oculocutaneous

syndrome associated with this agent. Topical ocular use of these agents has little clinical application, although it has been advocated for thyrotoxic lid retraction and glaucoma therapy. Propranolol given topically on the eye has a local anesthetic effect.

REFERENCES AND FURTHER READING

Almog Y, et al. The effect of oral treatment with beta blockers on the tear secretion. Metab Pediatr Syst Ophthalmol 6: 343, 1982.
Dennis KE, Froman D, Morrison AS, et al. Beta blocker therapy: identification and management of side effects. Heart & Lung 20(5 Pt 1): 459–463, 1991.
Dollery CT, et al. Eye symptoms in patients taking propranolol and other hypotensive agents. Br J Clin Pharmacol 4: 295, 1977.
Draeger J, Winter R. Corneal sensitivity and intraocular pressure. In: Glaucoma Update II, Krieglstein GK, Leydhecker W (eds), Springer-Verlag, New York, pp 63–67, 1983.
Felminger R. Visual hallucinations and illusions with propranolol. BMJ 1: 1182, 1978.
Holt PJA, Waddington E. Oculocutaneous reaction to oxprenolol. BMJ 2: 539, 1975.
Kaeser HE. Drug-induced myasthenic syndromes. Acta Neurol Scand 70(suppl. 100): 39, 1984.
Knapp MS, Galloway NR. Ocular reactions to beta blockers. BMJ 2: 557, 1975.
Lewis BS, Setzen M, Kokoris N. Ocular reaction to oxprenolol. A case report. S Afr Med J 50: 482, 1976.
Malm L. Propranolol as cause of watery nasal secretion. Lancet 1: 1006, 1981.
Ohrstrom A, Pandolli M. Regulation of intraocular pressure and pupil size by β-blockers and epinephrine. Arch Ophthalmol 98: 2182, 1980.
Pecori-Giraldi J, et al. Topical propranolol in glaucoma therapy and investigations on the mechanism of action. Glaucoma 6: 31, 1984.
Singer L, Knobel B, Itomem M. Influence of systemic administered beta blockers on tear secretion. Ann Ophthalmol 16: 728, 1984.
Weber JCP. Beta-adrenoreceptor antagonists and diplopia. Lancet 2: 826–827, 1982.
Yeomans SM, et al. Ocular inflammatory pseudotumor associated with propranolol therapy. Ophthalmology 90: 1422, 1983.

Generic name: Quinidine.

Proprietary names: Generic only.

Primary use
This isomer of quinine is effective in the treatment and prevention of atrial, nodal and ventricular arrhythmias.

Ocular side effects

Systemic administration
Certain
1. Decreased vision

Probable
1. Problems with color vision – color vision defect, red-green defect
2. Eyelids or conjunctiva
    a. Allergic reactions
    b. Hyperpigmentation
    c. Photosensitivity
    d. Angioneurotic edema
    e. Urticaria
3. Anterior granulomatous uveitis
4. Visual hallucinations

Possible

1. Keratoconjunctivitis sicca
2. Myasthenia gravis
   a. Diplopia
   b. Ptosis
   c. Paresis of extraocular muscles
3. Corneal deposits
4. Eyelids or conjunctiva
   a. Lupoid syndrome
   b. Exfoliative dermatitis
5. Subconjunctival or retinal hemorrhages secondary to drug-induced anemia

Clinical significance

Ocular side effects possibly associated with quinidine are rare and many are not well proven. While blurred vision has been reported in the literature and in the National Registry, this is seldom a significant problem and is reversible. There have been no reports of permanent blindness with quinidine. There are reports of optic neuritis, constricted visual fields, mydriasis, scotomas, night blindness, keratitis sicca, photophobia and toxic amblyopia, but a cause-and-effect relationship has not been proven. Zaidman (1984) reported fine gray epithelial opacities in a whorl-type pattern resembling those of chloroquine in a patient on quinidine for 2 years. These disappeared 2 months after stopping the drug. There are no reports in the National Registry. We are aware of nine cases of uveitis associated with this agent. This is probably an allergic or type I or II hypersensitivity reaction characterized by keratic precipitates, flare and cells in the anterior chamber. Koeppe nodules and elevation of intraocular pressure have been reported. Five of the nine cases were bilateral. While there are no rechallenge data, patients improved rapidly with treatment when the drug was discontinued. Recently, well-documented data from Edeki et al (1995) show that this agent blocks the action of cytochrome P_{450} enzyme CYPZD6 which metabolizes timolol. Higher plasma levels of this beta blocker have therefore occurred. Higginbotham (1996) has reviewed this in an ophthalmic editorial.

REFERENCES AND FURTHER READING

Birch J, et al. Acquired color vision defects. In: Congenital and Acquired Color Vision Defects, Pokorny J, et al. (ed), Grune & Stratton, New York, p 243–350, 1979.

Caraco Y, Arnon R, Raveh D, et al. Quinidine-induced uveitis. Isr J Med Sci 28: 741–743, 1992.

Edeki TI, He H, Wood AJJ. Pharmacogenetic explanation for excessive β-blockade following timolol eye drops: potential for oral-ophthalmic drug interaction. JAMA 27: 1611–1613, 1995.

Fisher CM. Visual disturbances associated with quinidine and quinine. Neurology 31: 1569, 1981.

Fraunfelder FW, Rosenbaum JT. Drug-induced uveitis. Drug Safety 1(3): 197–207, 1997.

Higginbotham EJ. Topical β-adrenergic antagonists and quinidine. Arch Ophthalmol 114: 745–746, 1996.

Hording M, Feldt-Rasmussen UF. Acute iridocyclitis with fever and liver involvement during quinidine therapy. Ugeskrift for Laeger 153(34): 2362–2363, 1991.

Hustead JD. Granulomatous uveitis and quinidine hypersensitivity. Am J Ophthalmol 112(4): 461–462, 1991.

Kaeser HE. Drug-induced myasthenic syndromes. Acta Neurol Scand 70(Suppl. 100): 39, 1984.

Mahler R, Sissons W, Watters K. Pigmentation induced by quinidine therapy. Arch Dermatol 122: 1062, 1986.

Naschitz JE, Yeshurun D. Quinidine induced sicca syndrome. J Toxicol Clin Toxicol 20: 367, 1983.

Spitzberg DH. Acute anterior uveitis secondary to quinidine sensitivity. Arch Ophthalmol 97: 1993, 1979.

Wittbrodt ET. Drugs and myasthenia gravis: an update. Arch Intern Med 157: 399–408, 1997.

Zaidman GW. Quinidine keratopathy. Am J Ophthalmol 97: 247, 1984.

CLASS: ANTIHYPERTENSIVE AGENTS

Generic names: 1. Acebutolol; 2. atenolol; 3. carvedilol; 4. labetolol hydrochloride; 5. metoprolol; 6. nadolol; 7. pindolol.

Proprietary names: 1. Sectral; 2. Tenormin; 3. Coreg; 4. Trandate; 5. Toprol-XL, Lopressor; 6. Corgard; 7. Visken.

Primary use

Systemic

These adrenergic blockers are used in the management of mild to severe hypertension, myocardial infarction and chronic stable angina pectoris.

Ophthalmic

These adrenergic blockers are used in the treatment of elevated intraocular pressure.

Ocular side effects

Systemic administration
Certain

1. Decreased vision
2. Visual hallucinations
3. Non-specific ocular irritation (labetalol, metoprolol)
   a. Photophobia
   b. Ocular pain

Probable

1. Eyelids or conjunctiva
   a. Hyperemia (metoprolol)
   b. Erythema
   c. Blepharoconjunctivitis (metoprolol)
   d. Urticaria (labetolol, metoprolol)
   e. Purpura (metoprolol)
   g. Eczema (metoprolol)
   h. Exacerbation psoriasis
2. Keratoconjunctivitis sicca

Possible

1. Decreased intraocular pressure
2. Myasthenia gravis
   a. Diplopia
   b. Ptosis
   c. Paresis of extraocular muscles
3. Subconjunctival or retinal hemorrhages secondary to drug-induced anemia
4. Enhances migraine scotoma
5. Eyelids or conjunctiva – lupoid syndrome (acebutolol, labetolol)

Local ophthalmic use or exposure
Certain

1. Decreased intraocular pressure
2. Irritation
   a. Lacrimation
   b. Burning sensation
3. Keratitis
4. Local anesthetic effect
5. Keratoconjunctivitis sicca
6. Blepharoconjunctivitis (nadolol)

Systemic side effects

Local ophthalmic use or exposure
Possible
1. Bradycardia
2. Hypotension

Clinical significance

Not all of the above listed ocular side effects have been associated with each of the beta blockers, but each drug has been associated with an ocular side effect. All appear to cause transitory minor visual disturbances, probably decrease tear production and possibly enhance migraine ocular scotoma. If a muscle imbalance or diplopia occurs, then an evaluation for myasthenia gravis may be necessary. These drugs can cause vivid visual hallucinations that are dosage dependent and may disappear at lower dosages. When these drugs are given systemically, rarely do they cause a lowering of intraocular pressure and if they do it is usually only minimal.

Topically applied medication may cause sicca symptoms, decreased tear film break-up times, corneal anesthesia and ocular irritation. Systemic side effects from these topical ophthalmic beta blockers appear to be minimal; measurements of plasma concentrations of these ocularly applied drugs were below those levels known to induce systemic beta-blockade. Regardless, one must be aware that some of these agents have been associated with systemic beta-blocker side effects after topical ocular application.

Ocular side effects

Systemic administration
Certain
1. Floppy iris syndrome (tamsulosin)
2. Amblyopia
3. Blurred vision

Clinical significance

Intraoperative floppy iris syndrome (IFIS) associated with tamsulosin was first reported by Chang and Campbell in 2005. They suggest that IFIS diagnosis should be based on three intraoperative findings: fluttering and billowing of the flaccid iris stroma, a propensity for iris prolapse, and progressive constriction of the pupil during surgery. Additional characteristics also include poor preoperative pupil dilation and elasticity of the pupil margin.

It is hypothesized that the alpha-1A blocking effect of tamsulosin is not purely selective for the prostate as it may also selectively block the receptors in the iris dilator muscle. Tamsulosin has a relatively long half-life, and it is possible that long-term receptor blockade could result in a type of disuse atrophy of the iris dilator smooth muscle. This may explain why some patients have permanent IFIS, even after the medication is discontinued.

Boehringer Ingelheim (2005) has subsequently changed the labeling on tamsulosin to reflect the possibility of IFIS in patients who may require cataract surgery.

REFERENCES AND FURTHER READING

Almog Y, et al. The effect of oral treatment with beta blockers on the tear secretion. Metab Pediatr Syst Ophthalmol 6: 343, 1982.
Cervantes R, Hernandez HH, Frati A. Pulmonary and heart rate changes associated with nonselective beta blocker glaucoma therapy. J Toxicol Cut Ocul Toxicol 5: 185–193, 1986.
Cocco G, et al. A review of the effects of β-adrenoceptor blocking drugs on the skin, mucosae and connective tissue. Curr Ther Res 31: 362, 1982.
Kaul S, et al. Nadolol and papilledema. Ann Intern Med 97: 454, 1982.
Kumar KL, Cooney TG. Visual symptoms after atenolol therapy for migraine. Ann Intern Med 112(1): 712–713, 1990.
Nielsen PC. et al. Metaprolol eyedrops 3%, a short-term comparison with pilocarpine and a five-month follow-up study. Acta Ophthalmol 60: 347, 1982.
Perell H, Campbell DG, Vela A, Henderson B. Choroidal detachment induced by a systemic beta blocker. Ophthalmol 95: 410–411, 1988.
Petounis AD, Akritopoulos P. Influence of topical and systemic beta blockers on tear production. Int Ophthalmol 13: 75–80, 1989.
Teicher A, Rosenthall T, Kissin E. Labetalol-induced toxic myopathy. BMJ 282(6): 1824–1825, 1981.
Weber JCP. Beta-adrenoreceptor antagonists and diplopia. Lancet 2: 826, 1982.
Wittbrodt ET. Drugs and myasthenia gravis: an update. Arch Intern Med 157: 399–408, 1997.

REFERENCES AND FURTHER READING

Arshinoff SA. Modified SST-USST for tamsulosin-associated intraocular floppy-iris syndrome. J Cataract Refract Surg 32: 559–561, 2006.
Boehringer Ingelheim. Important safety on intraoperative floppy iris syndrome (IFIS). Internet Document: 14 Oct 2005. Available from http://www.hc-sc.gc.ca.
Chang DF, Campbell JR. Intraoperative floppy iris syndrome associated with tamsulosin. J Cataract Refract Surg 31: 664–673, 2005.
Kershner RM. Intraoperative floppy iris syndrome associated with tamsulosin. J Cataract Refract Surg 31: 2239–2241, 2005.
Lawrentschuk N, Blysma GW. Intraoperative 'floppy iris' syndrome and its relationship to tamsulosin: a urologist's guide. Br J Urol Int 97: 2–4, 2006.
Nguyen DQ, Sebastian RT, Philip J. Intraoperative floppy iris syndrome associated with tamsulosin. Br J Urol Int 97: 197, 2006.
Osher RH. Association between IFIS and flomax. J Cataract Refract Surg 32: 547, 2006.
Parssinen O. The use of tamsulosin and iris hypotony during cataract surgery. Acta Ophthalmol Scand 83: 624–626, 2005.
Schwinn DA, Afshari NA. Alpha 1-adrenergic antagonists and floppy iris syndrome: tip of the iceberg? Ophthalmology 112: 2059–2060, 2005.
Tamsulosin Hydrochloride. [Package Insert]. Boehringer Ingelheim, Ridgefield, CT, 2005.

Generic name: 1. Alfuzosin hydrochloride; 2. doxazosin; 3. tamsulosin; 4. terazosin.

Proprietary name: 1. Uroaxatral; 2. Cardura, Cardura XL; 3. Flomax; 4. Hytrin.

Primary use

These alpha-adrenergic antagonists are used to treat benign prostatic hyperplasia and hypertension.

Generic names: 1. Captopril; 2. enalapril.

Proprietary names: 1. Capoten; 2. Vasotec.

Primary use

These angiotensin-converting enzyme inhibitors are used in the management of hypertension.

Ocular side effects

Systemic administration
Certain
1. Decreased vision
2. Eyelids
   a. Angioneurotic edema
   b. Brown discoloration
   c. Blepharoconjunctivitis
   d. Urticaria
   e. Pemphigoid lesion
3. Conjunctivitis
4. Photosensitivity reactions
5. Visual hallucinations

Possible
1. Eyelids or conjunctiva
   a. Lupoid syndrome
   b. Erythema multiforme
   c. Stevens-Johnson syndrome
   d. Exfoliative dermatitis
2. Subconjunctival or retinal hemorrhages secondary to drug-induced anemia

Clinical significance
The angiotensin-converting enzyme (ACE) inhibitors have a much higher incidence than most drugs of causing angioedema that includes the eye and orbit. This is often associated with a facial urticaria. Angioneurotic edema may occur within 2 months of starting the drug or 1 to 5 years after drug exposure. This resolves once the drug is discontinued. Conjunctivitis is the most common ocular adverse event. Ocular photosensitivity reactions are quite rare. Wizemann (1983) reported a case of necrotizing blepharitis as the first clinical signal of captopril-induced agranulocytosis. Balduf et al (1992) reported an unusual case of acute epiphora and rhinorrhea, usually unilateral but could alternate from side to side, which ceased when captopril was discontinued. The authors proposed that the possible pathogenesis is increased sensitivity of some reflexes due to the persistence of inflammatory mediators.

REFERENCES AND FURTHER READING

Ahmad S. Enalapril and reversible alopecia. Arch Intern Med 151: 404, 1991.
Balduf M, Steinkraus V, Ring J. Captopril associated lacrimation and rhinorrhoea. BMJ 305(6855): 693, 1992.
Carrington PR, Sanusi ID, Zahradka S, Winder PR. Enalapril-associated erythema and vasculitis. Cutis 51(2): 121–123, 1993.
Gianos ME, et al. Enalapril induced angioedema. Am J Emerg Med 8: 124–126, 1990.
Gonnering RS, Hirsch SR. Delayed drug-induced periorbital angioedema. Am J Ophthalmol 110(5): 566–568, 1990.
Goodfield MJ, Millard LG. Severe cutaneous reactions to captopril. BMJ 290: 1111, 1985.
Inman WHW, et al. Postmarketing surveillance of enalapril I: results of prescription-event monitoring. BMJ 297: 826–829, 1988.
Pillans PI, Coulter DM, Black P. Angioedema and urticaria with angiotensin converting enzyme inhibitors. Euro J Clin Pharm 51(2): 123–126, 1996.
Suarez M, et al. Angioneurotic edema, agranulocytosis and fatal septicemia following captopril therapy. Am J Med 81: 336, 1986.
Wizemann A. Nekrotisierende Blepharitis nach Captopril-induzierter Agranulozytose. Klin Monatsbl Augenheilkd 182: 82, 1983.

Generic name: Clonidine.

Proprietary names: Catapress, Catapress-TTS, Duraclon.

Primary use

Systemic
This alpha-adrenergic agonist is used in the management of hypertension.

Ophthalmic
Topical ocular clonidine has been used investigationally to reduce intraocular pressure.

Ocular side effects

Systemic administration
Certain
1. Decreased vision
2. Decreased intraocular pressure
3. Eyelids or conjunctiva
   a. Angioneurotic edema
   b. Urticaria
4. Non-specific ocular irritation – burning sensation
5. Visual hallucinations
6. Miosis – toxic states
7. Abnormal EOG

Probable
1. Decreased lacrimation – ocular sicca

Conditional/Unclassified
1. Phemphigoid

Local ophthalmic use or exposure
Certain
1. Blurred vision
2. Decreased intraocular pressure
3. Eyelids or conjunctiva
   a. Irritation – burning sensation
   b. Angioneurotic edema
   c. Urticaria
4. Miosis
5. Follicular conjunctivitis

Possible
1. Ocular sicca

Systemic side effects

Local ophthalmic use or exposure
Probable
1. Hypotension

Clinical significance
Ocular side effects associated with systemic clonidine have been inconsequential and ceased after discontinuation of the drug. Although miosis is the most commonly reported ocular sign in clonidine overdose, mydriasis may occasionally be a clinical feature. Clonidine-induced visual hallucinations may resolve with continued drug usage. Since systemic clonidine has been reported to cause vulval pemphigoid, one should be alert for ocular signs of pemphigoid.

Topical ocular clonidine has been found to reduce intraocular pressure up to 30%, while reducing systemic blood pressure up to 10%. The eyedrops are moderately well tolerated and produce miosis in the treated and contralateral eye. Local ophthalmic use of clonidine appears to be limited because of reduced ophthalmic arterial and episcleral venous pressure when concentrations are greater than 0.125%.

REFERENCES AND FURTHER READING

Banner W, Jr, Lund ME, Clawson L. Failure of naloxone to reverse clonidine toxic effect. Am J Dis Child 137: 1170, 1983.

Hodapp E, et al. The effect of topical clonidine on intraocular pressure. Arch Ophthalmol 99: 1208, 1981.

Kaskel D, Becker H, Itudolf H. Early effects of clonidine, epinephrine, and pilocarpine on the intraocular pressure and the episcleral venous pressure in normal volunteers. Graefes Arch Clin Exp Ophthalmol 213: 251, 1980.

Kosman ME. Evaluation of clonidine hydrochloride (Catapres). JAMA 233: 174–176, 1975.

Krieglstein GK, Langham ME, Leydhecker W. The peripheral and central neural actions of clonidine in normal and glaucomatous eyes. Invest Ophthalmol Vis Sci 17: 149, 1978.

Lee DA, Topper JE, Brubaker RF. Effect of clonidine on aqueous humor flow in normal human eyes. Exp Eye Res 38: 239, 1984.

Petursson G, Cole R, Hanna C. Treatment of glaucoma using minidrops of clonidine. Arch Ophthalmol 102: 1180, 1984.

Mathew PM, Addy DP, Wright N. Clonidine overdose in children. Clin Toxicol 18: 169, 1981.

Turacli ME. The clonidine side effect in the human eye. Ann Ophthalmol 6: 699, 1974.

Van Joost TN, Faber WR, Manuel HR. Drug-induced anogenital pemphigoid. Br J Dermatol 102: 715, 1980.

Generic name: Diazoxide.

Proprietary names: Hyperstat, Proglycem.

Primary use

This non-diuretic benzothiadiazine derivative is used in the emergency treatment of malignant hypertension.

Ocular side effects

Systemic administration
Certain
1. Lacrimation

Possible
1. Eyelids or conjunctiva
   a. Allergic reactions
   b. Erythema
2. Decreased vision
3. Oculogyric crises
4. Subconjunctival or retinal hemorrhages secondary to drug-induced anemia

Conditional/Unclassified
1. Optic nerve infarction
2. Transient lens changes

Clinical significance

Ocular side effects due to diazoxide are uncommon except for increased lacrimation, which occurs in up to 20% of patients taking this agent. In some instances, the lacrimation continued long after discontinued use of diazoxide. The cause of this unusual phenomenon is unknown. Cove et al reported (along with a case in the National Registry) blindness secondary to hypotension from a rapid decrease of blood pressure in malignant hypertension, with presumed ischemia of the optic nerve. An increase in eyelashes can occur with generalized hypertrichosis due to diazoxide. The 2006 Physicians' Desk Reference reports a transient cataract in an infant. Lens changes have been described in beagle dogs (Schiavo et al 1975).

REFERENCES AND FURTHER READING

Burton JL, et al. Hypertrichosis due to diazoxide. Br J Dermatol 93: 707–711, 1975.

Cove DH, et al. Blindness after treatment for malignant hypertension. BMJ 2: 245–246, 1979.

Crandall DC, Leopold IH. The influence of systemic drugs on tear constituents. Ophthalmology 86: 115, 1979.

McEvoy GK (ed). American Hospital Formulary Service Drug Information 87, American Society of Hospital Pharmacists, Bethesda, p 809–812, 1987.

Neary D, Thurston H, Pohl JEF. Development of extrapyramidal symptoms in hypertensive patients treated with diazoxide. BMJ 3: 474, 1973.

Physicians' Desk Reference, 60th edn, Thomson PDR, Montevale NJ, pp 3031–3032, 2006.

Schiavo DM, Field WE, Vymetal FJ. Cataracts in beagle dogs given diazoxide. Diabetes 24: 1041–1049, 1975.

Thomasen A et al. Clinical observations on an antihypertensive chlorothiazide analogue devoid of a diuretic activity. Can Med Assoc J 87: 1306, 1962.

Generic name: Guanethidine monosulfate.

Proprietary name: Ismelin.

Primary use
This adrenergic blocker is effective in the treatment of moderate to severe hypertension.

Ocular side effects

Systemic administration
Certain
1. Decreased vision
2. Non-specific ocular irritation
   a. Hyperemia
   b. Photophobia
   c. Edema
3. Horner's like syndrome
   a. Miosis
   b. Ptosis

Possible
1. Decreased intraocular pressure
2. Subconjunctival or retinal hemorrhages secondary to drug-induced anemia
3. Photophobia

Clinical significance
Ocular side effects from oral guanethidine are rare and seldom of clinical significance although Brest et al (1962) reported an incidence of 'blurring of vision' in 17% of patients taking 70 mg of this drug per day. Some patients have a slight transitory ptosis, miosis and conjunctival hyperemia. The drug is probably secreted in the tears.

REFERENCES AND FURTHER READING

Brest AN, Novack P, et al. Guanethidine. Dis Chest 42: 359–363, 1962.

Cant JS, Lewis DRH. Unwanted pharmacological effects of local guanethidine in the treatment of dysthyroid upper lid retraction. Br J Ophthalmol 53: 239–245, 1969.

Davidson SI. Reports of ocular adverse reactions. Trans Ophthalmol Soc UK 93: 495, 1973.

Gloster J. Guanethidine and glaucoma. Trans Ophthalmol Soc UK 94: 573, 1974.

Hoyng PhFJ, Dake CL. The aqueous humor dynamics and biphasic response to intraocular pressure induced by guanethidine and adrenaline in the glaucomatous eye. Graefes Arch Clin Exp Ophthalmol 214: 263, 1980.

Jones DEP, Norton DA, Davies DJG. Control of glaucoma by reduced dosage guanethidine-adrenaline formulation. Br J Ophthalmol 63: 813, 1979.

Krieglstein GK. The uses and side effects of adrenergic drugs in the management of intraocular pressure. In: Drance SM, Glaucoma: Applied Pharmacology in Medical Treatment. Neufeld AH (eds), Grune & Stratton, New York, p 255–276 1984.

Wright P. Squamous metaplasia or epidermalization of the conjunctiva as an adverse reaction to topical medication. Trans Ophthalmol Soc UK 99: 244, 1979.

Generic name: Hydralazine hydrochloride.

Proprietary names: Generic only.

Primary use

This phthalazine derivative is effective in the management of essential or malignant hypertension, hypertensive complications of pregnancy and hypertension associated with acute glomerulonephritis.

Ocular side effects

Systemic administration
Certain
1. Decreased vision
2. Non-specific ocular irritation
   a. Lacrimation
   b. Photophobia
   c. Ocular pain
3. Eyelids or conjunctiva
   a. Allergic reactions
   b. Erythema
   c. Conjunctivitis – non-specific
   d. Edema
   e. Urticaria

Probable
1. Periorbital edema

Possible
1. Colored flashing lights
2. Subconjunctival or retinal hemorrhages secondary to drug-induced anemia
3. Eyelids or conjunctiva – lupoid syndrome

Local ophthalmic use or exposure
Certain
1. Conjunctiva – hyperemia

Possible
1. Increased intraocular pressure – minimal

Clinical significance

All ocular side effects due to hydralazine are reversible, transient and seldom of clinical significance. A syndrome resembling systemic lupus erythematosus associated with hydralazine therapy is generally considered a benign condition that resolves without permanent sequelae. Several patients with hydralazine-induced lupus syndrome with ocular manifestations, including retinal vasculitis, episcleritis and exophthalmos, have been described.

Larsson et al (1995) studied topical ocular 0.1% hydralazine and found no clinically significant cardiovascular effects or significant ocular toxicity. Mild to moderate conjunctival hyperemia occurred in the series, and a small increase in intraocular pressure.

REFERENCES AND FURTHER READING

Crandall DC, Leopold IH. The influence of systemic drugs on tear constituents. Ophthalmology 86: 115, 1979.

Doherty M, Maddison PJ, Grey RHB. Hydralazine induced lupus syndrome with eye disease. BMJ 290: 675, 1985.

Johansson M, Manhem P. SLE-syndrome with exophthalmus after treatment with hydralazin. Lakartidningen 72: 153, 1975.

Larsson LI, Maus TL, Brubaker RF, et al. Topically applied hydralazine: effects on systemic cardiovascular parameters, blood-aqueous barrier, and aqueous humor dynamics in normotensive humans. J Ocul Pharmacol Ther 11(2): 145–156, 1995.

Mansilla-Tinoco R, et al. Hydralazine, antinuclear antibodies, and the lupus syndrome. BMJ 284: 936, 1982.

Peacock A, Weatherall D. Hydralazine-induced necrotising vasculitis. BMJ 282: 1121, 1981.

Sweetman SC (ed). Martindale: the Complete Drug Reference. 34th edn, Pharmaceutical Press, London, p 931–933, 2004.

Singh S. Hydralazine-induced lupus. South Med J 99: 6–7, 2006.

Generic name: Minoxidil.

Proprietary names: Loniten, Rogaine.

Primary use

This vasodilator is used in the treatment of severe hypertension resistant to other drugs and to treat alopecia.

Ocular side effects

Systemic administration
Certain
1. Eyelids or conjunctiva
   a. Hyperemia
   b. Erythema
   c. Conjunctivitis – non-specific
   d. Hyperpigmentation
   e. Discoloration of eyelashes or eyebrows
   f. Hypertrichosis
   g. Photodermatitis

Possible
1. Eyelids or conjunctiva – Stevens-Johnson syndrome

Conditional/Unclassified
1. Optic neuritis

Topical application
Certain
1. Keratitis
2. Decreased vision
3. Dry skin

Clinical significance

Minoxidil can cause an increase in the growth of fine hair that is darker and longer in up to 80% of the patients taking this drug. This usually occurs 3–6 weeks after exposure, and often occurs first between the eyebrows and on the forehead hairline. This side effect regresses and disappears 1–6 months after stopping the drug. There are more than 80 reports in the National Registry of non-specific conjunctivitis with or without ocular pain associated with the oral use of this agent. Gombos (1983) reported a case of bilateral optic neuritis associated with minoxidil usage.

Weinberg et al (1988) reported topical minoxidil in solution to treat alopecia can cause significant transitory ocular irritation with inadvertent ocular exposure.

REFERENCES AND FURTHER READING

Degreef H, et al. Allergic contact dermatitis to minoxidil. Contact Dermatitis 13: 194, 1985.

DiSantis DJ, Flanagan J. Minoxidil induced Stevens Johnson syndrome. Arch Intern Med 141: 1515, 1981.

Friedman ES, Friedman PM, Cohen DE, et al. Allergic contact dermatitis to topical minoxidil solution: etiology and treatment. J Am Acad Dermatol 46: 309–312, 2002.

Gombos GM. Bilateral optic neuritis following minoxidil administration. Ann Ophthalmol 15: 259, 1983.

Mitchell NC, Pettinger WA. Long-term treatment of refractory hypertensive patients with minoxidil. JAMA 239: 2131, 1978.

Trattner A, David M. Pigmented contact dermatitis from topical minoxidil 5%. Cont Derm 46: 246, 2002.

Traub YM, et al. Treatment of severe hypertension with minoxidil. Isr J Med Sci 11: 991, 1975.

Weinberg RS, Haynes JH, Ferry AP. Toxic keratitis following topical minoxidil use for baldness. In: The Cornea: Transactions of the World Congress on the Cornea III, Cavanagh HD (ed), Raven Press, New York, pp 141–145, 1988.

Generic name: Prazosin hydrochloride.

Proprietary names: Minipress, Minipress XL.

Primary use

This quinazoline derivative is used in the treatment of hypertension.

Ocular side effects

Systemic administration
Certain
1. Blurred vision
2. Eyelids or conjunctiva
   a. Erythema
   b. Conjunctivitis – non-specific
   c. Edema
   d. Urticaria
3. Visual hallucinations

Probable
1. Aggravate keratoconjunctivitis sicca

Conditional/Unclassified
1. Central serous retinopathy
2. Sclera – red discoloration

Clinical significance

Ocular side effects seen secondary to prazosin are uncommon and usually of little clinical significance. In some patients blurred vision occurs, primarily after the first dosage. Schachat (1981) reported two cases of retrobulbar optic neuritis possibly related to prazosin therapy. The National Registry has received several cases of aggravation of dry eyes following the administration of this agent. This is in conjunction with significant drying of the nose and mouth. The very unusual finding of reddening of the sclera is reported in the Physicians' Desk Reference (1999), and there are descriptions in the medical literature. While there have been various reports of central serous retinopathy to the National Registry, the data are soft and inconclusive.

REFERENCES AND FURTHER READING

Chin DKF, Ho AKC, Tse CY. Neuropsychiatric complications related to use of prazosin in patients with renal failure. BMJ 293: 1347, 1986.

McEvoy GK (ed). American Hospital Formulary Service Drug Information 87, American Society of Hospital Pharmacists, Bethesda, p 854–857 1987.

Physicians' Desk Reference, 53rd edn, Medical Economics, Montvale NJ, pp 2394, 1999.

Schachat A. Retrobulbar optic neuropathy associated with prazosin therapy. Ophthalmology 88(Suppl 9): 97, 1981.

Generic names: 1. Rescinnamine; 2. reserpine.

Proprietary names: 1. Moderil; 2. Serplan.

Primary use

These rauwolfia alkaloids are used in the management of hypertension and agitated psychotic states.

Ocular side effects

Systemic administration
Certain
1. Conjunctival hyperemia
2. Non-specific ocular irritation
   a. Lacrimation
   b. Hyperemia

Probable
1. Problems with color vision
   a. Color vision defect
   b. Objects have yellow tinge

Possible
1. Horner's syndrome
   a. Miosis
   b. Ptosis
   c. Increased sensitivity to topical ocular epinephrine preparations
2. Extraocular muscles
   a. Oculogyric crises
   b. Decreased spontaneous movements
   c. Abnormal conjugate deviations
   d. Jerky pursuit movements
3. Decreased vision
4. Decreased intraocular pressure
5. Mydriasis – may precipitate narrow-angle glaucoma

Clinical significance

Most of the preceding ocular side effects have been primarily due to reserpine instead of the other rauwolfia alkaloids. Ocular

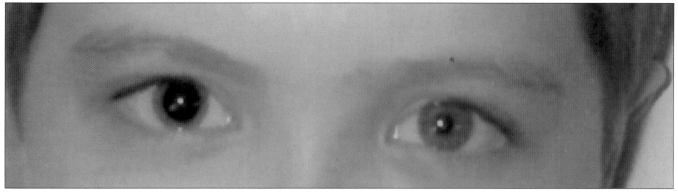

Fig. 7.6c Aniscoria after exposure to aerosol ipratropium. Photo courtesy of Weir REP, et al: Pupil blown by a puffer. Lancet 363: 1853, 2004.

conjunctival hyperemia is not uncommon with reserpine but is of no clinical importance. This is caused by a dilation of the conjunctival blood vessels. This may or may not be associated with increased lacrimation. Occasionally, there may be a slight decrease in intraocular pressure. On rare occasions, mydriasis may cause angle-closure glaucoma. Ocular side effects are otherwise rare and nearly all are reversible. Shimohira et al (2002) have shown rapid eye movements during sleep in infants on reserpine who have neonatal jitteriness.

REFERENCES AND FURTHER READING

Aceto ME, Harris LS. Effect of various agents on reserpine-induced blepharoptosis. Toxicol Appl Pharmacol 7: 329–336, 1965.

Alarcon-Segovia D. Drug-induced antinuclear antibodies and lupus syndromes. Drugs 12: 69, 1976.

Crandall DC, Leopold IH. The influence of systemic drugs on tear constituents. Ophthalmology 86: 115, 1979.

Freedman DX, Benton AJ. Persisting effects of reserpine in man. N Engl J Med 264: 529, 1961.

Fuldauer ML. Ocular spasma caused by reserpine. Ned Tijdschr Geneeskd 103: 110, 1959.

Peczon JD, Grant WM. Sedatives, stimulants and intraocular pressure in glaucoma. Arch Ophthalmol 72: 178–188, 1964.

Raymond LF. Ocular pathology in reserpine sensitivity: Report of two cases. J Med Soc NJ 60: 417, 1963.

Shimohira M, Iwakawa Y, Kohyama J. Rapid-eye-movement sleep in jittery infants. Early Him Dev 66: 25–31, 2002.

Spaeth GL, Nelson LB, Beaudoin AR. Ocular teratology. In: Ocular Anatomy, Embryology and Teratology, Jakobiec FA (ed), JB Lippincott, Philadelphia, p 955–975, 1982.

CLASS: BRONCHODILATORS

Generic name: Ipratropium.

Proprietary names: Atrovent, Atrovent HFA.

Primary use
An inhaled anticholinergic agent used for its bronchodilating and antisecretory properties in chronic obstructive pulmonary disease and asthmatics.

Ocular side effects

Systemic administration – solution, aerosols or nasal sprays
Certain
1. Blurred vision

2. Pupillary dilation (Fig. 7.6c)
   a. Precipitates angle-closure glaucoma
   b. Anisocoria
3. Decreased accommodation
4. Eyelids and conjunctiva
   a. Keratoconjunctivtis sicca
   b. Urticaria
   c. Angioedema
5. Non-specific ocular irritation

Clinical significance
This drug may be delivered to the eye via finger from the liquid, aerosol or spray formulation, which may confuse reactions from systemic exposure. Blurred vision, decreased accommodation and mydriasis are the most common ocular side effects seen. Anisocoria is clinically the most disturbing since it is an early sign of an impending neurological emergency. A unilateral exposure to ipratropium is more often seen in the pediatric age group due to an ill-fitting face mask (Woelfle et al 2000), an intensive care setting (Bisquerra et al 2005) or self-administered nebulizers (Weir et al 2004). There are reports of ipratropium induced angle-closure glaucoma (Ortiz-Rambla et al 2005; de Saint-Jean et al 2000; Lellouche et al 1999), but these are rare. This agent dries all mucous membranes, including the eye. Direct conjunctival drug contact may result in irritation and hypersensitivity reactions. Other than angle-closure glaucoma, all ocular side effects are transitory and reversible.

REFERENCES AND FURTHER READING

Bisquerra RA, Botz GH, Nates JL. Ipratropium-bromide-induced acute anisocoria in the intensive care setting due to ill-fitting face masks. Respir Care 50: 1662–1664, 2005.

Bond DW, Vyas H, Venning HE. Mydriasis due to self-administered inhaled iprotropium bromide. Eur J Pediatr 161: 178, 2002.

Cabana MD, Johnson H, Lee CK, et al. Transient anisocoria secondary to nebulized ipratropium bromide. Clin Pediatr 38: 318, 1999.

de Saint-Jean M, Bourcier T, Borderie V, et al. Acute closure-angle glaucoma after treatment with ipratropium bromide and salbutamol aerosols. J Fr Ophtalmol 23: 603–605, 2000.

Iosson N. Nebulizer-associated anisocoria. N Eng J Med 354: e8, 2006.

Kizer KM, Bess DT, Bedfor N. Blurred vision from ipratropium bromide inhalation. Am J Health Syst Pharm 56: 914, 1999.

Lellouche N, Guglielminotti J, de Saint-Jean M, et al. Acute glaucoma in the course of treatment with aerosols of ipratropium. Presse Med 28: 1017, 1999.

Lust K, Livingstone I. Nebulizer-induced anisocoria. Ann Intern Med 128: 327, 1998.

Ortiz-Rambla J, Hidalgo-Mora JJ, Gascon-Ramon G, et al. Acute angle-closure glaucoma and ipratropium bromide. Med Clin 124: 795, 2005.

Weir REP, Whitehead DEJ, Zaidi FH, et al. Pupil blown by a puffer. Lancet 363: 2004, 1853.

Woelfle J, Zielen S, Lentze MJ. Unilateral fixed dilated pupil in an infant after inhalation of nebulized ipratropium bromide. J Pediatr 136: 423–424, 2000.

Generic name: Salbutamol (albuterol).

Proprietary names: Accuneb, Proventil, Proair, Ventolin, Vospire.

Primary use

This sympathomimetic amine is primarily used as a bronchodilator in the symptomatic relief of bronchospasm.

Ocular side effects

Systemic administration – nebulizer
Certain
1. Decreased vision
2. Eyelids or conjunctiva
   a. Erythema
   b. Blepharoconjunctivitis
   c. Edema
   d. Angioneurotic edema
   e. Urticaria
3. Mydriasis – may precipitate angle-closure glaucoma
4. Ocular pain

Probable
1. Visual hallucinations

Clinical significance

Oral salbutamol has no reported adverse ocular effects. This beta-agonist only has significant ocular side effects if delivered via a nebulizer with the drug coming into direct contact with the eye. Methods to prevent ocular contact will completely prevent all ocular effects. Salbutamol can cause mydriasis and may increase intraocular pressure in predisposed narrow angles. This drug is often given also in nebulized form with ipratropium and will induce angle-closure glaucoma by its parasympathetic inhibitory effect. In a study by Kalra and Bone (1988), both salbutamol and ipratropium were administered simultaneously via nebulizers without eye protection and all patients with narrow angles had an increase in intraocular pressure. Transient angle closure occurred in 50% of them. This effect was completely prevented when protective eye goggles were worn. Contact of this drug with the eye and eyelids may occasionally cause transitory irritation and or ocular pain. Visual hallucinations have only been reported in children.

REFERENCES AND FURTHER READING

Basoglu OK, Emre S, Bacakoglu F, et al. Glaucoma associated with metered-dose bronchodilator therapy. Respir Med 95: 844–845, 2001.

Goldstein JB, Biousse V, Newman NJ. Unilateral pharmacologic mydriasis in a patient with respiratory compromise. Arch Ophthalmol 15: 806, 1997.

Kalra L, Bone MF. The effect of nebulized bronchodilator therapy on intraocular pressures in patients with glaucoma. Chest 93: 739–741, 1988.

Khanna PB, Davies R. Hallucinations associated with the administration of salbutamol via a nebulizer. BMJ 292: 1430, 1986.

Packe GE, Cayton RM, Mashhoudi N. Nebulised ipratropium bromide and salbutamol causing closed-angle glaucoma. Lancet 2: 691, 1984.

Rho DS. Acute angle-closure glaucoma after albuterol nebulizer treatment. Am J Ophthalmol 130: 123–124, 2000.

Shurman A, Passero MA. Unusual vascular reactions to albuterol. Arch Intern Med 144: 1771, 1984.

CLASS: DIURETICS

Generic names: 1. Bendroflumethiazide; 2. chlorothiazide; 3. chlortalidone; 4. hydrochlorothiazide; 5. hydroflumethiazide; 6. indapamide; 7. methyclothiazide; 8. metolazone; 9. polythiazide; 10. trichlormethiazide.

Proprietary names: 1. Naturetin-5; 2. Diuril; 3. Thalitone; 4. Esidrix, Microzide, Oretic; 5. Saluron; 6. Lozol; 7. Enduron; 8. Zaroxolyn; 9. Renese; 10. Metahydrin, Naqua, Trichlorex, Trichlormas.

Primary use

These thiazides and related diuretics are effective in the maintenance therapy of edema associated with chronic congestive heart failure, essential hypertension, renal dysfunction, cirrhosis, pregnancy, premenstrual tension and hormonal imbalance.

Ocular side effects

Systemic administration
Certain
1. Decreased vision
2. Myopia (Fig. 7.6d)
3. Problems with color vision
   a. Objects have yellow tinge (chlorothiazide)
   b. Large yellow spots on white background
4. Eyelids or conjunctiva
   a. Allergic reactions
   b. Conjunctivitis – non-specific
   c. Photosensitivity
   d. Urticaria
   e. Purpura
5. Visual hallucinations
6. Choroidal effusion
7. Increased anterior-posterior lens diameter
8. Shallow anterior chambers
9. Acute glaucoma

Probable
1. Retinal edema
2. Decreased lacrimation
3. Decreased intraocular pressure – minimal
4. Paralysis of accommodation

Possible
1. Eyelids or conjunctiva
   a. Lupoid syndrome
   b. Erythema multiforme
   c. Stevens-Johnson syndrome
   d. Lyell's syndrome
   e. Toxic epidermal necrolysis
2. Subconjunctival or retinal hemorrhages secondary to drug-induced anemia

Clinical significance

Ocular side effects due to these diuretics occur only occasionally and are usually transitory. It appears that most of these agents can cause transitory myopia. There are many different possible mechanisms involved in causing myopia. One is a change directly related to the crystalline lens and ciliary body, i.e. spasm of accommodation, altered sodium-chloride metabolism, ciliary body edema, inhibition of fluid by the lens or change in lenticular index

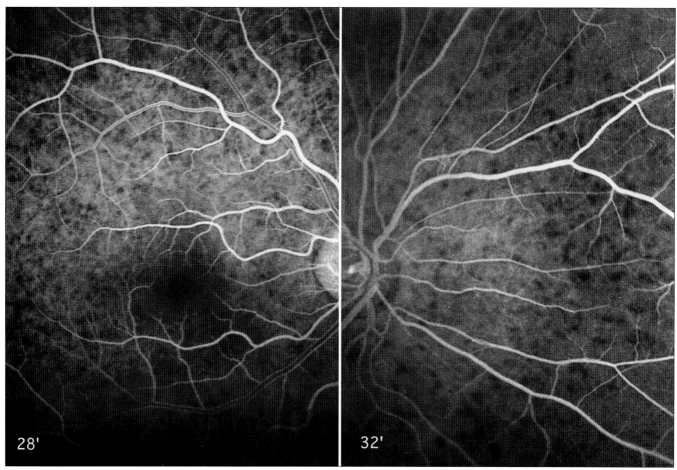

Fig. 7.6d Fluorescein angiogram showing islands of delayed filling. Photo courtesy of Blain P, et al: Acute transient myopia induced by indapamide. Am J Ophthalmol 129: 538-540, 2000.

of refraction. The second mechanism is related to changes in the media or sclera, i.e. changes in the refractive index of the media or stretching of the sclera (Jampolsky and Flom 1953). Blain et al (2000), using angiography, showed diffuse choroidal thickening during indapamide induced myopia. Some of the mechanisms proposed for inducing myopia are probably the cause of inducing angle-closure glaucoma. There are well-documented cases of unilateral or bilateral ciliary body edema or effusions, which produce anterior rotation of the ciliary body at the scleral spur, allowing laxity of the lens zonule and forward displacement of the iris-lens diaphragm. This increases the anterioposterior diameter of the lens, allowing for a shallowing of the anterior chamber with a resultant narrow angle. The cause of the ciliary body edema is unknown; however, Geanon and Perkins (1995) described a case they felt was due to a hypersensitivity reaction. Krieg and Schipper (1996) showed that prostaglandins and eicosanoids are involved. The management of this type of glaucoma is the same as with topiramate. Sponsel and Rapoza (1992) reported a posterior subcapsular cataract after indapamide therapy, but made no statement as to causation. Miller and Moses (1978) described a case of transient oculomotor nerve palsy associated with thiazide-induced glucose intolerance. Thiazide diuretics can also cause hypercalcemia, which may result in band keratopathy.

When thiazide diuretics are used in combination with carbonic anhydrase inhibitors, one should be alert for signs of hypokalemia. These diuretics are photosensitizers and Hartzer et al (1993) showed that in tissue culture hydrochlorothiazide will interact with UV-A radiation to produce toxic synergistic effects on human RPE cells. de la Mamierre et al (2003), in a case control study, concluded that drug-induced phototoxicity (thiazide diuretics in long-term treatment) may be involved in causing more severe neovascularization in age-related macular degeneration.

REFERENCES AND FURTHER READING

Ashraf N, Locksley R, Arieff AI. Thiazide-induced hyponatremia associated with death or neurologic damage in outpatients. Am J Med 70: 1163, 1981.

Beasley FJ. Transient myopia during trichlormethiazide therapy. Ann Ophthalmol 12: 705, 1980.

Bergmann MT, Newman BL, Johnson NC Jr. The effect of a diuretic (hydrochlorothiazide) on tear production in humans. Am J Ophthalmol 99: 473, 1985.

Birch J, et al. Acquired color vision defects. In: Congenital and Acquired Color Vision Defects, Pokorny J et al. (eds), Grune & Stratton, New York, p 243–350, 1979.

Blain P, Paques M, Massin P, et al. Acute transient myopia induced by indapamide. Am J Ophthalmol 129: 538–540, 2000.

de la Marnierre E, Guigon B, Quaranta M, et al. Phototoxic drugs and age-related maculopathy. J Fr Ophtalmol 26: 596–601, 2003.

Geanon JD, Perkins TW. Bilateral acute angle-closure glaucoma associated with drug sensitivity to hydrochlorothiazide. Arch Ophthalmol 113: 1231–1232, 1995.

Grinbaum A, Ashkenazi I, Avni I. Drug induced myopia associated with treatment for gynecological problems. Eur J Ophthalmol 5(2): 136–138, 1995.

Hartzer M, et al. Hydrochlorothiazide: increased human retinal epithelial cell toxicity following low-level UV-A irradiation. ARVO Invest Ophthalmol Vis Sci Annual Meeting Abstract (Issue), 3633–3640, May 1993.

Jampolsky A, Flom B. Transient myopia associated with anterior displacement of the crystalline lens. Am J Ophthalmol 36: 81–89, 1953.

Klein BEK, Klein R, Jensen SC, Linton KLP. Hypertension and lens opacities from the Beaver Dam eye study. Am J Ophthalmol 119: 640–646, 1995.

Krieg PH, Schipper I. Drug-induced ciliary body oedema: a new theory. Eye 10(pt 1): 121–126, 1996.

Miller NR, Moses H. Transient oculomotor nerve palsy. Association with thiazide-induced glucose intolerance. JAMA 240: 1887, 1979.

Palmer FJ. Incidence of chlorthalidone-induced hypercalcemia. JAMA 239: 2449, 1978.

Robinson HN, Morison WL, Hood AF. Thiazide diuretic therapy and chronic photosensitivity. Arch Dermatol 121: 522, 1985.

Söylev MF, Green RL, Feldon SE. Choroidal effusion as a mechanism for transient myopia induced by hydrochlorothiazide and triamterene. Am J Ophthalmol 120(3): 395–397, 1995.

Sponsel WE, Rapoza PA. Posterior subcapsular cataract associated with indapamide therapy. Arch Ophthalmol 110: 454, 1992.

REFERENCES AND FURTHER READING

Castel T, et al. Bullous pemphigoid induced by furosemide. Clin Exp Dermatol 6: 635, 1981.

Davidson SI. Reports of ocular adverse reactions. Trans Ophthalmol Soc UK 93: 495, 1973.

Lee AG, Anderson R, Kardon RH, et al. Presumed 'sulfa allergy' in patients with intracranial hypertension treated with acetazolamide or furosemide: cross-reactivity, myth or reality? Am J Ophthalmol 138: 114–118, 2004.

Peczon JD, Grant WM. Diuretic drugs in glaucoma. Am J Ophthalmol 66: 680, 1968.

Zugerman C, La Voo EJ. Erythema multiforme caused by oral furosemide. Arch Dermatol 116: 518, 1980.

CLASS: OSMOTICS

Generic name: Glycerol (glycerin).

Proprietary names: Colace infant/child, Computer eye drops, Eye lube-A, Fleet bablax, Osmoglyn, Sani-Supp.

Primary use

Systemic
This trihydric alcohol is a hyperosmotic agent used to decrease intraocular pressure in various acute glaucomas and in preoperative intraocular procedures.

Ophthalmic
This topical trihydric alcohol is a hyperosmotic used to reduce corneal edema for diagnostic procedures, increased comfort or improved vision.

Ocular side effects

Systemic administration
Certain
1. Decreased intraocular pressure
2. Subconjunctival or retinal hemorrhages
3. Visual hallucinations
4. Decreased vision

Possible
1. Retinal tears
2. Expulsive hemorrhage

Local ophthalmic use or exposure
Certain
1. Irritation
   a. Lacrimation
   b. Hyperemia
   c. Ocular pain
   d. Burning sensation
2. Vasodilation
3. Subconjunctival hemorrhages

Possible
1. Corneal endothelial damage
2. Contact allergy

Clinical significance

Systemic glycerin causes decreased intraocular pressure, which is an intended ocular response, and has surprisingly few other ocular effects. However, severe vitreal dehydration with resultant shrinkage of the vitreous may possibly cause traction on the adjacent retina,

Generic name: Furosemide.

Proprietary name: Lasix.

Primary use

This potent sulfonamide diuretic is effective primarily in the treatment of hypertension complicated by congestive heart failure or renal impairment.

Ocular side effects

Systemic administration
Certain
1. Decreased vision
2. Problems with color vision – objects have yellow tinge
3. Eyelids or conjunctiva
   a. Allergic reactions
   b. Photosensitivity
   c. Urticaria
   d. Purpura
   h. Pemphigoid lesion
4. Visual hallucinations

Probable
1. Decreased intraocular pressure – minimal
2. Decreased tolerance to contact lenses

Possible
1. Eyelids or conjunctiva
   a. Lupoid syndrome
   b. Erythema multiforme
   c. Exfoliative dermatitis
2. Subconjunctival or retinal hemorrhages secondary to drug-induced anemia
Ocular teratologic effects

Conditional/Unclassified
1. Blindness

Clinical significance

Furosemide has potent systemic side effects and is not commonly used. Ocular side effects are rare and seldom of significance. One instance of a baby born blind after the mother took 40 mg of furosemide three times daily during her second trimester has been reported. Lee et al (2004) found little clinical or pharmacologic evidence of sulfa allergy causing life-threatening cross-reaction with furosemide.

resulting in a tear. This principle has been described with cerebral dehydration as causing intracranial hemorrhages. Severe dehydration from systemic or topical ocular administration can rupture fine vessels, causing local bleeds. In addition, visual hallucinations are thought to occur, probably due to cerebral dehydration. There have been reports of expulsive hemorrhages occurring during intraocular surgery due to strong osmotic agents. The postulated mechanism is that a sudden drop in intraocular pressure may rupture sclerotic posterior ciliary arteries. Patients with renal, cardiovascular or diabetic disease are more susceptible to serious systemic side effects, particularly if they are elderly and already somewhat dehydrated. Kalin et al (1993) reported percutaneous retrogasserian glycerol injection to control intractable pain, where inadvertent orbital injection caused proptosis and vision loss. Mizuta et al (2000) reported a case of possible glycerol-induced asymmetry response to the inner ear, causing vertigo and a resultant vertical nystagmus.

REFERENCES AND FURTHER READING

Almog Y, Geyer O, Lazar M. Pulmonary edema as a complication of oral glycerol administration. Ann Ophthalmol 18: 38, 1986.
Chang S, Abramson DH, Coleman DJ. Diabetic ketoacidosis with retinal tear. Ann Ophthalmol 9: 1507, 1977.
Goldberg MN, et al. The effects of topically applied glycerin on the human corneal endothelium. Cornea 1: 39, 1982.
Havener WN. Ocular Pharmacology. 5th edn. Mosby, St Louis, 552–558, 1983.
Hovland KR. Effects of drugs on aqueous humor dynamics. Int Ophthalmol Clin 11(2): 99, 1971.
Kalin NS, et al. Visual loss after retrogasserian glycerol injection. Am J Ophthalmol 115(3): 396–398, 1993.
Mizuta K, Furuta M, Ito Y, et al. A case of Meniere's disease with vertical nystagmus after administration of glycerol. Auris Nasus Larynx 27: 271–274, 2000.

Generic name: Mannitol.

Proprietary names: Osmitrol, Resectisol.

Primary use

This hyperosmotic agent is used to decrease intraocular pressure in various acute glaucomas and in preoperative intraocular procedures. It is also used in the management of oliguria and anuria.

Ocular side effects

Systemic administration

Certain
1. Decreased intraocular pressure
2. Increased cells in the aqueous
3. Decreased vision
4. Subconjunctival or retinal hemorrhages
5. Visual hallucinations
6. Eyelids or conjunctiva
   a. Edema
   b. Urticaria

Probable
1. Retinal tears
2. Expulsive hemorrhage

Clinical significance

Probably all visual side effects are secondary to dehydration. An increase in aqueous flare but not cells has been caused by mannitol, especially in the elderly. Severe vitreal dehydration

with resultant shrinkage of the vitreous may cause traction on the adjacent retina, resulting in a tear. This principle has also been described with cerebral dehydration causing intracranial hemorrhage. Expulsive hemorrhages have been reported to occur during surgery in which strong osmotic agents were used. The postulated mechanism is the sudden decrease in intraocular pressure, which may rupture sclerotic posterior ciliary arteries. Isosorbide does not adversely affect blood glucose levels and is preferred in diabetics. Cardiovascular or renal disease may contraindicate use of isosorbide or mannitol. It has been suggested that these agents open the blood-retinal barrier and may give drugs or chemicals greater access to the retina and CNS.

REFERENCES AND FURTHER READING

Chang S, Abramson DH, Coleman DJ. Diabetic ketoacidosis with retinal tear. Ann Ophthalmol 9: 1507, 1977.
Grabie MT, et al. Contraindications for mannitol in aphakic glaucoma. Am J Ophthalmol 91: 265, 1981.
Lamb JD, Keogh JAM. Anaphylactoid reaction to mannitol. Can Anaesth Soc J 26: 435, 1979.
Mehra KS, Singh R. Lowering of intraocular pressure by isosorbide. Arch Ophthalmol 86: 623, 1971.
Millay RH, et al. Maculopathy associated with combination chemotherapy and osmotic opening of the blood-brain barrier. Am J Ophthalmol 102: 626–632, 1986.
Miyake Y, et al. Increase in aqueous flare by a therapeutic dose of mannitol in humans. Acts Soc Ophthalmol Jpn 93: 1149–1153, 1989.
Quon DK, Worthen DM. Dose response of intravenous mannitol on the human eye. Ann Ophthalmol 13: 1392, 1981.
Wood TO, et al. Effect of isosorbide on intraocular pressure after penetrating keratoplasty. Am J Ophthalmol 75: 221, 1973.

CLASS: PERIPHERAL VASODILATORS

Generic name: Phenoxybenzamine hydrochloride.

Proprietary name: Dibenzyline.

Primary use

This alpha-adrenergic blocking agent is used in the management of pheochromocytoma and sometimes in the treatment of vasospastic peripheral vascular disease other than the obstructive types.

Ocular side effects

Systemic administration
Certain
1. Miosis
2. Ptosis
3. Conjunctival hyperemia
4. Decreased intraocular pressure – minimal

Clinical significance

Although ocular side effects due to phenoxybenzamine are frequently seen, they are seldom clinically significant. Phenoxybenzamine is an alpha-adrenergic blocker so it can cause miosis. While this is rarely a problem, when it is associated with posterior subcapsular or central lens changes there may be a sudden decrease in vision. All adverse ocular reactions are reversible and transitory after discontinued drug use.

REFERENCES AND FURTHER READING

Drug Evaluations, 6th edn, American Medical Association, Chicago, pp 491–492, 529–530, 577, 1986.

Gilman AG, Goodman LS, Gilman A (eds). The Pharmacological Basis of Therapeutics. 6th edn. Macmillan, New York, pp 178-183, 1980.
Potter DE, Rowland JM. Adrenergic drugs and intraocular pressure. Gen Pharmacol 12: 1, 1981.
Walsh FB, Hoyt WF. Clinical Neuro-Ophthalmology, Vol. I, 3rd edn. Williams & Wilkins, Baltimore, p 447, 1969.

CLASS: VASOPRESSORS

Generic name: Ephedrine.

Proprietary names: Multi-ingredient preparations only.

Primary use

Systemic
This sympathomimetic amine is effective as a vasopressor, a bronchodilator and a nasal decongestant.

Ophthalmic
This topical sympathomimetic amine is used as a conjunctival vasoconstrictor.

Ocular side effects

Systemic administration
Probable
1. Mydriasis – may precipitate angle-closure glaucoma
2. Visual hallucinations
3. Decreased intraocular pressure

Possible
1. Acute macular neuroretinopathy

Local ophthalmic use or exposure
Certain
1. Conjunctival vasoconstriction
2. Decreased vision
3. Eyelids or conjunctiva
   a. Allergic reactions
   b. Conjunctivitis – non-specific
4. Irritation
   a. Lacrimation
   b. Rebound hyperemia
   c. Photophobia
5. Mydriasis – may precipitate angle-closure glaucoma
6. Aqueous floaters – pigment debris
7. Decreased intraocular pressure – minimal

Clinical significance
Ocular side effects from systemic administration of ephedrine are rare. O'Brien et al (1989) described an acute macular neuroretinopathy, possibly due to ephedrine. Dark red, outer retinal wedge-shaped lesions surrounding all or part of the central macula, with normal vision but permanent paracentral scotomas developed. This may be due to a direct retinal effect of the drug or an acute hypertensive effect.

Topical ocular ephedrine is not currently used by most ophthalmologists. The currently used concentration is rarely sufficient to cause significant side effects other than the intended response of vasoconstriction. Repeated use of topical ocular ephedrine, however, may cause rebound conjunctival hyperemia or loss of the drug's vasoconstrictive effect. The FDA gave a warning for drugs containing ephedrine: 'Pupils may become dilated. If you have narrow-angle glaucoma, do not use this product.'

REFERENCES AND FURTHER READING
Crandall DC, Leopold IH. The influence of systemic drugs on tear constituents. Ophthalmology 86: 115, 1979.
Drug Evaluations, 6th edn, American Medical Association, Chicago, pp 377, 404, 574–575, 1986.
Escobar JI, Karno M. Chronic hallucinosis from nasal drops. JAMA 247: 1982, 1859, 1982.
Havener WH. Ocular Pharmacology, 5th edn. Mosby, St Louis, p 299, 1983.
O'Brien DM, et al. Acute macular neuroretinopathy following intravenous sympathomimetics. Retina 9(4): 281-286, 1989.
Walsh FB, Hoyt WF. Clinical Neuro-Ophthalmology, Vol. I, 3rd edn, Williams & Wilkins, Baltimore, pp 446, 1969.

Generic name: 1. Epinephrine; 2. norepinephrine (levarterenol).

Proprietary names: 1. Epipen, Epipen Jr., Twinject, Twinject 0.3; 2. Levophed.

Primary use

Systemic
This sympathomimetic amine is effective as a vasopressor, a bronchodilator and a vasoconstrictor in prolonging the action of anesthetics.

Ophthalmic
Used in the management of open-angle glaucoma.

Ocular side effects

Systemic administration – injection
Certain
1. Mydriasis – may precipitate angle-closure glaucoma – transitory
2. Problems with color vision – transitory
   a. Color vision defect, red-green defect
   b. Objects have green tinge

Probable
1. Acute macular neuroretinopathy (epinephrine)
2. Increased aqueous production (epinephrine)
3. May precipitate an ocular vasoconstrictive vascular event (epinephrine)

Possible
1. Lacrimation (epinephrine)

Local ophthalmic use or exposure

Certain
1. Decreased intraocular pressure
2. Decreased vision
3. Mydriasis – may precipitate angle-closure glaucoma
4. Eyelids or conjunctiva
   a. Allergic reactions
   b. Blepharoconjunctivitis – follicular
   c. Vasoconstriction (epinephrine)
   d. Poliosis (epinephrine)
   e. Cicatrizing conjunctivitis – pseudo-ocular pemphigoid (epinephrine)

f. Hyperplasia of sebaceous glands (epinephrine)
g. Loss of eyelashes or eyebrows (epinephrine)
h. Rebound hyperemia
5. Irritation
   a. Lacrimation
   b. Photophobia
   c. Ocular pain
   d. Burning sensation
6. Adrenochrome deposits (epinephrine) (Fig. 7.6e)
   a. Conjunctiva
   b. Cornea
   c. Nasolacrimal system (cast formation)
7. Cystoid macular edema (epinephrine)
8. Cornea (epinephrine)
   a. Superficial punctuate keratitis
   b. Edema
9. Subconjunctival hemorrhages (epinephrine)
10. Paradoxical pressure elevation in open-angle glaucoma
11. Iris (epinephrine)
    a. Iritis
    b. Cysts
12. Black discoloration of soft contact lenses (epinephrine)
13. May aggravate herpes infections (epinephrine)
14. Narrowing or occlusion of lacrimal canaliculi (epinephrine)

Possible
1. Periorbital edema (epinephrine)

Systemic side effects

Local ophthalmic use or exposure – epinephrine

Certain
1. Headache
2. Sweats
3. Syncope
4. Arrhythmia
5. Tachycardia
6. Palpitations
7. Hypertension
8. Ventricular extrasystole

Clinical significance

Adverse events from systemic administration are heavily dose dependent or additive dependent on associated drug use. All events are rare since dosages used have been tested to be safe over time. O'Brien et al (1989) and Desai et al (1993) have reported cases of intravenous epinephrine causing acute macular neuroretinopathy. Savino et al (1990) described four patients with severe visual loss after intranasal anesthetic with epinephrine injections. The causes of the visual loss included retinal arterial occlusion and optic nerve ischemia, both of which the authors felt were due to secondary vasospasm induced by epinephrine. Patients undergoing ocular surgery with halothane anesthesia may experience tachycardia and arrhythmia from supplemental injection of local anesthetics containing epinephrine, from topical ophthalmic administration or intracameral injection of epinephrine.

Norepinephrine causes few ocular side effects from systemic exposure and those are transitory and reversible except in overdose situations. Jandrasits et al (2002) reported that high levels of circulating norepinephrine have little impact on retinal vascular tone or retinal blood flow.

In over 20% of patients, topical ocular epinephrine must be stopped after prolonged use because of ocular discomfort and rebound conjunctival hyperemia. Over 50% of patients develop reactive hyperemia with long-term use. Concomitant use of timolol and epinephrine therapy occasionally has an additive effect on reactive hyperemia, cardiac arrhythmia or elevated blood pressure. Long-term topical ocular epinephrine preparations can cause cicatrizing conjunctivitis, which clinically or pathologically may be difficult to distinguish from ocular pemphigoid. This may include shortening of the fornices. Most epinephrine-induced macular edema is reversible, but lack of early detection may cause irreversible cystoid macular changes. Cystoid maculopathy may require over 6 months to clear once the medication is discontinued. These changes occur more frequently in aphakic patients. This drug can cause conjunctival epidermalization, loss of eyelashes, blepharitis and meibomianitis. Most ocular adverse reactions due to epinephrine resolve or significantly improve with discontinuation of the drug. However, adrenochrome deposits in the cornea or conjunctiva may be exceedingly slow to absorb. Adrenochrome deposits in the lacrimal ducts may cause obstruction with epiphora. There are data to suggest that long-term topical ocular or intracameral epinephrine may cause significant corneal edema. This primarily occurs in corneas with damaged epithelium, which allows for increased penetration of this drug to reach the endothelium.

Norepinephrine is seldom given topically since epinephrine is much more effective and potent. Ocular side effects from norepinephrine are transitory and minimal. Systemic side effects are less potent then epinephrine, but norepinephrine may have greater effect on elevation of blood pressure.

REFERENCES AND FURTHER READING

Bealka N, Schwartz B. Enhanced ocular hypotensive response to epinephrine with prior dexamethasone treatment. Arch Ophthalmol 109: 346–348, 1991.

Bigger JF. Norepinephrine therapy in patients allergic to or intolerant of epinephrine. Ann Ophthalmol 11: 183, 1979.

Blondeau P, Cote M. Cardiovascular effects of epinephrine and dipivefrin in patients using timolol: a single-dose study. Can J Ophthalmol 19: 29, 1984.

Brummett R. Warning to otolaryngologists using local anesthetics containing epinephrine: potential serious reactions occurring in patients treated with beta-adrenergic receptor blockers. Arch Otolaryngol 110: 561, 1984.

Camras CB, et al. Inhibition of the epinephrine-induced reduction of intraocular pressure by systemic indomethacin in humans. Am J Ophthalmol 100: 169, 1985.

Desai UR, Sudhamathi K, Natarajan S. Intravenous epinephrine and acute macular neuroretinopathy. Arch Ophthalmol 111: 1026–1027, 1993.

Edelhauser HF, et al. Corneal edema and the intraocular use of epinephrine. Am J Ophthalmol 93: 327, 1982.

Jandrasits K, Luksch A, Söregi G, et al. Effect of noradrenaline on retinal blood flow in healthy subjects. Ophthalmology 109: 291–295, 2002.

Jay GT, Chow MS. Interaction of epinephrine and β-blockers. JAMA 274(23): 1830, 1995.

Kacere RD, Dolan JW, Brubaker RF. Intravenous epinephrine stimulates aqueous formation in the human eye. Invest Ophthalmol Vis Sci 33(10): 2861–2865, 1992.

Kaufman HE. Chemical blepharitis following drug treatment. Am Ophthalmol 95: 703, 1983.

Kerr CR, et al. Cardiovascular effects of epinephrine and dipivalyl epinephrine applied topically to the eye in patients with glaucoma. Br J Ophthalmol 66: 109, 1982.

Krejci L, Rezek P, Hoskovcova-Krejcova H. Effect of long-term treatment with antiglaucoma drugs on corneal endothelium in patients with congenital glaucoma: contact specular microscopy. Glaucoma 7: 81, 1985.

O'Brien DM, et al. Acute macular neuroretinopathy following intravenous sympathomimetics. Retina 9: 281–286, 1989.

Pollack IP, Rossi H. Norepinephrine in the treatment of ocular hypertension and glaucoma. Arch Ophthalmol 93: 173, 1975.

Sasamoto K, et al. Corneal endothelial changes caused by ophthalmic drugs. Cornea 3: 37, 1984.

Savino PJ, Burde RM, Mills RP. Visual loss following intranasal anesthetic injection. J Clin Neuro-ophthalmol 10(2): 140–144, 1990.

Stewart R, et al. Norepinephrine dipivalylate dose-response in ocular hypertensive subjects. Ann Ophthalmol 13: 1279, 1981.

Generic name: Phenylephrine.

Proprietary names: AH-chew D, Ak-Dilate, Children's nostril, Mydfrin, Neo-synephrine, Neofrin, Nostil, Ocu-phrin, Phenoptic, Prefin, Rectacaine, Relief, Rhinall, Sinex.

Primary use

Systemic

This sympathomimetic amine is effective as a vasopressor and is used in the management of hypotension, shock and tachycardia.

Ophthalmic

This topical sympathomimetic amine is used as a vasoconstrictor and a mydriatic.

Ocular side effects

Systemic administration – nasal application
Certain
1. Angle-closure glaucoma

Possible
1. Visual hallucinations
2. Facial and eyelid flushing

Local ophthalmic use or exposure
Certain
1. Pupil
   a. Mydriasis – may decrease vision
   b. Rebound miosis
2. Intraocular pressure
   a. Precipitate angle-closure glaucoma
   b. Transitory elevation of intraocular pressure – open angle
   c. Temporary decrease
3. Conjunctival vasoconstriction
4. Irritation
   a. Lacrimation
   b. Rebound hyperemia
   c. Photophobia
   d. Ocular pain
5. Cornea
   a. Punctate keratitis
   b. Edema
   c. Adenochrome deposits (Fig. 7.6e)
6. Eyelids or conjunctiva
   a. Allergic reactions
   b. Erythema
   c. Conjunctivitis – non-specific
   d. Blepharospasm
   e. Eczema
   f. Palpebral fissure – increase in width
   g. Pseudo-ocular pemphigoid

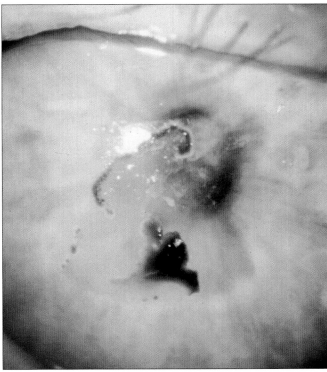

Fig. 7.6e Adenochrome deposits in cornea from topical ocular epinephrine treatment. Photos courtesy of Krachmer JH, Palay DA. Cornea Atlas, 2nd edn, Mosby Elsevier, London, 2006.

7. Aqueous floaters – pigment debris
8. Hydrogel keratoprothesis
   a. Surface spoliation
   b. Internal deposition/coloration

Possible
1. Optic nerve
   a. Worsen vaso-occlusive disease

Systemic side effects

Local ophthalmic use or exposure
Certain
1. Hypertension
2. Myocardial infarct
3. Tachycardia
4. Subarachnoid hemorrhage
5. Cardiac arrest
6. Cardiac arrhythmia
7. Coronary artery spasm
8. Headache
9. Syncope

Probable
1. Premature infants – pulmonary edema

Conditional/Unclassified
1. Premature infants – renal failure

Clinical Significance

Phenylephrine is given systemically primarily as sprays onto mucous membranes, i.e. nasal mucosa, therefore systemic side effects are essentially the same as for topical ocular exposure.

Ocular side effects due to topical ocular phenylephrine are usually of little significance unless the drug is used for prolonged periods of time. Phenylephrine used topically is one of the more toxic commercial drugs to the conjunctival and corneal epithelium. Soparkar et al (1997) have pointed out that even in low concentration in over-the-counter ophthalmic decongestants, acute and chronic conjunctivitis can go unrecognized. Unfortunately, signs and symptoms of these adverse effects of the drug may take 1–24 weeks to resolve. While the drug is used for pupillary dilation it may have a varied response on intraocular pressure. Initially, there may be a transitory decrease, later a transitory increase even with open angles. There may be no pressure change or in very rare instances angle-closure glaucoma may be precipitated. Pupillary dilatation lasting for prolonged periods has been reported, especially in patients on guanethidine. Mydriasis varies with iris pigmentation and depth of the anterior chamber. Blue irides and shallow anterior chambers produce the greatest mydriasis, and dark irides or deep chambers the least. A diminished mydriatic response has been seen after repeated use of phenylephrine. A 10% concentration of phenylephrine can cause significant keratitis and a reduction in the conjunctival PO_2, which may result in delayed wound healing by reducing aerobic metabolism of rapidly dividing cells. Blanching of the skin, particularly the lower eyelid, may occur secondary to topical ocular phenylephrine. Following ophthalmic examination with a combination of phenylephrine and cyclopentolate in neonates, an increased risk of feeding intolerance may result, which could be due to the mydriatic drugs, the physical stress applying eye medication or a combination of these factors. Pless and Friberg (2003) described four patients with non-arteritic ischemic optic neuropathy who experienced acute worsening of visual function after instillation of phenylephrine for a dilated fundus exam. Morrison et al (2006) pointed out the effects of topical ocular phenylephrine on hydrogel keratoprothesis, promoting hydrogel cloudiness and surface deposits. Chronic use of this drug may be one of the more common causes of contact dermatitis of the eyelids as per incidence of use. In fact, Villarreal (1998) reported that 93.5% of acute dermatitis from all eye drops was due to topical mydriatic drugs, primarily phenylephrine.

Over 100 plus articles support the finding that topical ocular phenylephrine can cause, in rare instances, severe stress on the cardiovascular system and marked elevation of blood pressure. This was first reported by Fraunfelder and Scafidi (1978), who reported 11 deaths. Numerous additional terminal cases have been reported to the National Registry. Phenylephrine 10% should be used with caution or not at all in patients with cardiac disease, significant hypertension, aneurysms and advanced arteriosclerosis. It also should be used with caution in the elderly and in patients on monoamine oxidase inhibitors, tricyclic antidepressants or atropine. Similar findings were reported in 11 patients (Fraunfelder et al 2002) to whom 10% phenylephrine was applied to the eye in pledget form.

Numerous reports in the National Registry and in the literature have associated unilateral and bilateral acute glaucoma, secondary to nasal drops containing phenylephrine (Khan et al 2002; Zenzen et al 2004). In a preterm infant, Berman and Deutsch (1994) postulate that 2.5% phenylephrine may have triggered a series of events to cause bilateral spontaneous pigment epithelial detachments. Also in infants, phenylephrine eye drops have been implicated in paralytic ileus (Lim et al 2003) and even renal failure (Shinomiya et al 2003). Baldwin and Morley (2002) reported interoperative pulmonary edema in a child following topical ocular application of numerous drops of both 2.5 and 10% phenylephrine. This was associated with cardiac arrhythmias and severe hypertension.

REFERENCES AND FURTHER READING

Baldwin FJ, Morley AP. Intraoperative pulmonary oedema in a child following systemic absorption of phenylephrine eyedrops. Br J Anaesth 88: 440–442, 2002.

Berman DH, Deutsch JA. Bilateral spontaneous pigment epithelial detachments in a premature neonate. Arch Ophthalmol 112(2): 161–162, 1994.

Fraunfelder FT. Pupil dilation using phenylephrine alone or in combination with tropicamide. Ophthalmology 106(1): 4, 1999.

Fraunfelder FT, Meyer SM. Possible cardiovascular effects secondary to topical ophthalmic 2.5% phenylephrine. Am J Ophthalmol 99: 362, 1985.

Fraunfelder FT, Scafidi AF. Possible adverse effects from topical ocular 10% phenylephrine. Am J Ophthalmol 85: 447–453, 1978.

Fraunfelder FW, Fraunfelder FT, Jensvold B. Adverse systemic effects from pledgets of topical ocular phenylephrine 10%. Am J Ophthalmol 134: 625, 2002.

Hanna C, et al. Allergic dermatoconjunctivitis caused by phenylephrine. Am J Ophthalmol 95: 703, 1983.

Hermansen MC, Sullivan LS. Feeding intolerance following ophthalmologic examination. Am J Dis Child 139: 367, 1985.

Isenberg SJ, Green BF. Effect of phenylephrine hydrochloride on conjunctival PO_2. Arch Ophthalmol 102: 1185, 1984.

Khan MAJ, Watt LL, Hugkulstone CE. Bilateral acute angle-closure glaucoma after use of Fenox nasal drops. Eye 16: 662–663, 2002.

Kumar SP. Adverse drug reactions in the newborn. Ann Clin Lab Sci 15: 195, 1985.

Kumar V, Packer AJ, Choi WW. Hypertension following phenylephrine 2.5% ophthalmic drops. Glaucoma 7: 131, 1985.

Kumar V, et al. Systemic absorption and cardiovascular effects of phenylephrine eyedrops. Am J Ophthalmol 99: 180, 1985.

Lim DL, Batilando M, Rajadurai VS. Transient paralytic ileus following the use of cyclopentolate-phenylephrine eyedrops during screening for retinopathy of prematurity. J Paediatr Child Health 39: 318–320, 2003.

Morrison DA, Gridneva Z, Chirila TV, et al. Screening for drug-induced spoliation of the hydrogel optic of the AlphaCor artifical cornea. Cont Lens Anterior Eye 29: 93–100, 2006.

Munden PM, et al. Palpebral fissure responses to topical adrenergic drugs. Am J Ophthalmol 111: 706–710, 1991.

Pless M, Friberg TR. Topical phenylephrine may result in worsening of visual loss when used to dilate pupils in patients with vas-occlusive disease of the optic nerve. Semin Ophthalmol 18: 218–221, 2003.

Powers JM. Decongestant-induced blepharospasm and orofacial dystonia. JAMA 247: 3244, 1982.

Rafael M, Pereira F, Faria MA. Allergic contact blepharoconjunctivitis caused by phenylephrine associated with persistent patch test reaction. Contact Derm 39: 143–144, 1997.

Resano A, Esteve C, Fernandez Benitez M. Allergic contact blepharoconjunctivitis due to phenylephrine eye drops. J Invest Allerg Clin Immun 9(1): 55–57, 1999.

Shinomiya K, Kajima M, Tajika H, et al. Renal failure caused by eyedrops containing phenylephrine in a case of retinopathy of prematurity. J Med Invest 50: 203–206, 2003.

Soparkar CN, Wilhelmus KR, Koch DD, et al. Acute and chronic conjunctivitis due to over-the-counter ophthalmic decongestants. Arch Ophthalmol 115(1): 34–38, 1997.

Villarreal O. Reliability of diagnostic tests for contact allergy to mydriatic eyedrops. Contact Derm 38: 150–154, 1998.

Wesley RE. Phenylephrine eyedrops and cardiovascular accidents after fluorescein angiography. J Ocular Ther Surg 2: 212, 1983.

Whitson JT, Love R, Brown RH, et al. The effect of reduced eyedrop size and eyelid closure on the therapeutic index of phenylephrine. Am J Ophthalmol 115: 357–359, 1993.

Zenzen CT, Eliott D, Balok EM, et al. Acute angle-closure glaucoma associated with intranasal phenylephrine to treat epistaxis. Arch Ophthalmol 122: 655–656, 2004.

HORMONES AND AGENTS AFFECTING HORMONAL MECHANISMS

CLASS: ADRENAL CORTICOSTEROIDS

Generic names: 1. Adrenal cortex injection; 2. beclomethasone dipropionate; 3. betamethasone; 4. cortisone acetate; 5. dexamethasone; 6. fludrocortisone acetate; 7. fluorometholone; 8. hydrocortisone; 9. medrysone; 10. methylprednisolone; 11. prednisolone; 12. prednisone; 13. rimexolone; 14. triamcinolone.

Proprietary names: 1. None; 2. Beconase AQ, Qvar, 40, Qvar 80; 3. Alphatrex, Celestone, Diprolene, Diprolene AF, Diproson, Luxiq, Taclonex; 4. generic only; 5. Decadron, Hexadrol, Maxidex, Mymethasone; 6. Florinef; 7. Flarex, FML, FML Forte, Fluor-op; 8. Ala-cort, Ala-Scalp, A-hydrocort, Anusol HC, Cetacort, Colocort, Cortef, Cortifoam, Dricort, Hi-Cor, Hydrocortone, Hytone, Locoid, Locoid lipocream, Micort HC, Nutracort, Orabase HCA, Pandel, Penecort, Sitecort, Sul-Cortef, Synacort, Texacort, Westcort; 9. HMS; 10. A-methapred, Depomedrol, Medrol, Solu-medrol; 11. Enconopred plus; Inflamase mild, Inflamase Forte, Orapred, Pediapred, Prelone, Pred Forte, Pred Mild; 12. generic only; 13. Vexol; 14. Aristocort, Aristocort A, Aristospan, Azmacort, Kenalog, Kenalog 10, Kenalog 40, Nasocort AQ, Nasocort HFA, Oracort, Triacet, Triderm.

Primary use

Systemic
These corticosteroids are effective in the replacement therapy of adrenocortical insufficiency and in the treatment of inflammatory and allergic disorders.

Ophthalmic
Used in the treatment of ocular inflammatory and allergic disorders.

Topical
These corticosteroids are effective for the relief of inflammatory and pruritic dermatoses.

Ocular side effects

Systemic administration
Certain
1. Decreased vision
2. Posterior subcapsular cataracts (early may be reversible) (Fig. 7.7b)
3. Increased intraocular pressure
4. Decreased resistance to infection
5. Mydriasis – may precipitate angle-closure glaucoma
6. Myopia
7. Exophthalmos
8. Papilledema secondary to intracranial hypertension
   a. Secondary to the drug
   b. Secondary to drug withdrawal
9. Myasthenic neuromuscular blocking effect
   a. Diplopia
   a. Ptosis
   b. Paresis of extraocular muscles

10. Problems with color vision
11. Delayed wound healing
12. Visual fields
    a. Scotomas
    b. Constriction
    c. Enlarged blind spot
    d. Glaucoma field defect
13. Visual hallucinations
14. Abnormal ERG or VEP
15. Retina
    a. Edema
    b. Hemorrhage
    c. Central serous retinopathy
16. Translucent blue sclera
17. Eyelids or conjunctiva
    a. Hyperemia
    b. Edema (Fig. 7.7a)
    c. Angioneurotic edema
18. Microcyst – non-pigment epithelium of ciliary body and pigment epithelium of iris
19. Subconjunctival hemorrhages
20. Decreased tear lysozymes
21. Toxic amblyopia
22. Retinopathy of prematurity – may increase
23. 'Rosecea-like' skin changes

Possible
1. Eyelids or conjunctiva – Lyell's syndrome

Local ophthalmic use or exposure – topical application, intralesional or subconjunctival or retrobulbar injection

Certain
1. Increased intraocular pressure
2. Decreased resistance to infection
3. Delayed wound healing
4. Mydriasis – may precipitate angle-closure glaucoma
5. Ptosis
6. Posterior subcapsular cataracts
7. Decreased vision
8. Enhances lytic action of collagenase
9. Paralysis of accommodation
10. Visual fields
    a. Scotomas
    b. Constriction
    c. Enlarged blind spot
    d. Glaucoma field defect
11. Problems with color vision
    a. Color vision defect
    b. Colored haloes around lights
12. Eyelids or conjunctiva
    a. Allergic reactions
    b. Persistent erythema
    c. Hyperemia
    d. Telangiectasia
    e. Depigmentation
    f. Poliosis
    g. Scarring (subconjunctival injection)
    h. Fat atrophy (retrobulbar or subcutaneous injection)
    i. Skin atrophy (subcutaneous injection)
    j. Necrosis (injection)
    k. Ptosis (injection)
    l. Ulceration (injection)

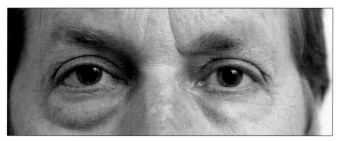

Fig. 7.7a Periorbital edema around the right eye in patient receiving systemic steroids.

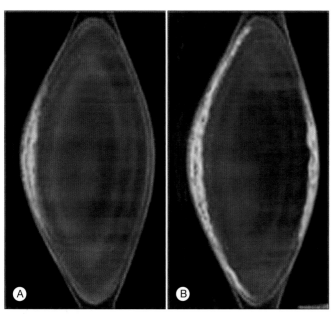

Fig. 7.7b A: Posterior subcapsular lens opacities (initial). B: Anterior lens opacities (late).

13. Cornea
    a. Punctate keratitis
    b. Superficial corneal deposits
    c. Thickness – increase initially and then decrease (Fig. 7.7b)
14. Irritation
    a. Lacrimation
    b. Photophobia
    c. Ocular pain
    d. Burning sensation
    e. Anterior uveitis
15. Scleral
    a. Thickness
        i. Increased – initial
        ii. Decreased
    b. Blue color – transient
16. Central serous retinopathy
17. Proptosis (retrobulbar injections)
18. Granulomas
19. May aggravate the following diseases
    a. Herpes simplex
    b. Bacterial infection
    c. Fungal infections
    d. Scleromalacia perforans
    e. Corneal 'melting' diseases
    f. Behçet's disease

g. Eales' disease
h. Presumptive ocular toxoplasmosis
i. Diabetes (periocular injection)
j. Facultative intraocular pathogens
20. Retinal embolic phenomenon (injection)

Probable
1. Cushing syndrome (infants and young children)

Possible
1. Scleritis (injection)

Intraocular injection
Certain
1. Ocular pain
2. Decreased vision
3. Cataracts
    a. Subscapular
    b. All layers of the lens
4. Intraocular pressure
    a. Increased – initial
    b. Decreased
5. Retina
    a. Hemorrhage
    b. Degeneration
    c. Necrosis
6. Ascending optic atrophy
7. Toxic amblyopia
8. Global atrophy
9. Endophthalmitis
    a. Sterile
    b. Enhances latent infections
    c. Pseudohyphoeon (crystalline drug deposition)

Periocular or intravitral injection
Certain
1. Increased intraocular pressure
2. Decreased resistance to infection
3. Delayed wound healing
4. Mydriasis – may precipitate angle-closure glaucoma
5. Ptosis
6. Posterior subcapsular cataracts
7. Decreased vision
8. Enhances lytic action of collagenase
9. Paralysis of accommodation
10. Visual fields
    a. Scotomas
    b. Constriction
    c. Enlarged blind spot
    d. Glaucoma field defect
11. Problems with color vision
    a. Color vision defect
    b. Colored haloes around lights
12. Eyelids or conjunctiva
    a. Allergic reactions
    b. Persistent erythema
    c. Hyperemia
    d. Telangiectasia
    e. Depigmentation
    f. Poliosis
    g. Scarring (subconjunctival injection)
    h. Fat atrophy (retrobulbar or subcutaneous injection)
    i. Skin atrophy (subcutaneous injection)
    j. Necrosis (injection)

13. Cornea
    a. Punctate keratitis
    b. Superficial corneal deposits
    c. Thickness – increases initially and then decreases
14. Irritation
    a. Lacrimation
    b. Photophobia
    c. Ocular pain
    d. Burning sensation
    e. Anterior uveitis
15. Scleral
    a. Thickness
        i. Increased – initial
        ii. Decreased
    b. Blue color – transient
16. Toxic amblyopia
17. Granulomas
18. May aggravate the following diseases
    a. Herpes simplex
    b. Bacterial infections
    c. Fungal infections
    d. Scleromalacia perforans
    e. Corneal 'melting' diseases
    f. Beçhet's disease
    g. Eales' disease
    h. Presumptive ocular toxoplasmosis
    i. Enhances facultative intraocular pathogens
19. Retinal embolic phenomenon (injection)
20. Migration of injection into anterior chamber from vitreous

Systemic absorption from topical application to the skin or nasal inhalants
Certain
1. Increased intraocular pressure
2. Decreased resistance to infection
3. Eyelids or conjunctiva
    a. Photosensitivity
    b. Urticaria
    c. Purpura
    d. Telangiectasia
    e. Depigmentation
    f. Skin atrophy
4. Papilledema secondary to intracranial hypertension
5. Cataracts

Ocular teratogenic effects
Certain
1. Cataracts

Clinical significance
This group of medicines is one of the most commonly used in all of ophthalmology. There are almost 1500 publications on ocular and periocular steroid complications and these data alone could fill a textbook. This section is only a brief and incomplete review. Steriod ocular side effects may vary with age (younger lenses being more susceptible to changes), type of steroid (fluorinated compounds), increased fat atrophy, race (glaucoma more common in Caucasians) and method of delivery (injections have a higher localized drug concentration so there is an increased frequency and severity of local adverse events).

A large study (Garbe et al 1998) clearly showed that oral and nasal spray steroids cause a statistically significant increase in cataract surgery in the elderly. This study infers that we significantly underestimate the importance of steroids as a co-factor in cataractogenesis. Smeeth et al (2003) confirmed that high-dose inhaled steroids are associated with an increased risk of lens changes. Jick et al (2001), in a retrospective observational cohort study, found that in individuals above the age of 40 years old there was an increased risk of inhaled steroids and cataracts. Lipworth (1999) found that while all inhaled steroids had increased risks of systemic side effects, fluticasone propionate exhibits greater dose-related systemic bioavailability, particularity at doses above 0.8 μg/dl. All forms of drug delivery and methods of administration are associated with lens changes if the drug gets into the eye. It has been shown that 50% of patients using 800 drops of topical ocular 0.1% dexamethasone will develop some lens changes. Generally, steroid-induced posterior subcapsular cataracts are irreversible, but data support the reversibility of cataracts in some early systemic steroid-induced changes of lenses, i.e. nephrotic children. Cekic et al (2005) have shown that single intravitreal triamcinolone injections can produce posterior subcapsular cataracts while multiple injections result in all layers of the lens having opacity progression. Thompson (2006) reported posterior subcapsular cataracts in 50% of patients; these are visually significant after 1 year with repeat intravitreal triamcinolone injections.

Topical ocular corticosteroid-induced glaucoma may take a number of weeks to develop and this occurs in about one-third of individuals. However, almost all those who are exposed to higher doses of topical ocular corticosteroids will develop some elevation in intraocular pressure if the drug is continued for more than 12 months. Inhaled steroid can cause or aggravate open-angle glaucoma, especially in patients with a family history of glaucoma (Mitchell et al 1999). Reports on various methods of injection, i.e. periorbital (Sahni et al 2004), sub-tenons (Levy et al 2004), intravitreal (Smithen et al 2004) and a host of others, confirm a strong association of injected corticosteroids with glaucoma. Intractable glaucoma after intravitreal triamcinolone injections has been well documented (Kaushik et al 2004; Quiram et al 2006). Early rapid rise of intraocular pressure may occur (Singh et al 2004) or be delayed even after more than 3 months (Quiram et al 2006). Although individual variation to steroid exposure may be marked, steroid responders with elevated intraocular pressure secondary to topical ocular corticosteroids have more field loss than steroid non-responders. Steroid-induced glaucoma patients will usually return to normal pressures after the drug is stopped. If optic damage has occurred, these patients can easily be confused with low-tension glaucoma patients. Rimexolone, a more recent topical ocular steroid, has the anti-inflammatory properties of the more potent steroids, but the glaucoma-inducing potential of mid-range steroids, such as fluorometholone (Leibowitz et al 1996).

A fatal reaction from complications of Cushing's syndrome following 3 months' treatment with corticosteroid eye drops and sub-Tenon's injection occurred in an 11-month-old child. Topical ocular corticosteroids are generally not associated with any significant risk of adrenal axis suppression, although extreme care must be exercised as to the amount prescribed in infants. Batton et al (1992) and Ehrenkranz (1992) felt there may be an association between increased retinopathy of prematurity and steroid exposure by the infant. Even the withdrawal of steroids can cause significant adverse effects, as seen in a 7-month-old child who developed benign intracranial hypertension with severe visual loss following withdrawal of topical cutaneous steroids. Liu et al (1994) reported this reaction in adults as well. Romano (2002) and Romano et al (1977) pointed out that, primarily in infants and young children, periocular injections or topical ocular steroids in high dosages can cause severe systemic reactions of hypertension, Cushing's syndrome, hypertensive encephalopathy and death.

The recent popularity of subconjunctival injections of steroids has been accompanied by additional ocular drug reactions. Subconjunctival injections of steroids placed over a diseased cornea or sclera can cause a thinning, and possibly a rupture, at the site of the injection. Zamir et al (2002) and Albini et al (2005) have shown that subconjunctival steroids in non-necrotizing anterior scleritis appear to be safe. Periocular injections may produce sclerosing lipogranuloma (Abel et al 2003). Posterior sub-tenon injections may cause ptosis associated with orbital fat prolapse (Dal Canto et al 2005), cutaneous hypopigmentation (Gallando and Johnson 2004), or retinal or choroidal vascular occlusion (Moshfeghi et al 2002). Feldman-Billard et al (2006) reported on a series of 25 patients with type-2 diabetes receiving subconjunctival or peribulbar injections of dexamethasone and found that this may induce a median doubling from baseline followed by a decrease in their blood glucose around 6 hours post injection. Intractable glaucoma can occur after subconjunctival depo-injections of steroids. The surgical removal of the steroids may be required to normalize the ocular pressure. Inadvertent intraocular steroid injections have caused blindness. This is probably due to the drug vehicle. Inadvertent intraocular depot injections are numerous and include a significant toxicity vehicle and the prolonged release of the steroid. While triamcinolone acetonide appears to be the least toxic of the steroid medications with inadvertent vitreous injections, often vitrectomy is required to remove the depot steroid, prevent tract bands and examine the penetration site. Pendergast et al (1995) reported a case of inadvertent depot betamethasone acetate and methasone sodium phosphate preserved with benzalkonium chloride that caused severe intraocular damage. The preservative, they feel, was the reason for the ocular changes. Most feel removal of deposteroids accidentally injected into the vitreous may be considered an emergency procedure. Keeping the patient prone before surgery to prevent the material from coming into contact with the macula is important. To date, all commercial deposteroids contain components that are toxic to the retina.

Multiple authors (Bouzas et al 1993; Haimovici et al 1997) have implicated corticosteroids as a causative factor in patients with central serous chorioretinopathy. This may occur for oral, intranasal sprays (Haimovici et al 1997), intrajoint or epidural injections (Iida et al 2001). Carvalho-Recchia et al (2002) did a prospective case-controlled study which identified corticosteroids as a significant risk factor for the development of acute exudative macular manifestation. Systemic steroids have been implicated in causing central serous chorioretinopathy (DeNijs et al 2003; Levy et al 2004) when injected intravenously or by epidural injection (Pizzimenti and Daniel 2005). Steroids effect changes in almost all ocular structures. This has been reconfirmed by showing that steroids can cause microcysts of the iris pigment epithelium and of the ciliary body non-pigment epithelium. The time required for onset of a major adverse effect from topical ocular steroids varies greatly. Effects to enhance epithelial herpes simplex may be days, while it may take years for posterior subcapsular cataracts to develop. Taravella et al (1994) have shown that the topical ocular phosphate preparations can cause a corneal band keratopathy, especially in patients with sicca. Huige et al (1991) stated that topical ocular beta blockers enhance superficial stromal deposits of the phosphated forms of steroid eye drops.

REFERENCES AND FURTHER READING

Abel AD, Carlson A, Bakri S, et al. Sclerosing lipogranuloma of the orbit after periocular steroid injection. Ophthalmology 110: 1841–1845, 2003.

Agrawal S, Agrawal J, Agrawal TP. Conjunctival ulceration following triamcinolone injection. Am J Ophthalmol 136: 538–540, 2003.

Albini TA, Zami E, Read RW, et al. Evaluation of subconjunctival triamcinolone for nonnecrotizing anterior scleritis. Ophthalmology 112: 1814–1820, 2005.

Batton DG, Roberts C, Trese M, Maisels MJ. Severe retinopathy of prematurity and steroid exposure. Pediatrics 90(4): 534–536, 1992.

Bouzas EA, Scott MH, Mastorakos G, et al. Central serous chorioretinopathy in endogenous hypercortisolism. Arch Ophthalmol 111: 1229–1233, 1993.

Bowie EM, Folk JC, Barnes CH. Corticosteroids, central serous chorioretinopathy, and neurocysticercosis. Arch Ophthalmol 122: 281–283, 2004.

Carvalho-Recchia CA, Yannuzzi LA, Negrão S, et al. Corticosteroids and central serous chorioretinopathy. Ophthalmology 109: 1834–1837, 2002.

Çekiç O, Chang S, Tseng JJ, et al. Cataract progression after intravitreal triamcinolone injection. Am J Ophthalmol 139: 993–998, 2005.

Chaine G, Haouat M, Menard-Molcard C, et al. Central serous chorioretinopathy and systemic steroid therapy. J Fr Opthalmol 24: 139–146, 2001.

Chen SDM, Lochhead J, McDonald B, et al. Pseudohypopyon after intravitreal triamcinolone injection for the treatment of pseudophakic cystoid macular oedema. Br J Ophthalmol 88: 843–844, 2004.

Cohen BA, et al. Steroid exophthalmos. J Comput Assist Tomogr 5: 907, 1981.

Dal Canto AJ, Downs-Kelly E, Perry JD. Ptosis and orbital fat prolapse after posterior sub-tenon's capsule triamcinolone injection. Ophthalmology 112: 1092–1097, 2005.

De Nijs E, Brabant P, De Laey JJ. The adverse effects of corticosteroids in central serous chorioretinopathy. Bull Soc Belge Ophtalmol 35: 35–41, 2003.

Ehrenkranz RA. Steroids, chronic lung disease, and retinopathy of prematurity. Pediatrics 90(4): 646–647, 1992.

Feldman-Billard S, Du Pasquier-Frediaevsky L, Héron E. Hyperglycemia after repeated periocular dexamethasone injections in patients with diabetes. Ophthalmology 113: 1720–1723, 2006.

Fischer R, Henkind P, Gartner S. Microcysts of the human iris pigment epithelium. Br J Ophthalmol 63: 750, 1979.

Fraunfelder FT, Meyer SM. Posterior subcapsular cataracts associated with nasal or inhalation corticosteroids. Am J Ophthalmol 109(4): 489–490, 1990.

Gallardo MJ, Johnson DA. Cutaneous hypopigmentation following a posterior sub-tenon triamcinolone injection. Am J Ophthalmol 137: 780–799, 2004.

Garbe E, Suissa S, Lelorier J. Association of inhaled corticosteroid use with cataract extraction in elderly patients. JAMA 280: 539–544, 1998.

Giangiacomo J, Dueker DK, Adelstein EH. Histopathology of triamcinolone in the subconjunctiva. Ophthalmology 94: 149, 1987.

Gilles MC, Simpson JM, Billson FA, et al. Safety of an intravitreal injection of triamcinolone. Arch Ophthalmol 122: 336–340, 2004.

Gilles MC, Kuzniarz M, Craig J, et al. Intravitreal triamcinolone-induced elevated intraocular pressure is associated with the development of posterior subcapsular cataract. Ophthalmology 112: 139–143, 2005.

Gupta V, Sharma SC, Gupta A. Retinal and choroidal microvascular embolization with methylprednisolone 22: 382–385, 2002.

Gupta OP, Boynton JR, Sabini P, et al. Proptosis after retrobulbar corticosteroid injections. Ophthalmology 110: 443–447, 2003.

Haimovici R, Gragoudas ES, Duker JS, et al. Central serous chorioretinopathy associated with inhaled or intranasal corticosteroids. Ophthalmology 104(10): 1653–1660, 1997.

Henderson RP, Lander R. Scleral discoloration associated with long-term prednisone administration. Cutis 34: 76, 1984.

Huige WM, Beekhuis WH, Rijneveld WJ, Schrage N. Unusual deposits in the superficial corneal stroma following combined use of topical corticosteroid and beta-blocking medication. Doc Ophthalmol 78(3-4): 169–175, 1991.

Iida T, Spaide RF, Negrao SG, et al. Central serous chorioretinopathy after epidural corticosteroid injection. Am J Ophthalmol 132: 423–425, 2001.

Jick SS, Vasilakis-Scaramozza C, Maier WC. The risk of cataract among users of inhaled steroids. Epidemiology 12: 229–234, 2001.

Jonas JB, Degenring RF, Kreissig I, et al. Intraocular pressure elevation after intravitreal triamcinolone acetonide injection. Ophthalmology 112: 593–598, 2005.

Jordan DR, Brownstein S, Lee-wing MW, et al. Orbital mass following injection with depot corticosteroids. Can J Ophthalmol 36: 153–155, 2001.

Kass MA, et al. Corticosteroid-induced iridocyclitis in a family. Am J Ophthalmol 93: 268, 1982.

Kaushik S, Gupta V, Gupta A, et al. Intractable glaucoma following intravitreal triamcinolone in central retinal vein occlusion. Am J Ophthalmol 137: 758–760, 2004.

Leibowitz HM, Bartlett JD, Rich R, et al. Intraocular pressure-raising potential of 1.0% rimexolone in patients responding to corticosteroids. Arch Ophthalmol 114: 933–937, 1996.

Levy J, Tessler Z, Klemperer I, et al. Acute intractable glaucoma after a single low-dose sub-Tenon's corticosteroid injection for macular edema. Can J Ophthalmol 39: 672–673, 2004.

Levy J, Marcus M, Belfair N, et al. Central serous chorioretinopathy in patients receiving systemic corticosteroid therapy. Can J Ophthalmol 40: 217–221, 2005.

Lipworth BJ. Systemic adverse effects of inhaled corticosteroid therapy. Arch Intern Med 159: 941–955, 1999.

Liu GT, Kay MD, Bienfang DC, Schatz NJ. Pseudotumor cerebri associated with corticosteroid withdrawal in inflammatory bowel disease. Am J Ophthalmol 117(3): 352–357, 1994.

Mabry RL. Visual loss after intranasal corticosteroid injection. Incidence, causes, and prevention. Arch Otolaryngol 107: 484, 1981.

Meyer CH, Mennel S, Schmidt JC. Intravitreal triamcinolone acetonide may increase the intraocular pressure even in vitrectomized eyes after more than 3 months. Am J Ophthalmol 140: 766–767, 2005.

Mills DW, Siebert LF, Climenhaga DB. Depot triamcinolone-induced glaucoma. Can J Ophthalmol 21: 150, 1986.

Mitchell P, Cumming RG, Mackey DA. Inhaled corticosteroids, family history, and risk of glaucoma. Ophthalmology 106: 2301–2306, 1999.

Moshfeghi DM, Lowder CY, Roth DB. Retinal and choroidal vascular occlusion after posterior sub-tenon triamcinolone injection. Am J Ophthalmol 134: 132–134, 2002.

Moshfeghi AA, Scott IU, Flynn HW. Pseudohypopyon after intravitreal triamcinolone acetonide injection for cystoid macular edema. Am J Ophthalmol 138: 489–492, 2004.

Parke DW. Intravitreal triamcinolone and endophthalmitis. Am J Ophthalmol 136: 918–919, 2003.

Pendergast SD, Eliott D, Machemer R. Retinal toxic effects following inadvertent intraocular injection of Celestone Soluspan. Arch Ophthalmol 113(10): 1230–1231, 1995.

Piccolino FC, Pandolfo A, Polizzi A, et al. Retinal toxicity from accidental intraocular injection of depo-medrol. Retina 22: 117–119, 2002.

Pizzimenti JJ, Daniel KP. Central serous chorioretinopathy after epidural steroid injection. Pharmacotherapy 25: 1141–1146, 2005.

Quiram PA, Gonzales CR, Schwartz SD. Severe steroid-induced glaucoma following intravitreal injection of triamcinolone acetonide. Am J Ophthalmol 141: 580–582, 2006.

Ramanathan R, Siassi B, deLemos RA. Severe retinopathy of prematurity in extremely low birth weight infants after short-term dexamethasone therapy. J Perinatology 15(3): 178–182, 1995.

Romano PE. Fluorinated ocular/periocular corticosteroids have caused death as well as glaucoma in children. Clin Experiment Ophthalmol 31: 278–279, 2002.

Romano PE, Traisman HS, Green OC. Fluorinated corticosteroid toxicity in infants. Am J Ophthalmol 84: 247–250, 1977.

Roth DB, Chieh J, Spirn MJ, et al. Noninfectious endophthalmitis associated with intravitreal triamcinolone injection. Arch Ophthalmol 121: 1279–1282, 2003.

Ruiz-Moreno JM, Montero JA, Artola A, et al. Anterior chamber tansit of triamcinolone after intravitreal injection. Arch Ophthalmol 123: 129–130, 2005.

Sahni D, Darley CR, Hawk JLM. Glaucoma induced by periorbital steroid use – a rare complication. Clin Exp Dermatol 29: 617–619, 2004.

Singh IP, Ahmad SI, Yeh D, et al. Early rapid rise in intraocular pressure after intravitreal triamcinolone acetonide injection. Am J Ophthalmol 138: 286–287, 2004.

Smeeth L, Boulis M, Hubbard R, et al. A population based case-control study of cataract and inhaled corticosteroids. Br J Ophthalmol 87: 1247–1251, 2003.

Smithen LM, Ober MD, Maranan L, et al. Intravitreal triamcinolone acetonide and intraocular pressure. Am J Ophthalmol 138: 740–743, 2004.

Srinivasan S, Prasad S. Conjunctival necrosis following intravitreal injection of triamcinolone acetonide. Cornea 24: 1027–1028, 2005.

Taravella MJ, et al. Calcific band keratopathy associated with the use of topical steroid-phosphate preparations. Arch Ophthalmol 112: 608–613, 1994.

Thompson JT. Cataract formation and other complications of intravitreal triamcinolone for macular edema. Am J Ophthalmol 141: 629–637, 2006.

Tognetto D, Zenoni S, Sanguinetti G, et al. Staining of the internal limiting membrane with intravitreal triamcinolone acetonide. Retina 25: 462–467, 2005.

Tsuchiya T, Ayaki M, Onishi T, et al. Three-year prospective randomized study of incidence of posterior capsule opacification in eyes treated with topical diclofenac and betamethasone. Ophthalmic Res 35: 67–70, 2003.

Zamir E, Read RW, Smith RE, et al. A prospective evaluation of subconjunctival injection of tiramcinolone acetonide for resistant anterior scleritis. Ophthalmology 109: 798–807, 2002.

CLASS: ANDROGENS

Generic name: Danazol.

Proprietary name: Generic only.

Primary use

This synthetic androgen is used to treat pelvic endometriosis, fibrocystic breast disease and hereditary angioneurotic edema.

Ocular side effects

Systemic administration
Certain
1. Decreased vision
2. Eyelids or conjunctiva
   a. Erythema
   b. Edema
   c. Photosensitivity
   d. Urticaria
   e. Purpura
   f. Loss of eyelashes or eyebrows

Possible
1. Eyelids or conjunctiva – Stevens-Johnson syndrome

Conditional/Unclassified
1. Diplopia
2. Optic nerve
   a. Papilledema secondary to intracranial hypertension
   b. Pallor
   c. Atrophy
3. Visual field defects
4. Cataracts

Clinical significance

Decreased vision, usually associated with headaches, is the most frequent ocular side effect reported secondary to danazol. This is reversible and may resolve while continuing to take the drug. There are at least 14 cases of intracranial hypertension with papilledema associated with this drug that were either published or reported to the National Registry. Intracranial hypertension may occur while taking this medication or shortly after stopping it. While intracranial hypertension was documented in at least half of the cases, only papilledema was mentioned in the rest. Causation is unknown, but may be due to danazol-induced weight gain, fluid retention or cerebral venous thrombosis. There are not enough data to prove a positive association. Presenile cataracts in young women treated with danazol have also been found in the absence of predisposed risk factors, but this is unsubstantiated.

REFERENCES AND FURTHER READING

Fanous M, et al. Pseudotumor cerebri associated with danazol withdrawal. Letter to the editor. JAMA 266(9): 1218–1219, 1991.

Hamed LM, et al. Pseudotumor cerebri induced by danazol. Am J Ophthalmol 107(2): 105–110, 1989.

McEvoy GK (ed). American Hospital Formulary Service Drug Information 87, American Society of Hospital Pharmacists, Bethesda, p 1616–1618, 1987.

Physicians' Desk Reference, 42nd edn, Medical Economics Co., Oradell, NJ, pp 2225–2226, 1988.

Pre-senile cataracts in association with the use of Danocrine (danazol). PMS News Quarterly April-June: 5, 1986.

Sandercock PJ. Benign intracranial hypertension associated with danazol. Pseudotumor cerebri: case report. Scottish Med J 35: 49, 1990.

Schmitz U, Honisch C, Zierz S. Pseudotumor cerebri and carpal tunnel syndrome associated with danazol therapy. J Neurol 238: 355, 1991.

Shah A, et al. Danazol and benign intracranial hypertension. BMJ 294: 1323, 1987.

Generic name: Leuprorelin acetate.

Proprietary names: Eligard, Lupron, Lupron Depot, Lupron Depot-3, Lupron Depot-4, Lupron Depot-PED, Viadur.

Primary use

This synthetic analogue of a gonadotrophin-releasing hormone is used in the management of sterility, endometriosis, precocious puberty or prostatic cancer.

Ocular side effects

Systemic administration
Certain
1. Blurring vision

Probable
1. Eye pain
2. Lid edema

Possible
1. Papilledema – intracranial hypertension
2. Retina
   a. Branch vein occlusions
   b. Retinal hemorrhage

Clinical significance

The most common adverse ocular event associated with leuprorelin acetate is blurred vision (Fraunfelder and Edwards 1995). In about half of the cases, this may be associated with headaches or dizziness, which may occur after each injection of the drug. These symptoms occur shortly after drug administration and rarely last more than 1–2 hours. There are rare instances of blurred vision lasting 2–3 weeks. Intracranial hypertension has also been seen with this drug, but a direct cause-and-effect relationship has not been established. If intracranial hypertension occurs while the patient is receiving leuprorelin, the decision to discontinue the drug may be based on the response of the intracranial hypertension to therapy, the severity of the intracranial hypertension and the severity of the underlying disease. Leuprorelin may be associated with thromboembolic phenomena, intraocular branch vein occlusion or hemorrhages. Ocular pain and lid edema may be drug related since these have been seen

elsewhere in the body due to this agent. Cases of ocular sicca or aggravation of ocular sicca have been reported to the National Registry, but a direct relationship has not been established.

REFERENCES AND FURTHER READING

Arber N, Fadila R, Pinkhas J, et al. Pseudotumor cerebri associated with leuprorelin acetate. Lancet 335: 668, 1990.

Boot JH. Pseudotumor cerebri as a side effect of leuprorelin acetate. Irish J Med Sci 165(1): 60, 1996.

Fraunfelder FT, Edwards R. Possible ocular adverse effects associated with leuprolide injections. JAMA 273(10): 773–774, 1995.

Plosker GL, Brogden RN. Leuprorein: a review of its pharmacology and therapeutic use in prostatic cancer, endometriosis and other sex hormone-related disorders. Drugs 48(6): 930–967, 1994.

CLASS: ANTITHYROID AGENTS

Generic names: 1. Iodide and iodine solutions and compounds; 2. radioactive iodides.

Proprietary names: 1. Bexxar, Iodopen, Iodotope, Pima, SSKI, Thyro-block.

Primary use

Systemic
Iodide and iodine are effective in the diagnosis and management of thyroid disease, and in the short-term management of respiratory tract disease and, in some instances, of fungal infections.

Ophthalmic
Topical iodide and iodine solutions are used primarily as a chemical cautery in the treatment of herpes simplex.

Ocular side effects

Systemic administration – oral
Certain
1. Non-specific ocular irritation
   a. Lacrimation
   b. Ocular pain
   c. Burning sensation
2. Eyelids or conjunctiva
   a. Allergic reactions
   b. Hyperemia
   c. Conjunctivitis – non-specific
   d. Edema
   e. Angioneurotic edema
   f. Urticaria
   g. Nodules

Probable
1. Decreased vision

Possible
1. Decreased accommodation
2. Exophthalmos
3. Keratoconjunctivitis sicca
4. Punctate keratitis
5. Hemorrhagic iritis
6. Hypopyon
7. Vitreous opacities
8. Scleral thinning
9. Eyelids or conjunctiva – exfoliative dermatitis

Systemic administration – intravenous

Probable

1. Problems with color vision
   a. Color vision defect
   b. Objects have green tinge
2. Visual hallucinations

Possible

1. Those mentioned for oral administration
2. Visual fields
   a. Scotomas
   b. Constriction
   c. Hemianopsia
3. Paralysis of accommodation
4. Mydriasis

Local ophthalmic use or exposure

Certain

1. Decreased vision
2. Eyelids or conjunctiva
   a. Allergic reactions
   b. Blepharoconjunctivitis
   c. Edema
   d. Urticaria
3. Irritation
   a. Lacrimation
   b. Hyperemia
   c. Ocular pain
   d. Edema
4. Brown corneal discoloration – transitory
5. Corneal vascularization
6. Stromal scarring
7. Delayed corneal wound healing

Possible

1. Keratitis bullosa

Probable

1. Ocular teratogenic effects (radioactive iodides)

Clinical significance

Few serious irreversible ocular side effects secondary to iodide preparations have been reported, except when these agents have been given intravenously. The severe retinal changes reported in the literature are secondary to a drug, septojod (iodines and iodates), that is no longer in use. It was the first drug recognized to cause retinal pigmentary degeneration (Duke-Elder and MacFaul 1972). When currently available products are given orally, retinal findings are probably non-existent. Allergic reactions to these agents are of rapid onset and not uncommon. They may occur at small doses with responses occurring within minutes. A delayed hypersensitivity reaction may occur, causing iododerma with tender pustules, vesicles and nodular eyelid lesions. This has been associated with keratoconjunctivitis sicca, hemorrhagic iritis and vitreous opacities.

REFERENCES AND FURTHER READING

Balazs G, Kincses E, Kosa C. Iatrogenic diseases caused by iodine. Orv Hetil 108: 407, 167.

Duke-Elder S, MacFaul PA. System of Ophthalmology, Vol. XIII, Duke-Elder S (ed.), Mosby, St Louis, p 957, 1972.

Gerber M. Ocular reactions following iodide therapy. Am J Ophthalmol 43: 879, 1957.

Goldberg HK. Iodism with severe ocular involvement. Report of a case. Am J Ophthalmol 22: 65, 1939.

Grant WM, Schuman JS. Toxicology of the Eye, 4th edn, Charles C. Thomas, Springfield, IL, pp 833–834, 1993.

Inman WHW. Iododerma. Pr J Dermatol 91: 709, 1974.

Kincaid MC, et al. Iododerma of the conjunctiva and skin. Ophthalmology 88: 1216, 1981.

CLASS: ERECTILE DYSFUNCTION AGENTS

Generic names: 1. Sildenafil citrate; 2. tadalafil; 3. vardenafil.

Proprietary names: 1. Revatio, Viagra; 2. Cialis; 3. Levitra.

Primary use

These agents are oral therapy used for erectile dysfunction.

Ocular side effects

Systemic administration

Certain

1. Problems with color vision
   a. Objects have colored tinges – usually blue or blue-green, may be pink or yellow
   b. Decreased color vision
   c. Dark colors appear darker
   e. Increased perception of brightness
   f. Flashing lights – especially when blinking
2. Blurred vision
   a. Central haze
   b. Transitory decreased vision
3. ERG changes
4. Conjunctival hyperemia
5. Ocular pain
6. Photophobia
7. Subconjunctival hemorrhage

Conditional/Unclassified

1. Non-arteritic ischemic optic neuropathy (NAION)
2. Central serous macular edema
3. Retinal vascular accidents

Clinical significance

Sildenafil (Viagra®) has been studied far more extensively than tadalafil and vardenafil, the two more recently released erectile dysfunction (ED) drugs. In pre-marketing clinical trials, all three agents have a similar incidence of visual side effects and all were proven transitory. Sildenafil citrate has been one of the largest-selling prescription drugs in the world. The ocular side effects most commonly associated with sildenafil are a transitory bluish tinge to objects, hypersensitivity to light and minimal hazy vision. These reversible side effects may last from a few minutes to hours, depending on drug dosage. Visual changes are seen in approximately 3% of men taking the standard 50 mg dose and 11% of men taking 100 mg, with the incidence rising to 40% at a dose of 200 mg. At four times the recommended dose (200 mg) sildenafil causes minimal reversible ERG changes in b2 wave amplitude, both in phototopic and scotopic conditions, but with a less than 10% decrease in photopic implicit times in a- and b-waves. Conjunctival hyperemia, ocular pain and photophobia may occur. Chandeclere et al (2004) has reported palpebral edema in one case with rechallenge data. Non-arteritic ischemic optic neuropathy (NAION) is a significant 'signal' to be watched for in patients on this group of drugs. There are approximately 25 cases of NAION published or unpublished, however many are not within the time lines of occurring within 4 hours for sildenafil and vardenafil or within 30 hours for tadalafil. Recovery times are within the range of normally occurring NAION. Presently it is premature to state that this group of drugs causes NAION. There are some neuropathologists who feel there is an association. McGwin et al (2006) stated that in men with a history of myocardial infarction or hypertension these agents may increase the risk of NAION. The association between this class of drugs and NAION is conditional/unclassified according to WHO criteria. This classification may well change as additional data become available. Laties and Siegel (2006), based on epidemiologic studies, showed that the incidences of NAION are about the same as in the normal population compared to the population taking sildenafil citrate. Escaravage et al (2005) reported a single well-documented rechallenge case associated with tadalafil use, which is the most compelling association between NAION and a phophodiesterase type 5 inhibitor. Hayreh (2005) has explained various mechanisms that could account for causation of NAION by these drugs. To date, however, no mechanism has been proven.

There are four published cases of macular edema (Allibhai et al 2004; Quiram et al 2005) and another seven in the National Registry (Fraunfelder and Fraunfelder 2007). Four of these cases have positive rechallenge of serous macular edema associated with erectile dysfunction drugs at normal or elevated dosages. Included are cases of chronic macular edema, which would not resolve until the drug was stopped. While these data are suggestive, the nature of non-drug-induced serous macular edema is recurrent and transitory. Further data are necessary.

Multiple reports of retinal vascular accidents associated with the use of these drugs are given in the National Registry. In elderly patients this is not an uncommon finding and a positive association is not possible.

Recommendations

1. Advise patient to stop use of all PDE-5 inhibitors and seek medical attention in the event of sudden loss of vision in one or both eyes. Even a transitory decrease in vision other than a mild haze should be a warning that an additional dose may cause a significant vascular ocular event.
2. Discuss with patient the possible increased risk of NAION in those who have already experienced NAION in one eye with the recommendation not to take this class of drugs.
3. Most reported cases of drug-related NAION have had a small cup:disc ratio. We do not feel it is necessary to screen patients for this prior to starting these drugs. Until more data are available, we do not feel informed consent is necessary.
4. In any patient on this class of drugs who develops idiopathic serous macular detachment , one should probably consider stopping these drugs to see if there is an association.

REFERENCES AND FURTHER READING

Allibhai ZA, Gale JS, Sheidow TS. Central serous chorioretinopathy in a patient taking sildenafil citrate. Ophthalmic Surg Las Imag 35: 165–167, 2004.

Bollinger K, Lee MS. Recurrent visual field defect and ischemic optic neuropathy associated with tadalafil rechallenge. Arch Ophthalmol 123: 400–401, 2005.

Chandeclerc M, Martin S, Petitpain N, et al. Tadalafil and palpebral edema. South Med J 97: 1142–1143, 2004.

Donahue SP, Taylor RJ. Pupil-sparing third nerve palsy associated with sildenafil citrate (Viagra). Am J Ophthalmol 126: 476–477, 1998.

Egan RA, Fraunfelder FW. Viagra and anterior ischemic optic neuropathy. Arch Ophthalmol 123: 709–710, 2005.

Egan R, Pomeranz H. Sildenafil (Viagra) associated anterior ischemic optic neuropathy. Arch Ophthalmol 118: 291–292, 2000.

Escaravage GK, Wright JD, Givre SJ. Tadalafil associated with anterior ischemic optic neuropathy. Arch Ophthalmol 123: 399–400, 2005.

Fraunfelder FW. An overview of visual side effects associated with erectile dysfunction agents. Am J Ophthalmol 140: 723–724, 2005.

Fraunfelder FW, Fraunfelder FT. Scientific challenges in postmarketing surveillance of ocular adverse drug reactions. Am J Ophthalmol 143: 145–149, 2007.

Fraunfelder FT, Laties A. Visual side effects possibly associated with Viagra®. J Toxicol Cut Ocular Toxicol 19(1): 21–25, 2000.

Hayreh SS. Erectile dysfunction drugs and non-arteritic anterior ischemic optic neuropathy: is there a cause and effect relationship. J Neuro-ophthalmol 25: 285–298, 2005.

Laties AM, Siegel RL. Ocular safety in patients using sildenafil citrate therapy for erectile dysfunction. J Sex Med 3: 12–27, 2006.

Lee AG, Newman NJ. Erectile dysfunction drugs and nonarteritic anterior ischemic optic neuropathy. Am J Ophthalmol 140: 707–708, 2005.

McGwin G, Vaphiades MS, Hall TA, et al. Non-arteritic anterior ischaemic optic neuropathy and the treatment of erectile dysfunction. Br J Ophthalmol 90: 154–157, 2006.

Pomeranz HD, Bhavsar AR. Nonarteritic ischemic optic neuropathy developing soon after use of sildenafil (Viagra): a report of seven new cases. J Neuroophthalmol 25: 9–13, 2005.

Pomeranz HD, Smith KH, Hart WM, Jr, Egan RA. Sildenafil-associated non-arteritic anterior ischemic optic neuropathy. Ophthalmology 109: 584–587, 2002.

Quiram P, Dumars S, Parwar B, Sarraf D. Viagra-associated serous macular detachment. Graefe's Arch Clin Exp Ophthalmol 243: 339–344, 2005.

Zrenner E. How should Viagra-induced vision disorders – especially retinal degeneration – be evaluated? Klinische Monatsblatter fur Augenheilkunde 212(6): aA12–13, 1998.

CLASS: ESTROGENS AND PROGESTOGENS

Generic names: 1. Combination products of estrogens and progestogens; 2. medroxyprogesterone acetate.

Proprietary names: 1. Allesse, Aranelle, Aviane-28, Balziva-21, Brevicon-28,Cyclessa, Cryselle, Demulen, Desogen, Diane 35, Enpresse-28, Estrostep FE, Femhrt, Gencept 10, Junel, Junel FE, Kariva, Kelnor, Lessina-28, Levora, Loestrin 21/24, Loestrin FE, Lo/orval-28, Low-ogestrel-21, Microgestrin FE, Mircette, Norethin, Norinyl, Nortdette-28, Nortrel, Nuvaring, Ogestrel, Ortho-cept, Ortho-cyclen, Ortho-Evra, Ortho-Novum, Ortho-Novum 77, Ortho-Tricyclen, Ortho-Tricyclen lo, Ovcon-35/50, Ovral birth control, Portia-28, Previfem, Seasonale, Seasonique, Select, Sprintec, Trinorinyl-28, Triphasil, Tri-previfem, Tri-Sprintec, Trivara-28, Velivet, Yasmin 28, Yaz, Zovia; 2. Depo-Provera, Provera.

Primary use

These hormonal agents are used in the treatment of amenorrhea, dysfunctional uterine bleeding, premenstrual tension, dysmenorrhea, hypogonadism and, most commonly, as oral contraceptives.

Ocular side effects

Systemic administration
Certain
1. Decreased vision
2. Decreased tolerance to contact lenses
3. Problems with color vision
   a. Color vision defect – red-green or yellow-blue defect
   b. Objects have blue tinge
   c. Colored haloes around lights – mainly blue
4. Eyelids or conjunctiva
   a. Allergic reactions
   b. Edema
   c. Hyperpigmentation
   d. Photosensitivity
   e. Angioneurotic edema
   f. Urticaria
5. Cornea – steeping of curvature

Probable

1. Retinal vascular disorders
   a. Occlusion
   b. Thrombosis
   c. Hemorrhage (Fig. 7.7c)
   d. Retinal or macular edema
2. Papilledema secondary intracranial hypertension
3. Decreased accommodation (diethylstilbestrol)
4. Macular edema

Possible

1. Retinal vascular disorders
   a. Acute macular neuroretinopathy (co-factor)
   b. Periphlebitis
2. Increased ocular mucous
3. Optic neuritis
4. Cataracts
5. Eyelids or conjunctiva
   a. Lupoid syndrome
   b. Erythema multiforme

Clinical significance

Over 150 million women have taken this group of drugs and still there is significant debate as to what side effects are real. This confusion is in large part due to their ever-changing formulation with newer contraceptives. A higher incidence of migraine, thrombophlebitis and intracranial hypertension probably occurs in women taking oral contraceptives than in a comparable population. There is some evidence that combination oral contraceptives, which contain more progestins, have fewer side effects than those that contain mainly estrogens. There is an increased risk of venous thrombosis in patients on these medications. Risk factors include personal history of venous thrombosis, gross obesity and abnormalities of the hemostatic mechanism (Vandenbroucke et al 2001). Arterial thrombosis may be less likely but aging, smoking and hypertension may increase patient risk. Schwartz et al (1999) reported that both ischemic and hemorrhagic stroke associated with the 'pill' were double over controls if the woman had a history of migraine headaches. In a few cases, the courts have ruled that there is a cause-and-effect relationship between the use of oral contraceptives and retinal vascular abnormalities. In selected patients with retinal vascular abnormalities there should probably be informed consent or even the consideration of not taking the drug. If retinal vascular abnormalities develop, the use of these drugs in that patient may need to be re-evaluated. With long-term use, there are data that suggest there can be decreased color perception, mainly blue and yellow, and prolonged photostress recovery times. This is seldom clinically identified. If a patient has a transient ischemic attack, the oral contraceptive may need to be discontinued since the incidence of strokes is significantly increased. In the National Registry and the literature there are cases that implicate these drugs in causing macular edema. A number of these patients have been rechallenged with recurrence of the edema. Rait and O'Day (1987) stated that most patients with acute macular neuroretinopathy have been taking oral contraceptive medication in addition to other possible causative factors. They postulate the 'pill' as a possible cofactor. There is a suggestion that pregnancy causes progression of retinitis pigmentosa. Since these oral contraceptives cause a pseudo-pregnancy, there is a question of whether they may also cause progression of this retinal disease. However, there is no proof of this and most researchers feel these agents are safe for the retinitis pigmentosa patient to use.

The National Registry has received numerous case reports of cataracts possibly related to the administration of oral contraceptives. Recent data by Klein et al (1994) show no evidence to support this. In fact, oral contraceptives may even have a modest protective effect on the lens. Benitez et al (1997) and Harding (1994) both support Klein's data in well-designed studies. However, recently Cumming and Mitchell (1997), in the Blue Mountain Eye Study, have supported the hypothesis that estrogen and/or progestin may be involved in cataract development. We are therefore not sure and can only settle on a possible association. The problem in part is the lack of an easy accurate way to grade lenses. There is a relationship of oral contraceptives and contact lens intolerance. Candela et al (1989) found increased tear mucus production in patients on these drugs. Tomlinson et al (2001) could not confirm this. Mayer (1944) found transitory decreased accommodation on diethylstilbestrol. There are a number of case reports in the literature and in the National Registry of retrobulbar and optic neuritis, optic nerve pathology with various visual field abnormalities, pupillary abnormalities, uveitis, transient myopia, exophthalmos, paralysis of extraocular muscles and nystagmus. A clear cause-and-effect relationship between these events and the drug is difficult to prove. Most of these reports were from patients who were in the age range usually associated with multiple sclerosis.

Having said all of the above, Vessey et al (1998) in two large UK cohort studies suggested that oral contraceptive use does not increase the risk of eye disease, with the possible exception of retinal vascular lesions. However, based on the literature and National Registry data, our classifications are our 'best guesses' at this time.

REFERENCES AND FURTHER READING

Benitez del Castillo JM, del Rio T, Garcia-Sanchez J. Effects of estrogen use on lens transmittance in postmenopausal women. Ophthalmology 104: 970–973, 1997.

Byrne E. Retinal migraine and the pill. Med J Aust 2: 659, 1979.

Candela V, Castagna I, et al. Modification of conjunctival mucus secretion by pregnancy and oral contraceptives. Boll Oculist 68(Suppl 1): 19–23, 1989.

Chakrapani K, et al. Ovulation-associated uveitis. Br J Ophthalmol 66: 320, 1982.

Chilvers E, Rudge P. Cerebral venous thrombosis and subarachnoid haemorrhage in users of oral contraceptives. BMJ 292: 524, 1986.

Corbett MC, O'Brat DP, Warburton FG, et al. Biologic and environmental risk factors for regression after photorefractive keratectomy. Ophthalmology 103: 1381–1391, 1966.

Cumming RG, Mitchell P. Hormone replacement therapy, reproductive factors, and cataract: the Blue Mountain Eye Study. Am J Epidemiol 145(3): 242–249, 1997.

Goren SB. Retinal edema secondary to oral contraceptives: their side effects and ophthalmological manifestations. Surv Ophthalmol 14: 90–105, 1969.

Harding JJ. Estrogens and cataract. Arch Ophthalmol 112: 1511, 1994.

Hartge P, et al. Case-control study of female hormones and eye melanoma. Ophthalmology 5(1): 18, 1990.

Klein BEK, Klein R, Ritter LL. Is there evidence of an estrogen effect on age-related lens opacities. Arch Ophthalmol 112: 85–91, 1994.

Lalive d'Epinay SF, Trub P. Retinale vaskulare komplikationen bei oralen kontrazeptiva. Klin Monatsbl Augenheilkd 188: 394, 1986.

Mayer L. Effect of diethylstilbestrol on accommodation. Arch Ophthalmol 32: 133–134, 1944.

Perry ND, Mallen FJ. Cilioretinal artery occlusion associated with oral contraceptives. Am J Ophthalmol 84: 56, 1977.

Petursson GJ, Fraunfelder FT, Meyer SM. Oral contraceptives. Ophthalmology 88: 368, 1981.

Rait JL, O'Day J. Acute macular neuroretinopathy. Aust NZ J Ophthalmol 15: 337–340, 1987.

Rock T, Dinar Y, Romen M. Retinal periphlebitis after hormonal treatment. Ann Ophthalmol 21: 75–76, 1989.

Schwartz SM, et al. Risk of stroke in users of oral contraceptives. JAMA 281(14): 1255, 1999.

Snir M, et al. Retinal manifestations of thrombotic thrombocytopenic purpura (TTP) following use of contraceptive treatment. Ann Ophthalmol 17: 109, 1985.

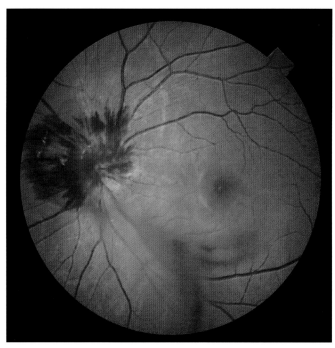

Fig. 7.7c Dense hemorrhage of the disc with vitreous hemorrhage. Photo courtesy of Higa A et al: Vitreous haemorrhage in a 19-year-old Japanese woman using an oral contraceptive. Acta Ophthalmol Scand 82(2): 244-246, 2004.

Stowe CC, III, Zakov ZN, Albert DM. Central retinal vascular occlusion associated with oral contraceptives. Am J Ophthalmol 86: 798, 1978.

Tagawa H, Yoshida A, Takahashi M. A case of bilateral branch vein occlusion due to long-standing use of oral contraceptives. Folia Ophthalmol Jpn 32: 1951, 1981.

Takahashi H, Sakai F, Sakuragi S. A case of retinal branch vein occlusion associated with oral contraceptives. Folia Ophthalmol Jpn 34: 2670, 1983.

Tomlinson A, Pearce EI, Simmons PA, et al. Effect of oral contraceptives on tear physiology. Ophthal Physiol Opt 21: 9–16, 2001.

Vandenbroucke JP, Rosing J, Bloemenkamp KWM, et al. Oral contraceptives and the risk of venous thrombosis. N Engl J Med 344: 1527–1535, 2001.

Vessey MP, et al. Oral contraception and eye disease: findings in two large cohort studies. Br J Ophthalmol 82: 538-542, 1998.

Generic name: Estradiol.

Proprietary names: Alora, Climara, Delestrogen, Estrace, Estraderm, Estrasorb, Estring, Estrogel, Femring, Femtrace, Gynodiol, Inofem, Menostar, Vagifem, Vivelle, Vivelle-Dot.

Primary use

This naturally occurring estrogen is administered in tablets, transdermal patches and vaginal creams, and used in the management of menopause, vulval and vaginal atrophy, ovarian failure, uterine bleeding, and prevention of osteoperosis.

Ocular side effects

Systemic administration – oral, transdermal patch or creams
Probable
1. Decreased vision
2. Decreased tolerance to contact lenses
3. Cornea
   a. Fluctuation of corneal curvature
   b. Increased steeping of cornea

4. Problems with color vision
   a. Color vision defect – red-green or yellow-blue defect
   b. Objects have blue tinge
   c. Colored haloes around lights – mainly blue
5. Eyelids or conjunctiva
   a. Allergic reactions
   b. Edema
   c. Hyperpigmentation
   d. Photosensitivity
   e. Angioneurotic edema
   f. Urticaria
   g. Ptosis

Possible
1. Retinal vascular disorders
   a. Occlusion
   b. Thrombosis
   c. Hemorrhage
   d. Retinal or macular edema
   e. Spasms
   f. Acute macular neuroretinopathy
   g. Periphlebitis
2. Papilledema secondary to intracranial hypertension
3. Eyelids or conjunctiva
   a. Lupoid syndrome
   b. Erythema multiforme

Clinical significance
This female hormone is largely responsible for the changes that take place at puberty in females and also provides their secondary sexual characteristics. These agents are infrequently given orally because of extensive first-pass hepatic metabolism and the resulting failure to produce high enough therapeutic blood levels. However, slow, sustained release from dermal patches or creams can produce systemic effects. Most ocular side effects are the same as those listed in Combination Products of Estrogens and Progestogens. Reports of fluctuation of corneal curvature, steepening of the cornea and intolerance of contact lens wear are probably real.

REFERENCES AND FURTHER READING

Gurwood AS, Gurwood I, Gubman DT, Brzezicki LJ. Idiosyncratic ocular symptoms associated with the estradiol transdermal estrogen replacement patch system. Optom Vis Sci 72(1): 29–33, 1995.

Physicians' Desk Reference, 60th edn, Thomson PDR, Montvale NJ, pp 795–800, 805–810, 2288–2293, 2340–2343, 3200–3205, 2006.

See also references of previous section, Combination Products of Estrogens and Progestogens.

Generic name: 1. Levonorgestrel; 2. norgestrel.

Proprietary names: 1. Mirena, Norplant II, Plan B; 2. multi-ingredient preparations only.

Primary use
Synthetic progestin given as an intradermal implant that acts as a long-term contraceptive agent.

Ocular side effects

Subdermal implantation
Probable
1. Decreased vision

Possible

1. Papilledema secondary to intracranial hypertension
2. Diplopia
3. Myasthenia gravis
   a. Diplopia
   b. Ptosis
   c. Paresis of extraocular muscles
4. Ocular porphyria

Clinical significance

Levonorgestrel is twice as potent as, and more commonly used than, norgestrel. Primarily, the documented side effects mentioned here are all for levonorgestrel. Alder et al (1995) reported 57 cases of intracranial hypertension or papilledema from a spontaneous reporting system and there are an additional 70 cases known to the manufacturer (Weber et al 1995), all possibly due to levonorgestrel. Alder's series of patients were female with a mean age of 23 years (range 16–34 years), with a mean levonorgestrel treatment of 175 days (range 9–616 days) before the onset of intracranial hypertension. Visual field defects were present in at least 12 cases, which were primarily enlarged blind spots. Diplopia, usually due to 6th nerve paresis, was present in 16 cases. However, there were at least 140 cases of blurred vision reported with patients taking this agent. The problem, of course, with this type of data is that intracranial hypertension occurs in this age group of persons without obesity at a rate of approximately 3.3 per 100 000 a year, therefore a report of 57 cases, with much of the data being incomplete, is suspect for causality. The drug first came on the market in 1991, and in 1994 the manufacturer first released the possible association of this drug with intracranial hypertension. They stated that in patients who have vision disturbances or headaches, especially headaches that change in frequency, pattern, severity or persistence, it is particularly important to view the optic nerves. Also, they suggest that patients who develop papilledema or intracranial hypertension have the implants removed. While not a proven association, one should probably remove the implants if optic nerve findings occur. Brittain and Lange (1995) reported myasthenia gravis occurring after insertion of a levonorgestrel implant and improving after its removal. Levonorgestrel has been associated with acute attacks of pophyria with various ocular and acute ocular findings. These include retinal edema, cotton wool spots, hemorrhages and scleral ulcers. Partial third nerve palsey, ptosis and mydriasis can occur.

REFERENCES AND FURTHER READING

Alder JB, Fraunfelder FT, Buchhalter JR. Levonorgestrel implants and intracranial hypertension. N Engl J Med 332(25): 1720–1721, 1995.

Brittain J, Lange LS. Myasthenia gravis and levonorgestrel implant. Lancet 346: 1556, 1995.

Physicians' Desk Reference, 60th edn, Thomson PDR, Montvale, NJ, pp 810–815, 2006.

Weber ME, et al. Levonorgestrel implants and intracranial hypertension. N Engl J Med 332: 1721, 1995.

CLASS: OVULATORY AGENTS

Generic name: Clomifene citrate.

Proprietary names: Clomid, Milophene, Serophene.

Primary use

This synthetic non-steroidal agent is effective in the treatment of anovulation.

Ocular side effects

Systemic administration
Certain

1. Visual sensations
   a. Flashing lights
   b. Scintillating scotomas
   c. Distortion of images secondary to sensations of waves or glare
   d. Various colored lights – mainly silver
   e. Phosphene stimulation
   f. Prolongation of after image
   g. Entoptic phenomenon
2. Decreased vision
3. Mydriasis
4. Visual fields
   a. Scotomas – central, paracentral, centrocecal
   b. Constriction
5. Photophobia
6. Eyelids or conjunctiva
   a. Allergic reactions
   b. Urticaria
   c. Loss of eyelashes or eyebrows

Probable

1. Decreased tolerance to contact lenses

Possible

1. Diplopia
2. Optic neuritis

Conditional/Unclassified

1. Cataracts
2. Retina
   a. Phebilitis
   b. Spasms
3. Increased intraocular pressure

Ocular teratogenic effects
Probable

1. Retinal aplasia
2. Cyclopia
3. Nystagmus

Clinical significance

Clomifene appears to have a unique effect on the retina that may occur in up to 10% of patients. This consists of any or all of the following: flashing lights, glare, various colored lines (often silver), multiple images, prolonged after images, 'like looking through heat waves', objects have 'comet' tails, phosphene stimulation and scintillating scotomas identical to migraine. These may occur as early as 48 hours after taking this agent and are reversible after stopping the medication. Transitory and prolonged decreased vision have also been reported. With prolonged use after years, vision loss in the 20/40 to 60 range may occur (etiology unknown), which may be slow to recover. Purvin reported three cases of irreversible prolonged visual disturbances (palinopsia), as described above. Cases in the National Registry support this. Bilateral acute reversible loss of vision, even in the light perception range, is a rare event. Mydriasis is common, but of a mild degree and reversible. Of major clinical significance are the unilateral or bilateral scotomas, and visual field constriction. It is of interest that classic scintillating scotoma seems to occur secondary to clomifene. In general, these side effects required discontinuing the medication. The causes of these are unclear but Padron Rivas et al (1994) and several cases in the National Registry suggest the possibility of an optic neuritis for some of these effects. These are in females in the multiple sclerosis age group and a cause-and-effect relationship is conjecture. Usually, the patient refuses to take further medication, and the long-term sequalae, if the drug is continued, are unclear. Decreased contact lens wear may be due to clomifene's ability to inhibit mucus production. Monocular and binocular diplopia have been reported but are not well documented. While the literature contains references to the cataractogenic potential of this agent, a drug-related cause has not been proven. There is one well-documented case in the National Registry of this agent causing bilateral elevated intraocular pressure. Lawton (1994) reported a case suggestive of anterior ischemic optic neuropathy on the basis that the drug may cause increased blood viscosity. If this were true, retinal vascular occlusions could also occur. This drug also has ocular teratogenic effects. It has been reported that about 1% of patients are forced to stop taking it secondary to ocular side effects.

REFERENCES AND FURTHER READING

Asch RH, Greenblatt RB. Update on the safety and efficacy of clomiphene citrate as a therapeutic agent. J Reprod Med 17: 175, 1976.

Kistner RW. The use of clomiphene citrate in the treatment of anovulation. Semin Drug Treatment 3(2): 159, 1973.

Kurachi K, Aono T, Minagawa J, Miyake A. Congenital malformations of newborn infants after clomiphene-induced ovulation. Fertil Steril 40(2): 187–189, 1983.

Laing IA et al. Clomiphene and congenital retinopathy. Lancet 2: 1107, 1981.

Lawton AW. Optic neuropathy associated with clomiphene citrate therapy. Fertil Steril 61(2): 390–391, 1994.

Padron Rivas VF, Sanchez Sanchez A, Lerida Arias MT et al. Optic neuritis appearing during treatment of clomiphene (letter). Atencion Primaria 14(7): 912–913, 1994.

Piskazeck VK, Leitsmann H. Uber die Behandlung derfunktionellen Sterilitat mit Clostylbegyt. Zentralbl Gynaekol 98: 904, 1976.

Purvin VA. Visual disturbance secondary to clomiphene citrate. Arch Ophthalmol 113(4): 482–484, 1995.

Roch LM, II et al: Visual changes associated with clomiphene citrate therapy. Arch Ophthalmol 77: 14, 1967.

Rock T, Dinar Y, Romen M. Retinal periphlebitis after hormonal treatment. Ann Ophthalmol 21: 75–76, 1989.

Van Der Merwe JV. The effect of clomiphene and conjugated oestrogens on cervical mucus. South Afr Med J 60(9): 347–349, 1981.

CLASS: THYROID HORMONES

Generic names: 1. Levothyroxine sodium; 2. liothyronine sodium; 3. thyroid.

Proprietary names: 1. Levolet, Levo-T, Levothroid, Levoxyl, Novothyrox, Synthroid, Unithroid; 2. Cytomel, Triostat; 3. Nature Throid.

Primary use

These thyroid hormones are effective in the replacement therapy of thyroid deficiencies such as hypothyroidism and simple goiter.

Ocular side effects

Systemic Administration

Certain
1. Decreased vision
2. Eyelids or conjunctiva
   a. Hyperemia
   b. Edema
3. Photophobia
4. Exophthalmos
5. Visual hallucinations

Probable
1. Eyelids or conjunctiva – angioneurotic edema
2. Papilledema secondary to intracranial hypertension

Possible
1. Myasthenia gravis
   a. Diplopia
   b. Ptosis
   c. Paresis of extraocular muscles
2. Open-angle glaucoma (levothyroxine)
3. Blepharospasm

Clinical significance

Lee et al (2004) found a possible association of glaucoma and thyroid disease in the Blue Mountains Eye Study. This was particularly true in patients currently treated with levothyroxine. They stated, however, that further evaluation of this potential association is warranted. There are numerous articles suggesting that this group of drugs can cause intracranial hypertension. Prepubertal and peripubertal hypothyroid children may be the most susceptible to intracranial hypertension when beginning this group of drugs. Sundaram et al (1985) reported petit mal status epilepticus with rapid rhythmic eyelid fluttering and blinking occurring in a patient approximately 1 week after starting levothyroxine therapy. Lledo Carreres et al (1992) reported a case of toxic internuclear ophthalmoplegia after the use of these agents for weight loss. Visual hallucinations have appeared soon after initiation of thyroid replacement therapy in hypothyroid patients, usually in patients with an underlying psychiatric disorder. Other than the CNS changes, most ocular findings clear within a few months of discontinuing the medication.

REFERENCES AND FURTHER READING

Hymes LC, Warshaw BL, Schwartz JF. Pseudotumor cerebri and thyroid-replacement therapy. N Engl J Med 309: 732, 1983.

Josephson AM, MacKensie TP. Thyroid-induced mania in hypothyroid patients. Br J Psychiatry 137: 222, 1980.

Kaeser HE. Drug-induced myasthenic syndromes. Acta Neurol Scand 70(Suppl. 100): 39, 1984.

Lee AJ, Rochtchina E, Wang JJ, et al. Open-angle glaucoma and systemic thyroid disease in an older population: the Blue Mountains Eye Study. Eye 28: 600–608, 2004.

Lledo Carreres M, Lajo Garrido JL, Gonzalez Rico M, et al. Toxic internuclear ophthalmoplegia related to antiobesity treatment. Ann Pharm 26(11): 1457–1458, 1992.

McVie R. Pseudotumor cerebri and thyroid-replacement therapy. N Engl J Med 309: 731, 1983.

Misra M, Khan GM, Rath S. Eltroxin induced pseudotumor cerebri? A case report. Indian J Ophthalmol 40(4): 117, 1992.

Raghavan S, DiMartino-Nardi J, Saenger P, Linder B. Pseudotumor cerebri in an infant after L-thyroxine therapy for transient neonatal hypothyroidism. J Ped 130(3): 478–480, 1997.

Sundaram MBM, Hill A, Lowry N. Thyroxine-induced petit mal status epilepticus. Neurology 35: 1792, 1985.

Van Dop C, et al. Pseudotumor cerebri associated with initiation of levothyroxine therapy for juvenile hypothyroidism. N Engl J Med 308:1076, 1983.

SECTION 8
AGENTS AFFECTING BLOOD FORMATION AND COAGULABILITY

CLASS: AGENTS USED TO TREAT DEFICIENCY ANEMIAS

Generic name: Cobalt.

Proprietary names: None.

Primary use
This agent is used in the treatment of iron-deficiency anemia.

Ocular side effects

Systemic administration
Probable
1. Eyelids or conjunctiva
   a. Allergic reactions
   b. Photosensitivity
   c. Urticaria
2. Uveitis (skin tattoo)

Possible
1. Decreased vision
2. Optic atrophy

Clinical significance
Cobalt is now only occasionally used since significant systemic side effects occur and safer drugs are available. Only rarely are ocular side effects due to cobalt therapy seen, and decreased vision is the most common complaint. Rorsman et al (1969) reported three cases of uveitis associated with cobalt skin tattooing. Each time a reaction at the tattoo site occurred, the uveitis exacerbated. Fraunfelder and Rosenbaum (1997) speculated that this is a type IV hypersensitivity reaction. There are two well-described cases of long-term cobalt treatment causing bilateral optic atrophy (Licht et al 1972; Meecham and Humphrey 1991).

REFERENCES AND FURTHER READING
Camarasa JG, Alomar A. Photosensitization to cobalt in a bricklayer. Contact Dermatitis 7: 154, 1981.
Fraunfelder FW, Rosenbaum JT. Drug-induced uveitis: incidence, prevention, and treatment. Drug Safety 17(3): 197–207, 1997.
Gilman AG, Goodman LS, Gilman A. (eds). The Pharmacological Basis of Therapeutics, 6th edn. Macmillan, New York, p 1326–1327, 1980.
Hjorth N. Contact dermatitis in children. Acta Derm Venereal 95(Suppl): 36, 1981.
Licht A, Oliver M, Rachmilewitz EA. Optic atrophy following treatment with cobalt chloride in a patient with pancytopenia and hypercellular marrow. Isr J Med Sci 8: 61–66, 1972.
Meecham HM, Humphrey P. Industrial exposure to cobalt causing optic atrophy and nerve deafness: a case report. J Neurol Neruosurg Psychiat 54: 374–375, 1991.
Rorsman H, et al. Tattoo granuloma and uveitis. Lancet 2: 27–28, 1969.
Smith JD, Odom RB, Maibach HI. Contact urticaria from cobalt chloride. Arch Dermatol 111: 1610, 1975.
Walsh FB, Hoyt WF. Clinical Neuro-Ophthalmology, Vol. III, 3rd edn, Williams & Wilkins, Baltimore, pp 2686–2687, 1969.

Generic name: Epoetin (erythropoietin).

Proprietary names: Epogen, Procrit.

Primary use
Recombinant human epoetin is used in the treatment of anemia in chronic renal failure in dialysis patients.

Ocular side effects

Systemic administration
Probable
1. Decreased vision
2. Iritis-like reaction
3. Retina
   a. Induces retinal angiogenesis
   b. Enhances retinopathy of prematurity
4. Conjunctiva – hyperemia

Possible
1. Visual hallucinations

Conditional/Unclassified
1. Recurrent post-operative lens capsule opacity

Clinical significance
Low birth weight premature infants are at higher risk for retinitis of prematurity and may undergo treatment with epoetin to prevent anemia of prematurity. Manzoni et al (2005) have reported this drug as an additional independent predictor of severe threshold retinopathy of prematurity, requiring urgent ablative surgery. This occurred in 31% of infants on this drug compared to 19.6% of those not receiving this agent. Kelley (2002) reported proliferation of lens capsular debris that may be due to epoetin. Beiran et al (1996) described 13 patients with an iritis-like reaction associated with the use of epoetin. They feel this may be related to epoetin's ability to alter prostaglandin levels, which may break the tight junctions of the iris and ciliary epithelium. Watanabe et al (2005) reported epoetin as a factor in inducing retinal angiogenesis in proliferative diabetic retinopathy. Patients on hemodialysis receiving epoetin may develop visual hallucinations.

REFERENCES AND FURTHER READING
Beiran I, Krasnitz I, Mezer E, et al. Erythropoietin induced iritis-like reaction. Eur J Ophthalmol 6(1): 14–16, 1996.
Kelley JS. Recurrent capsular opacity and erythropoietin. American Ophthalmological Society Meeting, 2002.
Manzoni P, Maestri A, Gomirato G. Erythropoietin as a retinal angiogenic factor. N Engl J Med 353: 782–792, 2005.
Stead R. Erythropoietin and visual hallucinations (reply). N Engl J Med 325(July 25): 285, 1991.
Steinberg H. Erythropoietin and visual hallucinations (letter). N Engl J Med 325: 285, 1991.
Steinberg H, Saravay SM, Wadhwa N, et al. Erythropoietin and visual hallucinations in patients on dialysis. Psychosomatics 37(6): 556–563, 1996.
Watanabe D, Suzuma K, Matsui S, et al. Erythropoietin as a retinal angiogenic factor in proliferative diabetic retinopathy. N Engl J Med 353: 782–792, 2005.

Generic names: 1. Ferrous fumarate; 2. ferrous gluconate; 3. ferrous sulfate; 4. iron dextran; 5. iron sucrose; 6. polysaccharide-iron complex.

Proprietary names: 1. Femiron, Feostat, Ferretts, Hemaspan, Hemocyte, Nephro-Fer, Vitron-C; 2. Fergon; 3. Ed-in-sol, Feosol, Fer-gen-sol, Fe-Iron, Feratab, Fero-Grad, Isospran, Slow-Fe; 4. Dexferrum, Infed, Proferdex; 5. Venofer; 6. Fe-Tinic, Ferrex, Ferrex Plus, Hytinic, Niferex, Nu-Iron, Poly-Iron.

Primary use

These iron preparations are effective in the prophylaxis and treatment of iron-deficiency anemias.

Ocular side effects

Systemic administration (toxic levels)
Certain
1. Decreased vision (iron dextran)
2. Yellow-brown discoloration
   a. Sclera
   b. Choroid
3. Eyelids or conjunctiva (iron dextran)
   a. Erythema
   b. Edema
   c. Angioneurotic edema
   d. Urticaria
   e. Photosensitivity reactions

Probable
1. Retinal degeneration – overdosage

Inadvertent ocular exposure
Certain
1. Irritation
   a. Hyperemia
   b. Photophobia
   c. Edema
2. Yellow-brown discoloration or deposits
   a. Eyelids
   b. Conjunctiva
   c. Cornea
   d. Sclera

Probable
1. Ulceration
   a. Eyelids
   b. Conjunctiva
   c. Cornea

Clinical significance

Systemically administered iron preparations seldom cause ocular side effects. Adverse ocular reactions have been reported after multiple blood transfusions (over 100), with unusually large amounts of iron in the diet or markedly prolonged iron therapy. A few cases of retinitis pigmentosa-like fundal degeneration have been reported. Hodgkins et al (1992) described a case of pigment epitheliopathy with an overlying serous retinal detachment following an infusion of iron dextran. Newer iron preparations make retinal degenerations less likely. Kawada et al (1996) described photosensitivity reactions due to sodium ferrous citrate.

Direct ocular exposure to acidic ferrous salts can cause ocular irritation, but significant ocular side effects rarely occur.

REFERENCES AND FURTHER READING

Appel I, Barishak YR. Histopathologic changes in siderosis bulbi. Ophthalmologica 176: 205, 1978.

Brunette JR, Wagdi S, Lafond G. Electroretinographic alterations in retinal metallosis. Can J Ophthalmol 15: 176, 1980.

Declercq SS. Desferrioxamine in ocular siderosis. Br J Ophthalmol 64: 626, 1980.

Hodgkins PR, Morrell AJ, Luff AJ, et al. Pigment epitheliopathy with serous detachment of the retina following intravenous iron dextran. Eye 6(Pt 4): 414–415, 1992.

Kawada A, Hiruma M, Noguchi H, et al. Photosensitivity due to sodium ferrous citrate. Contact Dermatitis 34(1): 77, 1996.

Kearns M, McDonald R. Generalized siderosis from an iris foreign body. Aust J Ophthalmol 8: 311, 1980.

Salminen L, Paasio P, Ekfors T. Epibulbar siderosis induced by iron tablets. Am J Ophthalmol 93: 660, 1982.

Syversen K. Intramuscular iron therapy and tapetoretinal degeneration. Acta Ophthalmol 57: 358, 1979.

Wolter JR. The lens as a barrier against foreign body reaction. Ophthalmic Surg 12: 42, 1981.

Generic name: Methylthioninium chloride (methylene blue).

Proprietary name: Urolene Blue.

Primary use

Systemic
Methylthioninium is a weak germicidal agent used as a urinary or gastrointestinal antiseptic. It is also given intravenously in the treatment of methemoglobinemia and 'cyanosis anemia'. It is also used as a dye to demonstrate cerebrospinal fluid fistulae or blocks.

Ophthalmic
Methylthioninium is used as a tissue marker during ocular or lacrimal surgery and has been applied to the conjunctiva to decrease glare during microsurgery.

Ocular side effects

Intrathecal and intraventricular injections
Certain
1. Decreased vision
2. Blue-gray discoloration
   a. Vitreous and retina
   b. Eyelids
3. Problems with color vision – objects have blue tinge

Probable
1. Decreased accommodation (intravenous)
2. Mydriasis (intravenous)

Possible
1. Papilledema
2. Diplopia
3. Paresis of extraocular muscles
4. Accommodative spasm
5. Optic atrophy
6. Subconjunctival or retinal hemorrhages secondary to drug-induced anemia

Intracameral injection
Certain
1. Cytotoxicity
   a. Corneal endothelium
   b. Iris

Local ophthalmic use or exposure
Certain
1. Irritation
    a. Lacrimation
    b. Edema
    c. Burning sensation
    d. Photosensitivity
2. Blue discoloration or staining
    a. Eyelid margins
    b. Conjunctiva
    c. Corneal nerves and epithelium
3. Cornea – endothelial toxicity

Clinical significance

Significant ocular side effects due to methylthioninium have only been reported with intrathecal or intraventricular injections and with intracameral injections at high concentrations. The most common ocular side effects after intravenous administration other than cyanopsia or blue-gray discoloration of ocular tissue are decreased vision, mydriasis and decreased accommodation. Porat et al (1996) have shown that this drug can be a photosensitizer, causing significant skin reactions with blue staining of tissues.

Infrequent use of topical ocular application of methylthioninium in low concentrations (1%) is almost free of ocular side effects. However, irritation and pain may be so severe that a local anesthetic may be required for the patient's comfort. Kushner (1993) reports a case in which this agent was used to irrigate the lacrimal system in a 2-year-old. The solution broke through to the periocular tissue, causing subcutaneous necrosis and marked edema along with bluish discoloration. Edema persisted for up to 2 years and amblyopia treatment was necessary. Staining of ocular and periocular tissue may be permanent if the dye is applied daily for years. Intracameral use appears safe if used in low concentration. Brouzas et al (2006) reported that inadvertent intracameral injection of 1% methylthioninium chloride may possibly cause extreme cytotoxicity of the corneal endothelium. Low concentrations may possibly aggravate already diseased endothelium, but this is theoretical.

REFERENCES AND FURTHER READING

Brouzas D, Droutsas S, Charakidas A. Severe toxic effect of methylene blue 1% on iris epithelium and corneal endothelium. Cornea 25: 470–471, 2006.

Chang YS, Tseng SY, Tseng SH, et al. Comparison of eyes for cataract surgery. Part 1: cytotoxicity to corneal endothelial cells in a rabbit model. J Cataract Refract Surg 31: 792–798, 2005.

Evans JP, Keegan HR. Danger in the use of intrathecal methylene blue. JAMA 174: 856, 1560.

Kushner BJ. Solutions can be hazardous for lacrimal system irrigation. Arch Ophthalmol 111: 904–905, 1993.

Lubeck MJ. Effects of drugs on ocular muscles. Int Ophthalmol Clin 11(2): 35, 1971.

Morax S, Limon S, Forest A. Exogenous conjunctival pigmentation by methylene blues. Arch Ophthalmol 37: 708A, 1977.

Norn MS. Methylene blue (Methylthionine) vital staining of the cornea and conjunctiva. Acta Ophthalmol 45: 347, 1967.

Pasticier-Florquin B, et al. Ocular tattooing from abuse of methylene blue collyrium. Bull Soc Ophtalmol Fr 77: 147, 1977.

Perry PM, Meinhard E. Necrotic subcutaneous abscesses following injections of methylene blue. Br J Clin Pract 8: 289–291, 1974.

Porat R, Gilbert S, Magilner D. Methylene blue-induced phototoxicity: an unrecognized complication. Pediatrics 97(5): 717–721, 1996.

Raimer SS, Quevedo EM, Johnston RV. Dye rashes. Cutis 63(2): 103–106, 1999.

Uttley SA. Methylene blue-associated corneal decompensation. Poster. AAO.

CLASS: ANTICOAGULANTS

Generic names: 1. Alteplase; 2. reteplase; 3. tenecteplase.

Proprietary names: 1. Activase, Cathflo activase; 2. Retavase; 3. TNKase.

Primary use

Systemic
These tissue plasminogen activators (t-PA) are produced by recombinant DNA technology and are primarily indicated for the management of acute myocardial infarctions. Alteplase is also used in the management of acute ischemic stroke and pulmonary embolism.

Ophthalmic
Used to treat submacular hemorrhages, post vitrectomy fibrin syndrome, fibrin lysis, lysis of blood clots, intravitreal t-PA and pneumatic displacement for submacular hemorrhages, central retinal artery occlusion.

Ocular side effects

Systemic administration – intravenous injections
Certain
1. Hemorrhages
    a. Hyphema
    b. Retinal
    c. Orbital
    d. Choroidal
    e. Vitreous
    f. Retrobulbar
    g. Subretinal

Probable
1. Eyelids or conjunctiva
    a. Allergic reactions
    b. Angioneurotic edema
    c. Rashes
    d. Urticaria

Intracrameral injections
Certain
1. Hemorrhages
    a. Subconjunctival
    b. Hyphemia
2. Cornea
    a. Band keratopahty
    b. Calcium phosphate precipitates
3. Retina – vitreous hemorrhage

Intravitreal injections
Certain
1. Retina toxicity (high dosages)
    a. Diffuse pigmentary changes
    b. Exudative retinal detachment
    c. Granular hyperfluorescent lesion (flourscein angiography) (Fig. 7.8a)
2. ERG (high dosage) – reduce scotopic and photoic a and b waves
3. Vitreous hemorrhages

Clinical significance
The major toxicity of tissue plasminogen activators (t-PAs) is hemorrhage. This results either from lysis of fibrin at the sites of vascular injury or a systemic lytic state from the formation of systemic plasmin, which produces fibrinogenolysis and the destruction of other coagulation factors.

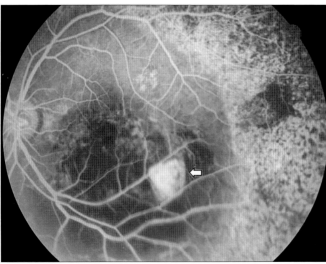

Fig. 7.8a Fluorescein angiography of diffuse granular hyperfluorescence. Photo courtesy of Chen S-N, et al. Retinal toxicity of intravitreal tissue plasminogen activator. Ophthalmology 110: 704–708, 2003.

Systemically administered t-PA for various illnesses can cause bleeding anywhere within the eye or periorbital tissues. This may occur in sites of recent ocular surgery (Khawly et al 1996; Roaf et al 1997) or be associated with the presence of exudative macular degeneration or retinal vascular diseases (Kaba et al 2005). Visual outcomes vary from no complications to blindness, or loss of the eye. Chorich et al (1998) emphasized that the onset of eye pain or vision loss after systemic t-PA should alert physicians to the possibility of an ocular or adnexal hemorrhage.

Intracameral injection complications are much more frequent in single dosage over 25 μg and/or multiple t-PA intracameral injections. Hyphemas (Tripathi et al 1991; Lundy et al 1996; Loffler et al 1997), subconjunctival hemorrhage (Lee et al 1995) and vitreous hemorrhages (Kim et al 1998) have all been reported. Rehfeldt and Hoh (1999), in their series of 185 intracameral t-PA injections, had a 5.4% incidence of hypema and a 3.2% incidence of transient corneal edema. This included one case of Fuch's dystrophy, which had irreversible corneal endothelial decompensation. Hesse et al (1999a) confirmed the temporary endothelial toxicity of t-PA. Damage to the corneal endothelium allows phosphate (buffer of t-PA) and calcium from the aqueous humour to distribute within the corneal stroma. The insoluble calcium phosphate may then be precipitated within the stroma. This results in irreversible corneal opacification. While this side effect is rare, it is easily produced in experimental animal models when the cornea endothelium is disturbed (Hesse et al 1999b).

Intravitreal injection complications increase with single dosages exceeding 50 μg and/or with repeat injections. Frequently, intravitreal t-PA is used along with pneumatic displacement, which adds a mechanical variable for possible ocular complications. Hesse et al (1999b) described four patients given 100 μg intravitreal t-PA who developed exudative retinal detachment followed by hyperpigmentation of the retinal pigment epithelium in the area of the detachment. Chen et al (2003) reported a case similar to the above after two successive injections of 50 μg intravitreal t-PA, 3 days apart with a minimal recovery of visual acuity. Because of numerous reports of retinal toxicity in animals and humans (Hrach et al 2000), Chen et al (2003) advocate not using an injection over 25 μg. Hassan et al (1999) varied

this by recommending 25–100 μg and Hesse et al (1999b) felt higher dosages were indicated. Intravitreal t-PA can cause sudden severe vitreous hemorrhages as an immediate complication (Kokame 2000).

REFERENCES AND FURTHER READING

Berry C, Weir C, Hammer H. A case of intraocular haemorrhage secondary to thrombolytic therapy. Acta Ophthalmol Scand 80: 561–562, 2002.

Chen S-N, Yang T-C, Cheng-Lien H, et al. Retinal toxicity of intravitreal tissue plasminogen activator: case report and literature review. Ophthalmology 110: 704–708, 2003.

Chorich LJ, Derick RJ, Chambers RB, et al. Hemorrhagic ocular complications associated with the use of systemic thrombolytic agents. Ophthalmology 105: 428–431, 1998.

Djalilian AR, Cantril HC, Samuelson TW. Intraocular hemorrhage after systemic thrombolytic therapy in a patient with exudative macular degeneration. Eur J Ophthalmol 13: 96–98, 2003.

Hassan AS, Johnson MW, Schneiderman TE, et al. Management of submacular hemorrhage with intravitreous tissue plasminogen activator injection and pneumatic displacement. Ophthalmology 106: 1900–1907, 1999.

Hesse L. Treating subretinal hemorrhage with tissue plasminogen activator. Arch Ophthalmol 120: 102–103, 2002.

Hesse L, Nebelin B, Kauffmann T. Etiology of corneal opacities after plasminogen activator-induced fibrinolysis of the anterior chamber. Ophthalmology 96: 448–452, 1999a.

Hesse L, Schmidt J, Kroll P. Management of acute submacular hemorrhage using recombinant tissue plasminogen activator and gas. Graefes Arch Clin Exp Ophthalmol 237: 273–277, 1999b.

Hrach CJ, Johson MW, Hassan AS, et al. Retinal toxicity of commercial intravitreal tissue plasminogen activator solution in cat eyes. Arch Ophthalmol 118: 659–663, 2000.

Kaba RA, Lewis A, Bloom P, et al. Intraocular haemorrhage after thrombolysis. Lancet 365: 330, 2005.

Khawly JA, Ferrone PJ, Holck DEE. Choroidal hemorrhage associated with systemic tissue plasminogen activator. Am J Ophthalmol 121: 577–578, 1996.

Kim MH, Koo TH, Sah WJ, et al. Treatment of total hyphema with relatively low dose tissue plasminogen activator. Ophthalmic Surg Laser 29: 762–766, 1998.

Kokame GT. Vitreous hemorrhage after intravitreal tissue plasminogen activator (t-PA) and pneumatic displacement of submacular hemorrhage. Am J Ophthalmol 129: 546–547, 2000.

Lee PF, Myers KS, Hsieh MM, et al. Treatment of failing glaucoma filtering cystic blebs with tissue plasminogen activator (t-PA). J Ocul Pharmacol Ther 11: 227–232, 1995.

Leong JK, Ghabrial R, McCluskey PJ. Orbital haemorrhage complication following postoperative thrombolysis. Br J Ophthalmol 87: 655–656, 2003.

Loffler KV, Meyer JH, Wollensak G, et al. Success and complications of rTPA treatment of the anterior eye segment. Opthalmologe 94: 50–52, 1997.

Lundy DL, Sidoti P, Winarko T, et al. Intracameral tissue plasminogen activator after glaucoma surgery. Ophthalmology 103: 274–282, 1996.

Rehfeldt K, Hoh H. Therapeutic and prophylactic application of TPA (recombinant tissue plasminogen activator) into the anterior chamber of the eye. Ophthalmologe 96: 587–593, 1999.

Roaf E, DaSilva C, Tsao K, et al. Orbital hemorrhage after thrombolytic therapy. Arch Intern Med 157: 2670–2671, 1997.

Skolnick CA, Fiscella RG, Tessles HH, et al. Tissue plasminogen activator to treat impending papillary block glaucoma in patients with acute fibrinous HLA-B27 positive iridocyclitis. Am J Ophthalmol 129: 363–366, 2000.

Smith MF, Doyle JW. Use of tissue plasminogen activator to revive blebs following intraocular surgery. Arch Ophthalmol 119: 809–812, 2001.

Tripathi RC, Tripathi BJ, Park JK, et al. Intracameral tissue plasminogen activator for resolution of fibrin clots after glaucoma filtering procedures. Am J Ophthalmol 111: 247–248, 1991.

Generic name: Heparin.

Proprietary names: Hepflush-10, Hep-lock, Hep-lock U/P.

Primary use

This complex organic acid inhibits the blood-clotting mechanism and is used in the prophylaxis and treatment of venous thrombosis.

Ocular side effects

Systemic administration
Certain
1. Subconjunctival, anterior chamber or retinal hemorrhages
   a. Secondary to drug-induced anticoagulation
   b. Secondary to drug-induced anemia
2. Eyelids or conjunctiva
   a. Allergic reactions
   b. Conjunctivitis – non-specific
   c. Angioneurotic edema
   d. Urticaria
   e. Necrosis

Probable
1. Lacrimation

Possible
1. Eyelids or conjunctiva – Lyell's syndrome

Local ophthalmic use or exposure – subconjunctival injection
Certain
1. Subconjunctival or periocular hemorrhages

Probable
1. Subconjunctival scarring
2. Decreased intraocular pressure (minimal)

Possible
1. Exacerbation of primary disease

Clinical significance

Ocular side effects due to systemic heparin are few and usually of little consequence. Ocular hemorrhage is the most serious adverse reaction and is probably more common in conditions with increased capillary fragility such as diabetes (Levartovsky et al 2003). Subconjunctival or periocular hemorrhage is the most common adverse reaction with subconjunctival heparin injections. It is more common after the third or fourth injection and seldom prevents continuous injections of heparin. Chang et al (1996) described two pregnant women who developed spontaneous orbital hemorrhages following treatment with subcutaneous heparin. Both women developed severe unilateral visual loss. Heparin-induced antiheparin platelet antibody leads to the thrombosis of ocular circulation (Nguyen et al 2003). Slusher et al (1975) reported hyphema in an otherwise normal eye seen 1 hour after 10 000 units of heparin were administered intravenously. The National Registry has received a single case each of sudden onset of severe keratoconjunctivitis sicca associated with the use of intravenous or subcutaneous heparin injections.

REFERENCES AND FURTHER READING

Aronson SB, Elliott JH. Ocular Inflammation. Mosby, St Louis, pp 91–92, 1972.

Chang WJ, Nowinski TS, Repke CS, et al. Spontaneous orbital hemorrhage in pregnant women treated with subcutaneous heparin. Am J Ophthalmol 122(6): 907–908, 1996.
Leung A. Toxic epidermal necrolysis associated with maternal use of heparin. JAMA 253: 201, 1985.
Levartovsky S, Reisin I, Reisin I, et al. Bilateral posterior segment intraocular hemorrhage in a diabetic patient after therapy with heparin. Isr Med Assoc J 5: 605, 2003.
Levine LE, et al. Heparin-induced cutaneous necrosis unrelated to injection sites. Arch Dermatol 119: 400, 1983.
Lipson ML. Toxicity of systemic agents. Int Ophthalmol Clin 11(2): 159, 1971.
Nguyen QD, Van DV, Feke GT, et al. Heparin-induced antiheparin-platelet antibody associated with retinal venous thrombosis. Ophthalmology 110: 600–603, 2003.
Slusher MM, Hamilon RW. Spontaneous hyphema during hemodialysis. N Engl J Med 293: 561, 1975.
Zurcher K, Krebs A. Cutaneous Side Effects of Systemic Drugs, S. Karger, Basel, pp 18–19, 300-303, 1980.

Generic name: Streptokinase.

Proprietary name: Streptase.

Primary use

This protein is used to dissolve thrombi in patients with myocardial infarction, pulmonary embolism and other thromboembolic occlusions of veins and arteries.

Ocular side effects

Systemic administration – intravenous
Certain
1. Bleeding
   a. Periocular
   b. Tenon's capsule
   c. Intraocular hemorrhage
   d. Total hyphema
   e. Choroidal hematoma
   f. Vitreous hemorrhage
   g. Postoperative ocular bleeding
2. Anterior uveitis
3. Eyelids and orbit
   a. Urticaria
   b. Rash
   c. Angioneurotic edema

Conditional/Unclassified
1. Central retinal artery occlusion

Clinical significance

There are a number of reports of streptokinase causing intraocular bleeding, hyphemas, vitreous hemorrhages or choroidal hematomas. Cahane et al (1990) reported a total hyphema secondary to streptokinase after cataract surgery. Marcus and Frederick (1994) described a case of streptokinase-induced tenon's capsule hemorrhage following retinal detachment surgery. The patient received intravenous streptokinase 2 hours after surgery when he developed a myocardial infarct. Potdar et al (2001) reported a case of unilateral central retinal artery occlusion following intravenous streptokinase, possibly due to an emboli leading to optic atrophy and blindness. There are a number of cases (Kinshuck 1992; Birnbaum et al 1993; Gray and Lazarus 1994; Proctor and Joondeph 1994; Fraunfelder and Rosenbaum 1997) of primarily bilateral anterior uveitis. Streptokinase-induced serum sickness, which Proctor and Joondeph (1994) felt occurs about 6% of the time, may occasionally exhibit a uveitis. Streptokinase-induced uveitis is most likely a result of an immune complex reaction, like serum sickness, and not due to any specific toxicity to the eye (Fraunfelder and Rosenbaum 1997). Anterior chamber injections of this agent for dissolution of fibrin exudates have had no detectable adverse intraocular effects (Cherfan et al 1991). Berger (1962) stated that there was intraocular irritation secondary to streptokinase, but it is possible that the drug used was not in as purified a form as is available now. Up to one-third of patients who have received repeat injections of this drug have become hypersensitive to it. This may present by periorbital swelling or angioneurotic edema.

REFERENCES AND FURTHER READING

Battershill PE, Benfield P, Goa KL. Streptokinse: a review of its pharmacology and therapeutic efficacy in acute myocardial infarction in older patients. Drugs & Aging 4(1): 63–86, 1994.

Beare N. 'Hyperacute' unilateral anterior uveitis and secondary glaucoma following streptokinase infusion. Eye 18: 111, 2004.

Bec P, Arne JL, et al. Choroidal and vitreous hemorrhage in the course of treatment of a thrombosis of the central retinal vein with streptokinase. Bull Soc Ophthalmol France 80: 607–609, 1980.

Berger B. The effect of streptokinase irrigation on experimentally clotted blood in the anterior chamber of human eyes. Acta Ophthalmol 40: 373–378, 1962.

Birnbaum T, et al. Acute iritis and transient renal impairment following thrombolytic therapy for acute myocardial infarction (letter). Ann Pharmacother 27(12): 1539–1540, 1993.

Boyer HK, et al. Studies on simulated vitreous hemorrhages. Arch Ophthalmol 59: 333–336, 1958.

Cahane M, et al. Total hyphaema following streptokinase administration eight days after cataract extraction. Br J Ophthalmol 74: 447, 1990.

Caramelli B, et al. Retinal haemorrhage after thrombolytic therapy. Lancet 337: 1356–1357, 1991.

Cherfan GM, et al. Dissolution of intraocular fibrinous exudate by streptokinase. Ophthalmology 98(6): 870–874, 1991.

Fraunfelder FW, Rosenbaum JT. Drug-induced uveitis: incidence, prevention, and treatment. Drug Safety 17(3): 197–207, 1997.

Glikson M, et al. Thrombolytic therapy for acute myocardial infarction following recent cataract surgery. Am Heart J 121: 1542–1543, 1991.

Gray MY, Lazarus JH. Iritis after treatment with streptokinase. Drug Points. BMJ 309: 97, 1994.

Kinshuck D. Bilateral hypopyon and streptokinase. Drug Points. BMJ 305(6865): 1332, 1992.

Lundgren B, Ocklind A, Holst A, Harfstrand A. Inflammatory response in the rabbit eye after intraocular implantation with poly(methyl methacrylate) and heparin surface modified intraocular lenses. J Cat Refract Surg 18(1): 65–70, 1992.

Manners TD, Turner DPJ, Galloway PH, Glenn AM. Heparinised intraocular infusion and bacterial contamination in cataract surgery. Br J Ophthalmol 81: 949–952, 1997.

Marcus DM, Frederick AR Jr. Streptokinase-induced tenon's hemorrhage after retinal detachment surgery. Am J Ophthalmol 118(6): 815–816, 1994.

Oliveira DC, Coelho OR, Paraschin K, et al. Angioedema related to the use of streptokinase. Arq Br Cardiol 85: 131–134, 2005.

Ortega-Carnicer J, Porras-Leal L, Fernandez-Ruiz A. Intraocular hemorrhage after intravenous streptokinase. Med Clin 115: 718–719, 2000.

Pick R, et al. Acute renal failure following repeated streptokinase therapy for pulmonary embolism. West J Med 138: 878–880, 1983.

Potdar NA, Shinde CA, Murthy GG, et al. Unilateral central retinal artery occlusion following intravenous streptokinase. J Postgrad Med 47: 262–263, 2001.

Proctor BD, Joondeph BC. Bilateral anterior uveitis. A feature of streptokinase-induced serum sickness. N Engl J Med 330: 576, 1994.

Steinemann T, et al. Acute closed-angle glaucoma complicating hemorrhagic choroidal detachment associated with parenteral thrombolytic agents. Am J Ophthalmol 106: 752–753, 1988.

Sunderraj P. Intraocular hemorrhage associated with intravenously administered streptokinase. Am J Ophthalmol 112(6): 734–735, 1991.

Van den Berg E, Lohmann N, Friedburg D, Rabe F. Report of general temporary anticoagulation in the treatment of acute cerebral and retinal ischaemia. Vasa 26(3): 222–227, 1997.

Winther-Nielson A, Johansen J, Pedersen GK, Corydon L. Posterior capsule opacification and neodymium: YAG capsulotomy with heparin-surface-modified intraocular lenses. J Cat Refract Surg 24(7): 940-944, 1998.

Generic name: Tranexamic acid.

Proprietary name: Cyklokapron.

Primary use

An antifibrinolytic agent used primarily for treatment of excessive fibrinolysis. It has been used to control uterine and gastrointestinal bleeding as well as traumatic hyphemas.

Ocular side effects

Systemic administration
Possible
1. Decreased vision
2. Abnormal color vision – transient
3. Retinal artery or venous occlusion
4. Decreased corneal thickness
   a. Post intraocular surgery
   b. Bullous keratopathy

Conditional/Unclassified
1. Conjunctivitis – ligneous
2. Retinal pigment epithelium disturbances

Clinical significance

This agent is not available in the USA, but is in Asia and Europe. Clinical trials have been done in the USA, and occasionally US ophthalmologists have used this drug. It is, however, not FDA approved. Its actions are similar to aminocaproic acid, but much more potent. In animals, at three to seven times human dosages, retinal degenerations were seen in a matter of days. These changes were both central and peripheral (Theil 1981). To date this has not been seen in humans. However, Kitamura et al (2003) with rechallenge data, showed that large dosages of tranexamic acid caused reversible decreased vision, probably due to malfunction of the pigment epithelium of the retina. The authors felt that reduction of renal function (where the drug is metabolized) was a factor. Pharmacia and UpJohn (unpublished) reported no retinal degenerative change in patients on therapeutic dosages for periods ranging from 15 months to 8 years. However, occasional cases of transient disturbances of color vision were seen. Theil (1981) confirmed this. Possible ocular side effects include arterial or venous occlusion, including venous stasis retinopathy (Snir et al 1990). Their two patients had venous stasis with disc edema, engorged veins, cotton-wool spots and hemorrhages. Findings resolved after stopping the drug with resultant 20/20 vision OU. Parsons et al (1988) described a case of branch retinal artery occlusion. There are six cases of central or branch venous occlusion associated with the use of this agent in the National Registry.

Bramsen et al (1978) found that this agent decreases corneal edema in both bullous keratopathy and post intraocular surgery in humans. Hull et al (1979) could not confirm this in rabbits. Diamond et al (1991) reported a possible case of ligneous conjunctivitis after exposure to this drug. Reports to the National Registry of decreased color vision, both transitory and possibly permanent, have come from Sweden.

REFERENCES AND FURTHER READING

Bramsen T, Ehlers N. Bullous keratopathy treated systemically with 4-trans-amino-cyclohexano-carboxylic acid. Acta Ophthalmol 55: 665–673, 1977.

Bramsen T, Corydon L, Ehlers N. A double-blind study of the influence of tranexamic acid on the central corneal thickness after cataract extraction. Acta Ophthalmol 56: 121–127, 1978.

Diamond JP, Chandna A, Williams C, et al. Tranexamic acid-associated ligneous conjunctivitis with gingival and peritoneal lesions. Br J Ophthalmol 75(12): 753–754, 1991.

Dunn CJ, Goa KL. Tranexamic acid: a review of its use in surgery and other indications. Drugs 57(6): 1005–1032, 1999.

Hull DS, Green K, Buyer JG. Tranexamic acid and corneal deturgescence. Acta Ophthalmol 57: 252–257, 1979.

Kitamura H, Matsui I, Itoh N. Tranexamic acid-induced visual impairment in a hemodialysis patient. Clin Exp Nephrol 7: 311–314, 2003.

Parsons MR, Merritt DR, Ramsay RC. Retinal artery occlusion associated with tranexamic acid therapy. Am J Ophthalmol 105(6): 688–689, 1988.

Snir M, Axer-Siegel R, Buckman G, Yassur Y. Tranexamic acid, antifibrinolytic agent, venous stasis retinopathy. Retina 10: 181, 1990.

Theil PL. Ophthalmological examination of patients in long-term treatment with tranexamic acid. Acta Ophthalmol 59: 237–241, 1981.

Generic name: Warfarin.

Proprietary name: Coumadin, Jantoven.

Primary use

This coumarin derivative is used as an anticoagulant in the prophylaxis and treatment of venous thrombosis.

Ocular side effects

Systemic administration
Certain
1. Bleeding
   a. Subconjunctiva
   b. Hyphema
   c. Retina
   d. Vitreous
   e. Periocular
   f. Choroidal
2. Eyelids or conjunctiva
   a. Allergic reactions
   b. Conjunctivitis – non-specific
   c. Urticaria
3. Problems with color vision – color vision defect

Probable
1. Lacrimation

Ocular teratogenic effects
Possible
1. Optic atrophy
2. Cataracts
3. Microphthalmia
4. Blindness

Clinical significance

Ocular side effects due to warfarin anticoagulant are uncommon. Massive retinal hemorrhages have been reported, especially in diseased tissue with possible capillary fragility, such as diabetic disciform degeneration of the macula (Lewis et al 1988). In addition, spontaneous hyphema can develop, which may be more common with iris fixed lenses. A potentially dangerous association between the onset of a herpes zoster infection and oral anticoagulant therapy has also been found. Even so, as extensively as this agent has been used, only a few major adverse ocular side effects have been reported. This drug probably should be discontinued before ocular surgery to prevent an increased incidence of hemorrhaging in patients with diabetes, hypertension, in some cases of exudative age-related macular degeneration (Tilanus et al 2000), atrial fibrillation with age-related macular degeneration (Ung et al 2003), exfoliative glaucoma with vasculized posterior synechia (Greenfield et al 1999), patients on fluconazole (Mootha et al 2002), and those with other hemopoetic deficiencies (Younger and McHenry 2006). In some cases there is a fear of stopping anticoagulant because it may give a period of transient, yet dangerous, hypercoagulable state. Retrobulbar hemorrhages may occur more frequently and normally occurring bleeds may be more extensive if the drug is suddenly discontinued (Konstantatos 2001). Parkin and Manner (2000) polled ocular plastic surgeons and over half have seen serious bleeding problems post-operatively in patients on this drug and about half considered stopping this agent pre-operatively.

There are data to suggest that this drug can cause teratogenic effects. Although the teratogenic effects appear to be most severe when warfarin is taken during the first trimester, the effects can occur any time during gestation. Conradi-Hunermann syndrome or chondrodysplasia punctata and Dandy-Walker syndrome with their associated ocular defects have been reported in the offspring of patients receiving warfarin therapy during their pregnancies. Caronia et al (1998) described a case of bilateral angle-closure glaucoma secondary to posterior segment intraocular hemorrhage due to anticoagulants in a nanophthalmic patient.

REFERENCES AND FURTHER READING

Blumenkopf B, Lockhart WS, Jr. Herpes zoster infection and use of oral anticoagulants. A potentially dangerous association. JAMA 250: 936, 1983.

Caronia RM, Sturm RT, Fastenberg DM, et al. Bilateral secondary angle-closure glaucoma as a complication of anticoagulation in a nanophthalmic patient. Am J Ophthalmol 126(2): 307–309, 1998.

Fenman SS, et al. Intraocular hemorrhage and blindness associated with systemic anticoagulation. JAMA 220: 1354–1355, 1972.

Gainey SP, et al. Ocular surgery on patients receiving long-term warfarin therapy. Am J Ophthalmol 108: 142–146, 1989.

Gordon DM, Mead J. Retinal hemorrhage with visual loss during anticoagulant therapy. J Am Geriat Soc 16: 99–100, 1968.

Greenfield DS, Liebmann JM, Ritch R. Hyphema associated with papillary dilation in a patient with exfoliation glaucoma and warfarin therapy. Am J Ophthalmol 128: 98–100, 1999.

Hall DL, Steen WH, Jr, Drummond JW. Anticoagulants and cataract surgery. Ann Ophthalmol 12: 759, 1980.

Harrod MJE, Sherro IPS. Warfarin embryopathy in siblings. Obstet Gynecol 57: 673, 1981.

Kaplan LC. Congenital Dandy Walker malformation associated with first trimester warfarin: a case report and literature review. Teratology 32: 333, 1985.

Kleinebrecht J. Zur Teratogenitat von Cumarin-Derivaten. Dtsch Med Wochenschr 107: 1929, 1982.

Koehler MP, Sholiton DH. Spontaneous hyphema resulting from warfarin. Ann Ophthalmol 1: 858, 1983.

Kostantatos A. Anticoagulation and cataract surgery: a review of the current literature. Anaesth Intensive Care 29: 553–554, 2001.

Leath MC. Coumarin skin necrosis. Texas Med 79: 62, 1983.

Lewis H, Sloan SH, Foos RY. Massive intraocular hemorrhage associated with anticoagulation and age-related macular degeneration. Graefes Arch Clin Exp Ophthalmol 226: 59–64, 1988.

Lumme P, Laatikainen LT. Risk factors for intraoperative and early postoperative complications in extracapsular cataract surgery. Eur J Ophthalmol 4(3): 151–158, 1994.

Mootha VV, Schluter ML, Das A, et al. Intraocular hemorrhages due to warfarin-fluconazole drug interaction in a patient with presumed candida endophthalmitis. Arch Ophthalmol 120: 94–95, 2002.

Parkin B, Manner R. Aspirin and warfarin therapy in oculoplastic surgery. Br J Ophthalmol 84: 1426–1427, 2000.

Robinson GA, Nylander A. Warfarin and cataract extraction. Br J Ophthalmol 73: 702–703, 1989.

Schiff FS. Coumadin related spontaneous hyphemas in patients with iris fixated pseudophakos. Ophthal Surg 16: 172–173, 1985.

Shaul WL, Hall JG. Multiple congenital anomalies associated with oral anticoagulants. Am J Obstet Gynecol 127: 191–198, 1977.

Superstein R, Gomolin JES, Hammouda W, et al. Prevalence of ocular hemorrhage in patients receiving warfarin therapy. Can J Ophthalmol 35: 385–389, 2000.

Taylor RH, Gibson JM. Warfarin, spontaneous hyphaemas, and intraocular lenses. Lancet 1: 762–763, 1988.

Tilanus MAD, Vaandrager W, Cuypers MHM, et al. Relationship between anticoagulant medication and massive intraocular hemorrhage in age-related macular degeneration. Graefe's Arch Clin Exp Ophthalmol 238: 482–485, 2000.

Ung T, James M, Gray RH. Long-term warfarin associated with bilateral blindness in a patient with atrial fibrillation and macular degeneration. Heart 89: 985, 2003.

Weir CR, Nolan DJ, Holding D, et al. Intraocular haemorrhage associated with anticoagulant therapy. Acta Ophthalmol Scand 78: 492–493, 2000.

Younger JR, McHenry JG. Visually disabling non-traumatic orbital hemorrhage in an anticoagulated patient with factor VII deficiency. J Neuro-Ophthalmol 26: 76–77, 2006.

CLASS: BLOOD SUBSTITUTES

Generic name: Dextran.

Proprietary names: Gentran 40, Gentran 70, Hyskon, Macrodex, Promit, Rheomacrodex.

Primary use

This water-soluble glucose polymer is used for early fluid replacement and for plasma volume expansion in the adjunctive treatment of certain types of shock.

Ocular side effects

Systemic administration
Certain
1. Eyelids or conjunctiva
   a. Erythema
   b. Conjunctivitis – non-specific
   c. Angioneurotic edema
   d. Urticaria
2. Non-specific ocular irritation
   a. Lacrimation
   b. Photophobia
   c. Edema
   d. Burning sensation
3. Keratitis

Clinical significance

The most common adverse ocular reaction due to dextran is ocular irritation, since this drug is secreted in the tears. An allergic keratitis, which disappeared when the drug was discontinued, has also been reported in several patients. A hypersensitivity reaction, including fever, nasal congestion, joint pain, urticaria, hypotension and ocular irritation, can occur. This is probably due to dextran-reactivated antibodies.

REFERENCES AND FURTHER READING

Blake J, Cassidy H. Ocular hypersensitivity to dextran. Ir J Med Sci 148: 249, 1979.

Fothergill R, Heaney GA. Reactions to dextran. BMJ 2: 1502, 1976.

Krenzelok EP, Parker WA. Dextran 40 anaphylaxis. Minn Med 58: 454, 1975.

Ledoux-Corbusier M. L'urticaire medicamenteuse. Brux Med 55: 629, 1975.

Richter W, et al. Adverse reactions to plasma substitutes: incidence and pathomechanisms. In: Adverse Response to Intravenous Drugs, Watkins J, Wand A (eds), Grune & Stratton, New York, p 49–70, 1978.

SECTION 9
HOMEOSTATIC AGENTS

CLASS: AGENTS USED TO TREAT HYPERGLYCEMIA

Generic names: 1. Acetohexamide; 2. chlorpropamide; 3. glibenclamide (glyburide); 4. glimepiride; 5. glipizide; 6. tolazamide; 7. tolbutamide.

Proprietary names: 1. Generic only; 2. Diabinese; 3. Diabeta, Gynase, Micronase; 4. Amaryl; 5. Glucotrol, Glucotrol XL; 6. Tolinase; 7. generic only.

Primary use

These oral hypoglycemic sulfonylureas are effective in the management of selected cases of diabetes mellitus.

Ocular side effects

Systemic administration
Certain
1. Decreased vision
2. Decreased accommodation (glibenclamide)
3. Eyelids or conjunctiva
   a. Allergic reactions
   b. Hyperemia
   c. Conjunctivitis – non-specific
   d. Edema
   e. Photosensitivity
   f. Purpura
4. Problems with color vision – color vision defect, red-green defect
5. Lens
   a. Osmotic changes
   b. Myopia
   c. Forward displacement iris lens diaphragm

Probable
1. May aggravate Wernicke's syndrome

Possible
1. Subconjunctival or retinal hemorrhages secondary to drug-induced anemia
2. Lens
   a. Opacities – irreversible
   b. Posterior subcapsular changes
3. Eyelids or conjunctiva
   a. Lupoid syndrome (tolazamide)
   b. Erythema multiforme
   c. Stevens-Johnson syndrome
   d. Exfoliative dermatitis

Conditional/Unclassified

1. Optic nerve
   a. Vascular events
   b. Neuritis

Clinical significance

While there are multiple reported adverse ocular effects due to these agents, the data, other than drug-induced hypoglycemia, are difficult to evaluate. Overall, chlorpropamide has a 6% incidence of untoward reactions, while the incidence with acetohexamide, tolazamide and tolbutamide is 3%. Isaac et al (1991) found an overall increased risk of cataracts in patients on antidiabetic agents. There are numerous reports of second-generation sulfonylureas (Hampson and Harvey 2000) causing lens changes, but this is not well proven. Skalka and Prchal (1981) found an increased incidence of posterior subcapsular lens changes in diabetic patients treated with oral hypoglycemics compared with diabetics controlled with diet and insulin. Transient myopia and decreased accommodation have been seen due to glibenclamide. While optic nerve disease has been reported in the literature (Wymore and Carter 1982) and to the National Registry, differentiation of which changes are due to diabetes and which are due to a toxic drug effect is difficult and may be impossible to determine. Reported optic or retrobulbar neuritis (Catros et al 1958; Givner 1961) with central or centrocecal scotoma has not been proven as a drug-related event. In some cases, the optic nerve damage may be secondary to the drug-induced hypoglycemia and related vascular events. In susceptible individuals who have low thiamine reserves, hypoglycemic agents may induce Wernicke's encephalopathy, including oculomotor disturbances such as ophthalmoplegia, ptosis and nystagmus.

REFERENCES AND FURTHER READING

Birch J, et al. Acquired color vision defects. In: Congenital and Acquired Color Vision Defects, Pokorny J, et al. (eds), Grune & Stratton, New York, p 243,1979.

Catros V, et al. Bilateral axial optic neuritis in the course of treatment with D860. Rev Otoneuropathol 30: 253–257, 1958.

D'arcy PF. Drug reactions and interactions. Int Pharm J 3: 220–222, 1989.

Garbe E, Lelorier J, Boivin JF, et al. Risk of ocular hypertension or open-angle glaucoma in elderly patients on oral glucocorticoids. Lancet 350: 979–982, 1997.

George CW. Central scotomata due to chlorpropamide (Diabenese). Arch Ophthalmol 69: 773, 1963.

Givner I. Centrocecal scotomas due to chlorpropamide. Arch Ophthalmol 66: 64, 1961.

Hamil MB, Suelflow JA, Smith JA. Transdermal scopolamine delivery system (Transderm-V) and acute angle closure glaucoma. Ann Ophthalmol 15: 1011–1012, 1983.

Hampson JP, Harvey JN. A systematic review of drug induced ocular reactions in diabetes. Br J Ophthalmol 84: 144–149, 2000.

Isaac NE, Walker AM, Jick H, Gorman M. Exposure to phenothiazine drugs and risk of cataract. Arch Ophthalmol 109: 256–260, 1991.

Kanefsky TM, Medoff SJ. Stevens-Johnson syndrome and neutropenia with chlorpropamide therapy. Arch Intern Med 140: 1543, 1980.

Kapetansky FM. Refractive changes with tolbutamide. Ohio State Med J 59: 275, 1963.

Kato S, Oshika T, Numaga J, et al. Influence of rapid glycemic control on lens opacity in patients with diabetes mellitus. Am J Ophthalmol 130: 354–355, 2000.

Kelly JT. Second generation oral hypoglycemia and lactic acidosis in a diabetic treated with chlorpromade and phenformin. South Med J 66: 190–192, 1973.

Kwee IL, Nakada T. Wernicke's encephalopathy induced by tolazamide. N Engl J Med 309: 999, 1983.

Lightman JM, Townsend JC, Selvin GJ. Ocular effects of second generation oral hypoglycemic agents. J Am Optom Assoc 60: 849–853, 1989.

Paice BJ, Paterson KR, Lavson DH. Undesired effects of the sulphonylurea drugs. Adverse Drug React Acute Poison Rev 4: 23, 1985.

Skalka HW, Prchal JT. The effect of diabetes mellitus and diabetic therapy on cataract formation. Ophthalmology 88: 117, 1981.

Teller J, Rasin M, Abraham FA. Accommodation insufficiency induced by glybenclamide. Ann Ophthalmol 88: 117, 1981.

Transient myopia from glibenclamide: Short-sightedness with glibenclamide. Int Pharm J 3: 221–222, 1989.

Wymore J, Carter JE. Chlorpropamide-induced optic neuropathy. Arch Intern Med 142: 381, 1982.

Generic name: Insulin.

Proprietary names: Apidra, Exubera, Humalog, Humalog Pen, Humulin 70/30, Humulin 50/50, Humulin L, Humulin, N, Humulin R, Humulin U, Lente, Levemir, Novolin 70/30, Novolin, N, Novolin, R, Novolog, Ultralente, Velosulin Human BR.

Primary use

This hypoglycemic agent is effective in the management of diabetes mellitus.

Ocular side effects

Systemic administration

Certain

1. Decreased vision
2. Extraocular muscles
   a. Paresis
   b. Nystagmus
   c. Diplopia
3. Eyelids or conjunctiva
   a. Allergic reactions
   b. Erythema
   c. Blepharoconjunctivitis
   d. Angioneurotic edema
   e. Urticaria
4. Decreased tear lysozymes

Probable

1. Angle-closure glaucoma

Possible

1. Immunogenic retinopathy
2. Myopia – transient

Clinical significance

The adverse ocular effects secondary to insulin are generally the result of insulin-induced hypoglycemia and not a direct toxic effect of the drug. This occurs due to an excessive dosage of insulin, omission of a meal by a patient or increased physical activity. Ocular symptoms are primarily decreased vision, blurred vision or double vision. While these effects are usually transitory, some cases may take many weeks to resolve. Blake and Nathan (2003) report on the exceedingly rare precipitation of acute angle-closure glaucoma following rapid correction of acute hyperglycemia. This is probably due to intralenticular glucose-sorbital, with a resultant swelling of the lens. It has been suggested that some diabetic retinopathy is insulin-induced and immunogenic in nature (Shabo and Maxwell 1976). While data in primates support this, it is difficult to prove in humans. Arun et al (2004) report that with initiation of insulin treatment in type II diabetes, clinically significant worsening of diabetic retinopathy over a 3-year period was uncommon in those with no retinopathy, but occurred in 31.8% of patients with retinopathy at baseline. They point out that the risk of serious worsening of retinopathy after the start of insulin therapy in all patients with type II diabetics may have been previously overestimated. Gold and Marshall (1996) point out cortical blindness and cerebral infarcts secondary to severe hypoglycemia. Insulin may cause or aggravate lipemic retinitis in a patient with possible hyperlipoproteinemia type V. Kitzmiller et al (1999) suggest that in pregnancy, when insulin lispro therapy is given, rapid acceleration of proliferative diabetic retinopathy, without background retinopathy, may occur. There are cases in the National Registry of up to 3 diopter changes of myopia with overdosage of insulin.

REFERENCES AND FURTHER READING

Arun CS, Pandit R, Taylor R. Long-term progression of retinopathy after initiation of insulin therapy in type 2 diabetes: an observational study. Diabetologia 47: 1380–1384, 2004.

Blake DR, Nathan DM. Acute angle closure glaucoma following rapid correction of hyperglycemia. Diabet Care 26: 3197–3198, 2003.

Gold AE, Marshall SM. Cortical blindness and cerebral infarction associated with severe hypoglycemia. Diabet Care 19(9): 1001–1003, 1996.

Gralnick A. The retina and intraocular tension during prolonged insulin coma with autopsy eye findings. Am J Ophthalmol 24: 1174, 1941.

Kitzmiller JL, Main E, Ward B, et al. Insulin lispro and the development of proliferative diabetic retinopahy during pregnancy. Diabet Care 22(5): 874–876, 1999.

Moses RA (ed). Adler's Physiology of the Eye, 6th edn, Mosby, St Louis, p 21, 1975.

Shabo AL, Maxwell DS. Insulin-induced immunogenic retinopathy resembling the retinitis proliferans of diabetes. Trans Am Acad Ophthalmol Otolaryngol 81: 497, 1976.

Vermeer BJ, Polano MK. A case of xanthomatosis and hyperlipoproteinemia type V probably induced by overdosage of insulin. Dermatologica 151: 43, 1975.

Walsh FB, Hoyt WF. Clinical Neuro-Ophthalmology, 3rd edn Vol. III, Williams & Wilkins, Baltimore pp 2684–2685, 1969.

Generic name: Metformin hydrochloride.

Proprietary names: Fortamet, Glucophage, Glucophage, XR, Glumetza, Riomet.

Primary use

A biguanide oral antidiabetic for the treatment of type II diabetes mellitus. This is the drug of choice for obese patients.

Ocular side effects

Systemic administration
Conditional/Unclassified
1. Lens – osmotic damage – transient (Fig. 7.9a)
2. Eyelids or conjunctiva – erythema multiforme
3. Periorbital edema

Clinical significance

Tangelder et al (2005) report a single case of a unique reversible lens change called 'sugar cracks'. These cracks were located primarily in the nucleus, running parallel to the nuclear curvature and in a straight band nearing both ends at the equator. This occurred with blurred vision in a newly diagnosed 62-year-old diabetic, 2 days after starting metformin. Two weeks later, the patient's vision was 20/80 OD and 20/33 OS. At 3 months, the lens changes vanished spontaneously and at 5 months vision was 20/20 OU. The authors felt these changes were related to a decrease in extracellular glucose and not a toxic effect of the drug.

REFERENCES AND FURTHER READING

Burger DE, Goyal S. Erythema multiforme from metformin. Ann Pharmacother 38: 1537, 2004.

Tangelder GJM, Dubbelman M, Ringens PJ. Sudden reversible osmotic lens damage ('sugar cracks') after initiation of metformin. N Engl J Med 353: 2621–2623, 2005.

Generic names: Rosiglitazone maleate; 2. pioglitazone hydrochloride.

Proprietary names: 1. Avandia; 2. Actos.

Primary use

Oral thiazolidinedione antidiabetic agents which act primarily by increasing insulin sensitivity.

Ocular side effects

Systemic administration – oral
Certain
1. Macula edema
2. Face
   a. Edema
   b. Periorbital edema
3. Decreased vision

Probable
1. Color vision defect
2. Decrease dark adaptation

Possible
1. Proptosis
2. Intracranial hypertension

Clinical significance

Glitazones can cause systemic peripheral edema in 5–7% of patients and up to 15% if pioglitazone and insulin are used in combination (package insert). Bresnick et al (1986) and others have shown that systemic fluid retention can aggravate diabetic macular edema and complicate its management. Systemic fluid retention is a possible mechanism for causing macular edema. Colucciello (2005) and Ryan et al (2006) found that stopping the drug allowed rapid resolution of the macular edema in about 25% of patients. In the other cases, the resolution was slower and may require laser treatment. The macular edema was more common in patients with peripheral edema and while its incidence is unknown, Ryan et al (2006) project approximately 3% of patients on this drug develop macular changes. Levin et al (2005) report proptosis due to adipogenesis properties of these agents and Starkey et al (2003) describe a case of aggravation of pre-existing thyroid eye disease. Dagdelen and Gedik (2006) describe a patient with intracranial hypertension, possibly due to rosiglitazone.

Recommendations

1. If peripheral edema (primarily lower extremity) occurs, patients should be warned that if any vision changes occur they should see an ophthalmologist to check for macular edema. Vision signs or symptoms include blurred or distorted vision, decreased dark adaptation and or decreased color sensation.

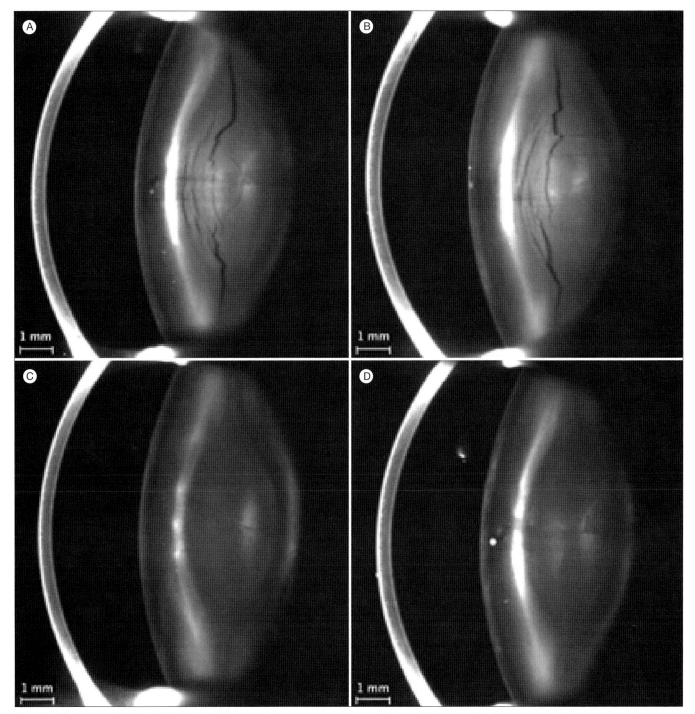

Fig. 7.9a Sugar cracks in right (A) and left (B) eye and spontaneous resolution (C and D) from metformin treatment. Photo courtesy of Tangelder GJM, et al. Sudden reversible osmotic lens damage (sugar cracks) after initiation of metformin. N Engl J Med 353: 2621–2623, 2005.

2. Consider recommending not using this agent if the patient has diabetic macular edema, congestive heart failure or nephropathy.
3. Recommend stopping the drug at the first signs of macular edema.

REFERENCES AND FURTHER READING

Bresnick GH. Diabetic macular edema. A review. Ophthalmology 93: 989–997, 1986.

Colucciello M. Vision loss due to macular edema induced by rosiglitazone treatment of diabetes mellitus. Arch Ophthalmol 123: 1273–1275, 2005.

Dagdelen S, Gedik O. Rosiglitazone-associated pseudotumor cerebri. Diabetologia 49: 207–208, 2006.

Kendall C, Wooltorton E. Rosiglitazone (Avandia) and macular edema. Can Med Assoc J 174: 623, 2006.

Levin F, Kazim M, Smith TJ, et al. Rosiglitazone-induced proptosis. Arch Ophthalmol 123: 119–121, 2005.

Pioglitazone. Package Insert, GlaxoSmithKline, Philadelphia, PA, 2005.

Ryan EH, Han DP, Ramsay RC, et al. Diabetic macular edema associated with glitazone use. Retina 26: 562–570, 2006.

Starkey K, Heufelder A, Baker G, et al. Peroxisome proliferator-activated receptor-gamma in thyroid eye disease: contraindication for thiazolidinedione use? J Clin Endocrinol Metab 88: 55–59, 2003.

SECTION 10
AGENTS USED TO TREAT ALLERGIC AND NEUROMUSCULAR DISORDERS

CLASS: AGENTS USED TO TREAT MYASTHENIA GRAVIS

Generic names: 1. Ambenonium chloride; 2. edrophonium chloride; 3. pyridostigmine bromide.

Proprietary names: 1. Mytelase; 2. Enlon, Tensilon; 3. Regonol, Mestinon.

Primary use
These anticholinesterase agents are effective in the treatment of myasthenia gravis. Edrophonium is primarily used as an antidote for curariform agents and as a diagnostic test for myasthenia gravis.

Ocular side effects

Systemic administration
Certain
1. Miosis – toxic states
2. Diplopia – toxic states
3. Lacrimation – toxic states
4. Blepharoclonus – toxic states
5. Nystagmus – toxic states
6. Paradoxical response (ptotic eye up and non-ptotic eye down)

Possible
1. Decreased vision
2. Oculogyric crisis (edrophonium)

Clinical significance
Ocular side effects due to these anticholinesterase agents are rare and seldom of clinical significance. All adverse ocular reactions are reversible with discontinued drug use. Overdose may lead to a cholinergic crisis, which includes miosis, ciliary spasm, nystagmus, extraocular muscle paresis and blepharoclonus. Blepharoclonus is seen only in overdose situations. In rare instances, edrophonium may cause a paradoxical response when used for myasthenia gravis testing. In these cases, the ptotic eyelid goes up, while the normal eyelid goes down. Serious systemic side effects from the edrophonium test for myasthenia gravis are relatively uncommon, especially if used with a preliminary small test dose to detect hypersensitive patients. Nucci and Brancato (1990) reported an episode of oculogyric crisis within a few minutes after performing a Tensilon test (edrophonium chloride).

REFERENCES AND FURTHER READING

Drug Evaluations, 6th edn, American Medical Association, Chicago, pp 224–226, 450, 1986.
Dukes MNG(ed). Meyer's Side Effects of Drugs, Vol. X, Excerpta Medica, Amsterdam, p 246, 1984.
Field LM. Toxic alopecia caused by pyridostigmine bromide. Arch Dermatol 116: 1103, 1980.
Havener WN. Ocular Pharmacology, 5th edn, Mosby, St Louis, pp 347–349, 1983.
McEvoy GK (ed). American Hospital Formulary Service Drug Information 87, American Society of Hospital Pharmacists, Bethesda, pp 520–521, 528–530, 1206–1208, 1987.
Nucci P, Brancato R. Oculogyric crisis after the Tensilon test. Graefes Arch Ophthalmol Clin Exp 228: 382–385, 1990.
Van Dyk HIL, Florence L. The Tensilon test. A safe office procedure. Ophthalmology 87: 210, 1990.

CLASS: ANTIHISTAMINES

Generic names: 1. Brompheniramine maleate; 2. chlorphenamine maleate; 3. dexchlorphenamine maleate; 4. triprolidine hydrochloride.

Proprietary names: 1. Generic only; 2. multi-ingredient preparations only; 3. Mylaramine; 4. multi-ingredient preparations only.

Primary use
These alkylamine antihistamines are used in the symptomatic relief of allergic or vasomotor rhinitis, allergic conjunctivitis and allergic skin manifestations.

Ocular side effects

Systemic administration
Certain
1. Decreased vision
2. Pupils
   a. Mydriasis – may precipitate angle-closure glaucoma
   b. Decreased or absent reaction to light – toxic states
   c. Anisocoria
3. Decreased tolerance to contact lenses
4. Decreased lacrimation
5. May aggravate keratoconjunctivitis sicca

Probable
1. Eyelids or conjunctiva
   a. Erythema
   b. Photosensitivity
   c. Urticaria
   d. Blepharospasm
   e. Angioneurotic edema
2. Visual hallucinations – toxic states
3. Abnormal critical flicker fusion (triprolidine)

Possible
1. Diplopia
2. Subconjunctival or retinal hemorrhages secondary to drug-induced anemia

Clinical significance
Ocular side effects due to these antihistamines are rare and may disappear even if use of the drug is continued. These antihistamines have a weak atropine action, which accounts for the pupillary changes. With chronic use, anisocoria, decreased accommodation and blurred vision can also occur. Chlorphenamine and others in this class have been found to decrease mucous and or tear production, which accounts for decreased contact lens tolerance and aggravation or transitory induction of keratoconjunctivitis sicca. Antihistamines in large dosages or with chronic therapy can produce facial dyskinesia, which may start with unilateral or bilateral blepharospasms. Lack of pupillary response occurs only in toxic states or with chronic use. The alkylamines seem to have a lower incidence of ocular side effects than other antihistamines, with dexchlorphenamine having the fewest reported side effects.

REFERENCES AND FURTHER READING

Davis WA. Dyskinesia associated with chronic antihistamine use. N Engl J Med 294: 113, 1976.

Farber AS. Ocular side effects of antihistamine-decongestant combinations. Am J Ophthalmol 94: 565, 1982.

Granacher RP Jr. Facial dyskinesa after antihistamines. N Engl J Med 296: 516, 1977.

Halperin M, Thorig L, van Haeringen NJ. Ocular side effects of antihistamine-decongestant combinations. Am J Ophthalmol 95: 563, 1983.

Koffler BH, Lemp MA. The effect of an antihistamine (chlorpheniramine maleate) on tear production in humans. Ann Ophthalmol 12: 217, 1980.

Miller D. Role of the tear film in contact lens wear. Int Ophthalmol Clin 13(1): 247, 1973.

Nicholson AN, Smith PA, Spencer MB. Antihistamines and visual function: Studies on dynamic acuity and the pupillary response to light. Br J Clin Pharmacol 14: 683, 1982.

Schuller DE, Turkewitz D. Adverse effects of antihistamines. Postgrad Med 79: 75, 1986.

Soleymanikashi Y, Weiss NS. Antihistaminic reaction: a review and presentation of two unusual examples. Ann Allergy 28: 486, 1970.

Sovner RD. Dyskinesia associated with chronic antihistamine use. N Engl J Med 294: 113, 1976.

Generic names: 1. Carbinoxamine maleate; 2. clemastine fumerate; 3. diphenyhramine; 4. doxylamine succinate.

Proprietary names: 1. Generic only; 2. generic only; 3. Benadryl; 4. Unisom Sleep tablets.

Primary use

These ethanolamine antihistamines are used in the symptomatic relief of allergic or vasomotor rhinitis, allergic conjunctivitis and allergic skin manifestations.

Ocular side effects

Systemic administration
Certain
1. Decreased tolerance to contact lenses
2. Decreased lacrimation
3. Visual hallucinations – toxic states
4. Nystagmus – toxic states
5. May aggravate keratoconjunctivitis sicca

Probable
1. Decreased vision
2. Pupils
   a. Mydriasis – may precipitate angle-closure glaucoma
   b. Decreased or absent reaction to light
   c. Anisocoria
3. Eyelids or conjunctiva
   a. Erythema
   b. Photosensitivity
   c. Urticaria
   d. Blepharospasm
4. Decrease or paralysis of accommodation

Possible
1. Diplopia
2. Subconjunctival or retinal hemorrhages secondary to drug-induced anemia

Clinical significance

Ocular side effects due to these antihistamines are rare and frequently disappear even if use of the drug is continued. These ethanolamines have a weak atropine action that accounts for the pupillary and ciliary body changes. However, with chronic long-term use, these effects can build so that unilateral or bilateral signs such as anisocoria, loss of accommodation and decreased vision may occur. A decrease in mucoid and or lacrimal secretions may account for contact lens intolerance and aggravation or induction of keratoconjunctivitis sicca. These drugs can all cause a dry mouth. In all probability, any drug that causes a dry mouth will cause or aggravate ocular sicca. It has been shown that these drugs in large dosages or with chronic therapy can produce facial dyskinesia. Many of these cases started with unilateral or bilateral blepharospasm. Lack of pupillary response, visual hallucinations and nystagmus usually occur in toxic states or with chronic high-dose therapy. Most of the ocular side effects in this group are attributed to diphenhydramine, which is the most commonly used drug. There are reports by both Walsh (1957) and Nigro (1968) of comas secondary to diphenhydramine ingestion in infants and teenagers where, on awakening, cortical blindness was evident. Over time vision reverted to normal. The National Registry has received two case reports of possible ocular teratogenic effects secondary to diphenhydramine or doxylamine.

REFERENCES AND FURTHER READING

Delaney WV Jr. Explained unexplained anisocoria. JAMA 244: 1475, 1980.

Drugs that cause photosensitivity. Med Lett Drugs Ther 28: 51, 1986.

Miller D. Role of the tear film in contact lens wear. Int Ophthalmol Clin 13:(1): 247, 1973.

Nigro SA. Toxic psychosis due to diphenhydramine hydrochloride. JAMA 203: 301, 1968.

Seedor JA, et al. Filamentary keratitis associated with diphenhydramine hydrochloride (Benadryl). Am J Ophthalmol 101: 376, 1986.

Walsh FB. Clinical Neuro-Ophthalmology, Williams & Wilkins, Baltimore, 1957.

Generic names: 1. Cetirizine hydrochloride; 2. desloratadine; 3. fexofenadine; 4. loratidine; 5. tripelennamine.

Proprietary names: 1. Zyrtec; 2. Clarinex, Clarinex D; 3. Allegra; 4. Alavert, Claritin, Travist ND; 5. Vaginex.

Primary use

These H_1 receptor antagonists are indicated for the treatment of allergic or vasomotor rhinitis, allergic conjunctivitis and allergic skin manifestations of urticaria and angioneurotic edema.

Ocular side effects

Systemic administration
Certain
1. Oculogyric crisis (cetirizine)
2. Decreased vision
3. May aggravate or cause keratoconjunctivitis sicca
4. Pupils
   a. Mydriasis
   b. Decreased or absent reaction to light
   c. Anisocoria
5. Decreased tolerance to contact lenses
6. Visual hallucinations – toxic states

7. Nystagmus (tripelennamine) – toxic states
8. Strabismus (tripelennamine) – toxic states

Probable
1. Eyelids or conjunctiva
   a. Erythema
   b. Photosensitivity
   c. Urticaria
   d. Blepharospasm

Possible
1. Decreased accommodation
2. Diplopia
3. Subconjunctival or retinal hemorrhages secondary to drug-induced anemia

Clinical significance

Ocular side effects due to these antihistamines are uncommon and frequently disappear even if the drug is continued. These antihistamines have a weak atropine action, which accounts for pupillary changes. However, with long-term use, these effects can accumulate, so that anisocoria, decreased accommodation or blurred vision can occur. The antimuscarine activity of H_1 antihistamines decreases basal tear production of the accessory and lacrimal glands, and decreases mucin production of the conjunctival goblet cells. This accounts for decreased contact lens tolerance and aggravation or induction of keratoconjunctivitis sicca. Ocular moisture returns once the drug is discontinued. These drugs all cause a dry mouth, so keratoconjunctivitis sicca is to be expected. Nine cases of oculogyric crisis due to cetirizine therapy (Fraunfelder and Fraunfelder 2004a), with eight occurring in the pediatric age group, have been reported. Dosage ranged from 5 to 10 mg orally, and time to onset of symptoms ranged from 3 to 184 days. Six cases of oculogyric crisis had positive rechallenge data. Eight cases had a complete neurological consultation, including radiographic studies. These drugs in large dosages or with chronic therapy can produce facial dyskinesia, which may start as a unilateral or bilateral blepharospasm. Total lack of pupillary response and visual hallucinations usually only occur in toxic states. There is a report of visual hallucinations occurring in a 5-year-old child after the third oral dose of tripelennamine (Hays et al 1980).

REFERENCES AND FURTHER READING

Abelson MB, Allansmith MR. Friedlaender MN. Effects of topically applied ocular decongestant and antihistamine. Am J Ophthalmol 90: 254, 1980.

Dukes MNG (ed). Meyler's Side Effects of Drugs, Vol. X, Excerpta Medica, Amsterdam, pp 286–287, 883, 1984.

Fraunfelder FW, Fraunfelder FT. Oculogyric crisis in patients taking cetirizine. Am J Ophthalmol 137: 355–357, 2004a.

Fraunfelder FW, Fraunfelder FT. Adverse ocular drug reactions recently identified by the national registry of drug-induced ocular side effects. Ophthalmology 111: 1275–1279, 2004b.

Grant WM, Loeb DR. Effect of locally applied antihistamine drugs on normal eyes. Arch Ophthalmol 39: 553–554, 1948.

Hays DP, Johnson BF, Perry R. Prolonged hallucinations following a modest overdose of tripelennamine. Clin Toxicol 16: 331, 1980.

Herman DC, Bartley GB. Corneal opacities secondary to topical naphazoline and antazoline (Albalon A). Am J Ophthalmol 103: 110–111, 1987.

Rinker JR, Sullivan JH. Drug reactions following urethral instillation of tripelennamine (Pyribenzamine). J Urol 91: 433, 1964.

Schipior PG. An unusual case of antihistamine intoxication. J Pediatr 71: 589, 1967.

Generic name: Cyproheptadine hydrochloride.

Proprietary name: Generic only.

Primary use

This antihistamine is used in the symptomatic relief of allergic or vasomotor rhinitis, allergic conjunctivitis and allergic skin manifestations.

Ocular side effects

Systemic administration
Certain
1. Decreased vision
2. Mydriasis
3. Decreased tolerance to contact lenses
4. Decreased lacrimation
5. Aggravate or cause transitory keratoconjunctivitis sicca

Probable
1. Eyelids or conjunctiva
   a. Erythema
   b. Edema
   c. Photosensitivity
   d. Urticaria
   e. Angioneurotic edema

Possible
1. Diplopia
2. Visual hallucinations
3. Subconjunctival or retinal hemorrhages secondary to drug-induced anemia

Clinical significance

Ocular side effects due to this agent are rare and may disappear even if use of the drug is continued. This agent has atropine-like effects, such as mydriasis and decreased secretions. Decreased lacrimal or mucoid secretion has been the cause of decreased tolerance to contact lenses and aggravation of keratoconjunctivitis sicca. Once the drug is discontinued, ocular moisture returns.

REFERENCES AND FURTHER READING

Drugs that cause photosensitivity. Med Lett Drugs Ther 28: 51, 1986.

Gilman AG, Goodman LS, Gilman A (eds).The Pharmacological Basis of Therapeutics, 6th edn, Macmillan, New York, p 639, 1980.

McEvoy GK (ed). American Hospital Formulary Service Drug Information 87, American Society of Hospital Pharmacists, Bethesda, pp 5–6, 14–15, 1987.

Miller D. Role of the tear film in contact lens wear. Int Ophthalmol Clin 13(1): 247, 1973.

CLASS: ANTIPARKINSONISM AGENTS

Generic name: Amantadine.

Proprietary name: Symmetrel.

Primary use

This synthetic antiviral agent is used in the treatment of Parkinson's disease, tardive dyskinesia and in the prophylaxis of influenza A2 (Asian) virus infections.

Ocular side effects

Systemic administration
Certain
1. Decreased vision
2. Visual hallucinations
3. Cornea
   a. Edema
   b. Punctate keratitis (Fig. 7.10a)
   c. Subepithelial opacities
4. Eyelids or conjunctiva
   a. Photosensitivity
   b. Purpura
   c. Eczema
   d. Loss of eyelashes or eyebrows

Probable
1. Oculogyric crises

Possible
1. Mydriasis – may precipitate angle-closure glaucoma
2. Cornea – abrasions

Clinical significance

Ocular side effects due to amantadine are rare except for decreased vision, which is transitory and seldom significant. All ocular effects appear to be dose related and are reversible with discontinued amantadine usage. A report of 23 cases of corneal lesions secondary to amantadine hydrochloride gave a pattern of diffuse, white, punctate subepithelial opacities, more prominent inferonasally, occasionally associated with a superficial punctate keratitis, corneal epithelial edema and markedly reduced visual acuity. This usually occurs within 1 to 2 weeks after starting the drug and clears between 2 to 6 days after stopping it. Amantadine was reinstituted in two patients, and the corneal deposits reoccurred (Fraunfelder and Meyer 1990). Nogaki and Morimatsu (1993) also noted corneal abrasion in a patient with superficial punctate keratitis. Blanchard (1990) and Hughes et al (2004) each reported one case and there are seven similar cases of corneal edema associated with amantadine use in the National Registry. The edema is more prominent in the palpebral aperture and involves the full thickness of the cornea, including epithelial blebs. This can occur anytime between a few weeks to a few years into therapy, and is reversible after the drug is discontinued. If this drug-related ocular side effect goes unrecognized, vision can go to only light perception. One case of sudden bilateral loss of vision in otherwise normal eyes has been reported secondary to amantadine. This sudden loss of vision was reversible after discontinuing the drug within several weeks. Visual hallucinations are often lilliputian and colored. While a few cases of mydriasis have been reported to the National Registry, causation is obscure.

REFERENCES AND FURTHER READING

Blanchard DL. Amantadine caused corneal edema. Letter to the Editor. Cornea 9(2): 181, 1990.

Drugs that cause psychiatric symptoms. Med Lett Drugs Ther 28: 81, 1986.

Fraunfelder FT, Meyer SM. Amantadine and corneal deposits. Am J Ophthalmol 110(1): 96–97, 1990.

Hughes B, Feiz V, Flynn SB, et al. Reversible amantadine-induced corneal edema in an adolescent. Cornea 23: 823–824, 2004.

Nogaki H, Morimatsu M. Superficial punctate keratitis and corneal abrasion due to amantadine hydrochloride (letter). J Neurol 240(6): 388–389, 1993.

Pearlman JT, Kadish AH, Ramseyer JC. Vision loss associated with amantadine hydrochloride use. JAMA 237: 1200, 1977.

Postma JU, Van Tilburg W. Visual hallucinations and delirium during treatment with amantadine (Symmetrel). J Am Geriatr Soc 23: 212, 1975.

Selby G. Treatment of parkinsonism. Drugs 11: 61, 1976.

van den Berg WHHW, van Ketel WG. Photosensitization by amantadine (Symmetrel). Contact Dermatitis 9: 165, 1983.

Wilson TW, Rajput AH. Amantadine–Dyazide interaction. Can Med Assoc J 129: 974, 1983.

Generic names: 1. Benzatropine mesilate; 2. biperiden; 3. procyclidine hydrochloride; 4. trihexyphenidyl hydrochloride.

Proprietary names: 1. Cogentin; 2. Akineton; 3. Kemadrin; 4. Artane, Trihexy-5.

Primary use

These anticholinergic agents are used in the management of Parkinson's disease and in the control of extrapyramidal disorders due to central nervous system drugs, such as reserpine or the phenothiazines.

Ocular side effects

Systemic administration
Certain
1. Pupils
   a. Mydriasis – may precipitate angle-closure glaucoma
   b. Decreased reaction to light
   c. Miosis – withdrawal
2. Decreased vision
3. Decrease or paralysis of accommodation
4. Visual hallucinations
5. Decreased critical flicker fusion (procyclidine)

Probable
1. Myasthenia gravis – exacerbates (trihexyphenidyl)
   a. Ptosis
   b. Diplopia
   c. Paresis of extraocular muscles

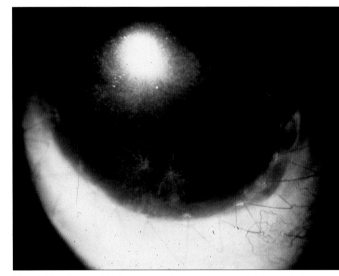

Fig. 7.10a Corneal lesions associated with superficial punctate keratitis in patient systemic amandatine.

Conditional/Unclassified
1. Retinal pigment changes

Clinical significance

The degree of anticholinergic activity induced ocular side effects varies with each agent. With benzatropine adverse ocular reactions are common, while with biperiden they are rare. In younger age groups decreased accommodation may cause considerable inconveniences and can be partially reversed by topical ocular application of a weak, long-acting anticholinesterase. There are a few cases in the literature and National Registry of these drugs precipitating glaucoma in patients at recommended dosages. Visual hallucinations are primarily of people who are normal in size and color, and they disappear if the dosage of the drug is reduced. Sharma et al (2002) showed that procyclidine reduced critical flicker fusion at therapeutic levels of 15 mg. Retinal pigmentary changes have been seen in patients taking these medications, but this has not been proven as a drug-related event.

REFERENCES AND FURTHER READING

Acute drug abuse reactions. Med Lett Drugs Ther 27: 77, 1985.
Anticholinergic drugs are abused. Int Drug Ther Newslett 20: 1, 1985.
Friedman Z, Neumann E. Benzhexol induced blindness in Parkinson's disease. BMJ 1: 605, 1972.
Gilbert GJ. Hallucinatons from levodopa. JAMA 235: 597, 1976.
McGucken RB, Caldwell J, Anthon B. Teenage procyclicline abuse. Lancet 1: 1514, 1985.
Medina C, Kramer MD, Kurland AA. Biperiden in the treatment of phenothiazine-induced extrapyramidal reactions JAMA 182: 1127–1129, 1962.
Selby G. Treatment of parkinsonism. Drugs 11: 61, 1976.
Sharma T, Galea A, Zachariah E, et al. Effects of 10 mg and 15 mg oral procyclidine on critical flicker fusion threshold and cardiac functioning in healthy human subjects. J Psychopharmacol 16: 183–187, 2002.
Thaler JS. The effect of multiple psychotropic drugs on the accommodation of pre-presbyopes. Am J Optom Physiol Optics 56: 259, 1979.
Thaler JS. Effects of benztropine mesylate (Cogentin) on accommodation in normal volunteers. Am J Optom Physiol Optics 59: 918, 1982.
Ueno S, Takahashi M, Kajiyama K, et al. Parkinson's disease and myasthenia gravis: adverse effect of trihexyphenidyl on neuonmuscular transmission. Neurology 37: 832-833, 1987.

Generic name: Levodopa.

Proprietary names: Multi-ingredient preparations only.

Primary use

This beta-adrenergic blocking agent is used in the management of Parkinson's disease.

Ocular side effects

Systemic administration
Certain
1. Pupils
   a. Mydriasis – may precipitate angle-closure glaucoma
   b. Miosis
2. Decreased vision
3. Diplopia
4. Blepharospasm
5. Blepharoclonus
6. Eyelids or conjunctiva
   a. Allergic reactions
   b. Edema

Probable
1. Widening of palpebral fissure
2. Extraocular muscles
   a. Paresis
   b. Abnormal involuntary movement
3. Oculogyric crisis
4. Amblyopia
   a. Increases visual acuity
   b. Decreases binocular suppression

Possible
1. Horner's syndrome
   a. Miosis
   b. Ptosis
2. Subconjunctival or retinal hemorrhages secondary to drug-induced anemia
3. Stimulation of malignant melanoma
4. Visual hallucinations
5. Eyelids or conjunctiva – lupoid syndrome

Clinical significance

While numerous ocular side effects due to levodopa are known, they appear to be dose dependent and reversible. Rarely is the drug given alone, so to determine causation is difficult. Pupillary side effects are variable. Initially, mydriasis may occur, which has been reported to precipitate angle-closure glaucoma. After a few weeks of levodopa therapy, miosis is not uncommon. Eyelid responses also appear to be variable. In some patients, levodopa produces ptosis, sometimes unilateral, while blepharospasm is reported in other patients. Apraxia of lid opening has been reported due to levodopa/carbidopa (Lamberti et al 2002; Lee et al 2004) but others feel this is not caused by levodopa per se, but more likely due to a fluctuation in the brain of dopamine levels during adjustment to levodopa/carbidopa therapy. Visual hallucinations are menacing and primarily of normal-size people and in color. These hallucinations can be stopped or decreased in frequency by reducing the drug dosage. Oculogyric crises have been precipitated by levodopa, primarily in patients with prior history of encephalitis. Gottlob et al (1992) reported that levodopa has improved contrast sensitivity, decreased the size of scotomas and improved vision in up to 70% of amblyopic eyes. This improvement is said to persist. Leguire et al (1991) reported a series of articles that suggest permanent improvement in some amblyopic eyes after administration of this drug. Procianoy et al (1999) also studied the effects of levodopa in children with strabismic amblyopia. One case of drug-induced intracranial hypertension occurred in a patient on carbidopa and levodopa. Since levodopa is an intermediate in melanin synthesis, there is a question of whether it might induce or stimulate the growth of melanomas (van Rens et al 1982). Although there are no proven data to support this, alternative forms of anti-Parkinsonian therapy have been suggested for susceptible patients.

REFERENCES AND FURTHER READING

Abramson DN, Rubenfield MR. Choroidal melanoma and levodopa. JAMA 252: 1011, 1984.
Barbeau A. L-Dopa therapy in Parkinson's disease: a critical review of nine years' experience. Can Med Assoc J 101: 791–800, 1969.
Barone DA, Martin HL. Causes of pseudotumor cerebri and papilledema. Arch Intern Med 139: 830, 1979.
Casey DE. Pharmacology of blepharospasm-oromandibular dystonia. Neurology 30: 690–695, 1980.
Cotzias GC, Papavasilliou PS, Gellene R. Modifications of Parkinsonism – chronic treatment with L-dopa. N Engl J Med 280: 337–345, 1969.

Glantz R, et al. Drug-induced asterixis in Parkinson disease. Neurology 32: 553, 1982.

Goetz CG, Leurgans S, Papper EJ, et al. Prospective longitudinal assessment of hallucinations in Parkinson's disease. Neurology 57: 2078–2082, 2001.

Gottlob I, Charlier J, Reinecke RD. Visual acuities and scotomas after one week levodopa administration in human amblyopia. Invest Ophthalmol Vis Sci 33(9): 2722–2727, 1992.

Lamberti P, De Mari M, Zenzola A, et al. Frequency of apraxia of eyelid opening in the general population and in patients with extrapyramidal disorder. Neurol Sci 23(Suppl 2): S81–S82, 2002.

Lee KC, Finley R, Miller B. Apraxia of lid opening: dose-dependent response to carbidopa-levodopa. Pharmacotherapy 24: 401–403, 2004.

Leguire LE, et al. Levodopa treatment for childhood amblyopia. Invest Ophthalmol Vis Sci 32(Suppl): 820, 1991.

Lequire LE, Walson PD, Roger GL, et al. Longitudinal study of levodopa/carbidopa for childhood amblyopia. J Pediatr Ophthalmol Strabismus 30(6): 354–360, 1993.

Lequire LE, Walson PD, Roger GL, et al. Levodopa/carbidopa for childhood amblyopia. Invest Ophthalmol Vis Sci 34(11): 3090–3095, 1993.

Lequire LE, Walson PD, Rogers GL, et al. Levodopa/carbidopa treatment of amblyopia in older children. J Pediatr Ophthalmol Strabismus 32(3): 143–151, 1995.

LeWitt PA. Conjugate eye deviations as dyskinesias induced by levodopa in Parkinson's disease. Mov Disord 13(4): 731–734, 1998.

Linazasoro F, Van Blercom N, Lasa A. Levodopa-induced ocular dyskinesias in Parkinson's disease. Mov Disord 17: 186–220, 2002.

Martin WE. Adverse reactions during treatment of Parkinson's disease with levodopa. JAMA 216: 1979–1983, 1971.

Procianoy E, Fuchs FD, Procianoy L, Procianoy F. The effect of increasing doses of levodopa on children with strabismic amblyopia. J Am Assoc Pediatr Ophthalmol Strabismus 3(6): 337–340, 1999.

Shimizu N, et al. Ocular dyskinesias in patients with Parkinson's disease treated with levodopa. Ann Neurol 1: 167, 1977.

van Rens GN, et al. Uveal malignant melanoma and levodopa therapy in Parkinson's disease. Ophthalmology 89: 1464, 1982.

Weiner WJ, Nausieda PA. Meige's syndrome during long-term dopaminergic therapy in Parkinson's disease. Arch Neurol 39: 451, 1982.

Generic name: Selegiline hydrochloride.

Proprietary names: Eldepryl, Emsam, Zelapar.

Primary use

This is a selective inhibitor of monoamine oxidase type B which enhances the effects of levodopa and is used in the management of Parkinson's disease.

Ocular side effects

Systemic administration
Certain
1. Blurred vision
2. Blepharospasm

Probable
1. Photophobia

Possible
1. Chromatopsia
2. Visual hallucinations
3. Vortex keratopathy
4. Diplopia

Clinical significance

This drug has had only a few ocular adverse events reported with its use. It is an agent that increases dopaminergic activity, thereby acting as a sympathomimetic. To date, all of the above side effects are reversible once the drug is discontinued. Buttner et al (1993) postulated a color perception problem with Parkinson's disease, so the drug may not be implicated. Rarely are any of the above side effects a reason to discontinue the drug, except in patients with diplopia or severe blepharospasm. A disagreement of whether or not selegiline causes visual hallucinations is in the literature (Kamakura et al 2004; Papapetropoulos and Argyriou 2005). There is only one case of bilateral vortex keratopathy in a patient on this medication for 1 month. This cleared after the drug was discontinued.

REFERENCES AND FURTHER READING

Buttner T, Kuhn W, Klotz P, et al. Disturbance of colour perception in Parkinson's disease. J Neural Transmission Parkinsons Dis Dementia Sect 6(1): 11–15, 1993.

Kamakura K, Mochizuki H, Kaida K, et al. Therapeutic factors causing hallucination in Parkinson's disease patients, especially those given selegiline. Parkinsonism Relat Disord 10: 235–242, 2004.

Papapetropoulos S, Argyriou AA. Administration of selegiline is not associated with visual hallucinations in advanced Parkinson's disease. Parkinsonism Relat Disord 11: 265–266, 2005.

Physicians' Desk Reference, 60th edn, Thomson PDR, Montvale, NJ, pp 3209–3211, 2006.

Sweetman SC (ed). Martindale: The Complete Drug Reference, 34th edn, Pharmaceutical Press, London, pp 1214–1215, 2004.

CLASS: CHOLINESTERASE REACTIVATORS

Generic name: Pralidoxime.

Proprietary name: Protopam.

Primary use

This cholinesterase reactivator is used as an antidote for poisoning due to organophosphate pesticides or other chemicals that have anticholinesterase activity. It is also of value in the control of overdosage by anticholinesterase agents used in the treatment of myasthenia gravis.

Ocular side effects

Systemic administration
Certain
1. Decreased vision
2. Diplopia
3. Decreased accommodation

Local ophthalmic use or exposure – subconjunctival injection
Certain
1. Irritation
   a. Hyperemia
   b. Burning sensation
2. Iritis
3. Reverses miosis
4. Reverses accommodative spasms

Possible
1. Subconjunctival hemorrhages

Clinical significance

Pralidoxime commonly causes adverse ocular reactions after systemic administration. These effects are of rapid onset, last from a few minutes to a few hours, and are completely reversible. In one series, up to 60% of patients using the agent complained of misty vision, heaviness of the eye, blurred near vision or decreased accommodation, especially after sudden head movement. Ocular side effects from subconjunctival injection are also transitory and reversible.

REFERENCES AND FURTHER READING

Bryon HM, Posner H. Clinical evaluation of Protopam. Am J Ophthalmol 57: 409, 1964.
Dekking HM. Stopping the action of strong miotics. Ophthalmologica 148: 428, 1964.
Drug Evaluations, 6th edn, American Medical Association, Chicago, pp 1647–1648, 1986.
Holland P, Parkes DC. Plasma concentrations of the oxime pralidoxime mesylate (P25) after repeated oral and intramuscular administration. Br J Ind Med 33: 43, 1676.
Jager BV, Stagg GN. Toxicity of diacetyl monoxime and of pyridine-2-aldoxime methiodide in man. Bull Johns Hopkins Hosp 102: 203, 1958.
Taylor WJR, et al. Effects of a combination of atropine, metaraminol and pyridine aldoxime methanesulfonate (AMP therapy) on normal human subjects. Can Med Assoc J 93: 957, 1965.

CLASS: MUSCLE RELAXANTS

Generic name: Dantrolene sodium.

Proprietary name: Dantrium.

Primary use

This skeletal muscle relaxant is effective in controlling the manifestations of clinical spasticity resulting from serious chronic disorders, such as spinal cord injury, stroke, cerebral palsy or multiple sclerosis.

Ocular side effects

Systemic administration
Certain
1. Decreased vision
2. Visual hallucinations

Possible
1. Eyelids or conjunctiva
   a. Photosensitivity
   b. Urticaria
2. Diplopia
3. Lacrimation

Clinical significance

Ocular side effects due to dantrolene are transient and seldom of clinical significance. Decreased vision, diplopia and excessive lacrimation are the most common adverse ocular effects. Visual hallucinations associated with the use of this drug usually subside on drug withdrawal, but this may take several days.

REFERENCES AND FURTHER READING

Andrews LG, Muzumdar AS, Pinkerton AC. Hallucinations associated with dantrolene sodium therapy. Can Med Assoc J 112: 148, 1975.
McEvoy GK (ed). American Hospital Formulary Service Drug Information 87. American Society of Hospital Pharmacists, Bethesda, pp 652–655, 1987.
Pembroke AC, et al. Acne induced by dantrolene. Br J Dermatol 104: 465, 1981.
Silverman HI, Harvie RJ. Adverse effects of commonly used systemic drugs on the human eye – Part III. Am J Optom Physiol Optics 52: 275, 1975.
Sweetman SC (ed). Martindale: The Complete Drug Reference. 34th edn. Pharmaceutical Press, London, pp 1393–1394, 2004.

Generic name: Orphenadrine citrate.

Proprietary name: Norflex.

Primary use

This antihistaminic agent is used in the treatment of skeletal muscle spasm and the associated pain of Parkinsonism.

Ocular side effects

Systemic administration
Probable
1. Pupils
   a. Mydriasis – may precipitate angle-closure glaucoma
   b. Decreased or absent reaction to light (toxic states)
2. Decreased vision
3. Decrease or paralysis of accommodation

Possible
1. Diplopia
2. Visual hallucinations
3. Subconjunctival or retinal hemorrhages secondary to drug-induced anemia
4. Decreased tolerance to contact lenses

Clinical significance

Ocular side effects due to orphenadrine are transient and probably the result of its weak anticholinergic effect. These are seldom a significant clinical problem, although angle-closure glaucoma has been precipitated secondary to drug induced mydriasis. Non-reactive dilated pupils are only seen in overdose situations.

REFERENCES AND FURTHER READING

Bennett NB, Kohn J. Case report: orphenadrine overdose. Cerebral manifestations treated with physostigmine. Anaesth Intens Care 4: 67, 1976.
Davidson SI. Reports of ocular adverse reactions. Trans Ophthalmol Soc UK 93: 495–510, 1973.
Furlanut M, et al. Orphenadrine serum levels in a poisoned patient. Hum Toxicol 4: 331, 1985.
Heinonen J, et al. Orphenadrine poisoning. A case report supplemented with animal experiments. Arch Toxicol 23: 264, 1968.
Selby G. Treatment of parkinsonism. Drugs 11: 61, 1976.
Stoddart JC, Parkin JM, Wytne NA. Orphenadrine poisoning. A case report. Br J Anaesth 40: 786, 1968.

SECTION 11
ONCOLYTIC AGENTS

CLASS: ANTINEOPLASTIC AGENTS

Generic names: 1. Bleomycin; 2. dactinomycin; 3. daunorubicin; 4. doxorubicin; 5. mitomycin.

Proprietary names: 1. Blenoxane; 2. Cosmegen; 3. Cerubidine, Daunoxome; 4. Adriamycin PFS, Doxil, Rubex; 5. Mutamycin, Mytozytrex.

Primary use

Systemic

These antibiotics are used in a variety of malignant conditions. Bleomycin is a polypeptide antibiotic used in the management of squamous cell carcinomas, lymphomas and testicular carcinomas. Dactinomycin is an antibiotic used in the management of choriocarcinoma, rhabdomyosarcoma, Wilms' tumor, testicular neoplasms and carcinoid syndrome. Daunorubicin is used in the treatment of acute leukemia, and doxorubicin is used in sarcomas, lymphomas and leukemia. Mitomycin is useful in the therapy of disseminated adenocarcinoma of the stomach or pancreas.

Ophthalmic

Mitomycin is used as an adjunct in the surgical treatment of pterygia and glaucoma. It may also be used in the management of carcinoma in situ and primary acquired melanosis.

Ocular side effects
Systemic administration
Certain
1. Eyelids or conjunctiva
   a. Conjunctivitis
   b. Allergic reactions
   c. Erythema
   d. Edema
   e. Hyperpigmentation
   f. Angioneurotic edema
   g. Urticaria
   h. Loss of eyelashes or eyebrows
2. Decreased vision
3. Lacrimation

Probable
1. May aggravate herpes infections
2. Ocular teratogenic effects

Possible
1. Eyelids or conjunctiva – erythema multiforme
2. Subconjunctival or retinal hemorrhages secondary to drug-induced anemia

Inadvertent ocular exposure (doxorubicin)
Certain
1. Keratoconjunctivitis
2. Chemosis
3. Subepithelial dot infiltrates
4. Transitory anterior uveitis

Local ophthalmic use or exposure – mitomycin
Certain
1. Irritation
   a. Lacrimation
   b. Hyperemia
   c. Photophobia
   d. Ocular pain
2. Eyelids or conjunctiva
   a. Allergic or irritative reactions
   b. Hyperemia
   c. Erythema
   d. Blepharitis
   e. Conjunctivitis
   f. Edema
   g. Granuloma
   h. Avascularity
   i. Symblepharon (Fig. 7.11a)
3. Cornea
   a. Punctate keratitis
   b. Edema
   c. Delayed wound healing
   d. Erosion (epithelial and stromal)
   e. Perforation
   f. Crystalline epithelial deposits
   g. Recurrence of herpes simplex
   h. Astigmatism
   i. Ulceration
4. Sclera
   a. Erosion
   b. Delayed wound healing
   c. Perforation
   d. Avascularity
   e. Necrotizing scleritis
   f. Calcium deposits
   g. Yellowish plaques
   h. Scleritis (anterior and posterior)
5. Uvea
   a. Iridocyclitis
   b. Hypopigmentation of iris
   c. Hyperemia
6. Glaucoma
7. Punctal occlusion
8. Hypotony – occasionally persistent
9. Filtering blebs
   a. Thinned wall
   b. Excessive size
   c. Overfiltration
   d. Spontaneous leaks
   e. Late bleb infections
10. Cataract formation
11. Choroidal effusions

Clinical significance

All of these agents are antimetabolites and, when given systemically, may be concentrated in the tears and cause irritation of the conjunctiva, cornea and lid margin. This usually occurs within a few days after drug exposure and may return to normal a few days after the drug is stopped. Conjunctivitis and blurred vision are the most frequent drug-induced side effects. Blum (1975) stated that up to 25% of patients on doxorubicin may have increased lacrimation. The cause may be secondary to ocular irritation. Which drug causes which ocular side effect is often difficult to determine because these agents are often used in combination. Megadoses of mitomycin and carmustine (Cruciani et al 1994) cause changes in the tear film in all patients with changes to the corneal and conjunctival epithelium. Young et al (1993) described transient cortical blindness due to bleomycin along with other drugs. These drugs may be cofactors in cataractogenesis. In most instances, this group of drugs is only given systemically for cancer therapy and their systemic side effects are often so severe that ocular side effects may be insignificant to the overall clinical disability.

Inadvertent topical ocular exposure causes only transitory ocular effects. Keratoconjunctivitis, with or without punctate subepithelial dot infiltrates, may occur. These effects resolve after a few days without sequelae. McLoon et al (1988) reported muscle loss secondary to direct injection of doxorubicin in the management of blepharospasm.

The topical ocular use of these drugs is limited to mitomycin, which has been in clinical use for over two decades. During this time much has been learnt about how to limit local side effects and improve the risk-benefit ratio of this potent agent. This drug is used in glaucoma filtering surgery to inhibit wound healing, in pterygium surgery to limit recurrence, in dacryocystorhinostomy to decrease fibrous tissue growth, scarring and granulation, in refractive surgery to limit post-operative corneal haze, in cicatrical ocular surface disease to limit scaring, and for treatment of ocular surface malignancies. The ocular complications that occur are due directly to the concentration, duration of application and the surface to which it is applied. Patient acceptance of the frequency and extent of the ocular complications is dependent on the severity of the disease being treated. Mitomycin action on ocular tissue mimics that of ionizing radiation with probable resultant lifelong effects on tissue. A major characteristic of this chemical is that some side effects are immune mediated and may manifest themselves months after exposure. Irritative signs and symptoms are usually short-lived and seldom last more than a few weeks after discontinuing the drug. The most serious side effects are probably immune mediated. Although these may affect many areas, a long-term effect on both fibroblast activity and vascular endothelial cells is most evident. This could account for severe non-responsive corneal and scleral melts that may mimic scleromalacia perforans and/or necrotizing scleritis. Cases in the literature report perforation and, in some instances, the loss of the eye. Porcelainization of the conjunctiva and sclera (avascularity) has been permanent. As with systemic exposure, local recurrence of herpes simplex and calcification of tissue in direct contact with mitomycin can occur. Robin et al (1997) pointed out that the length of exposure may be more important than the concentration of the drug. In their series, the most important complications were cataract formation and persistent choroidal effusion, which are secondary to hypotony. There are more than 60 papers in the literature describing various aspects of complications from topical ocular application of mitomycin. The Higginbotham (1997) editorial summarizes and gives perspective on its use in glaucoma surgery. Abraham et al (2006) give a complete review of this drug's use in ophthalmology. What role mitomycin C has in corneal dysplasias and primary acquired melanosis is still being developed. The complications for high-dose or frequent application seem acceptable to date, if the bare scleral is not exposed. Gebhardt (1998) pointed out these agents as a potential carcinogenic hazard. See references for additional information on specific side effects.

REFERENCES AND FURTHER READING

Abraham LM, Selva D, Casson R, et al. Mitomycin: clinical application in ophthalmic practice. Drugs 66: 321–340, 2006.

Al-Hazmi A, Zwaan J, Awad A, et al. Effectiveness and complications of mitomycin C use during pediatric glaucoma surgery. Ophthalmology 105(10): 1915–1919, 1998.

Billing K, Karagiannis A, Selva D. Punctal-canalicular stenosis associated with mitomycin-C for corneal epithelial dysplasia. Am J Ophthalmol 136: 746–747, 2003.

Bindish R, Condon GP, Schlosser JD, et al. Efficacy and safety of mitomycin-c in primary trabeculectomy. Ophthalmology 109: 1336–1342, 2002.

Blum R. An overview of studies with adriamycin in the United States. Cancer Chemother Rep 6: 247–251, 1975.

Carrasco MA, Rapuano CJ, Cohen EJ, et al. Scleral ulceration after preoperative injection of mitomycin c in the pterygium head. Arch Ophthalmol 120: 1585–1586, 2002.

Cartsburg O, Kallen C, Hillenkamp J, et al. Topical mitomycin c and radiation induce conjunctival DNA-polyploidy. Anal Cell Pathol 23: 65–74, 2001.

Cruciani F, Tamanti N, Abdolrahimzadeh S, et al. Ocular toxicity of systemic chemotherapy with megadoses of carmustine and mitomycin. Ann Ophthalmol 26: 97–100, 1994.

Dafgard-Kopp E, Seregard S. Epiphora as a side effect of topical mitomycin c. Br J Ophthalmol 88: 1422–1424, 2004.

Danias J, Rosenbaum J, Podos SM. Diffuse retinal heorrhages (ocular decompression syndrome) after trabeculectomy with mitomycin c for neovascular glaucoma. Acta Ophthalmol Scand 78: 468–469, 2000.

Daugelience L, Yamamoto T, Kitazawa Y. Cataract development after traveculectomy with mitomycin c: a 1-year study. Surv Ophthalmol 45: 165, 2000.

DeBry PW, Perkins TW, Heatley G, et al. Incidence of late-onset bleb-related complications following trabeculectomy. Arch Ophthalmol 120: 297–300, 2002.

Dev S, Herndon L, Shields MB. Retinal vein occlusion after trabeculectomy with mitomycin C. Am J Ophthalmol 122(4): 574–575, 1996.

Dudney BW, Malecha M. Limbal stem cell deficiency following topical mitomycin c treatment of conjunctival-corneal intraepithelial neoplasia. Am J Ophthalmol 137: 950–951, 2004.

Fourman S. Scleritis after glaucoma filtering surgery with mitomycin C. Ophthalmology 102(10): 1569–1571, 1995.

Gebhardt DOE. Topical mitomycin C for the treatment of conjunctival and corneal epithelial dysplasia and neoplasia. Am J Ophthalmol 125(3): 416–417, 1998.

Gupta S, Basti S. Corneoscleral, ciliary body, and vitreoretinal toxicity after excessive instillation of mitomycin C [letter]. Am J Ophthalmol 114: 503–504, 1992.

Higginbotham EJ. Adjunctive use of mitomycin in filtration surgery: is it worth the risk? Arch Ophthalmol 115(8): 969–974, 1068–1069 , 1997.

Khong JJ, Muecke J. Complications of mitomycin c therapy in 100 eyes with ocular surface neoplasia. Br J Ophthalmol 90: 819–822, 2006.

Kirschen McLoon L, Wirtschafter JD, Cameron JD. Muscle loss from doxorubicin injections into the eyelids of a patient with blepharospasm. Am J Ophthalmol 116(5): 646–648, 1993.

Knowles RS, Virden JE. Handling of injectable antineoplastic agents. BMJ 2: 589, 1980.

Kymionis GD, Tsiklis NS, Ginis H, et al. Dry eye after photorefractive keratectomy with adjuvant mitomycin c. J Refract Surg 22: 511–513, 2006.

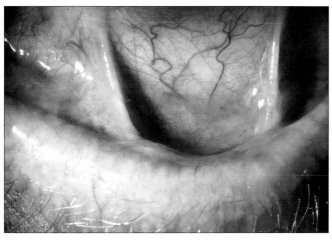

Fig. 7.11a Topical ocular mitomycin-induced symblepharon.

McDermott ML, Wang J, Shin DH. Mitomycin and the human corneal endothelium. Arch Ophthalmol 112: 533–537, 1994.

McLoon LK, Wirtschafter J. Doxorubicin chemomyectomy: injection of monkey orbicularis oculi results in selective muscle injury. Inv Ophthalmol Vis Sci 29(12): 1854–1859, 1988.

Mietz H, Roters S, Krieglstein GK. Bullous keratopathy as a complication of trabeculectomy with mitomycin c. Grafes Arch Clin Exp Ophthalmol 243: 1284–1287, 2005.

Oram O, et al. Necrotizing keratitis following trabeculectomy with mitomycin. Arch Ophthalmol 113: 19–20, 1995.

Pfister RR. Permanent corneal edema resulting from the treatment of PTK corneal haze with mitomycin. Cornea 23: 744–747, 2004.

Price FW Jr. Corneal endothelial damage after trabeculectomy with mitomycin c in two patients with glaucoma with cornea guttata. Cornea 21: 733, 2002.

Robin AL, Ramakrishnan R, Krishnadas R, et al. A long-term dose response study of mitomycin in glaucoma filtration surgery. Arch Ophthalmol 115: 969–974, 1997.

Rubinfeld RS, Pfister RR, Stein RM, et al. Serious complications of topical mitomycin-C after pterygium surgery. Ophthalmology 99(11): 1647–1654, 1992.

Sacu S, Ségur-Eltz N, Horvat R, et al. Intumescent cataract after topical mitomycin-C for conjunctival malignant melanoma. Am J Ophthalmol 136: 375–377, 2003.

Sauder G, Jonas JB. Limbel stem cell deficiency after subconjunctival mitomycin c injection for trabeculectomy. Am J Ophthalmol 141: 1129–1130, 2006.

Sihota R, Dada T, Gupta SD, et al. Conjunctival dysfunction and mitomycin c-induced hypotony. J Glaucoma 9: 392–397, 2000.

Suner IJ, Greenfield DS, Miller MP, et al. Hypotony maculopathy after filtering surgery with mitomycin C. Ophthalmology 104(2): 207–215, 1997.

Vizel M, Oster MW. Ocular side effects of cancer chemotherapy. Cancer 49: 1999–2002, 1982.

Wu SC. Central retinal vein occlusion after trabeculectomy with mitomycin c. Can J Ophthalmol 36: 37–39, 2001.

You Y, Gu Y-S, Fang C-T, et al. Long-term effects of simultaneous subconjunctival and subscleral mitomycin C application in repeat trabeculectomy. J Glaucoma 11: 110–118, 2002.

Young DC, Mitchell A, Kessler J, et al. Cortical blindness and seizures possibly related to cisplatin, vinblastine, and bleomycin treatment of ovarian dysgerminoma. J Am Osteopath Assoc 93: 502–504, 1993.

Zarnowski T, Haszcz D, Rakowska E, et al. Corneal astigmatism after trabeculectomy. Klinika Oczna 99(5): 313–315, 1997.

Generic name: Busulfan.

Proprietary names: Busulfex, Myleran.

Primary use

This alkylating agent is used in the palliative treatment of chronic granulocytic leukemia and other blood dyscrasias.

Ocular side effects

Systemic administration – intravenous
Certain
1. Decreased vision
2. Cataracts
   a. Posterior subcapsular
   b. Punctate cortical opacities
3. Eyelids
   a. Hyperpigmentation
   b. Angioneurotic edema
   c. Loss of eyelashes or eyebrows
4. Visual hallucinations

Probable
1 Keratoconjunctivitis sicca

Possible
1 Subconjunctival or retinal hemorrhages secondary to drug-induced anemia
2. Myasthenia gravis
   a. Diplopia
   b. Ptosis
   c. Paresis of extraocular muscles
3. Eyelids or conjunctiva
   a. Erythema multiforme
   b. Exfoliative dermatitis

Ocular teratogenic effects
Possible
1. Retinal degeneration
2. Microoophthalmia

Clinical significance

Blurred vision, eyelid changes and a sicca-like syndrome may be seen and are reversible (Sidi et al 1977). Busulfan-induced cataract is not reversible. This anticancer agent characteristically causes posterior subcapsular lens opacities after 4–5 years of therapy or a cumulative amount of 2000 mg of the drug (Honda et al 1993). These lens changes are often associated with scattered punctate cortical opacities and/or a polychromatic sheen to the posterior capsule of the lens. The incidence and severity increases with duration and total dosage. Kaida et al (1999) reported one case of a 42-year-old who was treated with 212 mg per day for 4 days and developed posterior sub-capsular opacities. Al-Tweigeri et al (1996) suggested that the mechanism of busulfan-induced cataracts is related to decreased DNA synthesis in the lens epithelium. Holmström et al (2002) reported a series of children who received total body radiation and busulfan. The incidence of cataracts increased along with the cataractogenic additive cofactor effects of corticosteroids and other cytostatic drugs. Holmström et al stress early diagnosis by observing lens changes to prevent the development of amblyopia.

Rare reports suggest that this agent can cause teratogenic effects such as microoophthalmia or retinal degeneration.

REFERENCES AND FURTHER READING

Al-Tweigeri T, Nabholtz JM, Mackey JR. Ocular toxicity and cancer chemotherapy. Cancer 78: 1359–1373, 1996.

Dahlgren S, Holm G, Svanborg N, et al. Clinical and morphological side-effects of busulfan (myleran) treatment. Acta Med Scand 192: 129–135, 1972.

Fraunfelder FT, Meyer SM. Ocular toxicology. In: Clinical Ophthalmology, Vol. 5, Duane TD (ed), Harper and Row, Philadelphia, ch. p 37, 1987.

Grimes P, von Sallmann L, Frichette A. Influence of Myleran on cell proliferation in the lens epithelium. Invest Ophthalmol 3: 566–576, 1965.

Holmström G, Borgström B, Calissendorff B. Cataract in children after bone marrow transplantation: relation to conditioning regimen. Acta Ophthalmol Scand 80: 211–215, 2002.

Honda A, Dake Y, Amemiya T. Cataracts in a patient treated with busulfan (Mablin powder) for eight years. Nippon Ganka Gakkai Zasshi Acta Societatis 97(1): 1242–1245, 1993.

Imperia PS, Lazarus HM, Lass JH. Ocular complication of systemic cancer chemotherapy. Surv Ophthalmol 34: 209–230, 1989.

Kaida T, Ogawa T, Amemiya T. Cataract induced by short term administration of large doses of busulfan: a case report. Ophthalmologica 213: 397–399, 1999.

Podos SM, Canellos GP. Lens changes in chronic granulocytic leukemia. Am J Ophthalmol 68: 500–504, 1969.

Ravindranathan MP, Paul VJ, Kuriakose ET. Cataract after busulphan treatment. BMJ 1: 218–219, 1972.

Schmid KE, Kornek GV, Scheithauer W, et al. Update on ocular complications of systemic cancer chemotherapy. Surv Ophthalmol 51: 19–40, 2006.

Sidi Y, Douer D, Pinkhas J. Sicca syndrome in a patient with toxic reaction to busulfan. JAMA 238: 1951, 1977.

Smalley RV, Wall RL. Two cases of busulfan toxicity. Ann Intern Med 64: 154–164, 1966.
Soysal T, Bavunoglu I, Baslar Z, et al. Cataract after prolonged busulphan therapy. Acta Haematol 90: 213, 1993.

Generic name: Capecitabine.

Proprietary name: Xeloda.

Primary use

This antimetabolite is an orally administered fluoropyrimadine carbamate used for the treatment of metastatic breast and colon rectal cancers.

Ocular side effects

Systemic administration
Certain
1. Ocular irritation
2. Cornea
   a. Superficial punctate keratitis
   b. Superficial corneal deposits (Fig. 7.11b)
   c. Keratoconjunctivitis
3. Photophobia
4. Conjunctiva
   a. Chemosis
   b. Erythema
   c. Conjunctivitis
5. Decreased vision
6. Lacrimation increased

Clinical significance

This anticancer agent is probably secreted in the tears and therefore various degrees of ocular irritation may occur. In rare cases it appears to be associated with a superficial punctate keratitis, decreased vision and marked photophobia. Walkhom et al (2000) reported two cases of bilateral superficial white corneal deposits in a whorl pattern. Both cases were in ocular sicca patients with incapacitating visual and ocular symptoms. In one case there were two positive rechallenges with complete clearing in between. These signs and symptoms may take 4–6 weeks to develop and take an equal amount of time to resolve. These

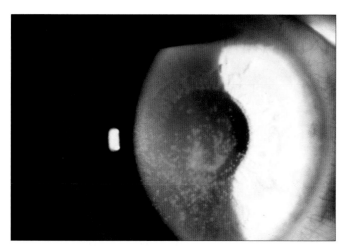

Fig. 7.11b Corneal deposits from systemic capecitabine.

findings appear to be totally reversible when the drug is discontinued or lessens if the dosage is decreased.

REFERENCES AND FURTHER READING

Drug Information for the Health Care Professional, 20th edn, Micromedex, Englewood, CO, pp 768–771, 2000.
Physicians' Desk Reference, 60th edn, Thomson PDR, Montvale, NJ, pp 2825–2834, 2006.
Waikhom B, Fraunfelder FT, Henner WD. Severe ocular irritation and corneal deposits associated with capecitabine use. N Engl J Med 343: 1428, 2000.

Generic name: Carmustine (BCNU).

Proprietary name: BiCNU, Gliadel.

Primary use

This nitrosourea is used in the treatment of brain tumors and various malignant neoplasms.

Ocular side effects

Systemic administration – intraveneous
Certain
1. Blurred vision
2. Orbit
   a. Vasodilatation
   b. Proptosis
   c. Pain
   d. Edema
3. Eyelids and conjunctiva
   a. Allergic reactions
   b. Hyperemia (Fig. 7.11cA)
   c. Blepharoconjunctivitis
   d. Chemosis
   e. Hyperpigmentation-skin
4. Non-specific ocular irritation
   a. Lacrimation
   b. Photophobia
   c. Burning sensation

Possible
1. Optic nerve
   a. Neuritis
   b. Atrophy
2. Subconjunctival or retinal hemorrhages secondary to drug-induced anemia
3. May aggravate
   a. Herpes infections
   b. Keratitis sicca
4. Cornea
   a. Edema
   b. Opacities (Fig. 7.11cB)
5. Arteriovenous shunting

Systemic administration – intracarotid injection
Certain
1. Blurred vision
2. Orbit
   a. Vasodilatation
   b. Proptosis

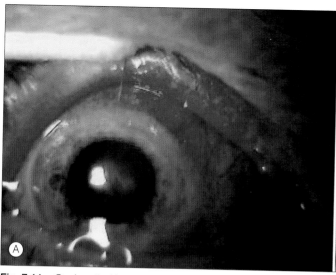
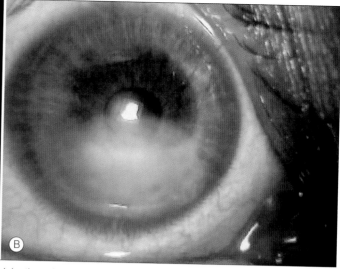

Fig. 7.11c Conjunctival hyperemia (A) and opacity (B) after intravenous injection of carmustine. Photo courtesy of Schmid KE, et al. Update on ocular complications of systemic cancer therapy. Surv Ophthalmol 51: 19–40, 2006.

c. Pain
d. Edema
3. Eyelids and conjunctiva
a. Hyperemia
b. Blepharoconjunctivitis
c. Chemosis
4. Non-specific ocular irritation
a. Lacrimation
b. Photophobia
c. Burning sensation
5. Optic nerve
a. Neuritis
b. Atrophy
6. Retinal vascular disorders
a. Occlusion
b. Thrombosis
c. Hemorrhages
d. Exudates
7. Cornea
a. Edema
b. Opacities
8. Extraocular muscle
a. Fibrosis of recti muscles
b. Internal ophthalmoplegia
9. ERG abnormalities
10. Viterous opacities

Possible

1. Subconjunctival or retinal hemorrhages secondary to drug-induced anemia
2. May aggravate
a. Herpes infections
b. Keratitis sicca
3. Arteriorvenous shunting
4. Secondary glaucoma

Clinical significance

Due to this agent's ability to penetrate the blood-retinal barrier, increased neuro-retinal toxicity may occur. It can also cause ischemic changes (Wang et al 2000) with vascular narrowing. Side effects are related to dose, injection site, frequency of injections and speed of infusion. Many side effects are delayed, possibly implying long-lasting active metabolites. This drug is given intravenously as well as intracarotid and ocular side effects are much more severe with the later. Ocular side effects of intracarotid injections can be limited by advancing the intracarotid catheter beyond the origin of the ophthalmic artery. Applying pressure on the eye with a Honan balloon during the infusion may decrease the amount of drug getting to the eye (Imperia et al 1989). If these measures are not done, up to 70% of patients' eyes, within 2–14 weeks, will have significant ocular side effect from intracarotid infusions. Even with proper placement of the catheter, various degrees of blurred vision, retrobulbar pain, conjunctival hyperemia, corneal edema and opacities, secondary glaucoma, internal ophthalmoplegia, vitreous opacities, various orbital vascular pathologies, optic neuropathy, bleeding, retinal arterial narrowing, nerve fiber layer infarcts and intraretinal hemorrhages can occur. Like most anticancer agents, this agent causes a transitory irritative conjunctivitis. This is probably due to an irritative or toxic antimetabolic effect since the drug is secreted in the tears. These effects may aggravate ocular sicca. This drug is often used in combination with various other antimetabolites as well as in combination with bone marrow transplantation. Various reports (Singleton et al 1982; Miller et al 1985; Johnson et al 1999) have shown a variety of the same ocular side effects associated with carmustine, including blindness.

REFERENCES AND FURTHER READING

Barrada A, Peyman GA, et al. Toxicity of antineoplastic drugs in vitrectomy infusion fluids. Ophthalmic Surg 14: 845–847, 1983.

Chrousos GA, Oldfield EH, et al. Prevention of ocular toxicity of carmustine (BCNU) with supraophthalmic intracarotid infusion. Ophthalmology 93: 1471–1475, 1986.

Elsas T, Watne K, et al. Ocular complications after intracarotid BCNU for intracranial tumors. Acta Ophthalmol 67: 83–86, 1989.

Greenberg HS, et al. Intra-arterial BCNU chemotherapy for treatment of malignant gliomas of the central nervous system. J Neurosurg 61: 423–429, 1984.

Imperia PS, Lazarus HM, Lass JH. Ocular complications of systemic cancer chemotherapy. Surv Ophthalmol 34(3): 209–230, 1989.

Johnson DW, Cagnoni PJ, Schossau TM, et al. Optic disc and retinal microvasculopathy after high-dose chemotherapy and autologous hematopoietic progenitor cell support. Bone Marrow Transplant 24: 785–792, 1999.

Khawly JA, Rubin P, Petros W, et al. Retinopathy and optic neuropathy in bone marrow transplantation for breast cancer. Ophthalmology 103: 87–95, 1996.

Kupersmith MJ, Frohman LP, et al. Visual toxicity following intraarterial chemotherapy. Neurology 38: 284–289, 1988.

Mahaley MS. Commentary on ocular toxicity following intracarotid chemotherapy. J Clin Neuro-Ophthalmol 7: 92, 1987.

McLennan R, Taylor HR. Optic neuroretinitis in association with BCNU and procarbazine therapy. Med Pediatr Oncol 4: 43–48, 1978.

Miller DF, Bay JW, et al. Ocular and orbital toxicity following intracarotid injection of BCNU (Carmustine) and cisplatinum for malignant gliomas. Ophthalmology 92: 402–406, 1985.

Pickrell L, Purvin V. Ischemic optic neuropathy secondary to intracarotid infusion of BCNU. J Clin Neuro-Ophthalmol 7: 87–91, 1987.

Schmid KE, Kornek GV, Scheithauer W, et al. Update on ocular complication of systemic cancer chemotherapy. Surv Ophthalmol 51: 19–40, 2006.

Shingleton BJ, Bienfang DC, et al. Ocular toxicity associated with highdose carmustine. Arch Ophthalmol 100: 1766–1772, 1982.

Wilson WB, Perez GM, Kleinschmidt-Demasters BK. Sudden onset of blindness in patients treated with oral BCNU and low-dose cranial irradiation. Cancer 59: 901–907, 1987.

Wang MY, Arnold AC, Vinters HV, et al. Bilateral blindness and lumbosacral myelopathy associated with highdose carmustine and cisplatin therapy. Am J Ophthalmol 120: 297–368, 2000.

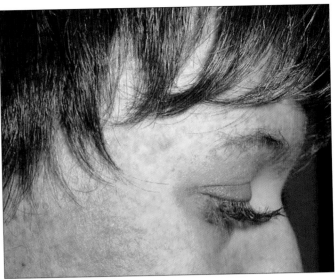

Fig. 7.11d Growth of eyelashes after treatment with Irinotecan and cetuximab. Photo courtesy of Dueland S, et al. Epidermal growth factor receptor inhibition induces trichomegaly. Acta Oncol 42: 345–346, 2003.

Generic name: Cetuximab.

Proprietary name: Erbitux.

Primary use

This monoclonal antibody binds to epidermal growth factor receptors (EGFR) and is used in the treatment of metastatic colorectal cancer, solid cancers and cancers of the head and neck.

Ocular side effects

Systemic administration – intravenous
Probable
1. Eyelids or conjunctiva
   a. Hyperemia
   b. Conjunctivitis
   c. Squamous blepharitis
2. Non-specific ocular irritation
   a. Photophobia
   b. Epiphoria
   c. Itching

Possible
1. Eyelids or conjunctiva – exfoliative dermatitis
2. Trichomegaly (Fig. 7.11d)

Clinical significance

All ocular side effects are listed as probable because there are so few reports. There is one well-documented case (Tonini et al 2005) of squamous blepharitis and associated ocular discomfort with a positive rechallenge. The adverse ocular events occurred within 3 weeks of starting cetuximab and recovery happened within 1 week after stopping the drug. Tonini et al (2005) postulated that EGFR is expressed in the epidermis, the sweat glands and hair follicular epithelium. This drug directly interferes with the EGFR signaling pathway. It also targets the EGFR-expressing cells of the meiboman glands and may consequently lead to altered secretion functions.

Bouché et al (2005) and Dueland et al (2003) reported trichomegaly without hypertrichosis. This occurred within a few months of therapy and required the cutting of the lashes to allow for ocular comfort. Surprisingly, the regulation of hair growth in these patients was only limited to the eyelid. This adverse event resolved 1 month after stopping the drug.

REFERENCES AND FURTHER READING

Bouché O, Brixi-Benmansour H, Bertin A, et al. Trichomegaly of the eyelashes following treatment with cetuximab. Ann Oncol 16: 1711–1712, 2005.

Dueland S, Sauer T, Lund-Johansen F, et al. Epidermal growth factor receptor inhibition induces trichomegaly. Acta Oncol 42: 345–346, 2003.

Tonini G, Vincenzi B, Santini D, et al. Ocular toxicity related to cetuximab monotherapy in an advanced colorectal cancer patient. J Natl Cancer Inst 97: 606–607, 2005.

Generic name: Cisplatin (cisplatinum).

Proprietary names: Platinol, Platinol-AQ.

Primary use

This platinum-containing antineoplastic agent is used for the treatment of metastatic testicular or ovarian tumors, advanced bladder carcinoma and a wide variety of other neoplasms.

Ocular side effects

Systemic administration – intravenous
Certain
1. Blurred vision
2. Color blindness – blue-yellow axis
3. Abnormal ERG, EOG or VEP
4. Loss of contrast sensitivity
5. Macular pigment changes – mild
6. Eyelids or conjunctiva
   a. Erythema
   b. Conjunctivitis – non-specific
   c. Edema
   d. Urticaria
   e. Loss of eyelashes or eyebrows
7. Orbital pain

Probable

1. Optic nerve
   a. Edema
   b. Neuritis
   c. Retrobulbar neuritis
2. Cortical blindness
3. Visual fields
   a. Central visual constricted
   b. Hemianopsia
4. May aggravate herpes infections

Possible

1. Myasthenic neuromuscular blocking effect
   a. Diplopia
   b. Ptosis
   c. Paresis of extraocular muscles
2. Oculogyric crises
3. Nystagmus
4. Subconjunctival or retinal hemorrhages secondary to drug-induced anemia

Systemic administration – intracarotid injections
Certain

1. Ipsilateral vision loss
2. Ipsilateral orbital pain
3. Periorbital erythema and edema
4. Cavernous sinus-like syndrome
5. Blindness
6. ERG – abnormal
7. Optic nerve degeneration
8. Retina (Fig. 7.11e)
   a. Pigmentary maculopathy
   b. Cotton-wool spots
   c. Intraretinal hemorrhage
   d. Neovascularization

Possible

1. Nystagmus

Clinical significance

Cisplatin (cisplatinum) is given by intravenous or intracarotid arterial injection often with other chemotherapeutic agents, which makes it difficult to define which drug causes ocular toxicity.

Intravenous cisplatin ocular side effects differ significantly from intracarotid injections. With intravenous injections,

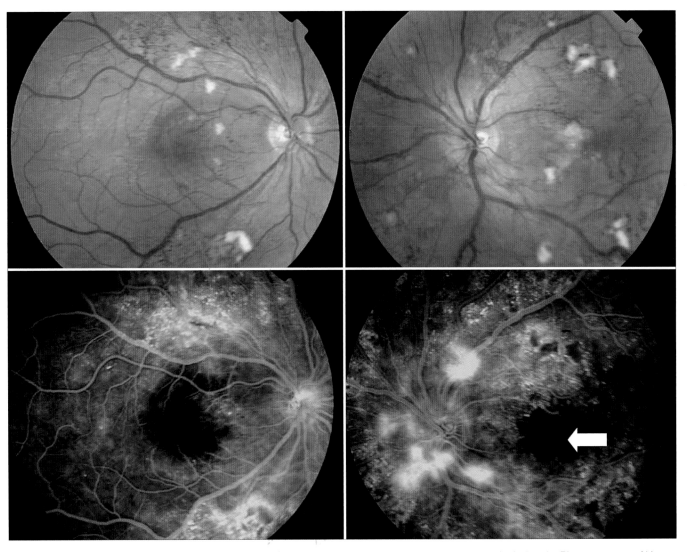

Fig. 7.11e Color photographs and fluorescein angiogram of retinal ischemia with arrow pointing to macular ischemia. Photo courtesy of Kwan ASL, et al. Retinal ischemia with neovascularization in cisplatin related retinal toxicity. Am J Ophthalmol 141: 196–197, 2006.

the more significant ocular side effects are neuro-retinal with blurred vision, color vision defects and ERG changes. Changes in the optic nerve include edema, neuritis and retrobulbar neuritis. These side effects are dose dependent and unless given over two to three courses are seldom significant in dosages of 60–100 mg/m^2 (Einhorn and Donahue 1977; Young et al 1979). Ozols et al (1983) felt advancing age and being female to be risk factors for increased ocular toxicity. In patients taking dosages above 200 mg/m^2 divided into five daily dosages, blurred vision occurred in 62% of patients, decreased color vision (blue-yellow axis) in 23%, and 84% of patients had some cone dysfunction demonstrated by color vision testing or ERG (Wilding et al 1985). Both Caruso et al (1985) and Wilding et al (1985) showed mild, irregular macular pigmentary changes in many patients with blurred vision rarely worse than 20/25. Blurred vision returns to normal after discontinuing the drug, but persistent color defects may continue for up to 16 months. There are also numerous single case reports of optic neuritis, retrobulbar neuritis and disc edema (Katz et al 2003). It is felt that this drug can cause reversible segmented nerve demyelination, similarly to heavy metal CNS toxicity. High-dose cisplatin (85–200 mg/m^2) alone or with other antimetabolites has been associated with reversible cortical blindness. Prim et al (2001) reported nystagmus secondary to cisplatin-induced vestibular pathology. Metastases, infarcts, infections, bleeding, etc., may mimic drug toxicity.

The side effects from intra-arterial injection differ in part because many of the effects are due to the high drug concentration in the eye, resulting in direct chemical retinal toxicity (Khawly et al 1996; Gonzales et al 2001; Kwan et al 2006). Retinal pathology, besides pigmentary disturbances, also includes ischemic changes such as cotton wool spots, intraretinal hemorrhages and neovascularization. These are clearly dose related and include ipsilateral visual loss in 15–60% of patients. Some patients (Kupersmith et al 1992) also received carmustine, which may also be toxic to ocular pigment epithelium. Miller et al (1985) described a patient who, after the second intracarotid injection of cisplatin and carmustine, developed ophthalmoplegia and only light perception within a few days. To limit these side effects, the intra-arterial catheter can be advanced beyond the ophthalmic artery; however, this appears to increase the risk of cerebral toxicity. Margo and Murtagh (1993) described a patient who had infusion of intra-arterial cisplatin distal to the ophthalmic artery and in a matter of days had unilateral massive orbital edema, uveal effusion, exudative retinal detachment, ophthalmoplegia, non-reactive pupil and irreversible loss of vision. Wu et al (1997) reported a case of extreme facial periorbital edema, proptosis and chemosis. This was followed by permanent unilateral loss of vision (light perception) and complete ophthalmoplegia with retinal change. They felt this was due to a combination of chemotherapeutic agents, including cisplatin.

Barr-Hamilton et al (1991) reported increased ototoxicity secondary to cisplatin in patients with darker irises. The melanin content of the inner ear is related to eye color. Melanin accumulates cisplatin, which is toxic to the vestiubular area, hence a pathology of nystagmus.

REFERENCES AND FURTHER READING

Bachmeyer C, Decroix Y, Medioni J, et al. Hypomagnesemic and hypocalcemic coma, convulsions, and ocular motility disorders after chemotherapy with platinum compounds. Revue de Medecine Interne 17(6): 467–469, 1996.

Barr-Hamilton RM, Matheson LM, Keay DG. Ototoxicity of cisplatinum and its relationship to eye color. J Laryngol Otol 105(1): 7–11, 1991.

Caraceni A, Martini C, Spatti G, et al. Recovering optic neuritis during systemic cisplatin and carboplatin chemotherapy. Acta Neurol Scand 96(4): 260–261, 1997.

Caruso R, Wilding G, Ballintine E, et al. Cis-platinum retinopathy. Invest Ophthalmol Vis Sci 26: 34, 1985.

Chalam KV, Tsao K, Malkani S, et al. Cisplatin causes neuroretinal toxicity. J Toxicol Cut Ocular Toxicol 18: 270, 1999.

Cohen RJ, et al. Transient left homonymous hemianopsia and encephalopathy following treatment of testicular carcinoma with cisplatinum, vinblastine, and bleomycin. J Clin Oncol 1: 392, 1983.

Diamond SB, et al. Cerebral blindness in association with cis-platinum chemotherapy for advanced carcinoma of the fallopian tube. Obstet Gynecol 59: 845, 1982.

Einhorn LH, Donahue J. Cis-diamminedichloroplatinum, vinblastine and bleomycin combination chemotherapy in disseminated testicular cancer. Ann Intern Med 87: 293–298, 1977.

Feun LG, et al. Intracarotid infusion of cis-diammine-dichloroplatinum in the treatment of recurrent malignant brain tumors. Cancer 54: 794, 1984.

Gonzalez F, Menedez D, Gomez-Ulla F. Monocular visual in a patient undergoing cisplatin chemotherapy. Int Ophthalmol 24: 301–304, 2001.

Hilliard LM, Berkow RL, Watterson J, et al. Retinal toxicity associated with cisplatin and etoposide in pediatric patients. Med Pediatr Oncol 28: 310–313, 1997.

Katz BJ, Ward JH, Digre KB, et al. Persistent severe visual and electroretinographic abnormalities after intravenous cisplatin therapy. J Neuro-ophthalmol 23: 132–135, 2003.

Khawly JA, Rubin P, Petros W, et al. Retinopathy and optic neuropathy in bone marrow transplantation for breast cancer. Ophthalmology 103(1): 87–95, 1996.

Kupersmith MJ, Seiple WH, Holopigian K, Noble K, et al. Maculopathy caused by intra-arterially administered cisplatin and intravenously administered carmustine. Am J Ophthalmol 113(4): 435–438, 1992.

Kwan ASL, Sahu A, Palexes G. Retinal ischemia with neovascularization in cisplatin related retinal toxicity. Am J Ophthalmol 141: 196–197, 2006.

Margo CE, Murtagh FR. Ocular and orbital toxicity after intracarotid cisplatin therapy. Am J Ophthalmol 116(4): 508–509, 1993.

Miller DF, et al. Ocular and orbital toxicity following intracarotid injection of BCNU (carmustin) and cisplatinum for malignant gliomas. Ophthalmology 92: 402, 1985.

Ozols RF, et al. Treatment of poor prognosis nonseminomatous testicular cancer with a 'high dose' platinum combination chemotherapy regimen. Cancer 51: 1803–1807, 1983.

Pollera CF, et al. Sudden death after acute dystonic reaction to high-dose metoclopramide. Lancet 2: 460, 1984.

Prim MP, de Diego JI, de Sarria MJ, et al. Vestibular and oculomotor changes in subjects with cisplatin. Acta Otorrinolaringol Esp 52: 370–397, 2001.

Shimamur Y, Chikama M, Tanimoto T, et al. Optic nerve degeneration caused by supraophthalmic carotid artery infusion with cisplatin and ACNU. J Neuro-surg 72: 285–288, 1990.

Solak Y, Dikbas O, Altundag K, et al. Myasthenic crisis following cisplatin chemotherapy in a patient with malignant thymoma. J Exp Clin Cancer Res 23: 343–344, 2004.

Swan I, Gatehouse S. Cisplatinum ototoxicity and eye colour. J Laryngol Otol 105(1): 294, 1992.

Tang RA, et al. Ocular toxicity and cisplatin. Invest Ophthalmol Vis Sci 24(Suppl.): 284, 1983.

Walsh TJ, et al. Neurotoxic effects of cisplatin therapy. Arch Neurol 39: 719, 1982.

Wilding G, et al. Retinal toxicity after high-dose cisplatin therapy. J Clin Oncol 3: 1683–1689, 1985.

Wu H, Lee A, Lehane D, et al. Ocular and orbital complications of intraarterial cisplatin: a case report. J Neuro-ophthalmol 17(3): 195–198, 1997.

Young RC, VonHoff DD, Gormley P, et al. Cis-diammine-dichlorplatinum (II) for the treatment of advanced ovarian cancer. Cancer Treat Rep 63: 1539–1544, 1979.

Generic name: Cyclophosphamide.

Proprietary names: Cytoxan, Lyophilized Cytoxan, Neosar.

Primary use

This alkylating agent is used in the treatment of various malignant diseases, including lymphoma, myeloma and a variety of solid tumors.

Ocular side effects

Systemic administration

Certain
1. Blurred vision
2. Non-specific ocular irritation
   a. Lacrimation
   b. Hyperemia
   c. Photophobia
   d. Burning sensation
3. Eyelids and conjunctiva
   a. Allergic reactions
   b. Hyperemia
   c. Blepharoconjunctivitis
   d. Angioneurotic edema
4. Keratitis sicca
5. Visual hallucinations
6. Pupils – pinpoint
7. Loss of eyelashes and eyebrows

Possible
1. Accommodative spasm
2. Subconjunctival or retinal hemorrhages secondary to drug-induced anemia
3. Myopia – transient
4. May aggravate
   a. Cytomegalovirus retinitis
   b. Cataract formation
5. Graft versus host disease
6. Eyelids or conjunctiva
   a. Stevens-Johnson syndrome
   b. Erythema multiforme
   c. Toxic epidermal necrosis

Clinical significance

This anticancer drug is generally used in combination with others, which makes it difficult to specify the ocular side effects. Transitory blurred vision is common, and occurs minutes to within 24 hours of receiving high-dose intravenous therapy (Kende et al 1979). This resolves within 1 to 14 days. Keratoconjunctivitis sicca has been reported in up to 50% of patients. Blepharoconjunctivitis, or conjunctivitis, may occur secondary to the antimetabolite effects or to a direct toxic effect of the drug in the tears (Johnson and Burns 1965). Pinpoint pupils are probably secondary to the parasympathomimetic effects of this drug, which may rarely include accommodative spasms and transient myopia (Arranz et al 1992). Other adverse ocular effects may be graft versus host disease, Stevens-Johnson syndrome and possibly enhancement of lens changes. Agrawal et al (2003) reported on four patients on long-term cyclophosphamine for collagen vascular disease who developed cytomegalovirus retinitis. Cyclophosphamide's main systemic toxicity is bone marrow depression, so subconjunctival and retinal hemorrhages can occur.

REFERENCES AND FURTHER READING

Agrawal A, Dick AD, Olson JA. Visual symptoms in patients on cyclophosphamide may herald sight threatening disease. Br J Ophthalmol 87: 122–123, 2003.
Anonymous. Drug-induced myopia. Prescrire Int 12: 22–23, 2003.
Arranz JA, et al. Cyclophosphamide-induced myopia. Ann Intern Med 116: 92–93, 1992.
Bressler RB, Huston DP. Water intoxication following moderate-dose intravenous cyclophosphamide. Arch Intern Med 145: 548–549, 1985.
Fraunfelder FT, Meyer SM. Ocular toxicity of antineoplastic agents. Ophthalmology 90: 1–3, 1983.
Jack MK, Hicks JD. Ocular complications in high dose chemoradiotherapy and marrow transplantation. Ann Ophthalmol 13: 709–711, 1981.
Johnson DR, Burns RP. Blepharoconjunctivitis associated with cancer therapy. Trans Pac Coast Oto-Ophthalmol 46: 43–49, 1965.
Kende G, Sirkin S, et al. Blurring of vision – a previously undescribed complication of cyclophosphamide therapy. Cancer 44: 69–71, 1979.
Lennan RM, Taylor HR. Optic neuroretinitis in association with BCNU and procarbazine therapy. Med Pediatr Oncol 4: 43–48, 1978.
Porter R. Acute necrotizing retinitis in a patient receiving immunosuppressive therapy. Br J Ophthalmol 56: 555–558, 1972.
Porter R, Crombie AL. Cataracts after renal transplantation. BMJ 3(829): 766, 1972.

Generic name: Cytarabine (Ara-C, cytosine arabinoside).

Proprietary names: Cytosar-U, Depocyt.

Primary use

Systemic
This antimetabolite is effective in the management of acute granulocytic leukemia, polycythemia vera and malignant neoplasms.

Ophthalmic
This topical pyrimidine nucleoside is used in the treatment of herpes simplex keratitis.

Ocular side effects

Systemic administration

Certain
1. Decreased vision
2. Cornea
   a. Punctate keratitis
   b. Subepithelial granular deposits
   c. Refractive microcysts (Fig. 7.11f)
   d. Stromal edema
   e. Stria in Descemet's membrane
3. Non-specific ocular irritation
   a. Lacrimation
   b. Hyperemia
   c. Photophobia
   d. Ocular pain
   e. Burning sensation
4. Eyelids or conjunctiva
   a. Allergic reactions
   b. Erythema
   c. Conjunctivitis – hemorrhagic
   d. Hyperpigmentation
   e. Urticaria
   f. Purpura
   g. Edema
5. Extraocular muscles – intrathecal
   a. Paresis
   b. Diplopia
   c. Nystagmus

Probable
1. Optic atropy (intrathecal or intravenous)

Possible
1. Intracranial hypertension
2. Uveitis

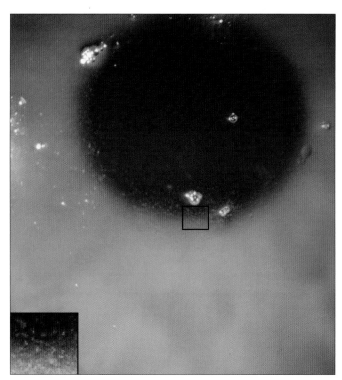

Fig. 7.11f Corneal cyst from systemic cytarabine. Photo courtesy of Krachmer JH, Palay DA. Cornea Atlas. 2nd edn, Mosby Elsevier, London, 2006.

3. Subconjunctival or retinal hemorrhage secondary to drug-induced anemia
4. Eyelids or conjunctiva – toxic epidermal necrolysis

Local ophthalmic use or exposure
Certain
1. Ocular pain
2. Iritis
3. Corneal opacities
4. Corneal ulceration
5. Delayed corneal wound healing
6. Decreased resistance to infection

Clinical significance
Ocular toxicity from systemic cytarabine is the most frequent side effect of the drug. The frequency of the ocular toxicity is both time and dose dependent. The most common ocular side effects are blurred vision and keratoconjunctivitis. The keratitis may occur in 100% of patients on high dosages, regardless of the method of administration. Barletta et al (1992) reported corneal and conjunctival changes even on low-dose systemic cytosine arabinoside. Cytarabine-induced ocular toxicity usually occurs after 5–7 days of therapy and is associated with pain, lacrimation, foreign body sensation and blurred vision. Clinically, one sees central punctate corneal opacities, subepithelial granular deposits, refractile microcysts, superficial punctate keratitis and, rarely, mild corneal edema with stria in Descemet's membrane. Symptoms improve after a few days off the drug, vision improves in 1–2 weeks and the corneal opacities within 4 weeks. The cause of these adverse effects may primarily be due to the non-selective inhibition of DNA synthesis by this drug. This explains the 5- to 7-day delay in onset of corneal changes (i.e. the length of time it takes the basal cells of the corneal epithelium to reach the surface). Cytarabine can be found in the tears from systemic administration, which can account for

immediate ocular and periocular symptoms. Weak topical ocular steroids and frequent preservative-free artificial tears often improve these ocular symptoms. Anterior uveitis has been reported by Planer et al (2004) and there are a few cases in the National Registry but a clear-cut association has not been established.

Adverse effects associated with high-dose intravenous regimens may also include cerebral or cerebellar dysfunction, which is usually reversible. Ocular manifestations of this CNS toxicity may include lateral gaze nystagmus, diplopia and lateral rectus palsy. Neurotoxicity following intrathecal injection and intravenous cytarabine have been associated with optic atrophy and blindness (Hoffman et al 1993; Schwartz et al 2000). Wiznia et al (1994) and Lopez et al (1991) pointed to an additive effect of cytarabine and low-dosage radiation on occlusive microvascular retinopathy in patients with leukemia.

Topical cytarabine causes significant corneal toxicity, and therefore has been replaced by equally effective and less toxic antiviral agents.

REFERENCES AND FURTHER READING
Barletta JP, Fanous MM, Margo CE. Corneal and conjunctival toxicity with low-dose cytosine arabinoside [letter]. Am J Ophthalmol 113(5): 587–588, 1992.
Friedland S, Loya N, Shapiro A. Handling punctate keratitis resulting from systemic cytarabine. Ann Ophthalmol 25: 290–291, 1993.
Gressel MG, Tomsak RL. Keratitis from high dose intravenous cytarabine. Lancet 2: 273, 982.
Hoffman DL, Howard JR, Sarma R, Riggs JE. Encephalopathy, myelopathy, optic neuropathy, and anosmia associated with intravenous cytosine arabinoside. Clin Neuropharmacol 16(3): 258–262, 1993.
Hopen G, Mondino BJ, Johnson BL, et al. Corneal toxicity with systemic cytarabine. Am J Ophthalmol 91: 500–504, 1981.
Hwang TL, et al. Central nervous system toxicity with high-dose Ara-C. Neurology 35: 1475, 1985.
Imperia PS, Lazarus HM, Lass JH. Ocular complications of systemic cancer chemotherapy. Surv Ophthalmol 34(3): 209–230, 1989.
Lass JH, et al. Topical corticosteroid therapy for corneal toxicity from systemically administered cytarabine. Am J Ophthalmol 94: 617, 1982.
Lazarus HM, et al. Comparison of the prophylactic effects of 2-deoxycytidine and prednisolone or high-dose intravenous cytarabine-induced keratitis. Am J Ophthalmol 104: 476, 1987.
Lochhead J, Salmon JF, Bron AJ. Cytarabine-induced corneal toxicity. Eye 17: 677–678, 2003.
Lopez JA, Agarwal RP. Acute cerebellar toxicity after high-dose cytarabine associated with CNS accumulation of its metabolite, uracil arabinoside. Cancer Treat Rep 68: 1309, 1984.
Lopez PF, Sternberg P, Dabbs CK, et al. Bone marrow transplant retinopathy. Am J Ophthalmol 112(6): 635–646, 1991.
Matteucci P, Carlo-Stella C, di Nicola M, et al. Topical prophylaxis of conjunctivitis induced by high-dose cytosine arabinoside. Hematologica 91: 255–257, 2006.
Planer D, Cukirman T, Liebster D, et al. Anterior uveitis as a complication of treatment with high dose cytosine-arabinoside. Am H Hematol 76: 304–306, 2004.
Ritch PS, Hansen RM, Heuer DK. Ocular toxicity from high-dose cytosine arabinoside. Cancer 51: 430, 1983.
Schwartz J, Alster Y, Ben-Tal O, et al. Visual loss following high-dose cytosine arabinoside (ara-c). Eur J Hematol 64: 208–209, 2000.
Wiznia RT, Rose A, Levy AL. Occlusive microvascular retinopathy with optic disc and retinal neovascularization in acute lymphocytic leukemia. Retina 14(3): 253–255, 1994.

Generic name: Denileukin diftitox.

Proprietary name: Ontak.

Primary use
A recombinant DNA-derived cytotoxic agent used in persistent or recurrent cutaneous T-cell lymphoma as well as some systemic cancers. These are monoclonal antibodies that recognize a specific antigen.

Ocular side effects

Systemic administration – intravenous
Possible
1. Visual loss
2. Decreased color vision
3. Retinal pigment mottling

Clinical significance

This intravenous cancer agent in post-marketing reports has been implicated in causing irreversible visual side effects. No published reports are yet available, but the manufacturer has sent out a 'healthcare professional' warning letter, 'Loss of visual acuity, usually with loss of color vision, with or without retinal pigment mottling has been reported following administration of ONTAK. Recovery was reported in some of the affected patients; however, most patients reported persistent visual impairment.' This drug can cause vascular leak syndrome characterized by two or more of the following signs and/or symptoms: hypotension, hypoalbumimia or edema. This may, in part, be the cause of the retinal visual problems. There are no data available as to the incidence and causality has not been fully established.

REFERENCES AND FURTHER READING

Changes in the Ontak (denileukin diftitiox) package insert to include a desctiption of ophthalmologic adverse events [letter]. Available at: http://www.fda.gov/cder/offices/oodp/whatsnew/denileukin.htm. Accessed August 28, 2006.

Ontak. Package Insert. San Diego, CA, Ligand Pharmaceuticals, Inc., 2006.

Generic name: Etoposide.

Proprietary name: Vepesid.

Primary use

This antineoplastic agent is used for various systemic malignancies and irreversibly inhibits CMV replication.

Ocular side effects

Systemic administration – intracarotid injection
Possible
1. Uveal effusion
2. Orbital inflammation
3. Proptosis
4. Decreased vision
5. Anterior uveitis
6. Macular pigmentary changes
7. Cortical blindness – transient
8. Optic neuritis

Clinical significance

The acute ocular-orbital inflammatory responses above are based on one well-documented case (Lauer et al 1999). However, the patient was also given carboplatin. Etopside phosphate is seldom given alone via intracarotid injections. While most of the above are probably due to a drug-related event, it is hard to discern if etoposide was singularly associated or if a combination of drugs was the cause. However, other antineoplastic agents given intracarotid have also caused drug-induced acute orbital and ocular inflammation syndromes. Other reported side effects are rare and unproven.

REFERENCES AND FURTHER READING

Hilliard LM, Berkow RL, Watterson J, et al. Retinal toxicity associated with cisplatin and etoposide in pediatric patients. Med Pediatr Oncol 28: 310–313, 1997.

Lauer AK, Wobig JL, Shults WT, et al. Severe ocular and orbital toxicity after intracarotid etoposide phosphate and carboplatin therapy. Am J Ophthalmol 127(2): 230–233, 1999.

Luke C, Bartz-Schmidt KU, Walter P, et al. Effects of etoposide (VP 16) on vertebrate retinal function. J Toxicol Cut Ocular Toxicol 18(1): 23–32, 1999.

Peyman GA, Greenberg D, Fishman GA. Evaluation of toxicity of intravitreal antineoplastic drugs. Ophthalmic Surg 15: 411, 1984.

Generic name: Fluorouracil (5FU).

Proprietary names: Carac, Efudex, Fluuroplex.

Primary use

Systemic
This fluorinated pyrimidine antimetabolite is used in the management of carcinoma of the colon, rectum, breast, stomach and pancreas. Fluorouracil is also used topically for actinic keratoses and intradermally for skin cancer.

Ophthalmic
It is also used topically and subconjunctivally to enhance glaucoma filtration surgery.

Ocular side effects

Systemic administration
Certain
1. Non-specific ocular irritation
   a. Lacrimation
   b. Photophobia
   c. Ocular pain
2. Decreased vision
3. Eyelids or conjunctiva
   a. Cicatricial ectropion
   b. Occlusion of lacrimal canaliculi or punctum
   c. Erythema
   d. Blepharoconjunctivitis
   e. Edema
   f. Hyperpigmentation
   g. Photosensitivity
   h. Ankyloblepharon
   i. Loss of eyelashes or eyebrows
   j. Keratinization lid margin
   k. Dermatitis
4. Cornea
   a. Superficial punctate keratitis
   b. Epithelial erosion
   c. Opacity
5. Circumorbital edema

Probable
1. Nystagmus (coarse)
2. Decreased convergence or divergence

3. Diplopia
4. Blepharospasm
5. May aggravate herpes infections

Possible

1. Decreased accommodation
2. Subconjunctival or retinal hemorrhages secondary to drug-induced anemia
3. Optic neuritis

Local ophthalmic use or exposure – (fluorouracil) subconjunctival

Certain

1. Irritation
   a. Lacrimation
   b. Ocular pain
   c. Edema
   d. Burning sensation
2. Conjunctiva
   a. Edema
   b. Hyperpigmentation
   c. Keratinization
   d. Cicatricial changes
   e. Delayed wound healing
3. Periorbital edema
4. Cornea
   a. Superficial punctate keratitis
   b. Ulceration
   c. Scarring – stromal
   d. Keratinized plaques
   e. Delayed wound healing
   f. Striate melanokeratosis
   g. Endothelial damage
   h. Limbal stem cell deficiency
   i. Crystalline keratopathy
   j. Pannus
5. Filtering blebs
   a. Delayed leaks
   b. Giant blebs
   c. Thin walled
   d. Infections
   e. Cystic blebs
   f. Ectasia
6. Anterior uveitis
7. Hypotonous maculopathy

Injection into the eyelid (fluorouracil)

Certain

1. Eyelid
   a. Edema
   b. Erythema
   c. Cicatricial reaction
   d. Ectropion
   e. Lid necrosis if followed by cryotherapy
   f. Hyperpigmentation
   g. Allergic or toxic reaction
2. Conjunctival
   a. Chemosis
   b. Erythema
   c. Cicatricial reaction

Possible

1. Loss of eyelashes
2. Crystalline keratopathy

Clinical significance

Fluorouracil (5FU) is one of the more commonly used cytotoxic drugs in the palliative treatment of solid tumors. Since its therapeutic dose is often close to its toxic level, 25–35% of patients on systemic therapy have some ocular side effects. One of the more complete reviews of anterior segment 5FU complications is by Eiseman et al (2003). They point out that adverse effects can be divided into those occurring in the first 3 months (early) of therapy and those occurring with chronic therapy. The most common early adverse ocular effects, besides blurred vision, are low-grade blepharitis and conjunctival irritation with symptoms well out of proportion to the clinical findings. These reactions usually peak in the second and third weeks of therapy and, in rare instances, are severe enough to cause discontinuation of treatment. The reason for discomfort is multifactorial, including 5FU or its antimetabolite secreted in the tears, decrease in basal cell secretion and excessive lacrimation. Eiseman et al (2003) found epiphoria to be the most common adverse ocular event with the highest incidence among African Americans. With long-term therapy, up to one-third of patients may have a cicatricial reaction occurring in the conjunctiva, punctum, canaliculi or lacrimal sac. If recognized early, this may be reversed, but if unrecognized, the scarring is irreversible with resulting epiphora (Hassan et al 1998). There are a number of reports (Brink and Beex 1995; Prasad et al 2000; Stevens and Spooner 2001) of irreversible punctual, canalicular or lacrimal sac stenosis as well as cicatricial changes in the fornices. Agarwal et al (2002) reported severe squamous metaplasia in the lacrimal canalicui. A toxic effect to the cornea can occur for the same reasons as above. Fortunately, other than corneal sloughs, this uniformly resolves within a few weeks of the drug being discontinued. Corneal opacities can occur. Neurotoxicity, which possibly affects the brain stem and causes oculomotor disturbance, has been reported. This may include various ocular motor defects, including blepharospasm, nystagmus (Prasad et al 2000) and diplopia. Delval and Klastersky (2002) reported a case of bilateral anterior optic neuropathy in a patient with dihydropyrimidine dehydrogenase deficiency. Bixenman et al (1968) reported diplopia heralding the onset of further cerebral dysfunction. Sato et al (1988) reported that injections of 5FU in the superficial temporal artery caused complete bilateral visual loss. There are several cases of possible optic nerve toxicity secondary to fluorouracil in the literature and in the National Registry.

Direct injection of fluorouracil into the eyelids for the treatment of basal cell carcinoma can cause cicatricial ectropion and hyperpigmentation. This drug should be used with caution in patients with pre-existent corneal pathology, and in diabetics. Lid necrosis has been reported in one patient receiving cryotherapy for trichiasis when the patient was also on 5FU.

Fluorouracil has gained increasing popularity in the management of difficult glaucoma patients requiring filtration surgery. Initially, significant ocular side effects occurred but with the method of application and the ideal concentration of the drug being determined, this has decreased. 5FU is most commonly given as a subconjunctival injection, which enhances bleb formation. However, adverse ocular effects, most reversible, occur in up to 50% of cases. The most common is superficial keratitis, which may rarely become ulcerated. Hayashi et al (1994) reported a permanent corneal opacity requiring a lamellar keratoplasty when this agent was used after a trabeculectomy. Patitsas et al (1991) reported an infectious and Rothman et al (1999) a non-infectious reversible crystalline keratopathy secondary to subconjunctival 5FU injections in post-operative filtering surgery. Libre (2003) reported a profound transient cataract secondary to subconjunctival 5FU in after filtering surgery. Pires et al (2000) reported a late complication of limbal stem cell deficiency in two patients after 5FU subconjunctival injections. These required stem cell transplantation to correct. Other defects include conjunctival wound leaks, excessive filtration with shallow to flat anterior chambers and conjunctival or corneal keratnization. Ticho et al (1993) reviewed long-term complications and incidences with 8.6% mild iridocyclitis, 3.8% endophthalmitis, 2.9% hypotony and 1.9% transient leaking blebs. Stamper et al (1992) reported on hypotonous maculopathy, while Oppenhein and Ortiz (1993) suggested that some of these may be due to drug-induced ciliary body shutdown. Hickey-Dwyer and Wishart (1993) felt that 5FU subconjunctival injections should be used with great care in diabetic patients due to potential corneal complications and may be contraindicated in corneas with band keratopathy.

Topical 5FU has had some popularity in the management of conjunctival and corneal neoplasia (Yeatts et al 2000). Ocular irritation and other side effects are directly related to concentration, dose and length of treatment. All the signs of severe ocular toxicity of the anterior segment may be seen, including corneal erosions, opacities (permanent), pannus and scleral melts.

Recommendations

1. Ocular symptoms may be decreased by preservative-free topical ocular artificial tears or mild steroids during peak serum levels of 5FU.
2. If patients are given the drug intravenously or intra-arterially, ocular ice packs should be applied for 30 minutes in total, starting 5 minutes prior to injection. This significantly decreases ocular symptoms (Loprinzi et al 1994).
3. If chronic therapy is necessary, a prophylactic silastic intubation of the lacrimal system is advised (Imperia et al 1989; Agrawal et al 2002).
4. If topic ocular 5FU is used, consider using punctual plugs.
5. Pires et al (2000) found amniotic membrane transplants or conjunctival limbal autografts to be of value for limbal cell deficiency induced by 5FU post glaucoma surgeries.
6. Use with caution in diabetic patients.

REFERENCES AND FURTHER READING

Adams JW, et al. Recurrent acute toxic optic neuropathy secondary to 5-FU. Cancer Treat Rep 68: 565, 1984.

Agarwal MR, Esmaeli B, Burnstine MA. Squamous metaplasia of the canaliculi associated with 5-fluorouracil: a clinicopathologic case report. Ophthalmology 109: 2359–2361, 2002.

Alward WLM, Farrell T, Hayreh S, et al. Fluorouracil filtering surgery study one-year follow-up. Am J Ophthalmol 108(6): 625–635, 1989.

Baldassare RD, Brunette I, Desjardine DC, et al. Corneal extasia secondary to excessive ocular massage following trabeculectomy with 5-fluorouracil. Can J Ophthalmol 31(5): 252–254, 1996.

Bixenman WW, Nicholls JVV, Warwick OH. Oculomotor disturbances associated with 5-fluorouracil chemotherapy. Am J Ophthalmol 83: 604–608, 1968.

Brink HM, Beex LV. Punctal canalicular stenosis associated with systemic fluorouracil therapy. Doc Ophthalmol 90: 1–6, 1995.

Caravella LP Jr, Burns JA, Zangmeister M. Punctal-canalicular stenosis related to systemic fluorouracil therapy. Arch Ophthalmol 99: 284, 1981.

Delval L, Klastersky J. Optic neuropathy in cancer patients. Report of a case possibly related to 5-fluorouracil toxicity and review of the literature. J Neurooncol 60: 165–169, 2002.

Eiseman AS, Flanagan JC, Brooks AB, et al. Ocular surface, ocular adnexal, and lacrimal complications associated with the use of systemic 5-fluorouracil. Ophthal Plast Reconstr Surg 19: 216–224, 2003.

Esmaeli B, Golio D, Lubecki L, et al. Canalicular and nasolacrimal duct blockage: an ocular side effect associated with the antineoplastic drug s-1. Am J Ophthalmol 140: 325–327, 2005.

Forbes JE, Brazier DJ, Spittle M. 5-Fluorouracil and ocular toxicity. Letters to the editor. Br J Ophthalmol 77(7): 465–466, 1993.

Galentine P, et al. Bilateral cicatricial ectropion following topical administration of 5-fluorouracil. Ann Ophthalmol 13: 575, 1981.

Hassan A, Hurwitz JJ, Burkes RL. Epiphora in patients receiving systemic 5-fluorouracil therapy. Can J Ophthalmol 33: 14–19, 1998.

Hayashi M, Ibaraki N, Tsuru T. Lamellar keratoplasty after trabeculectomy with 5-fluorouracil. Am J Ophthalmol 117(2): 268–269, 1994.

Hickey-Dwyer M, Wishart PK. Serious corneal complication of 5-fluorouracil. Br J Ophthalmol 77: 250–251, 1993.

Hurwitz BS. Cicatricial ectropion: a complication of systemic fluorouracil. Arch Ophthalmol 111: 1608–1609, 1993.

Imperia PS, Lazarus HM, Lass JH. Ocular complications of systemic cancer chemotherapy. Surv Ophthalmol 34: 209–230, 1989.

Knapp A, et al. Serious corneal complications of glaucoma filtering surgery with postoperative 5-fluorouracil. Am J Ophthalmol 103: 183, 1987.

Lemp MA. Striate melanokeratosis. Arch Ophthalmol 109(7): 917, 1991.

Libre PE. Transient, profound cataract associated with intracameral 5-fluorouracil. Am J Ophthalmol 135: 101–102, 2003.

Loprinzi CL, Wender DB, Veeder MH, et al. Inhibition of 5-fluorouracil-induced ocular irritation by ocular ice packs. Cancer 74: 945–948, 1994.

Mannis MJ, Sweet EH, Lewis RA. The effect of fluorouracil on the corneal endothelium. Arch Ophthalmol 106: 816–817, 1988.

Ophir A, Ticho U. Subconjunctival 5-fluorouracil and herpes simplex keratitis. Ophthalmic Surg 22(2): 109–110, 1991.

Oppenheim B, Ortiz JM. Hypotonous maculopathy after trabeculectomy with subconjunctival 5-fluorouracil. Am J Ophthalmol 115(4): 546–547, 1993.

Patitsas C, Rockwood EJ, Meisler DM, et al. Infectious crystalline keratopathy occurring in an eye subsequent to glaucoma filtering surgery with postoperative subconjunctival 5-fluorouracil. Ophthalmic Surg 22(7): 412–413, 1991.

Pires RTF, Chokshi A, Tseng SCG. Amniotic membrane transplantation or conjunctival limbal autograft for limbal stem cell deficiency induced by 5-fluorouracil in glaucoma sugeries. Cornea 19: 284–287, 2000.

Prasad S, Kamath GG, Phillips RP. Lacrimal canalicular stenosis associated with systemic 5-fluorouracil therapy. Acta Ophthalmol 78: 110–113, 2000.

Rothman RF, Liebmann JM, Ritch R. Noninfectious crystalline keratopathy after postoperative subconjunctival 5-fluorouracil. Am J Ophthalmol 128(2): 236–237, 1999.

Sato K, Watanabe J, Nakayama T, Seki R. Clinical investigation of corneal damage induced by 5-fluorouracil. Folia Ophthalmol 39(1): 1754–1760, 1988.

Schmid KE, Kornek GV, Scheithauer W, et al. Update on ocular complications of systemic cancer chemotherapy. Surv Ophthalmol 51: 19–40, 2006.

Solomon LM. Plastic eyeglass frames and topical fluorouracil therapy. JAMA 253: 3166, 1985.

Stamper RL, McMenemy MG, Lieberman MF. Hypotonous maculopathy after trabeculectomy with subconjunctival 5-fluorouracil. Am J Ophthalmol 114(5): 544–553, 1992.

Stank TM, Krupin T, Feitl ME. Subconjunctival 5-fluorouracil-induced transient striate melanokeratosis. Arch Ophthalmol 108: 1210, 1990.

Stevens A, Spooner D. Lacrimal duct stenosis and other ocular toxicity associated with adjuvant cyclophosphamide, methotrexate and 5-fluorouracil combination chemotherapy for early stage breast cancer. Clin Oncol 13: 438–440, 2001.

Ticho U, Ophir A. Late complications after glaucoma filtering surgery with adjunctive 5-fluorouracil. Am J Ophthalmol 115: 506–510, 1993.

Yeatts RP, Engelbrecht NE, Curry CD, et al. 5-fluorouracil for the treatment of intraepithelial neoplasia of the conjunctiva and cornea. Ophthalmology 107: 2190–2195, 2000.

Generic name: Imatinib mesilate.

Proprietary name: Gleevec.

Primary use

This selective inhibition of the bcr-abl and platelet-derived growth factor receptor (PDGFR) tyrosine kinase is a new form of targeted therapy for the management of myelogenous leukemia and gastrointestinal stromal tumors.

Ocular side effects

Systemic administration
Certain
1. Blurred vision
2. Edema
   a. Orbital (Fig. 7.11g)
   b. Eyelid
   c. Conjunctiva
3. Epiphoria

Possible
1. Eyelids and conjunctiva
   a. Blepharoconjunctivitis
   b. Stevens-Johnson syndrome
   c. Toxic epidermal necroylsis
   d. Hypopigmentation
2. Retina – edema
3. Optic disc – leakage
4. Vitreous – haze
5. Extra ocular muscles
   a. Palsy
   b. Ptosis

Conditional/Unclassified
1. Intracranial hypertension

Clinical significance

This antimetabolite causes various degrees of edema in up to 70% of patients taking this drug. The orbit is one of the more common sites of edema and the swelling may be so severe that it causes visual obstruction that requires surgical debulking or topical steroids (Esmaeli et al 2002 and 2004). Fraunfelder et al (2003) and Demetri et al (2002) found in 70–74% of patients taking the standard dose of 400 mg/day that orbital edema occurred. This reaction is dose dependent. Edema is mild to moderate in most patients and may occur within a few weeks of starting therapy. Orbital edema is twice as common as peripheral edema (Fraunfelder et al 2003). Epiphoria is the primary complaint in some patients according to Esmaeli et al (2004). The cause of the epiphoria is multifactorial and includes severe chemosis and secretion

of an irritating drug or its by-products in the tears. Conjunctival chalasis may occlude the punctum or severe orbital edema may interfere with the lacrimal pump (Fraunfelder et al 2003).

Kusumi et al (2004) reported a case of retinal macular edema (between the pigment epithelium and the neurosensory retina), causing a significant decrease in vision, occurring within 2 months of starting imatinib and completely resolving within 2 weeks of stopping this drug. Imatinib may block the PDGF receptors in the retina, allowing edema to occur (Kusumi et al 2004). Caccavale et al (2002) reported leakage from the optic discs with the resultant posterior vitreous haze and decrease in vision.

Recommendations

1. Orbital edema can be managed conservatively by either observation alone or, in more symptomatic patients, with low dose diuretics in short pulses. Surgical excision of periocular soft tissue may, in rare instances, be necessary to improve visual function.
2. Epiphoria is not improved by probing or irrigating the nasal lacrimal system. Topical steroids or, rarely, conjunctivo-chalasis surgery may be considered.

REFERENCES AND FURTHER READING

Caccavale A, Ferrari D, Girmenia G, et al. Optic nerve head leakage in chronic myeloid leukemia treated with imatinib mesylate: successful therapy with antiangiotensin converting enzyme. Blood 100: 329–330, 2002.

Demetri G, vonMehren M, Blank CD, et al. Efficacy and safety of imatinib mesylate in advanced gastrointestinal stromal tumors. N Engl J Med 347: 472–480, 2002.

Esmaeli B, Diba R, Ahmadi MA, et al. Periorbital oedema and epiphoria as ocular side effects of imatinib mesylate (Gleevec). Eye 18: 760–762, 2004.

Esmaeli B, Prieto VG, Butler CE, et al. Severe periorbital edema secondary to STI571 (Gleevec). Cancer 95: 881–887, 2002.

Fraunfelder FW, Solomon J, Druker BJ, et al. Ocular side effects associated with imatinib mesylate (gleevec). J Ocul Pharmacol Ther 19: 371–375, 2003.

Grossman WJ, Wilson DB. Hypopigmentation from imatinib mesylate (gleevec). J Pediatr Hematol Oncol 26: 214, 2004.

Kusumi E, Arakawa A, Kami M, et al. Visual disturbance due to retinal edema as a complication of imatinib. Leukemia 18: 1138–1139, 2004.

Pavithran K, Thomas M. Imatinib induced Stevens-Johnson syndrome: lack of recurrence following rechallenge with a lower dose. Indian J Dermatol Venerol Leprol 71: 288–289, 2005.

Schaich M, Schakel K, Illmer T, et al. Severe epidermal necrolysis after treatment with imatinib and consecutive allogeneic hematopoietic stem cell transplantation. Ann Hematol 82: 303–304, 2003.

Tsao AS, Kantarjian H, Cortes J, et al. Imatinib mesylate causes hypopigmentation of the skin. Cancer 98: 2483–2487, 2003.

Valeyrie L, Basuji-Garin S, Revuz J, et al. Adverse cutaneous reactions to imatinib (STI571) in Philadelphia chromosome-positive leukemias: a prospective study of 54 patients. J Am Acad Dermatol 48: 201–206, 2003.

Vidal D, Puig L, Sureda A, et al. STI571-induced Stevens-Johnson syndrome. Br J Haematol 119: 274–275, 2002.

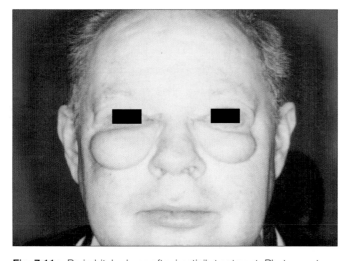

Fig. 7.11g Periorbital edema after imatinib treatment. Photo courtesy of Esmaeli B, et al. Severe periorbital edema secondary to STI571 (Gleevec). Cancer 95: 881–887, 2002.

Generic name: Interferon (alpha, beta, gamma or PEG).

Proprietary names: 1. Actimmune, Alferon N, Avonex, Betaseron, Infergen, Intron A, Pegasys, Peg-intron, Rebif, Roferon-A.

Primary use

These proteins and glycoproteins have antiviral, antiproliferative and immunomodulatory activity. They are therefore used in a variety of diseases, including chronic viral infections, chronic blood diseases and various malignancies.

Ocular side effects

Systemic administration (intramuscular, subcutaneous or intravenous injections)
Certain
1. Decreased vision
2. Ocular pain
3. Diplopia
4. Eyelids or conjunctiva
   a. Conjunctivitis – non-specific
   b. Subconjunctival hemorrhage
   c. Increased eyelash growth
5. Retina – choroid
   a. Hemorrhages
   b. Cotton wool spots (Fig. 7.11h)
   c. Microaneurysm
   d. Vascular tortuosity
   e. Vascular occlusion
   f. Vascular dilation
   g. Macular edema
6. Abnormal VEP
7. Visual hallucinations
8. Photophobia

Probable
1. Myasthenia gravis
   a. Diplopia
   b. Ptosis
   c. Paresis of extraocular muscles
2. Graves ophthalmopathy
3. Cornea
   a. Sicca
   b. Squamous metaplasia
   c. Epithelial cysts

Possible
1. May aggravate herpes infections

Conditional/Unclassified
1. Optic nerve
   a. Anterior ischemic optic neuropathy
   b. Neuritis
2. Oculomotor nerve palsy
3. Uveitis
4. Ocular sicca
5. Nystagmus

Clinical significance
Most adverse interferon-related drug effects have been due to interferon alpha, but beta, gamma and PEG side effects may be similar. Interferon is given in various forms of administration and dosages for various moderate to life-threatening diseases. The most common adverse ocular effect is a change in vision followed by a non-specific conjunctivitis and ocular pain. While ocular side effects are uncommon, they have been blinding. They are more commonly seen with diabetics, hypertensive patients and at higher dosages. Ocular side effects may occur within 15 minutes after first exposure or not for many months. Decreased vision is usually transitory. It may occur after each drug exposure and in very rare instances may be permanent. This may be based on an ischemic event, although in many cases the cause

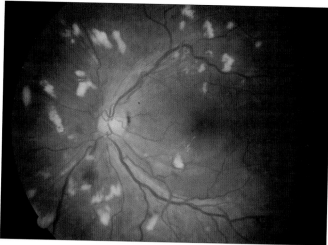

Fig. 7.11h Multiple cotton-wool spots and hemorrhage in patient taking systemic interferon. Photo courtesy of Esmaeli B, et al. Interferon-induced retinopathy in asymptomatic cancer patients. Ophthalmology 108: 858–860, 2001.

is unclear. The drug or underlying disease causes various blood dyscrasias, including anemia, and this may also be the cause of the adverse event. Visual changes may include bright afterimages that are reversible. Ocular or orbital pain can occur, with the cause unknown, and can be intense. The drug can cause conjunctivitis, subconjunctival hemorrhages (without blood dyscrasias) or corneal changes (Fracht et al 2005) since the drug is secreted in the tears. Deng-Huang et al (2005) reported impairment of tear dynamic and squamous metaplastic changes on the ocular surface in patients with chronic hepatitis C receiving long-term interferon and ribavirin. While these changes were reversible, abnormal tear function and metaplasia persisted for up to 6 months after the drugs were discontinued. There are a number of reports (Foon and Dougher 1984) of eyelash growth, requiring up to twice-weekly trimming. Myasthenia and Grave's disease can be associated with drug-associated development of autoimmune-induced pathology.

The greatest clinical interest is the drug's effect on the retina. The ocular side effects characteristically occur between 2 weeks and 3 months after drug exposure. These changes occur in less than 1% of patients treated and may spontaneously regress on the drug or when it is stopped. The primary complication is retinal ischemic changes, both in large vessels and capillaries, as shown by fluorescein angiography. Retinal capillary nonperfusion and/or cotton wool spots due to vascular occlusion can occur, but usually good central vision remains. There are a number of reports of branch arterial or venous obstruction. Only a small percentage of patients have permanent changes. Why these retinal changes occur is open to debate. Anything from deposition of immune complexes, leukocyte infiltrates, anemia and exacerbation of autoimmune disease have been postulated.

About 15 published cases suggest these agents, on rare occasions, may affect the optic nerve. A cause-and-effect relationship is not established since the underlying diseases may also affect the optic nerve directly or decrease its blood supply. These cases are made up of ischemic optic neuropathy as well as optic neuritis.

Recommendations
Hayasaka et al (1998) suggested retinal examination prior to starting interferon, and if any retinal ischemic changes are seen the drug should probably not be used. They suggest following the

patient for retinal problems on a monthly basis. Assessing the risk factors, i.e. high dosage, diabetics, hypertension and a patient's underlying disease, will help the clinician to decide how best to monitor these patients.

REFERENCES AND FURTHER READING

Adams F, Quesada JR, Gutterman JU. Neuropsychiatric manifestations of human leukocyte interferon therapy in patients with cancer. JAMA 252(7): 938–941, 1984.

Borgia G, Reynaud L, Gentile I, et al. Myasthenia gravis during low-dose IFN-α therapy for chronic hepatitis C. J Interferon Cytokine Res 21: 469–470, 2001.

Cuthbertson FM, Davies M, McKibbin M. Is screening for interferon retinopathy in hepatitis C justified? Br J Ophthalmol 88: 1518–1520, 2004.

Deng-Huang S, Ying-Chun C, Shu-Lang L, Tien-Chun C. Lanreotide treatment in a patient with interferon-associated Grave's ophthalmology. Graefe's Arch Clin Exp Ophthalmol 243: 269–272, 2005.

Esmaeli B, Koller C, Papadopoulos N, Romaguera J. Interferon-induced retinopathy in asymptomatic cancer patients. Ophthalmology 108: 858–860, 2001.

Farkkila M, et al. Neurotoxic and other side effects of high-dose interferon in amyotrophic lateral sclerosis. Acta Neurol Scand 70: 42, 1984.

Foon KA, Dougher G. Increased growth of eyelashes in a patient given leukocyte A interferon. N Engl J Med 111: 1259, 1984.

Fracht HU, Harvey TJ, Bennett TJ. Transient corneal microcysts associated with interferon therapy. Cornea 24: 480–481, 2005.

Gupta R, Singh S, Tang R, Blackwell TA. Anterior ischemic optic neuropathy caused by interferon alpha therapy. Am J Med 112: 683–684, 2002.

Hayasaka S, Nagaki YU, Matsumoto M, Sato S. Interferon associated retinopathy. Br J Ophthalmol 82: 323–325, 1998.

Hejny C, Sternber P, Lawson DH, et al. Retinopathy associated with high-dose interferon alfa-2b therapy. Am J Ophthalmol 131: 782–787, 2001.

Huang F, Shih M, Tseng S, et al. Tear function changes during interferon and ribavirin treatment in patients with chronic hepatitis C. Cornea 24: 561–566, 2005.

Isler M, Akhan G, Bardak Y, Akkaya A. Dry cough and optic neuritis: two rare complications of interferon treatment in chronic viral hepatitis. Am J Gastroenterol 96: 1302–1303, 2001.

Lohmann CP, Preuner J, Kroher G, Bogenrieder T. Scientific Poster 41. Permanent Loss of Vision During Interferon-Alfa Treatment for Malignant Melanoma. Academy and PAAO Scientific Posters, Annual Meeting, American Academy of Ophthalmology, Oct, 1999.

Rohatiner AZS, et al. Central nervous system toxicity of interferon. Br J Cancer 47: 419, 1983.

Rubio JE, Charles S. Interferon-associated combined branch retinal artery and central retinal vein obstruction. Retina 23: 546–548, 2003.

Scott GM, Secher DS, Flowers D, et al. Toxicity of interferon. BMJ 282(25): 1345–1348, 1981.

Tokai R, Ikeda T, Miyaura T, Sato K. Interferon-associated retinopathy and cystoid macular edema. Arch Ophthalmol 119: 1077–1079, 2001.

Vardizer Y, Linhart Y, Loewenstein A, et al. Interferon-α-associated bilateral simultaneous ischemic optic neuropathy. J Neuro-ophthalmol 23: 256–259, 2003.

Generic name: Interleukin 2, 3 and 6.

Proprietary name: Proleukin.

Primary use

Interleukin is used in the treatment of various neoplasms, notably metastatic renal cell carcinoma and malignant melanomas.

Ocular side effects

Systemic administration (interleukin 2)
Possible
1. Eyelids
   a. Pruritus
   b. Macular erythema
   c. Desquamative rash
   d. Angioneurotic edema
   e. Urticaria
   f. Subcutaneous lymphomas (transient)
   g. Toxic epidermal necrolysis
2. Visual hallucinations
3. Visual field defects (transient)
   a. Scintillating scotoma
   b. Binocular negative scotoma
   c. Quadratic defects
   d. Total loss
4. Diplopia
5. Palinopsia
6. Amaurosis fugax

Subcutaneous administration (interleukin 3 and 6)
Conditional/Unclassified
1. Anterior uveitis

Clinical significance

The most striking ophthalmic effects of this agent are neuro-ophthalmic, but there are only limited reports and little data available. Scotomas appear to be dose-related and are usually prevented by non-steroidal anti-inflammatory agents (Friedman et al 1991). The cause of these transient migraine-like symptoms may be prolonged hypotensive episodes. It has also been suggested that there is alteration in the permeability of the blood-brain barrier by interleukin 2, which may be responsible for some of these side effects. It is not apparent that any of the visual ophthalmic side effects prevent the continued use of this agent (Friedman et al 1991). Palinopsia is an object seen in the functioning visual area that is drawn to a non-functioning (blind) area and may be persistently visible. These side effects appear to be dose related, occurring within 3–4 hours after a single bolus of interleukin 2. Bernard et al (1990) describe two patients, one with complete monocular loss of vision for 1 month and the other with a superior quadratic loss lasting 1–2 hours. Both resolved after stopping the drug but reoccurred on two separate rechallenges.

Wu et al (1995) reported a case with positive rechallenge data of interleukin 3 in combination with interleukin 6 that caused bilateral anterior uveitis, which resolved in 3 weeks with intensive topical ocular steroids. Interleukin 6 has been found in the aqueous humor in patients with uveitis (Murray et al 1990; Hoekzema et al 1991) and in the experimental model of uveitis (Rosenbaum 1995). Interleukin 1 is well known to cause capillary leak syndrome.

REFERENCES AND FURTHER READING

Bernard JT, et al. Transient focal neurologic deficits complicating interleukin-2 therapy. Neurology 40: 154–155, 1990.

Friedman DI, Hu EH, Sadun AA. Neuro-ophthalmic complications of interleukin 2 therapy. Arch Ophthalmol 109: 1679–1680, 1991.

Gambacorti-Passerini C, Radrizzani M, et al. In vivo activation of lymphocytes in melanoma patients receiving escalating doses of recombinant interleukin 2. Int J Cancer 41: 700–706, 1988.

Gaspari AA, et al. Dermatologic changes associated with interleukin 2 administration. JAMA 258(12): 1624–1629, 1987.

Hoekzema R, Murray PI, van Haren MAC, et al. Analysis of interleukin 6 in endotoxin-induced uveitis. Invest Ophthalmol Vis Sci 32: 88–95, 1991.

Murray PI, Hoekzema R, van Haren MAC, et al. Aqueous humor interleukin 6 levels in uveitis. Invest Ophthalmol Vis Sci 31: 917–920, 1990.

Rosenbaum JT. Towards cytokine insight in sight. Br J Ophthalmol 79: 970–971, 1995.

Thompson JA, Lee DJ, Cox WW, et al. Recombinant interleukin 2 toxicity, pharmacokinetics, and immunomodulatory effects in a phase I trial. Cancer Res 47: 4202–4207, 1987.

Whittington R, Faulds D. Interleukin 2: a review of its pharmacological properties and therapeutic use in patients with cancer. Drugs 46(3): 446–514, 1993.

Wu WC-S, Mannion B, Stone RM, et al. Uveitis associated with interleukin 3 and interleukin 6 therapy. Arch Ophthalmol 113: 408–409, 1995.

Generic names: 1. Mercaptopurine; 2. tioguanine.

Proprietary names: 1. Purinethol; 2. Tabloid.

Primary use

These purine analogs are used in the treatment of acute and some forms of chronic leukemias.

Ocular side effects

Systemic administration
Certain
1. Eyelids or conjunctiva
   a. Hyperpigmentation
   b. Icterus

Possible
1. Problems with color vision – color vision defect, red-green defect
2. May aggravate herpes infections
3. Subconjunctival or retinal hemorrhages secondary to drug-induced anemia

Ocular teratogenic effects
Possible
1. Microphthalmia
2. Corneal opacities

Clinical significance

Ocular side effects due to these antimetabolites are seldom of clinical importance. Between 10 and 40% of patients with acute leukemia receiving mercaptopurine may develop conjunctival icterus. Diamond et al (1960) reported ocular abnormalities in a live birth secondary to mercaptopurine.

REFERENCES AND FURTHER READING

Apt L, Gaffney WL. Congenital eye abnormalities from drugs during pregnancy. In: Symposium on Ocular Therapy, Vol. VII, Leopold IH (ed), Mosby, St Louis, pp 1–22, 1974.

Birch J, et al. Acquired color vision defects. In: Congenital and Acquired Color Vision Defects, Pokorny J et al. (eds), Grune & Stratton, New York, pp 243–350, 1979.

Buscema J, Stern JL, Johnson TRB Jr. Antineoplastic drugs and pregnancy. In: Drug Use in Pregnancy, Niebyl JR et al. (ed), Lea & Febiger, Philadelphia, pp 89–108, 1988.

Diamond J, Anderson MM, McCreadie SR. Transplacental transmission of busulfan (Myleran) in a mother with leukemia: production of fetal malformation and cytomegaly. Pediatrics 25: 85–90, 1960.

Sweetman SC (ed). Martindale: The Complete Drug Reference, 34th edn, Pharmaceutical Press, London, pp 567–568, 2004.

Generic name: Methotrexate.

Proprietary name: Trexall.

Primary use

This folic acid antagonist is effective in the treatment of certain neoplastic diseases, rheumatoid arthritis, psoriasis and uveitis.

Ocular side effects

Systemic administration
Certain
1. Eyelids or conjunctiva
   a. Allergic reactions
   b. Erythema
   c. Blepharoconjunctivitis
   d. Seborrheic blepharitis
   e. Depigmentation
   f. Hyperpigmentation
   g. Urticaria
   h. Loss of eyelashes or eyebrows
2. Decreased vision
3. Non-specific ocular irritation
   a. Lacrimation
   b. Hyperemia
   c. Photophobia
   d. Ocular pain
   e. Burning sensation
4. Periorbital edema
5. Keratitis (Fig. 7.11i)
6. Retinal pigmentary changes (intrathecal or carotid artery infusion)

Possible
1. Subconjunctival or retinal hemorrhages secondary to drug-induced anemia
2. Decreased lacrimation
3. Paralysis of extraocular muscles (intrathecal or carotid artery infusion with mannitol)
4. Optic nerve (intrathecal or carotid artery infusion)
   a. Neuritis
   b. Atrophy
5. May aggravate
   a. Herpes infections
   b. Molluscum contagiosum
6. Eyelids or conjunctiva
   a. Erythema multiforme
   b. Lyell's syndrome

Clinical significance

Ocular side effects such as periorbital edema, blepharitis, conjunctival hyperemia, increased lacrimation or photophobia may occur in about 25% of patients on methotrexate (Fraunfelder

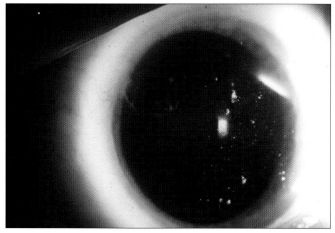

Fig. 7.11i Methotrexate-induced keratitis.

1980). Despite minimal drug-related blepharoconjunctivitis, some patients have marked subjective complaints. The drug is secreted in the tears, and probably causes a direct irritation and interferes with the metabolism of the meibomian glands as well as the corneal and conjunctival epithelium. Lacrimation is increased initially and is probably secondary to ocular irritation, but some have reported a decrease in lacrimation. Peak methotrexate drug levels were measured in tears and found to be equivalent to plasma levels 48 hours after therapy, in both symptomatic and asymptomatic patients. O'Neill et al (1993) reported a small vessel vasculitis in the skin after low-dose methotrexate. Cursiefen and Holbach (1998) reported that methotrexate-induced immunosuppression that may be associated with multiple bilateral eyelid molluscum contagiosum. Also, in an immunosuppressed patient, Rizkalla et al (2005) reported a case of intraocular lymphoma, possibly due to this agent. A case of transient bilateral ophthalmoplegia with exotropia has been reported from intrathecal administration of methotrexate in combination with radiation for the treatment of lymphoma.

Methotrexate-induced retinal or optic nerve pathology is not clear cut. Oral methotrexate, given on a weekly basis for 8.5 years to a 13-year-old, had shown partially reversible decreased vision and abnormal ERG findings 3 years after stopping the drug. There are eight cases of optic neuritis after methotrexate exposure reported in the National Registry. For the number of patients exposed to this agent, the number of adverse reports makes a cause-and-effect relationship doubtful and could probably be only normal background noise. Millay et al (1986) reported that retinal pigmentary epithelial changes developed ipsilateral to carotid arterial infusion of mannitol and methotrexate in patients with intracranial malignant neoplasms. A mannitol-induced 'opening' of the blood-retina barrier may have potentiated these changes. Intrathecal or intracarotid injections of methotrexate suggest the potential for optic nerve toxicity. There are only a few case reports of neurotoxicity and many are complicated by the co-administration of other anticancer drugs and/or radiation. Clare et al (2005) reported a case of possible low-dose methotrexate causing irreversible optic neuropathy. Balachandran et al (2002) gave a single case of possible methotrexate-induced central scotoma, reduction in vision and optic atrophy. Boogerd et al (1990) described a case with histology of intraventricular methotrexate and cytarabine showing major CNS and optic nerve damage. Epstein et al (2001) described a case of see-saw nystagmus after intrathecal methotrexate and other complicating factors. In children with acute leukemia, intrathecal methotrexate in conjunction with radiation therapy has been associated with reports of optic nerve atrophy at radiotherapy doses below those usually associated with such toxicity.

REFERENCES AND FURTHER READING

Balachandran C, McCluskey PJ, Champion GD, et al. Methotrexate-induced optic neuropathy. Clin Exp Ophthalmol 30: 440–441, 2002.

Boogerd W, Moffie D, Smets LA. Early blindness and coma during intrathecal hemotherapy for meningeal carcinomatosis. Cancer 65: 452–457, 1990.

Clare G, Colley S, Kennett R, et al. Reversible optic neuropathy associated with low-dose methotrexate therapy. J Neuroophthalmol 25: 109–112, 2005.

Cursiefen C, Holbach LM. Molluscum contagiosum in immunosuppression with methotrexate: multiple warts with central depressions of the eyelids. Linische Monatsblatter fur Augenheilkunde 212(2): 123–124, 1998.

Cursiefen C, Grunke M, Dechant C, et al. Multiple bilateral eyelid molluscum contagiosum lesions associated with TNFα-antibody and methotrexate therapy. Am J Ophthalmol 134: 270–271, 2002.

Doroshow JH, et al. Ocular irritation from high-dose methotrexate therapy: Pharmacokinetics of drugs in the tear film. Cancer 482: 158, 1981.

Epstein JA, Moster ML, Spiritos M. Seesaw nystagmus following whole brain irradiation and intrathecal methotrexate. J Neuroophthalmol 21: 264–265, 2001.

Fishman ML, Beati SC, Cogan DC. Optic atrophy following prophylactic chemotherapy and cranial radiation for acute lymphocytic leukemia. Am J Ophthalmol 82: 571, 1976.

Fraunfelder FT. Interim report: National Registry of Drug-Induced Ocular Side Effects. Ophthalmology 87: 87, 1980.

Hussain MI. Ocular irritation from low-dose methotrexate therapy. Cancer 50: 605, 1982.

Imperia PS, Lazarus HM, Lass JH. Ocular complications of systemic cancer chemotherapy. Surv Ophthalmol 34(3): 209–230, 1989.

Johansson BA. Visual field defects during low-dose methotrexate therapy. Doc Ophthalmol 79(1): 91–94, 1992.

Knowles RS, Virder JE. Handling of injectable antineoplastic agents. BMJ 281: 589, 1980.

Lepore FE, Nissenblatt MJ. Bilateral internuclear ophthalmoplegia after intrathecal chemotherapy and cranial irradiation. Am J Ophthalmol 92: 851, 1981.

Margileth DA, et al. Blindness during remission in two patients with acute lymphoblastic leukemia. A possible complication of multimodality therapy. Cancer 39: 58, 1977.

Millay RH, et al. Maculopathy associated with combination chemotherapy and osmotic opening of the blood-brain barrier. Am J Ophthalmol 102: 626, 1986.

Nelson RW, Frank JT. Intrathecal methotrexate-induced neurotoxicities. Am J Hosp Pharm 38: 65, 1981.

O'Neill T, et al. Porphyria cutanea tarda associated with methotrexate therapy. Br J Rheumatol 32: 411–412, 1993.

Oster MW. Ocular side effects of cancer chemotherapy. In: Toxicity of Chemotherapy, Perry MC, Yarbro JW. (eds), Grune & Stratton, New York, pp 181–197, 1984.

Ponjavic V, Gränse L, Stigma EB, et al. Reduced full-field electroretinogram (ERG) in a patient treated with methotrexate. Acta Ophthalmol Scand 82: 96–99, 2004.

Rizkalla K, Rodrigues S, Proulx A, et al. Primary intraocular lymphoma arising during methotrexate treatment of temporal arteritis. Can J Ophthalmol 40: 585–592, 2005.

Generic name: Mitoxantrone hydrochloride.

Proprietary name: Novantrone.

Primary use

This is a synthetic anthracycline derivative used for its antineoplastic properties to treat acute leukemias and various malignant neoplasms of the breast and ovary.

Ocular side effects

Systemic administration
Certain
1. Blurred vision
2. Sclera
   a. Blue pigmentation
   b. Blue-green pigmentation
3. Eyelids and conjunctiva
   a. Edema
   b. Blue or blue-green pigmentation
   c. Conjunctivitis

Possible
1. Alopecia primarily in areas of white hair

Clinical significance

As with most antineoplastic drugs, this agent is probably secreted via the lacrimal gland, causing color changes in the conjunctiva, eyelid and sclera. The drug, either mechanically or chemically, is the probable reason for conjunctivitis. The conjunctivitis is self-limiting and resolves once therapy is stopped. Pigmentation of the sclera and eyelids is transitory and secondary to the deposition of the dark-blue drug. All ocular side effects are transitory and of no major clinical significance.

REFERENCES AND FURTHER READING

Kumar K, Kochipillai V. Mitoxantrone induced hyperpigmentation. N Z Med J 103: 55, 1990.
Leyden MJ, Sullivan JR, Cheng ZM, et al. Unusual side effect of mitoxantrone. Med J Aust 2(10): 514, 1983.
Sweetman SC (ed). Martindale: The Complete Drug Reference, 34th edn, Pharmaceutical Press, London, pp 575–576, 2004.

Generic name: Nilutamide.

Proprietary name: Nilandron.

Primary use

This antiandrogen is used in the treatment of prostatic cancer.

Ocular side effects

Systemic administration
Certain
1. Photostress – slow recovery
2. Decreased dark adaptation
3. Chromatopsia

Clinical significance

The most common adverse drug-related effects of nilutamide are visual. Multiple, well-controlled clinical trials state that, after roughly 2 weeks, anywhere from 12 to 65% of patients receiving this drug experienced delayed adaptation to darkness after exposure to bright illumination (sun, television or bright light). In general, photostress recovery time values were from 9 to 25 minutes, where the normal upper limit was 1.3 minutes. In one double-blind placebo control trial, 30% of patients had this adverse event versus 6% of those taking placebos. This delayed adaptation to dark reversed on discontinuation of therapy, dosage reduction and spontaneously in some patients despite continuation of therapy. Dukman et al (1997b) noted that in their experience the 'transient visual disturbance' that occurred at entrance into a dark area was seldom troublesome and only mild in nature. Dole (1997), however, feels that this adverse event is a reason to discontinue the medication. Patients may take up to a year before recovery is complete after the drug is discontinued. Theoretically, this may be due to a delayed regeneration of the visual pigments. Anatomically, no retinal changes, clinical or histological, can be found. In a randomized double-blind study, Namer et al (1990) showed a 3% incidence of chromatopsia, 1% incidence of diplopia and 1% incidence of abnormal accommodation in which the placebo group showed none of these adverse events. There is one case report in the National Registry of bilateral magenta anterior subcapsular cataracts in a patient after 7 years of nilutamide therapy.

REFERENCES AND FURTHER READING

Brisset JM, et al. Ocular toxicity of Anandron. Br J Ophthalmol 71: 639, 1987.
Dole EJ. Comment: Clinical experiences of visual disturbances with nilutamide (author's reply). Ann Pharmacother 31: 1551–1552, 1997.
Dukman GA, Klotz LH, Diokno AC, et al. Clinical experiences of visual disturbances with nilutamide (comment). Ann Pharmacother 31(12): 1550–1552, 1997a.
Dukman GA, Klotz LH, Diokno AC, et al. Comment: clinical experiences of visual disturbances with nilutamide. Ann Pharmacother 31: 1550–1551, 1997b.
Harnois C, et al. Ocular toxicity of Anandron I patients treated for prostatic cancer. Br J Ophthalmol 70: 471–473, 1986.
Harris MG, et al. Nilutamide: a review of its pharmacodynamic and pharmacokinetic properties, and therapeutic efficacy in prostate cancer. Drugs Aging 3(1): 9–25, 1993.
Kuhn JM, et al. Prevention of the transient adverse effects of a gonadotropin releasing hormone analogue (buserelin) in metastatic prostatic carcinoma by administration of an antiandrogen (nilutamide). N Engl J Med 321: 413–418, 1989.
Migliari R, et al. Evaluation of efficacy and tolerability of nilutamide and buserelin in the treatment of advanced prostate cancer. Arch It Urol 63: 147–153, 1991.
Namer M, et al. A randomized double-blind study evaluating anandron associated with orchiectomy in stage D prostate cancer. J Steroid Biochem Molec Biol 37(6): 909–915, 1990.

Generic name: Oprelvekin.

Proprietary name: Neumega.

Primary use

Oprelvekin is a recombinant form of interleukin engineered by combining the antibody with a toxin. It is primarily used to treat chemotherapy-related thrombocytopenia and Wiskott-Aldrich syndrome.

Ocular adverse effects

Systemic administration
Certain
1. Conjunctiva – hyperemia
2. Optic discs
   a. Papilledema
   b. Peripapular exudates

Probable
1. Blurred vision (mild)
2. Subconjunctival hemorrhages
3. Periorbital edema

Clinical significance

Rarely is this drug given in isolation so adverse events are difficult to evaluate. In the manufacturer's clinical trials 13% of patients had conjunctival injections compared to 2% in the placebo group. Edema anywhere in the body was 41% on drug versus 10% in the control group. In the manufacturer's clinical trials, bilateral disk edema occurred in 1% of adults and 16% of children. In a letter to healthcare professionals, 25% of pediatric patients on 100 μg/kg/day developed papilledema. None of the nine patients at 75 μg developed this complication. Peterson et al (2005) reported a well-documented case of oprelvekin-associated bilateral optic disk edema in a 38-year-old male, which resolved when the drug was discontinued. The National Registry has eight cases of disc edema, some with peripapular exudates. One case had a positive rechallenge. Most of the disc edema improved markedly when the drug was discontinued. The Physicians' Desk Reference states that in a primate model this disc edema was also reversible. To date, all ocular signs and symptoms from this drug are reversible on stopping the drug.

Recommendations

As per the manufacturer, use this drug with caution if the patient has pre-existing papilledema, known increased intracranial pressure or tumors involving the central nervous system.

REFERENCES AND FURTHER READING

Data on file (Protocol C9504-14, Final Clinical Study Report 1998). Genetics Institute, Inc.

Peterson DC, Inwards DJ, Younge BR. Oprelvekin-associated bilateral optic disk edema. Am J Ophthalmol 139: 367–368, 2005.

Physicians' Desk Reference, 60th edn, Thomson PDR, Montevale, NJ, pp 3433–3438, 2006.

Generic name: Plicamycin (mithramycin).

Proprietary names: Mithracin.

Primary use

This cytostatic antibiotic is used primarily in the treatment of testicular neoplasms.

Ocular side effects

Systemic administration
Probable
1. Subconjunctival or retinal hemorrhages

Possible
1. Periorbital pallor
2. May aggravate herpes infections
3. Inhibits wound healing

Clinical significance

The main adverse reaction to plicamycin is severe thrombocytopenia, which may affect the eye by causing bleeding. Oster (1984) reported that a striking, periorbital pallor in the absence of anemia may occur in patients taking this drug. Lee et al (1990) suggested that the use of plicamycin topically to enhance filtration procedures for glaucoma may be associated with conjunctival or retinal hemorrhages.

REFERENCES AND FURTHER READING

Drug Evaluations, 6th edn, American Medical Association, Chicago, p 1203, 1986.

Lee DA, Lee TC, Cortes AE, Kitada S. Effects of mitramycin, mitomycin, daunorubicin, and bleomycin on human subconjunctival fibroblast attachment and proliferation. Invest Ophthalmol Vis Sci 31(10): 2136–2144, 1990.

Oster MW. Ocular side effects of cancer chemotherapy. In: Toxicity of Chemotherapy. Perry MC, Yarbro JW. (eds), Grune & Stratton, New York, p 181–197, 1984.

Sweetman SC (ed). Martindale: The Complete Drug Reference, 34th edn, Pharmaceutical Press, London, p 580, 2004.

Generic names: Tamoxifen.

Proprietary names: Nolvadex, Soltamox.

Primary use

Tamoxifen is a first-generation and raloxifene a second-generation selective estrogen receptor inhibitor in the palliative treatment of breast carcinoma, ovarian cancer, pancreatic cancer and malignant melanoma. It is also used as an adjuvant therapy for early and late stage breast cancer.

Ocular side effects

Systemic administration
Certain
1. Decreased vision
2. Corneal opacities
   a. Whorl-like, subepithelial
   b. Calcium
   c. Map dot
3. Retina or macula (Fig. 7.11j)
   a. Yellow-white refractile opacities
   b. Edema
   c. Degeneration
   d. Pigmentary changes
   e. Hemorrhages
4. Posterior subcapsular cataracts
5. Decreased color vision

Probable
1. Visual fields
   a. Constriction
   b. Paracentral scotoma

Clinical significance

Tamoxifen has 30-plus years of clinical use, and there is an extensive, ever-changing adverse ocular profile for it. Gallicchio et al (2004) reported an incidence of 13% of tamoxifen users having an adverse ocular side effect. They have shown that women who complain of visual side effects have high serum blood levels of tamoxifen and its metabolite N-desmethyltamoxifen compared to those without visual complaints. Gorin et al (1998 and 2005)

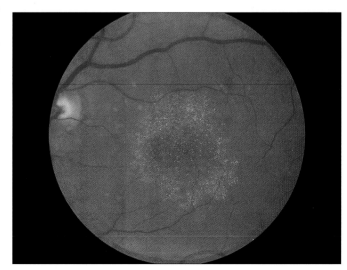

Fig. 7.11j Tamoxifen retinopathy with intraretinal white deposits. Photo courtesy of Spalton DJ, Hitchings RA, Hunter PA. Atlas of Clinical Ophthalmology, 3rd edn, Mosby Elsevier, London, 2005.

has reported the largest series of more detailed ocular studied patients. While it is clear that tamoxifen can affect vision and the eye, serious side effects are rare and primarily at high doses. Serious effects are seldom seen at total dosages of less than 10 g. However, in highly susceptive individuals, at only a few grams, ocular side effects have been seen. More extensive retinal and corneal findings were evident when the drug was given at daily doses of up to 180 mg per day (standard dosage is 20 mg per day or less). At lower dosages, the severity, incidence and reversibility of ocular complications are significantly lower. In a prospective study by Pavlidis et al (1992) at higher doses, 6.3% of patients developed keratopathy or retinopathy due to tamoxifen. However, most incidence levels in the literature are in the 1–2% range. Tamoxifen is secreted in the tears, which may cause reduced vision, photophobia and ocular irritation. Corneal deposits are seldom of major clinical significance and are typically white, whorl-like subepithelial corneal deposits. These deposits are similar to other amphiphilic-like compounds (chloroquine, amiodarone, etc.) and are reversible. Hollander and Aldave (2004) felt these are usually dose related. On rare occasions, hypercalcemia developed with associated corneal changes.

Gorin et al (1998 and 2005) were the first to do a long-term follow-up study that included a tamoxifen exposed and unexposed group. This study included a standardized clinical examination of the lens. They found a markedly elevated risk for posterior subcapsular cataracts. Fisher et al (1998) reported an increased risk of cataract surgery for women on tamoxifen versus women on placebo. Paganini-Hill and Clark (2000) found a 70% increase in cataracts for long-term users of tamoxifen compared to those never exposed to this drug. Bradbury et al (2004), in a large matched case-controlled study done by family practitioners, found no increased risk of cataracts, but no systematic ophthalmic examinations were performed. Gorin et al (1998 and 2005) were also the first to describe subclinical color discrimination in women on long-term tomoxifen. Eisner et al (2004, 2006a and 2006b) studied these phenomena using various sophisticated electrophysiological techniques, showing changes in both the peripheral and central retina. To date, all changes are reversible and subclinical.

Typical tamoxifen retinopathy (i.e. striking white-to-yellow refractile bodies perimacular and temporal to the macula) most commonly occur after 1+ years of therapy with at least 100+ g of the drug (Kaiser-Kupfer et al 1981). There are, however, a number of cases in the National Registry and literature of minimal retinal pigmentary changes without visual loss, occurring after a few months and only a few grams of tamoxifen. Retinal deposits may be associated with cystoid macular edema, punctate macular retinal pigment epithelial changes, parafoveal hemorrhages and peripheral reticular pigment changes. These deposits are refractile bodies located in the inner retina and histologically may be the products of axonal degeneration. Gualino et al (2005) suggested that tamoxifen maculopathy may include cystoid space different from macular edema. The lesions do not appear to regress if the drug is discontinued. Gorin et al (1998), using a single-masked treatment and placebo cohort study, showed a low risk for tamoxifen-related retinal toxicity. Loss of visual acuity in this chronic form of maculopathy is often progressive, dose dependent and irreversible unless the cystoid macular edema or hemorrhage is the cause of the visual loss. Retinopathy due to tamoxifen can be seen without refractile bodies being present. Kalina and Wells (1995) pointed out that idiopathic juxtafoveal retinal telangiectasis can also be confused with tamoxifen retinopathy.

Gorin et al (2005) showed that tamoxifen is associated with thromboembolic events in large vessels, but they found little evidence for this occurring in small vessels as in the eye. The incidence of retinal occlusive disease due to tamoxifen in their study was consistent with chance.

What effect tamoxifen has on the optic nerve is uncertain. In the literature, and in the National Registry, there are reports of unilateral and bilateral optic neuritis or neuropathy. It is uncertain if this is a drug-related event. Two cases in the literature have associated optic nerve pallor. Eisner et al (2006) have documented some subclinical swelling of the optic nerve in women with small optic cups, possibly secondary to the action of this drug on estrogen receptors. There is no evidence of any clinical effect in the optic nerve due to tamoxifen from this edema.

Raloxifene is a second-generation selective estrogen receptor modulator with limited data as to its ocular side effects. Vogel et al (2006) reported a 21% lower rate of cataract development and an 18% lower rate of cataract surgery than compared to patients on tamoxifen. There may be a slight increase in non-specific conjunctivitis and venous thromboembolism during the first 4 months of therapy. There are no data yet to support raloxifene as causing corneal lens or retinal changes.

Recommendations for following patients on tamoxifen

There are many who believe that low-dose tamoxifen (less than 10 g cumulative) causes few to no significant ocular side effects. They recommend not seeing an ophthalmologist until visual symptoms occur. At that point, even with retinal crystals, just see the patient every 3 months and stay in close contact with the oncologist (Heier et al 1994). Gianni et al (2006), through the American Cancer Society, do not recommend stated times for ocular examinations. Rather they recommend the patient should be told the ocular signs and symptoms due to tamoxifen, 'so that they may seek prompt ophthalmic evaluation for ocular complaints'.

Guidelines for management (modified after Gorin et al 1998 and 2005)

1. If requested, do a baseline examination within the first year of starting tamoxifen. This should include slit lamp biomicroscopy of the anterior and posterior segments in combination with a handheld indirect or contact lens. Baseline color vision testing should be done. Warn the patient to contact you at the first signs of any change in vision. Unexplained visual loss may require temporary cessation of therapy to evaluate cause and reversibility.
2. In keeping with the American Academy of Ophthalmology's current recommendations, in normal adults, do a complete eye examination at least every 2 years. More frequent examinations are recommended if ocular symptoms occur.
3. The discovery of a limited number of intraretinal crystals in the absence of macular edema or visual impairment does not seem to warrant discontinuation of the drug.
4. Significant color loss may be a valid reason to consider discontinuing the drug. Gorin et al (1998 and 2005) recommend considering stopping the drug for 3 months (in patients on prophylactic therapy) and retesting. If the color vision returns to normal, restart the drug and retest in 3 months. If, at any time, there is no rebound from stopping the drug, or continued progression, then one may need to consult the oncologist and re-evaluate the risk-benefit ratio.
5. The presence of posterior subcapsular cataracts is not an indication to stop the drug since the condition usually progresses even if the drug is discontinued.

6. The presence of age-related maculopathy is not a contra-indication to the use of tamoxifen. However, informed consent may be advisable in our litigious society.
7. Consultation with the oncologist is recommended if significant ocular findings occur.

REFERENCES AND FURTHER READING

Ah-Song R, Sasco AJ. Tamoxifen and ocular toxicity. Rev Cancer Detect Prevent 21: 522–531, 1997.

Alwitry A, Gardner I. Tamoxifen maculopathy. Arch Ophthalmol 120: 1402, 2002.

Ashford AR, et al. Reversible ocular toxicity related to tamoxifen therapy. Cancer 61: 33, 1988.

Bradbury BD, Lash TL, Kaye JA, et al. Tamoxifen and cataracts: a null association. Breast Cancer Res Treat 87: 189–196, 2004.

Chang T, Gonder JR, Ventresca MR. Case report: Low-dose tamoxifen retinopathy. Can J Ophthalmol 27: 148–149, 1992.

Colley SM, Elston JS. Tamoxifen optic neuropathy. Clin Exp Ophthalmol.

Eisner A, Incognito LJ. The color appearance of stimuli detected via short-wavelength-sensitive cones for breast cancer survivors using tamoxifen. Vis Res 46: 1816–1822, 2006a.

Eisner A, Austin DF, Samples JR. Short wavelength automated perimetry and tamoxifen use. Br J Ophthalmol 88: 125–130, 2004.

Eisner A, O'Malley JP, Incognito LJ, et al. Small optic cup sizes among women using tamoxifen: assessment with scanning laser ophthalmoscopy. Curr Eye Res 31: 367–379, 2006b.

Fisher B, Costantino JP, Wickerham L, et al. Tamoxifen for prevention of breast cancer: report of the national surgical adjuvant breast and bowel project P-1 study. J Natl Cancer Inst 90: 1371–1388, 1998.

Gallicchio L, Lord G, Tkaczuk K, et al. Association of tamoxifen (TAM) and TAM metabolite concentrations with self-reported side effects of TAM in women with breast cancer. Breast Cancer Res Treat 85: 89–97, 2004.

Gianni L, Panzini I, Li S, et al. Ocular toxicity during adjuvant chemoendocrine therapy for early breast cancer. Cancer 106: 505–513, 2006.

Gorin MB, Day R, Costantino JP, et al. Long-term tamoxifen citrate use and potential ocular toxicity. Am J Ophthalmol 125: 493–501, 1998.

Gorin MB, Costantino JP, Kulacoglu DN, et al. Is tamoxifen a risk factor for retinal vaso-occlusive disease. Retina 25: 523–526, 2005.

Griffiths MFP. Tamoxifen retinopathy at low dosage. Am J Ophthalmol 104: 185–186, 1987.

Gualino V, Cohen SY, Dalyfer M-N, et al. Optical coherence tomography findings in tamoxifen retinopathy. Am J Ophthalmol 140: 757–758, 2005.

Heier JS, Dragoo RA, Enzenauer RW, et al. Screening for ocular toxicity in asymptomatic patients treated with tamoxifen. Am J Ophthalmol 117: 772–775, 1994.

Hollander DA, Aldave AJ. Drug-induced corneal complications. Curr Opin Ophthalmol 15: 541–548, 2004.

Imperia PS, Lazarus HM, Lass JH. Ocular complications of systemic cancer chemotherapy. Surv Ophthalmol 34(3): 209–230, 1989.

Kaiser-Kupfer MI, Kupfer C, Rodrigues MM. Tamoxifen retinopathy. A clinicopathologic report. Ophthalmology 88: 89, 1981.

Kalina RE, Wells CG. Screening for ocular toxicity in asymptomatic patients treated with tamoxifen. Am J Ophthalmol 119: 112–113, 1995.

McKeown CA, et al. Tamoxifen retinopathy. Br J Ophthalmol 65: 177, 1981.

Nayfield SG, Gorin MB. Tamoxifen associated eye disease: a review. J Clin Oncol 14: 1018–1026, 1996.

Paganini-Hill A, Clark LJ. Eye problems in breast cancer patients treated with tamoxifen. Breast Cancer Res Treat 60: 167–172, 2000.

Pavlidis NA, et al. Clear evidence that long-term, low-dose tamoxifen treatment can induce ocular toxicity. A prospective study of 63 patients. Cancer 69(12): 2961–2964, 1992.

Pugesgaard T, von Eyben F. Bilateral optic neuritis evolved during tamoxifen treatment. Cancer 58: 383, 1986.

Robinson E, Kimmick GG, Muss HB. Tamoxifen in postmenopausal women, a safety perspective. Review 8: 329–337, 1996.

Sadowski B, Kriegbaum C, Apfelstedt-Sylla E. Tamoxifen side effects, age-related macular degeneration (AMD) or cancer associated retinopathy (CAR)? Eur J Ophthalmol 11: 309–312, 2001.

Tamoxifen and venous thromboembolism. WHO ADR Newslett 2: 3, 1999.

Tang R, Shields J, Schiffman J, et al. Retinal changes associated with tamoxifen treatment for breast cancer. Rev Eye 11: 295–297, 1997.

Tsai D-C, Chen S-J, Chiou S-H, et al. Should we discontinue tamoxifen in a patient with vision-threatening ocular toxicity related to low-dose tamoxifen therapy? Eye 17: 276–278, 2003.

Vinding T, Nielsen NV. Retinopathy caused by treatment with tamoxifen in low dosage. Acta Ophthalmol 61: 45, 1983.

Vogel VG, Costantino JP, Wickerman DL, et al. Effects of tamoxifen vs raloxifene on the risk of developing invasive breast cancer and other disease outcomes. JAMA 295: 2727–2741, 2006.

Zinchuk O, Watanabe M, Hayashi N, et al. A case of tamoxifen keratopathy. Arch Ophthalmol 124: 10461048, 2006.

Generic name: Thiotepa.

Proprietary name: Generic only.

Primary use

Systemic

This ethylenimine derivative is used in the management of carcinomas of the breast and ovary, lymphomas, Hodgkin's disease and various sarcomas.

Ophthalmic

This topical agent is used to inhibit pterygium recurrence and possibly to prevent corneal neovascularization after chemical injuries.

Ocular side effects

Systemic administration (intravenous, intramuscular)
Certain
1. Eyelids or conjunctiva
   a. Erythema
   b. Angioneurotic edema
   c. Urticaria
   d. Periorbital depigmentation

Possible
1. Eyelids or conjunctiva – loss of eyelashes or eyebrows
2. Hyperpigmentation
3. Ocular teratogenic effects (intravenous, intramuscular only)
4. Subconjunctival or retinal hemorrhages secondary to drug-induced anemia

Local ophthalmic use or exposure
Certain
1. Irritation
2. Eyelids or conjunctiva
   a. Allergic reactions
   b. Conjunctivitis – non-specific
   c. Depigmentation
   d. Poliosis
3. Delayed corneal wound healing
4. Keratitis
5. Corneal edema
6. Occlusion of lacrimal punctum

Possible
1. Corneal ulceration

Clinical significance

Thiotepa is seldom given systemically because it has been replaced by more effective drugs. It is still used for mucosal neoplasia (i.e. bladder). The primary ocular side effect from systemic use is periorbital pigmentation (Horn et al 1989). While various other eyelid and conjunctival side effects have been reported, these are rare and seldom of clinical importance. Grant and Schuman (1993) reported a single case of acute bilateral plastic uveitis. We have no other cases like this in the National Registry.

Topical ocular thiotepa is still of clinical value in ophthalmology. Its use may be contraindicated in dark-skinned individuals since permanent depigmentation of the eyelid or eyelashes can occur. Depigmentation may occur within a few weeks or at various times up to 6 years after exposure (Berkow et al 1969; Howitt and Karp 1969; Hornblass et al 1974). The depigmentation effect seems to be enhanced by excessive sunlight exposure (Asregadoo 1972) and in rare cases can be permanent in heavenly pigmented skin. Irritative reactions are common and dependent on dosage. Allergic reactions are rare. Use of thiotepa for many months in dosages 4–6 times daily has caused keratitis. There are reports in the literature and in the National Registry of punctal occlusion due to topical ocular use of this drug. Thiotepa probably retards wound healing and possibly retards corneal blood vessel ingrowth. It has been implicated in either causing or enhancing pre-existing corneal ulceration. Thiotepa can enter the bloodstream through the mucous membrane. Since the drug is potentially mutagenic and teratogenic, topical ocular application is contraindicated in pregnancy. The drug has also been shown to be carcinogenic.

REFERENCES AND FURTHER READING

Asregadoo ER. Surgery, thiotepa, and corticosteroid in the treatment of pterygium. Am J Ophthalmol 74: 960, 1972.
Berkow JW, Gill JP, Wise JB. Depigmentation of eyelids after topically administered thiotepa. Arch Ophthalmol 82: 415–420, 1969.
Cooper JC. Pterygium: prevention of recurrence by excision and postoperative thiotepa. Eye Ear Nose Throat Monthly 45: 59–61, 1966.
Dunigan WG. Dermatologic toxicity. In: Toxicity of Chemotherapy, Perry MC, Yarbro JW (eds), Grune & Stratton, New York, pp 125–154, 1984.
Grant WM, Schuman JS. In: Toxicology of the Eye, 4th edn, Charles C Thomas, Springfield, IL, pp 1412–1414, 1993.
Greenspan EM, Jafrrey I, Bruckner H. Thiotepa, cutaneous reactions, and efficacy. JAMA 237: 2288, 1977.
Harben DJ, Cooper PH, Rodman OG. Thiotepa-induced leukoderma. Arch Dermatol 115: 973, 1979.
Horn TD, et al. Observations and proposed mechanism of N, N′, N″-triethylenethiophosphoramide (thiotepa)-induced hyperpigmentation. Arch Dermatol 125: 524–527, 1989.
Hornblass A, et al. A delayed side effect of topical thiotepa. Ann Ophthalmol 6: 1155, 1974.
Howitt D, Karp EJ. Side effects of topical thiotepa. Am J Ophthalmol 68: 473–474, 1969.
Olander K, Haik KG, Haik GM. Management of pterygia. Should thiotepa be used? Ann Ophthalmol 10: 853, 1978.
Weiss RB, Bruno S. Hypersensitivity reactions to cancer chemotherapeutic agents. Ann Intern Med 94: 66, 1981.

Generic names: 1. Vinblastine; 2. vincristine.

Proprietary names: Generic only.

Primary use

These vinca alkaloids are often used in conjunction with other antineoplastic agents. Vinblastine is primarily used for inoperable malignant neoplasms of the breast, the female genital tract, the lung, the testis and the gastrointestinal tract. Vincristine is primarily used in Hodgkin's disease, lymphosarcoma, reticulum cell sarcoma, rhabdomyosarcoma, neuroblastoma and Wilms' tumor.

Ocular side effects

Systemic administration (vincristine unless stated)
Certain
1. Eyelids
   a. Ptosis (Fig. 7.11k)
   b. Photosensitivity
2. Extraocular muscles
   a. Paresis or paralysis
   b. Diplopia
   c. Nystagmus (vinblastine)
3. Visual hallucinations
4. Decreased corneal reflex

Probable
1. Visual fields
   a. Scotomas – central or centrocecal
   b. Constriction
   c. Hemianopsia
2. Retrobulbar or optic neuritis
3. Abnormal ERG
4. Cortical blindness

Possible
1. Loss of eyelashes or eyebrows
2. Decreased accommodation
3. Problems with color vision – color vision defect, red-green defect
4. Decreased dark adaptation
5. Subconjunctival or retinal hemorrhages secondary to drug-induced anemia
6. Optic atrophy
7. Ocular signs of gout

Inadvertent ocular exposure – vinblastine
Certain
1. Irritation – generalized
   a. Lacrimation
   b. Hyperemia
   c. Photophobia
   d. Edema
2. Cornea
   a. Keratitis
   b. Superficial gray opacities
   c. Edema
   d. Decreased corneal reflex
   e. Ulceration
   f. Subepithelial scarring
3. Blepharospasm
4. Decreased vision
5. Keratitis sicca

Possible
1. Astigmatism

Clinical significance

These plant alkaloids can be used together or singularly. Except for vestibular and auditory damage with resultant nystagmus or topical ocular toxicity due to vinblastine, all data present here are for vincristine. The most recent overall review of vincristine is by Schmid et al (2006). Vincristine neurotoxicity is dose related and, if recognized, at least 80% of the drug-induced side effects are reversible. The most common ocular side effect involves the cranial nerves and may be manifested by ptosis, extraocular

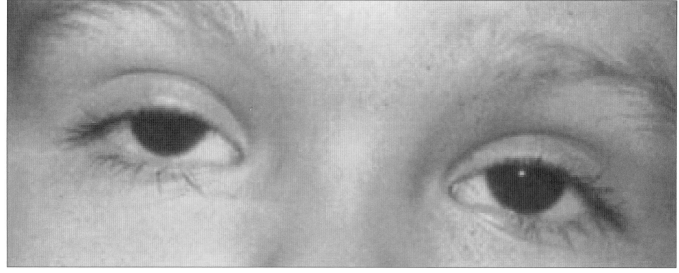

Fig. 7.11k Bilateral ptosis after treatment with vincristine. Photo courtesy of Müller, et al. Treatment of vincristine-induced bilateral ptosis with pyridoxine and pyridostigmine. Paediatr Blood Cancer 42: 287–288, 2004.

muscle palsies, internuclear opthalmoplegia, corneal anesthesia and lagophthalmos occuring in one form or another in up to 50% of the cases (Albert et al 1967). Lash et al (2004) and Toker et al (2004) reported reversible 6th nerve palsy associated with vincristine use. Müller et al (2004) reported the benefits of pyridoxine and pyridostigmine therapy to improve vincristine-induced ptosis. Optic neuropathy has been reported with vincristine, which can improve if the drug is discontinued in most cases (Sanderson et al 1976; Norton et al 1979). However, irreversible blindness has been reported (Margileth et al 1977). Retinal damage can occur based on autopsy findings (Sanderson et al 1976; Munier et al 1992). Transient cortical blindness has also been reported, with recovery in 1 to 14 days (Byrd et al 1981; Schouten et al 2003). The later case showed transient neuroradiological lesions in the occipital cortex. The ocular signs of gout that may occur include conjunctival hyperemia, uveitis, scleritis and corneal deposits or ulcerations. Ripps et al (1984) extensively studied a patient who developed night blindness after vincristine therapy. They felt that this drug interfered in the process of synoptic transmission between the photoreceptors and their second order neurons.

The accidental splashing of vinblastine causes a characteristic keratopathy, which includes microcystic edema, superficial punctate keratitis and corneal erosion with or without low-grade anterior uveitis. Corneal epithelial damage is usually apparent within the first few days along with decreased vision. The keratitis resolves within weeks to months. There is one report of increased astigmatism after inadvertent drug exposure. Most cases develop keratoconjunctivitis sicca and some show opacities in the area of Bowman's layer - both of which appear to be permanent. Chowers et al (1996) postulated that sicca is caused by severe initial inflammation or vinblastine-induced neuropathy. Steroids experimentally had no effect on improving these toxic reactions.

REFERENCES AND FURTHER READING

Albert DM, Wong V, Henderson ES. Ocular complications of vincristine therapy. Arch Ophthalmol 78: 709–713, 1967.

Awidi AS. Blindness and vincristine. Ann Intern Med 93: 781, 1980.

Birch J, et al. Acquired color vision defects. In: Congenital and Acquired Color Vision Defects, Pokorny J, et al. Grune & Stratton, New York, p 243–350, 1979.

Byrd RL, et al. Transient cortical blindness secondary to vincristine therapy in childhood malignancies. Cancer 47: 37, 1981.

Chowers I, Frucht-Pery J, Siganos CS, et al. Vinblastine toxicity to the ocular surface. Anti-Cancer Drugs 7(7): 805–808, 1996.

Cohen RJ, et al. Transient left homonymous hemianopsia and encephalopathy following treatment of testicular carcinoma with cisplatinum, vinblastine, and bleomycin. J Clin Oncol 1: 392, 1983.

Elomaa I, Pajunen M, Virkkunen P. Raynaud's phenomenon progressing to gangrene after vincristine and bleomycin therapy. Acta Med Scand 216: 323, 1984.

Holland JF, et al. Vincristine treatment of advanced cancer: a cooperative study of 392 cases. Cancer Res 33: 1258–1264, 1973.

Imperia PS, Lazarus HM, Lass JH. Ocular complications of systemic cancer chemotherapy. Surv Ophthalmol 34(3): 209–230, 1989.

Kaplan RS, Wiernik PH. Neurotoxicity of antineoplastic drugs. Semin Oncol 9: 103, 1982.

Lash SC, Williams CP, Marsh CS, et al. Acute sixth-nerve palsy after vincristine therapy. J Aapos 8: 67–68, 2004.

Margileth DA, Polplack DG, Tizzo PA, et al. Blindness during remission in two patients with acute lymphoblastic leukemia: a possible complication of multimodality therapy. Cancer 39: 58–61, 1977.

McLendon BF, Bron AJ. Corneal toxicity from vinblastine solution. Br J Ophthalmol 62: 97, 1978.

Müller L, Kramm C, Tenenbaum T. Treatment of vincristine-induced bilateral ptosis with pyridoxine and pyridostigmine. Pediatr Blood Cancer 42: 287–288, 2004.

Munier F, Uffer S, Herbort CP, et al. Loss of ganglion cells in the retina secondary to vincristine therapy. Klinische Monatsblatter fur Augenheilkunde 200(5): 550–554, 1992.

Norton SW, Stockman JA III. Unilateral optic neuropathy following vincristine chemotherapy. J Pediatr Ophthalmol Strabismus 16: 190, 1979.

Ripps H, et al. Functional abnormalities in vincristine-induced night blindness. Invest Ophthalmol Vis Sci 25: 787, 1984.

Sanderson PA, Kuwabara T, Cogan DG. Optic neuropathy presumably caused by vincristine therapy. Am J Ophthalmol 81: 146–150, 1976.

Schmid KE, Kornek GV, Scheithauer W, et al. Update on ocular complications of systemic cancer chemotherapy. Surv Ophthalmol 51: 19–40, 2006.

Schouten D, de Fraff SSN, Verrips A. Transient cortical blindness following vincristine therapy. Med Pediatr Oncol 41: 470, 2003.

Shurin SB, Rekate HL, Annable W. Optic atrophy induced by vincristine. Pediatrics 70: 288, 1982.

Spaeth GL, Nelson LB, Beaudoin AR. Ocular teratology. In: Ocular Anatomy, Embryology and Teratology, Jakobiec FA (ed), JB Lippincott, Philadelphia, p 955–975, 1982.

Teichmann KD, Dabbagh N. Severe visual loss after a single dose of vincristine in a patient with spinal cord astrocytoma. J Ocular Pharmacol 4: 149–151, 1988. Surv Ophthalmol 34: 149–150, 1989.

Toker E, Yenice O, Ogut MS. Isolated abducens nerve palsy induced by vincristine therapy. J Aapos 8: 69–71, 2004.

SECTION 12
HEAVY METAL ANTAGONIST AND MISCELLANEOUS AGENTS

CLASS: AGENTS TO TREAT ALCOHOLISM

Generic name: Disulfiram.

Proprietary name: Antabuse.

Primary use
This thiuram derivative is used as an aid in the management of chronic alcoholism.

Ocular side effects

Systemic administration – implantation
Certain
1. Decreased vision
2. Optic nerve
   a. Hyperemia
   b. Edema
   c. Neuritis
   d. Retrobulbar neuritis
   e. Pallor
3. Scotomas – central or centrocecal
4. Problems with color vision – color vision defect, red-green defect
5. Eyelids or conjunctiva
   a. Allergic reactions
   b. Erythema
   c. Urticaria
6. Visual hallucinations

Probable
1. Toxic amblyopia

Possible
1. Extraocular muscles – paresis or paralysis

Clinical significance
Disulfiram has been in use for over 55 years as a 'psychological threat' to treat alcoholism because of the severity of the disulfiram-ethanol interaction. When this interaction occurs, blurred vision may be marked, but serious adverse ocular side effects due to disulfiram are uncommon. Retrobulbar and optic neuritis have been well documented by numerous authors. In general, the vision loss secondary to retrobulbar or optic neuritis occurs 1–5 months after disulfiram is discontinued. These ocular side effects may be more common at higher dosages, in the elderly or in patients with impaired hepatic function. There are a few reports of optic disc hyperemia or optic nerve pallor. Neuropathy elsewhere occurs in 1 in 15 000 patients (Beveilacqua et al 2002) therefore optic nerve disorders are plausible. Other ocular side effects are reversible and seldom of importance. There is a case report in the National Registry of sisters on disulfiram who experienced transient repeating episodes of vertical diplopia. They were not related to time, day or activity and lasted only a matter of minutes then spontaneously resolved. Acheson and Howard (1988) reported a case of decreased and delayed visual evoked potential in a patient with bilateral optic neuropathy with recovery after 8 months off disulfiram.

REFERENCES AND FURTHER READING

Acheson JF, Howard RS. Reversible optic neuropathy associated with disulfiram. A clinical and electrophysiological report. J Neuroophthalmol 8: 175–177, 1988.
Bevilacqua JA, Diaz M, Diaz V, et al. Disulfiram neuropathy. Report of 3 cases. Rev Med Chil 130: 1037–1042, 2002.
Birch J, et al. Acquired color vison defects. In: Congenital and Acquired Color Vision Defects, Pokorny J et al. (eds), Grune & Stratton, New York, pp 243–350, 1979.
Gardner RJM, Clarkson JE. A malformed child whose previously alcoholic mother had taken disulfiram. N Z Med J 93: 184, 1981.
Geffray L, Dao T, Cevallos R, et al. Retrobulbar optic neuritis caused by disulfiram. Revue de Medecine Interne 16(12): 973, 1995.
Graveleau J, Ecoffet M, Villard A. Les neuropathies peripheriques dues au disulfirame. Nouv Presse Med 9: 2905, 1980.
Mokri B, Ohnishi A, Dyck PJ. Disulfiram neuropathy. Neurology 31: 730–735, 1981.
Morcamp D, Boudin G, Mizon JP. Complications neurologiques inhabituelles du disulfirame. Nouv Presse Med 10: 338, 1981.
Norton AL, Walsh FB. Disulfiram-induced optic neuritis. Trans Am Acad Ophthal Otol 76: 1263–1265, 1972.

CLASS: CALCIUM-REGULATING AGENTS

Generic names: 1. Alendronate sodium; 2. disodium etidronate; 3. disodium pamidronate; 4. risedronate sodium; 5. sodium ibandronate; 6. tiludronate sodium; 7. zolendronic acid.

Proprietary names: 1. Fosamax; 2. Didronel; 3. Aredia; 4. Actonel; 5. Boniva; 6. Skelid; 7. Zometa.

Primary use
These biphosphonate calcium regulating agents are used primarily in the management of hypercalcemia of malignancy, metastasis bone pain, osteoporosis and Paget's disease of bone.

Ocular side effects

Systemic administration (disodium pamidronate)
Certain
1. Blurred vision
2. Conjunctiva – transitory
   a. Lacrimation
   b. Hyperemia
   c. Ocular pain
   d. Burning sensation
   e. Gritty sensation
   f. Irritation
   g. Angioneurotic edema
3. Anterior uveitis
4. Episcleritis
5. Scleritis

Possible
1. Visual hallucinations
2. Orbital inflammation
3. Color vision abnormalities
4. Eyelid or conjunctiva
   a. Stevens-Johnson syndrome
   b. Toxic epidermal necrolysis

Conditional/Unclassified
1. Optic neuritis

Clinical significance
It is rare in ophthalmology to get such a clear-cut positive rechallenge data of a drug-induced ocular side effect as with this class

of drugs. Fraunfelder and Fraunfelder (2003) reported that all bisphosphonates can cause blurred vision and photophobia. Supported by multiple cases in the literature and positive rechallenge data, almost all bisphosphonates can cause non-specific conjunctivitis, blurred vision and anterior uveitis. More rarely, they have been associated with posterior non-granulomatous uveitis, scleritis, episcleritis, ocular pain and photophobia. The authors suggest that probably any bisphosphonate can cause any of these adverse effects, but these adverse effects have not been proven for all bisphosphonates. There have been multiple papers supporting a causal relationship of these effects secondary to this class of drugs.

Non-specific conjunctivitis usually occurs within 6–48 hours after drug exposure. This conjunctivitis is transitory and seldom requires treatment. Cases of anterior or posterior uveitis (Haverbeke et al 2003) may occur unilaterally or bilaterally within 24–48 hours after drug exposure, and episcleritis or scleritis can occur as early as 1 to 6 days after. The onset is more rapid and intense with intravenous medication. Fraunfelder et al (2003) reported 17 cases of unilateral and one case of bilateral scleritis after IV pamidronate with the first positive rechallenge data for any drug causing scleritis. The cause of the uveitis, scleritis and episcleritis is conjecture but, since this is a high molecular weight drug, the potential for an immune complex formation has been suggested. The cause for the non-specific conjunctivitis is also unknown, but the pattern suggests that the drug is secreted into the tears by the lacrimal gland and then causes transitory irritation to the mucous membranes. If patients develop a uveitis, episcleritis or scleritis, one needs to monitor these patients more closely, and in some cases discontinue the drug. Xanthopsia (red vision-look up) occurs with positive rechallenge within 2 hours of drug exposure, but only in two single case reports. Des Grottes et al (1997) described a patient with porphyria who developed reversible retrobulbar neuritis after intravenous pamidronate. Ghose et al (1994) also reported a case with orbital pain, proptosis, ptosis, chemosis and partial 3rd and 4th nerve palsy. The patient had a negative neurologic work-up that resolved after a course of oral steroids. Stach and Tan (2006) reported a case of possible optic neuritis due to alendronte, however the National Registry has no other cases.

Subramanian et al (2003) reported two cases and Ryan and Sampath (2001) a third, which suggest intravenous pamidronate may cause unilateral or bilateral significant orbital inflammation. No rechallenge data are available. With the absence of another clinical cause and close temporal relation with positive dechallenge, the authors suggest this drug as the probable cause. Each case developed diplopia. Meaney et al (2004) reported a case with positive rechallenge of a possible early phase orbital inflammation with bilateral chemosis, lid edema, erythema and vertical diplopia 2 hours after intravenous pamidronate.

Recommendations

1. Any patients on this group of drugs who report any change in vision or ocular pain should see an ophthalmologist.
2. Non-specific conjunctivitis seldom requires treatment and usually decreases in intensity with repeat exposure to the drug. Use of preservative-free artificial tears may give temporary relief.
3. One needs to be aware that multiple ocular side effects may occur in the same patients so a complete dilated ophthalmic exam is necessary. In some instances the drug may need to be discontinued for severe uveitis to resolve, but in the main uveitis can be controlled with topical steroids.
4. In our experience, for the slceritis to resolve, even with the patient on full medical therapy, the bisphosphonate must be discontinued.

REFERENCES AND FURTHER READING

Adverse Drug Reactions Advisory Committee. Bisphosphonates and ocular inflammation. Aust Adv Drug React Bull 23: 7–8, 2004.

Coleman CI, Perkerson KA, Lewis A. Alendronate-induced hallucinations and visual disturbance. Pharmacotherapy 24: 799–802, 2004.

De S, Meyer P, Crisp AJ. Pamidronate and uveitis (letter to the editor). Br J Rheumatol 34(5): 479, 1995.

Des Grottes JM, Schrooyen M, Dumon JC, et al. Retrobulbar optic neuritis after pamidronate administration in a patient with a history of cutaneous porphyria. Clin Rheum 16(1): 93–95, 1997.

Fraunfelder FW, Fraunfelder FT. Bisphosphonates and ocular inflammation. N Engl J Med 348: 1187–1188, 2003.

Fraunfelder FW, Fraunfelder FT, Jensvold B. Scleritis and other ocular side effects associated with pamidronate disodium. Am J Ophthalmol 135: 219–222, 2003.

Ghose K, Waterworth R, Trolove P, et al. Uveitis associated with pamidronate. Aust N Z J Med 24: 320, 1994.

Haverbeke G, Pertile G, Claes C, et al. Posterior uveitis: an under-recognized adverse effect of pamidronate: 2 case reports. Bull Soc Belge Ophthalmol 290: 71–76, 2003.

Leung S, Ashar BH, Miller RG. Bisphosphonates-associated scleritis: a case report and review. South Med J 98: 733–735, 2005.

Macarol V, Fraunfelder FT. Disodium pamidronate and adverse ocular drug reactions. Am J Ophthalmol 118: 220–224, 1994.

Mbekeani JN, Slamovits TL, Schwartz BH, Sauer HL. Ocular inflammation associated with alendronate therapy. Arch Ophthalmol 117: 837–838, 1999.

Meany TPJ, Musadiq M, Corridan PGJ. Diplopia following intravenous administration of pamidronate. Eye 18: 103–104, 2004.

MHRA. Final report on TGN1412 clinical trial. Media release: 25 May 2006. Available from: http://www.mhra.gov.uk.

Morton AR, et al. Disodium pamidronate (APD) for the management of single-dose versus daily infusions and of infusion duration. In: Disodium Pamidronate (APD) in the Treatment of Malignancy-Related Disorders, Hans Huber Publishers, Toronto, pp 85–100, 1989.

O'Donnell NP, Rao GP, Aguis-Fernandez A. Paget's Disease: ocular complications of disodium pamidronate treatment. Br J Clin Pract 49(5): 272–273, 1995.

Ryan PJ, Sampath R. Idiopathic orbital inflammation following intravenous pamidronate. Rheumatology 40: 956–957, 2001.

Siris ES. Bisphophonates and iritis. Lancet 342: 436–437, 1993.

Stach R, Tarr K. Drug-induced optic neuritis and uveitis secondary to bisphosphonates. N Z Med J 119: 74–76, 2006.

Stewart GO, Stuckey BG, Ward LC, et al. Iritis following intravenous pamidronate. Aust N Z J Med 26(3): 414–415, 1996.

Subramanian PS, Kerrison JB, Calvert PC, et al. Orbital inflammatory disease after pamidronate treatment for metastatic prostate cancer. Arch Ophthalmol 121: 1335–1336, 2003.

Vinas G, Olive A, Holgado S, et al. Episcleritis secondary to risedronate. Med Clin 118: 598–599, 2002.

CLASS: CHELATING AGENTS

Generic name: Deferoxamine mesilate.

Proprietary name: Desferal.

Primary use

Systemic

This chelating agent is used in the treatment of iron-storage diseases and acute iron poisoning.

Ophthalmic

This topical agent is used in the treatment of ocular siderosis and hematogenous pigmentation of the cornea.

Ocular side effects

Systemic administration

Certain

1. Decreased vision
2. Problems with color vision
3. Decreased dark adaptation
4. Retina
   a. Pigment epithelium (Fig. 7.12a)
      i. Opacitification
      ii. Loss of transparency
      iii. Molting
   b. Bullege maculopathy
   c. Vitellifrom maculopathy
   d. Cystoid macular edema
5. Optic nerve
   a. Disc edema
   b. Pallor
   c. Atrophy
6. Abnormal – ERG, EOG or VEP
7. Visual field defects
   a. Scotoma – central, centrocecal and ring
   b. Constriction
8. Eyelids and conjunctiva
   a. Allergic reactions
   b. Urticaria
   c. Angioneurotic edema

Possible

1. Cataracts
2. Optic neuritis

Local ophthalmic use or exposure
Certain

1. Eyelids or conjunctiva
   a. Allergic reactions
   b. Hyperemia

Clinical significance

Deferoxamine has been used clinically for almost 40 years and with expanded therapeutic uses, additional ocular toxicity reports are occurring. Ocular toxicity usually occurs with long-term therapy, although acute toxicity may occur with rechallenge exposure

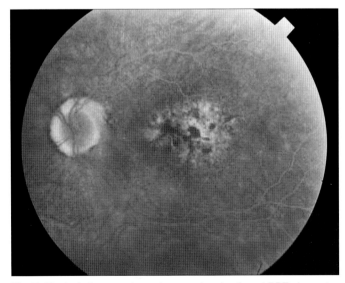

Fig. 7.12a Late flourescein angiogram showing foveal RPE pigment clumping after deferoxamine treatment. Photo courtesy of Haimovici R, et al. The expanded clinical spectrum of deferoxamine retinopathy. Ophthalmology 109: 164–171, 2002.

(Bene et al 1989; Yaqoob et al 1991; Mehta et al 1994), in dialysis patients (Blake et al 1985) or in endstage renal disease (Davies et al 1983; Rubinstein et al 1985; Cases et al 1988). The acute reactions are no different to those found in patients on long-term deferoxamine therapy and may be irreversible, even with only a single dose (Bene et al 1989; Pengloan et al 1990). While ocular toxicity is rare, it varies from minimal reversible changes in approximately two-thirds of cases to irreversible changes, including blindness, in approximately one-third of cases. Acute adverse ocular effects are seen most frequently in high dosages while low-dose chronic exposure over a 20-year period does not appear to appear to show retinal toxicity (Elison et al 2005).

No clear-cut relationship between drug dosage and retinopathy has been established for deferoxamine, a drug for which there are no alternative medications. The earliest signs of retinal toxicity include blurred or decreased night vision. Retinal pigment epithelial mottling changes are only seen after the onset of visual color abnormalities or after nyctalopia occurs. Hiamovici et al (2002) reported that the earliest fundus findings are subtle opacifications or loss of transparency of the outer retina and retinal pigment epithelium. Fluorescein angiography in the earliest stage of toxicity is variable. During the transition stage, there is often block fluorescence and then late fluorescence in the late stage. This occurs before retinal pigment epithelium molting. If vitelliform maculopathy develops, permanent visual loss may occur (Mehta et al 1994; Gonzales et al 2004). Gonzales et al (2004) pointed out that persistent hyperfluorescence within the macula may represent a poor prognostic finding due to irreversible retinal pigment epithelium damage. This molting is primarily foveal, but with time may extend to the paramacular, papullomacular and peripapillar areas. Electrophysiologic studies suggest widespread retinal involvement, not just focal areas as seen on funduscopic examination (Haimovici et al 2002). Albalate et al (1996) studied 24 patients and controls on dialysis with chronic renal failure with aluminum intoxication. Thirty-three per cent had macular changes, often with good vision. After 1 year the retinal changes persisted, but only one patient continued to have a significant decrease in vision that did not improve. These pigmentary changes may be progressive for many months, even if the drug is discontinued. ERG, EOG and dark adaptation may also be abnormal.

Toxic cerebral and optic neuropathy with central or centrocecal scotomas and peripheral constriction of visual fields has also been reported in patients receiving deferoxamine (Lakhanpal et al 1984; Blake et al 1985; Pinna, et al 2001). Various symmetrical or asymmetrical disc changes have been described, including edema and atrophy. While these events may well be drug related, there are a few with no clear pattern or mechanism. While this drug can cause cataracts in animals, there are few reports of this in humans (Jacobs et al 1965; Ciba 1969; Bloomfield et al 1978). These reports were before 1978; more recently Popescu et al (1998) suggested that deferoxamine may even be protective against cataracts. To date therefore there is no evidence that this drug is cataractogenic in humans, and at worst there is possibly only a weak association. The exact mechanism of deferoxamine toxicity to the eye is unknown and varies, in part, according to the condition that is being treated. However, in some cases it is probably due to the drug's capacity to chelate the essential trace elements required for normal enzymatic activity and cellular function.

Recommendations

There are no universally accepted ophthalmic guidelines for following patients on deferoxamine. It is clear that with low dose-ages, very few ocular side effects are seen. However, in patients

SECTION 12 • Heavy metal antagonist and miscellaneous agents susceptible to retinal toxicity, such as diabetics, and patients with rheumatoid arthritis, metabolic encephalopathy and renal failure the following should be considered.

1. Baseline ocular exam, including dilated funduscopy, color vision testing, visual fields, dark adaptometry and angiography. An electrophysiologic study is ideal and it is possible to include multifocal ERG (Kertes et al 2004).

2. Frequent serum ferritin levels (<0.025) should probably be taken. If intravenous deferoxamine is necessary, the patient should undergo an ophthalmic exam with visualization of the fundus (Lai et al 2006).

3. Patients should be told to see an ophthalmologist at the first signs of a change in vision, color perception or night vision.

4. Late hyperfluorescence on fluorescein angiography seems to be a reliable indicator of active retinopathy. Retinal pigment epithelium molting does not resolve with stopping deferoxamine. ERG and EOG are confirmatory tests and may show more widespread dysfunction then seen by fundoscopy alone (Haimovici et al 2002).

5. The frequency of ophthalmic examination is dependent on the dosage and method of administration. At the first signs of toxicity to the retina, the risk-benefit ratio needs to be called to the attention of the treating physician.

6. As Arora et al (2004) point out, even using the above guidelines and stopping the drug early, some patients will develop significant visual loss.

7. Pinna et al (2001) suggest oral zinc sulfate for presumed optic neuropathy and hearing loss.

REFERENCES AND FURTHER READING

Albalate M, Velasco L, Ortiz A, et al. High risk of retinal damage by desferrioxamine in dialysis patients [letter]. Nephron 73(4): 726–727, 1996.

Arden GB, Wonke B. Desferrioxamine (DFX) and ocular toxicity. Invest Ophthalmol Vis Sci 25(Suppl): 336, 1984.

Arora A, Wren S, Evans KG. Desferrioxamine related maculopathy: a case report. Am J Hematol 76: 386–388, 2004.

Bansal V, Elgarbly I, Ghanchi FD, et al. Bull's eye maculopathy with deferoxamine. Eur J Haematol 70: 420–421, 2003.

Bene C, et al. Irreversible ocular toxicity from single 'challenge' dose of deferoxamine. Clin Nephrol 31(1): 45–48, 1989.

Bentur Y, McGuigan M, Koren G. Deferoxamine (Desferrioxamine) new toxicities for an old drug. Drug Safety 6(1): 37–46, 1991.

Blake DR, et al. Cerebral and ocular toxicity induced by desferrioxamine. Q J Med 56: 345, 1985.

Bloomfield SE, Markenson AL, Miller DR, et al. Lens opacities in thalassemia. J Pediatr Ophthalmol Strabismus 15: 154–156, 1978.

Borgna-Pignatti C, de Stefano P, Broglia AM. Visual loss in patient on high-dose subcutaneous desferrioxamine. Lancet 1: 681, 1984.

Cases A, Kelly J, Sabater J, et al. Acute visual and auditory neurotoxicity in patients with end-stage renal disease receiving desferrioxamine. Clin Nephrol 29(4): 176–178, 1988.

Ciba Pharmaceutical Company. Official literature on new drugs: deferoxamine mesylate. Clin Pharmacol Ther 10: 595–596, 1969.

Davies SC, et al. Ocular toxicity of high-dose intravenous desferrioxamine. Lancet 2: 181, 1983.

Elison JR, Liss JA, Lee TC, et al. Effects of long-term deferoxamine on retinal function. Scientific poster 184. American Academy of Ophthalmology Meeting, 2005.

Gonzales CR, Lin AP, Engstrom RE, et al. Bilateral vitelliform maculopathy and deferoxamine toxicity. Retina 24: 464–467, 2004.

Haimovici R. The Deferoxamine Retinopathy Study Group: the expanded clinical spectrum of deferoxamne retinopathy. IOVS 39(4): S1133, March 15, 1998.

Haimovici R, D'Amico DJ, Gragoudas ES, et al. The expanded clinical spectrum of deferoxamine retinopathy. Ophthalmology 109: 164–171, 2002.

Jacobs J, Greene H, Grendel BR. Acute iron intoxication. N Engl J Med 273: 1124–1127, 1965.

Kertes PJ, Lee TKM, Couplan SG. The utility of multifocal electroretinography in monitoring drug toxicity: deferoxamine retinopathy. Can J Ophthalmol 39: 656–661, 2004.

Lai TYY, Lee GKY, Chan W-M, et al. Rapid development of severe toxic retinopathy associated with continuous intravenous deferoxamine infusion. Br J Ophthalmol 90: 243–244, 2006.

Lakhanpal V, Schocket SS, Jiji R. Deferoxamine (Desferal)-induced toxic retinal pigmentary degeneration and presumed optic neuropathy. Ophthalmology 91: 443, 1984.

Marciani MG, Stefani N, Stefanini F, et al. Visual function during longterm desferrioxamine treatment [letter]. Lancet 341(8843): 491, 1993.

Mehta AM, Engstrom RE, Kreiger AE. Deferoxamine-associated retinopathy after subcutaneous injection. Am J Ophthalmol 118(2): 260–262, 1994.

Olivieri NF, et al. Visual and auditory neurotoxicity in patients receiving subcutaneous deferoxamine infusions. N Engl J Med 314: 869, 1986.

Orton RB, de Veber LL, Sulh HMB. Ocular and auditory toxicity of long-term, high-dose subcutaneous deferoxamine therapy. Can J Ophthalmol 20: 153, 1985.

Pengloan J, Dantal J, Rossazza C, et al. Ocular toxicity after a single intravenous dose of desferrioxamine. Nephron 56: 19–23, 1990.

Pinna A, Corda L, Carta F. Rapid recovery with oral zinc suphate in deferoxamine-induced presumed optic neuropathy and hearing loss. J Neuroophthalmol 21: 32–33, 2001.

Popescu C, Siganos D, Zanakis E, Padakis A. The mechanism of cataract formation in persons with beta-thalassemia. Oftalmologia 45(4): 10–13, 1998.

Porter JB. A risk-benefit assessment of iron chelation therapy. Drug Safety 17: 407–421, 1997.

Rubinstein M, Dupont P, Doppee JP, et al. Ocular toxicity of desferrioxamine. Lancet 1: 817, 1985.

Simon P, et al. Desferrioxamine, ocular toxicity, and trace metals. Lancet 2: 512, 1983.

Yaqoob M, Prabhu P, Ahmad R. Comment on 'Irreversible ocular toxicity from single challenge dose of desferrioxamine' by Bene C, et al. Clin Nephrol 36(3): 155, 1991.

Generic name: Hexachlorophene.

Proprietary names: Phisohex, Pre-Op, Pre-Op II.

Primary use

This chlorinated biphenol is a topical germicide with high bacteriostatic activity that is commonly used to disinfect the skin.

Ocular side effects

Systemic administration – inadvertent oral ingestion
Certain

1. Decreased vision
2. Blindness
3. Pupils
   a. Miosis
   b. Mydriasis
   c. Absence of reaction to light
4. Optic atrophy
5. Toxic amblyopia
6. Papilledema secondary to intracranial hypertension

Systemic absorption from topical application
Certain

1. Eyelids
   a. Erythema
   b. Photosensitivity
2. Extraocular muscles
   a. Paresis
   b. Diplopia
3. Mydriasis – may precipitate angle-closure glaucoma
4. Papilledema secondary to intracranial hypertension
5. Retinal hemorrhages

Local ophthalmic use or exposure – inadvertent ocular exposure

Certain
1. Irritations
   a. Conjunctivitis
   b. Lacrimation
   c. Hyperemia
   d. Photophobia
   e. Burning sensation
2. Decreased vision
3. Cornea
   a. Keratitis
   b. Edema

Clinical significance

Hexachlorophene is toxic by the oral route, and in overdose situations can be toxic to any and all areas of the visual system. Case reports, both published and in the National Registry, confirm a predilection of the toxic effect for the optic nerve. There are large numbers of reports in animals (rats, dogs, sheep, calves, monkeys) of hexachlorophene producing cerebral edema, papilledema, mydriasis, no pupillary reaction to light and optic nerve atrophy. Histologically, widespread 'status spongiosus', vacuolation of the white matter of the central nervous system, was evident in animals and in one human case (Martinez et al 1974). The clinical finding in animals was identical to a human outbreak of hexachlorophene nervous system toxicity when given orally (Martinez et al 1974; Slamovits et al 1980), from systemic absorption through excoriated skin (Goutieres and Aicardi 1977; Martin-Bouyer et al 1982) or by infant exposure when this agent is used as a vaginal disinfectant (Strickland et al 1983). This agent, in toxic amounts, can cause selective damage to any and all parts of the visual systems from the retina to the cerebral cortex. There is a dose-response curve with reversibility in mild exposure to irreversibility in high doses or chronic exposure.

Inadvertent ocular exposure of this agent can produce severe keratitis involving all layers of the human cornea. A marked reduction of visual acuity has been reported to occur initially, but seldom are these changes irreversible.

REFERENCES AND FURTHER READING

Goutieres F, Aicardi J. Accidental percutaneous hexachlorophene intoxication in children. BMJ 2: 663, 1977.
Leopold IH, Wong EK Jr. The eye: Local irritation and topical toxicity. In: Cutaneous Toxicity, Drill VA, Lazar P (eds), Raven Press, New York, pp 99–108, 1984.
MacRae SM, Brown B, Edelhauser HF. The corneal toxicity of presurgical skin antiseptics. Am J Ophthalmol 97: 221, 1984.
Martin-Bouyer G, et al. Outbreak of accidental hexachlorophene poisoning in France. Lancet 1: 91, 1982.
Martinez AJ, Boehm R, Hadfield MG. Acute hexachlorophene encephalopathy: clinico-neuopathological correlation. Acta Neuropathol 28: 93, 1974.
Slamovits TL, Burde RM, Klingele TG. Bilateral optic atrophy caused by chronic oral ingestion and topical application of hexachlorophene. Am J Ophthalmol 89: 676, 1980.
Strickland D, et al. Vaginal absorption of hexachlorophene during labor. Am J Obstet Gynecol 147: 769, 1983.

Generic name: Methoxsalen.

Proprietary names: 8-Mop, Oxsoralen, Oxsoralen-Ultra, Uvadex.

Primary use

This psoralen is administered orally or topically for the treatment of psoriasis. The drug is administered before long-wave (320—400 nm) ultraviolet light source exposure (PUVA therapy).

Ocular side effects

Systemic administration or absorption from topical application without UV blocking goggles

Certain
1. Eyelids
   a. Hyperpigmentation
   b. Erythema
   c. Phytodermatitis
2. Conjunctival hyperemia
3. Keratitis
4. Photophobia

Probable
1. Eyelids and periocular skin – increased incidence of malignancies

Possible
1. Eyelids – hypertrichosis
2. Decreased lacrimation
3. Cataracts

Conditional/Unclassified
1. Pigmentary glaucoma

Clinical significance

This medication is given orally as a photosensitizing agent prior to ultraviolet A therapy (PUVA) for treatment of various skin disorders. Wrap-around UV protecting sunglasses are given to the patient during and for at least 12 hours post treatment. To date, this regimen has had little to no ocular side effects other than a photosensitizing effect on the periocular skin. Most ocular adverse effects are transitory and reversible, and have been due to inadvertent light exposure or not wearing protective lenses. Other than the typical photosensitivity reaction of the anterior segment (conjunctival hyperemia, keratitis photophobia), occasionally a patient may also complain of sicca-like symptoms for 48–72 hours following therapy. In a study of 82 patients who refused goggles and post-treatment UV blocking lenses over a 2- to 4-year period, about one-quarter had transitory conjunctival hyperemia and decreased lacrimation. Souêtre et al (1989) reported increased sensitivity of the retina to visible light. Reported visual field changes (Fenton and Wilkinson 1983) are transitory and probably functional rather than drug related. There are a few case reports of pigmentary glaucoma after PUVA therapy in the National Registry, but this is not a proven drug-related event. Since this therapy causes proliferation of pigment epithelial cells, this association may not be coincidental. The increased incidence of skin cancers is probable (Forman et al 1989; Lever and Farr 1994).

The area of greatest controversy is whether PUVA therapy causes cataracts. It has been shown in animals without UV ocular protection that systemic psoralens can cause anterior inferior cortical cataracts. Lerman et al (1980) detected methoxsalen in the lens for at least 12 hours after oral administration. Lerman et al (1980) as well as Woo et al (1985) state that this drug is photobound in the lens and may be cumulative with additional therapy. Van Deenen and Lamers (1988) reported transitory punctiform opacities in the nucleus and cortex of patients undergoing PUVA treatment. There have been numerous reports both supporting and denying lens changes in patients with proper eye protection after long-term PUVA therapy. Glew and Nigra (1992) have written a comprehensive review of a series of patients undergoing PUVA therapy followed up for 14 years. With proper UV-blocking lenses, they found no evidence of a higher incidence of lens changes, even with long-term therapy, versus that expected with normal aging change. Stern et al (1985) reported the results of 1235 patients enrolled in the PUVA Follow-up Study with an average follow-up of 10 years. Although they showed an increase in posterior subcapsular cataracts and a four times higher incidence of cataract extraction in the PUVA cohorts, the authors concluded that these differences may be attributable to variations in the lens abnormalities, non-uniform examination techniques or exposure to other agents. A review of the literature, the FDA data and more than 40 cases in the National Registry of lens changes associated with psoralen use seems to support the following conclusions. Usually a drug causes a certain type of cataract. To date, no characteristic pattern of lens abnormalities have been associated with psoralen use. Few, if any, lens changes occur with proper UV-blocking lenses. Theoretically, PUVA therapy without UV-blocking lenses could cause cataracts in humans, and while a definite cause-and-effect relationship has not been proven in humans, it is prudent to always wear UV blocking goggles as prescribed and eye protection for 12 hours post treatment.

REFERENCES AND FURTHER READING

Bartley GB. Ocular lens findings in patients treated with PUVA. Am J Ophthalmol 119(2): 252–253, 1995.

Calzavara-Pinton PG, Carlino A, Manfred E, et al. Ocular side effects of PUVA-treated patients refusing eye sun protection. Acta Derm Venereol (Stockh) 186: 164–165, 1994.

Farber EM, Abel EA, Cox AJ. Long-term risks of psoralens and UV-A therapy for psoriasis. Arch Dermatol 119: 426, 1983.

Fenton DA, Wilkinson JD. Dose-related visual-field defects in patients receiving PUVA therapy. Lancet 1: 1106, 1983.

Forman AB, et al. Long-term follow-up of skin cancer in the PUVA-48 cooperative study. Arch Dermatol 125: 515–519, 1989.

Glew WB, Nigra TP. PUVA and the eye. In: Photochemotherapy in Dermatology, Elizabeth AA (ed), Stanford, California, IGAKU-SHOIN Medical Publishers, Inc., pp. 241–253, 1992.

Lafond G, Roy PE, Grenier R. Lens opacities appearing during therapy with methoxsalen and long-wavelength ultraviolet radiation. Can J Ophthalmol 19: 173, 1984.

Lerman S, et al. Potential ocular complications from PUVA therapy and their prevention. J Invest Dermatol 74: 197–199, 1980.

Lever LR, Farr PM. Skin cancers or premalignant lesions occur in half of high-dose PUVA patients. Br J Dermatol 131: 215–219, 1994.

Souêtre E, et al. 5-Methoxypsoralen increases the sensitivity of the retina to light in humans. Eur J Clin Pharmacol 36: 59–61, 1989.

Stern RS. Photochemotherapy follow-up study: ocular lens findings in patients treated with PUVA. Am J Ophthalmol 119(2): 252–253, 1995.

Stern RS, Parrish JA, Fitzpatrick TB. Ocular findings in patients treated with PUVA. J Invest Dermatol 85: 269, 1985.

Van Deenen WL, Lamers WPMA. PUVA therapy and the lens reconsidered. Doc Ophthalmol 70: 179–184, 1988.

Woo TY, et al. Lenticular psoralen photoproducts and cataracts of a PUVA treated psoriatic patient. Arch Dermatol 121: 1307, 1985.

Generic name: Penicillamine.

Proprietary names: Cuprimine, Depen.

Primary use

This amino acid derivative of penicillin is a potent chelating agent effective in the management of Wilson's disease, cystinuria and copper, iron, lead or mercury poisonings. It is also a second-line drug in the management of rheumatoid arthritis.

Ocular side effects

Systemic administration
Certain
1. Myasthenia gravis
   a. Diplopia
   b. Ptosis
   c. Paresis of extraocular muscles
2. Eyelids or conjunctiva
   a. Blepharoconjunctivitis
   b. Urticaria
   c. Pemphigoid lesion with symblepharon
   d. Trichomegaly
   e. Yellowing and wrinkling of eyelids
   f. Chalazion
3. Problems with color vision – color vision defect, red-green defect

Possible
1. Extraocular muscles
   a. Decreased convergence
   b. Nystagmus
   c. Internuclear ophthalmoplegia
2. Non-specific ocular irritation
   a. Lacrimation
   b. Hyperemia
   c. Photophobia
   d. Edema
3. Retina
   a. Pigmentary changes
   b. Hemorrhages
   c. Serous detachment
4. Retrobulbar or optic neuritis
5. Visual fields
   a. Scotomas – centrocecal
   b. Constriction
6. Eyelids or conjunctiva
   a. Lupoid syndrome
   b. Lyell's syndrome

Clinical significance

Adverse ocular reactions to penicillamine are rare. Myasthenia gravis is a well-documented complication from long-term penicillamine therapy (Delamere et al 1983). Ptosis, diplopia or extraocular muscle paresis may be the first signs of this drug-related event. The onset usually occurs within 6–7 months, but in some cases it may take years to become manifest (Katz et al 1989). These side effects usually resolve spontaneously once the drug is stopped, but some patients require anticholinesterase therapy. This adverse drug event may be more common in the immunosuppressed or in those with a genetic predisposition to developing myasthenia.

The drug appears to affect the nervous system so neuroophthalmic complications seem plausible but to date none have been proven. Damaske and Althoff (1972), Klingele and Burde (1984) and cases in the National Registry suggest retrobulbar or optic neuritis may be associated with the use of penicillamine. The unmarketed DL and L forms of penicillamine probably cause optic nerve changes. Pless and Sandson (1997) reported chronic internuclear ophthalmoplegia secondary to D-penicillamine cerebral vasculitis. There are cases both in the literature (Peyri et al 1986) and the National Registry that suggest that this drug can cause an ocular pemphigoid clinical picture. Penicillamine has been implicated in delayed corneal wound healing, decreased proliferation of connective tissue and corneal superficial punctate keratitis. Penicillamine-induced zinc deficiency may be the cause of keratitis, blepharitis and loss of eyelashes, but this is unproven. Retinal pigment epithelial defects, serous detachments of the macula and subretinal or choroidal hemorrhages have also been reported with this agent.

REFERENCES AND FURTHER READING

Atcheson SG, Ward JR. Ptosis and weakness after start of D-penicillamine therapy. Ann Intern Med 89: 939, 1978.

Bigger JF. Retinal hemorrhages during penicillamine therapy of cystinuria. Am J Ophthalmol 66: 954–955, 1968.

Birch J, et al. Acquired color vision defects. In: Congenital and Aquired Color Vision Defects, Pokorny J, et al. (eds), Grune & Stratton, New York, pp 243–350, 1979.

Damaske E, Althoff W. Optic neuritis in a child with Wilson's disease. Klin Monatsbl Augenheilkd 160: 168–175, 1972.

Delamere JP, et al. Penicillamine-induced myasthenia in rheumatoid arthritis: its clinical and genetic features. Ann Rheum Dis 42: 500, 1983.

Dingle J, Havener WH. Ophthalmoscopic changes in a patient with Wilson's disease during long-term penicillamine therapy. Ann Ophthalmol 10: 1227, 1978.

Fenton DA. Hypertrichosis. Semin Dermatol 4: 58, 1985.

George J, Spokes E. Myasthenic pseudo-internuclear ophthalmoplegia due to penicillamine. J Neurol Neurosurg Psychiatry 47: 1044, 1984.

Haviv YS, Safadi R. Rapid progression of scleroderma possibly associated with penicillamine therapy. Clin Drug Invest 15(1): 61–63, 1998.

Katz LJ, et al. Ocular myasthenia gravis after d-penicillamine administration. Br J Ophthalmol 73: 1015–1018, 1989.

Kimbrough RL, Mewis I, Stewart RH. D-penicillamine and the ocular myasthenic syndrome. Ann Ophthalmol 13: 1171, 1981.

Klepach GL, Way SH. Bilateral serous retinal detachment with thrombocytopenia during penicillamine therapy. Ann Ophthalmol 13: 201, 1981.

Klingele TG, Burde RM. Optic neuropathy associated with penicillamine therapy in a patient with rheumatoid arthritis. J Clin Neuro-Ophthalmol 4: 75–78, 1984.

Loffredo A, et al. Hepatolenticular degeneration. Acta Ophthalmol 61: 943, 1983.

Marti-Huguet T, Quintana M, Cabiro I. Cicatricial pemphigoid associated with D-penicillamine treatment. Arch Ophthalmol 107: 115, 1989.

Moore AP, Williams AC, Hillenbrand P. Penicillamine induced myasthenia reactivated by gold. BMJ 288: 192, 1984.

Peyri J, et al. Cicatricial pemphigoid in a patient with rheumatoid arthritis treated with D-penicillamine. J Am Acad Dermatol 14: 681, 1986.

Pless M, Sandson T. Chronic internuclear ophthalmoplegia. A manifestation of D-penicillamine cerebral vasculitis. J Neuro-Ophthalmol 17(1): 44–46, 1997.

CLASS: DIAGNOSTIC AIDS

Generic name: Adipiodone (iodipamide meglumine).

Proprietary names: Cholografin meglumine.

Primary use

This radiographic contrast medium is used for intravenous cholecystography and cholangiography.

Ocular side effects

Systemic administration
Certain
1. Eyelids or conjunctiva
   a. Allergic reactions
   b. Erythema
   c. Edema
   d. Angioneurotic edema
   e. Urticaria

Conditional/Unclassified
1. Corneal infiltrates
2. Lateral rectus palsy

Clinical significance

Adverse ocular reactions to intravenous cholangiography or cholecystography with adipiodone are rare. Neetans and Buroenich (1979) reported a patient who developed corneal infiltrates following intravenous adipiodone. The corneal lesion disappeared with corticosteroid treatment. Bell et al (1990) reported a case of transient lateral rectus palsy, which is not unlike those reported with other contrast media. While it appears to be a direct toxic event of the contrast agent, the role the procedure plays is unknown.

REFERENCES AND FURTHER READING

Bell JA, Dowd TC, McIlwaine GG, et al. Postmyelographic abducent nerve palsy in association with the contrast agent iopamidol. J Clin Neuro-Ophthalmol 10(2): 115–117, 1990.

McEvoy GK (ed). American Hospital Formulary Service Drug Information 86, American Society of Hospital Pharmacists, Bethesda, pp 1253–1255, 1986.

McMahon KA, et al. Adverse reactions to drugs: a 12-month hospital survey. Aust N Z J Med 7: 382, 1977.

Neetans A, Buroenich H. Anaphylactic marginal keratitis. Bull Soc Belge Ophthalmol 186: 69, 1979.

Sweetman SC (ed). Martindale: The Complete Drug Reference, 34th edn, Pharmaceutical Press, London, p 1060, 2004.

Generic name: Amidotrizaote (diatrizoate meglumine and/or sodium).

Proprietary names: Cystografin, Gastrografin, Hypaque, Hypaque-76, MD-76R, MD-Gastroview, Reno-30, Reno-60, Renocal-76, Reno-Dip, Renografin 60, Renografin 76.

Primary use

This organic iodide is used in excretion urography, aortography, pediatric angiocardiography and peripheral arteriography.

Ocular side effects

Systemic administration
Certain
1. Decreased vision
2. Eyelids or conjunctiva
   a. Allergic reactions
   b. Hyperemia
   c. Erythema
   d. Conjunctivitis – follicular
   e. Edema
   f. Angioneurotic edema
   g. Urticaria
3. Non-specific ocular irritation
   a. Lacrimation
   b. Photophobia
   c. Ocular pain
   d. Burning sensation
4. Corneal infiltrates
5. Cortical blindness

Possible
1. Visual fields
   a. Scotomas – paracentral
   b. Hemianopsia

2. Retinal vascular disorders
   a. Hemorrhages
   b. Thrombosis
   c. Occlusion

Conditional/Unclassified
1. Acute macular neuroretinopathy

Clinical significance

Ocular complications associated with radiopaque contrast media arteriography have been well documented. These complications usually result from either the toxic irritative or hypersensitivity responses on blood vessels or emboli. A number of hypersensitivity responses have occurred with these agents, especially perilimbal corneal infiltrates (Baum and Bierstock 1978; cases in the National Registry), not unlike those seen with staphylococcal hypersensitivity reactions. These may or may not be associated with ocular pain, hyperemia and chemosis. These infiltrates clear on application of topical ocular steroids without complication. There are cases in the National Registry where amidotrizaote has layered out in the anterior chamber, like a hypopyon, in postoperative cataract surgery patients. No complications from this occurred. In the absence of pathologic confirmation, retinal or cerebral emboli with resultant secondary complications have been variously interpreted as cholesterol crystals, fat, air, dislodged atheromatous plaques and the injected contrast media. These have caused various degrees of retinal, choroidal or optic nerve infarcts with permanent loss of vision. Lantos (1989) described four cases of acute cortical blindness after the use of these agents, including hemianopic or complete visual loss. All cases reverted to normal in hours or days. Guzak et al (1983) described two cases of acute macular neuroretinopathy in a young woman after intravenous diatrizoate. Findings included swollen macules and subtle opacification of the parafoveal retina. Deep retinal lesions developed later.

REFERENCES AND FURTHER READING

Baum JL, Bierstock SR. Peripheral corneal infiltrates following intravenous injection of diatrizoate meglumine. Am J Ophthalmol 85: 613, 1978.

Guzak SV, Kalina RE, Chenoweth RG. Acute macular neuroretinopathy following adverse reaction to intravenous contrast media. Retina 3: 312–317, 1983.

Haney WP, Preston RE. Ocular complications of carotid arteriography in carotid occlusive disease. Arch Ophthalmol 67: 127–137, 1962.

Junck L, Marshall WH. Neurotoxicity of radiological contrast agents. Ann Neurol 13: 469, 1983.

Lantos G. Cortical blindness due to osmotic disruption of the blood-brain barrier by angiographic contrast material: CT and MRI studies. Neurology 39: 567–571, 1989.

McMahon KA, et al. Adverse reactions to drugs: A 12-month hospital survey. Aust N Z J Med 7: 382, 1977.

Priluck IA, Buettner H, Robertson DM. Acute macular neuroretinopathy. Am J Ophthalmol 86: 775, 1978.

Generic names: Iotalamic acid (iothalamate meglumine and/or sodium).

Proprietary names: Conray, Conray-30, Conray-43, Cysto-conray, Glofil-125.

Primary use

This radiopaque contrast medium is used for excretion urography, contrast enhancement of CT of the brain, aortography, selective renal arteriography, angiocardiography and selective coronary arteriography.

Ocular side effects

Systemic administration
Certain
1. Decreased vision
2. Eyelids or conjunctiva
   a. Allergic reactions
   b. Erythema
   c. Conjunctivitis – non-specific
   d. Edema
   e. Angioneurotic edema
   f. Urticaria
3. Non-specific ocular irritation
   a. Lacrimation
   b. Photophobia
4. Cortical blindness

Probable
1. Myasthenia gravis
   a. Diplopia
   b. Ptosis
   c. Paresis of extraocular muscles
   d. Divergent strabismus
2. Cornea
   a. Superficial, cloudy peripheral infiltrates

Possible
1. Scotomas – paracentral
2. Retina or macular
   a. Edema
   b. Wedge-shaped lesions
3. Lowers intraocular pressure (transitory)

Clinical significance

Potential complications of cerebral angiography may include temporary disturbances in vision and neuromuscular disorders. Visual field losses are usually transient, although permanent changes have been reported after intravenous iothalamate. Guzak et al (1983) reported two cases of acute macular neuroretinopathy associated with scotoma, metamorphopsia, macular swelling and typical wedge-shaped retinal lesions. Neetens and Buroenich (1979) reported a rapid onset of anaphylactic corneal perilimbal superficial marginal infiltrates, which cleared in a few days on topical ocular steroid application. Smith and Carlson (1994) reported a 20–45% decrease in intraocular pressure after intravenous iothalamate sodium. The peak effect is at 30 minutes and returns to baseline in 120 minutes. Lantos (1989) reported four cases of cortical blindness secondary to this agent, all recovering within 1 month. He postulated that the cause of the clinical manifestations of cortical blindness could be the drug passing through the blood-brain barrier along with toxic effects of the contrast agent on neural elements.

REFERENCES AND FURTHER READING

Canal N, Francesci M. Myasthenic crisis precipitated by iothalamic acid. Lancet 1: 1288, 1983.

Guzak SV, Kalina RE, Chenoweth RG. Acute macular neuroretinopathy following adverse reaction to intravenous contrast media. Retina 3: 312: 1983.

Junck L, Marshall WH. Neurotoxicity of radiological contrast agents. Ann Neurol 13: 469, 1983.

Lantos G. Cortical blindness due to osmotic disruption of the blood-brain barrier by angiographic contrast material. CT and MRI studies. Neurology 39: 567–571, 1989.

McEvoy GK (ed). American Hospital Formulary Service Drug Information 87, American Society of Hospital Pharmacists, Bethesda, pp 1258–1270, 1987.

Neetens A, Buroenich H. Anaphylactic marginal keratitis. Bull Soc Belge Ophthalmol 186: 69–72, 1979.

Smith RE, Carlson DW. Intravenous pyelography contrast media acutely lowers intraocular pressure. Invest Ophthalmol Vis Sci 35(4): 1387, 1994.

Sweetman SC (ed). Martindale: The Complete Drug Reference, 34th edn, Pharmaceutical Press, London, pp 1065–1066, 2004.

CLASS: IMMUNOSUPPRESSANTS

Generic name: Azathioprine.

Proprietary names: Azasan, Imuran.

Primary use
This imidazolyl derivative of mercaptopurine is used as an adjunct to help prevent rejection in homograft transplantation and to treat various autoimmune diseases.

Ocular side effects

Systemic administration
Probable
1. Decrease activation of resistance to infection
2. Delayed corneal wound healing

Possible
1. Subconjunctival or retinal hemorrhages secondary to drug-induced anemia
2. Brow and eyelash loss

Conditional/unclassified
1. Fine macular pigmentation

Ocular teratogenic effects
Possible
1. Cataracts

Clinical significance
Ocular side effects are uncommon and are reversible on withdrawing the drug. There are reports of activation of ocular viral disease, such as cytomegalic inclusion disease (Scott et al 2004), vaccinia (Thomas 1976), and bacterial and herpes zoster (Speerstra et al 1982; Lawson et al 1984). There is evidence that this drug impedes corneal wound healing (Elliott and Leibowitz 1966; Francois and Feher 1972). This drug has been implicated in numerous blood dyscrasias. Sudhir et al (2002) reported bilateral macular hemorrhages due to azathioprine-induced aplastic anemia. Miserocchi et al (2002) reported blood dyscrasias in patients treated with this drug for ocular cicatricial pemphigoid. Apaydin et al (1992), along with two cases in the National Registry, show an increase in macular pigment while on azathioprine. Patients were on multiple other drugs and an association cannot be made without more cases being reported.

REFERENCES AND FURTHER READING
Apaydin C, Gur B, Yakupoglu G, Saka O. Ocular and visual side effects of systemic cyclosporine. Ann Ophthalmol 24(12): 465–469, 1992.

Drug Evaluations, 6th edn, American Medical Association, Chicago, pp 1074–1075, 1151–1152, 1986.

Elliot JH, Leibowitz HM. The influence of immunosuppressive agents upon corneal wound healing. Arch Ophthalmol 76: 334–337, 1966.

Francois J, Feher J. The effect of azathioprine and chlorpromazine on corneal regeneration. Exp Eye Res 14: 69–72, 1972.

Knowles RS, Virden JE. Handling of injectable antineoplastic agents. BMJ 2: 589, 1980.

Lawson DH, et al. Adverse effects of azathioprine. Adverse Drug React Acute Poison Rev 3: 161, 1984.

Miserocchi E, Baltatzis S, Roque MR, et al. The effect of treatment and its related side effects in patients with severe ocular cicatricial pemphigoid. Ophthalmology 109: 111–118, 2002.

Schneider F. Progressive multifocal leukoencephalopathy as a cause of neurologic symptoms in Sharp syndrome. Zeitschrft fur Rheumatologie 50(4): 222–224, 1991.

Scott WJ, Giangiacoma J, Hodges KE, et al. Accelerated cytomegalovirus retinitis secondary to immunosuppressive therapy. Arch Ophthalmol 104: 1117–1118. 1124, 2004.

Speerstra F, et al. Side-effects of azathioprine treatment in rheumatoid arthritis: analysis of 10 years of experience. Ann Rheum Dis 41(Suppl): 37, 1982.

Sudhir RR, Rao SK, Shanmugam MP, et al. Bilateral macular hemorrhage caused by azathioprine-induced aplastic anemia in a corneal graft recipient. Cornea 21: 712–714, 2002.

Sweetman SC (ed). Martindale: The Extra Pharmacopoeia, 28th edn, Pharmaceutical Press, London, pp 1348–1349, 2004.

Thomas MH. Azathioprine and severe vaccinia. Arthritis Rheum 19: 270, 1976.

Tuchmann-Duplessis H, Mercier-Parot L. Dissociation of antitumor and teratogenic properties of a purine antimetabolite, azathioprine. C R Soc Biol 159: 2290–2294, 1965.

Generic name: Ciclosporin (cyclosporine).

Proprietary names: Gengraf, Neoral, Restasis, Sandimmune.

Primary use

Systemic
This immunosuppressive agent is used for prevention of kidney, liver or heart allografts. Disorders of the skin, blood, gastrointestinal tract, liver, neurologic system and kidney, as well as collagen vascular diseases have been treated with this agent.

Ophthalmic
This agent has also been used in the management of uveitis, Behçet's syndrome, corneal disease, scleritis and various severe conjunctivitis cases.

Ocular side effects

Systemic administration
Certain
1. Decreased vision
2. Eyelids or conjunctiva
   a. Erythema
   b. Conjunctivitis – non-specific
   c. Urticaria
   d. Edema
   e. Ptosis
3. Visual hallucinations
4. Cortical blindness (posterior leukoencephalopathy syndrome)
5. Optic nerve
   a. Edema (with or without intracranial hypertension)
   b. Neuropathy
6. Extraocular muscles
   a. 6th nerve palsy
   b. Ocular flutter
   c. External ophthalmoplegia
   d. Nystagmus

7. Trichomegaly
8. Ocular pain

Possible
1. Retinal and optic nerve ischemia (with total body radiation)
   a. Cotton wool spots
   b. Hemorrhages
   c. Lipid deposits
2. Increased lymphoproliferative ocular disease
3. Intracranial hypertension

Local ophthalmic use or exposure
Certain
1. Irritation
   a. Burning sensation
   b. Pain, itching

Possible
1. Cornea
   a. Superficial punctate keratitis
   b. Superficial deposits (Fig. 7.12b)
2. Eyelids and conjunctiva
   a. Edema
   b. Hyperemia

Clinical significance

This drug is used systemically for medical conditions of some complexity where multiple medications and procedures (i.e. bone marrow transplants, total body radiation, leukemias, etc.) are complicating factors in determining specific drug side effects. However, with the drug now in clinical use for over 30 years, drug-induced ocular side effects are fairly well understood.

Bone marrow transplantation patients seem to have some unique ocular toxicity due to ciclosporin and associated drugs. Avery et al (1991) describe eight cases of optic disc edema which resolved after discontinuing or decreasing the dosage of this drug. Optic disc edema due to ciclosporin may be a direct toxic effect of the drug on the optic nerve or papilledema secondary to increased intracranial pressure. This drug rarely affects the optic nerve in renal transplant patients (Rodriguez et al 1992) but it is not uncommon in bone marrow transplantation (Walter et al 2000). Bernauer et al (1991) described retinal and optic nerve ischemia in 13 patients, including bilateral disc edema, cotton wool spots, retinal hemorrhages and lipid deposits. This occurred within the first 6 months of ciclosporin therapy after bone marrow transplantation and was reversible in nine of the 13 cases after the drug was discontinued. The authors concluded that this adverse event was due to a combined effect of ciclosporin along with total body radiation. In this group of patients and others

ciclosporin has a neurotoxic effect. This includes cortical blindness, increased intracranial pressure and papilledema. There are a few reports of intracranial hypertension (Cruz et al 1996; Büschen et al 2004) with this drug, but a clear-cut cause-and-effect relationship is not proven. There are four cases (Openshaw et al 1997; Openshaw 2001) of unilateral or bilateral 6th nerve palsy with or without ptosis in patients on both ciclosporin and ganciclovir. An MRI showed this was due to abnormalities in the region of the sixth nerve nucleus rather than a localized ocular neuromuscular event. The palsies reverted to normal in a matter of days once ciclosporin was stopped. The MRI findings also resolved. Ocular flutter in bone marrow transplant patients taking ciclosporin has been described by Apsner et al (1997). Porges et al (1998) reported a case of ciclosporin-induced optic neuropathy, ophthalmoplegia and nystagmus in a patient with Crohn's disease. Palmer et al (1995) showed that in renal allograft patients, systemic ciclosporin increased tear flow even when no lacrimal autoimmune disease exists. This drug may cause trichomegaly.

Ciclosporin causes a syndrome with various degrees of visual loss, including blindness, encephalopathy, white matter changes and seizures. The presentation of these findings is termed a 'posterior leukoencephalopathy'. These changes usually return to near normal after stopping ciclosporin. There are at least 40 well-documented cases of this syndrome, primarily in bone marrow or liver transplant cases, but also in patients with leukemia or aplastic anemia. Visual abnormalities have a variable presentation, but most commonly occur within the first 2 months after starting ciclosporin. The retinal exam is negative, although Estel et al (1996) described yellow retinal exudates. When this syndrome is discovered, one must reduce or discontinue the drug. Recovery of vision is often directly proportional to the severity of the syndrome (DeGroen et al 1987). While complete recovery is the standard, there are cases of permanent blindness (Estel et al 1996; Casanova et al 1997). There have been reports of positive rechallenge (Knower et al 2003).

With systemic administration, severe ocular pain may occur for unexplained reasons with or without evidence of an ocular abnormality. This may occur while taking the drug, or when the drug is discontinued. Various irritative reactions may occur around the eye, but these are seldom of major clinical significance. Visual hallucinations may be so severe that they require ciclosporin to be discontinued. Cho et al (2001) suggested the possibility that ciclosporin may increase post-transplant lymphoproliferative disorder uveitis and iris nodules. These four cases were without systemic involvement.

Commercial topical ocular ciclosporin (0.05%) may, in up to 17% of patients, cause some burning or stinging on application. Occasionally patients may develop lid irritation, superficial punctate keratitis and erythema of the lids and/or conjunctiva. Sall et al (2000) reported few ocular side effects other than burning and stinging. Kachi et al (2000) reported a patient developing corneal deposits bilaterally within 5 days of starting topical ocular ciclosporin (2%) three times daily. She had severe disturbances of her corneal epithelial and decrease tear production. After 12 months, other than some peripheral clearing, no improvement in the density of the opacities was seen. Barber et al (2005) found no associated systemic side effects when using a 0.1% ophthalmic emulsion for up to 3 years.

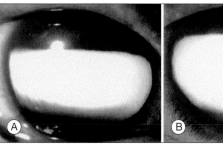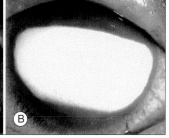

Fig. 7.12b Dense white deposits after topical ocular ciclosporin treatment. Photo courtesy of Kachi S, et al: Unusual corneal deposit after the topical use of cyclosporine as eyedrops. Am J Ophthalmol 130: 667–669, 2000.

REFERENCES AND FURTHER READING

Ahern MJ, et al. A randomized double-blind trial of cyclosporin and azathioprine in refractory rheumatoid arthritis. Aust N Z J Med 21: 844–849, 1991.

Apsner R, Schulenburg A, Steinhoff N, et al. Cyclosporin A induced ocular flutter after marrow transplantation. Bone Marrow Transplant 20(3): 255–256, 1997.

Avery R, et al. Optic disc edema after bone marrow transplantation. Ophthalmology 98: 1294–1301, 1991.

Barber LD, Pflugfelder SC, Tauber J, et al. Phase III safety evaluation of cyclosporine 0.1% ophthalmic emulsion administered twice daily to dry eye disease patients for up to 3 years. Ophthalmology 112: 790–1794, 2005.

BenEzra D, et al. Cyclosporine eyedrops for the treatment of severe vernal keratoconjunctivitis. Am J Ophthalmol 101: 278, 1986.

Bernauer W, Gratwohl A, Keller A, et al. Microvasculopathy in the ocular fundus after bone marrow transplantation. Ann Int Med 115(12): 925–930, 1991.

Büscher R, Vij O, Hudde T, et al. Pseudotumor cerebri following cyclosporine A treatment in a boy with tubulointerstitial nephritis associated with uveitis. Pediatr Nephrol 19: 558–560, 2004.

Casanova B, Prieto M, Deya E. Persistent cortical blindness after cyclosporine leukoencephalopathy. Liver Transplant Surg 3: 638–640, 1997.

Cho AS, Holland GN, Glasgow BJ, et al. Ocular involvement in patients with posttransplant lymphoproliferative disorder. Arch Ophthalmol 119: 183–189, 2001.

Cruz OA, Fogg SG, Roper-Hall G. Pseudotumor cerebri associated with cyclosporine use. Am J Ophthalmol 122(3): 436–437, 1996.

Dawson DG, Trobe JD. Blindness after liver transplant. Surv Ophthalmol 47: 387–391, 2002.

DeGroen PC, Aksamit AJ, Rakela J, et al. Central nervous system toxicity after liver transplantation: the role of cyclosporine and cholesterol. N Engl J Med 317: 861–866, 1987.

Estel RM, Gupta N, Garvin PJ. Permanent blindness after cyclosporine neurotoxicity in a kidney-pancreas transplant recipient. Clin Neuropharmacol 19: 259–266, 1996.

Filipec M, et al. Topical cyclosporine A and corneal wound healing. Cornea 11: 546–552, 1992.

Ghalie R, et al. Cortical blindness: a rare complication of cyclosporine therapy. Bone Marrow Transplant 6: 147–149, 1990.

González-Vincent M, Díaz MA, Madero L. 'Pseudotumor cerebri' following allogeneic bone marrow transplantation (BMT). Ann Hematol 80: 236–237, 2001.

Kachi S, Hirano K, Takesue Y, et al. Unusual corneal deposit after the topical use of cyclosporine as eyedrops. Am J Ophthalmol 130: 667–669, 2000.

Katirji MB. Visual hallucinations and cyclosporine. Transplantation 43: 768, 1987.

Knower MT, Pethke SD, Valentine VG. Reversible cortical blindness after lunch transplantation. South Med J 96: 606–612, 2003.

Laibovitz RA, et al. Pilot trial of cyclosporine 1% ophthalmic ointment in the treatment of keratoconjunctivitis sicca. Cornea 12: 315–323, 1993.

Marchiori PE, Mies S, Scaff M. Cyclosporine A-induced ocular opsoclonus and reversible leukoencephalopathy after orthotopic liver transplantation. Clin Neuropharmacol 27: 195–197, 2004.

Meyers-Elliott RH, Chitjian PA, Billups CB. Effects of cyclosporine A on clinical and immunological parameters in herpes simplex keratitis. Invest Ophthalmol Vis Sci 28: 1170–1180, 1987.

Noll RB, Kulkarni R. Complex visual hallucinations and cyclosporine. Arch Neurol 41: 329, 1984.

Obermoser G, Weber F, Sepp N. Discoid lupus erythematosus in a patient receiving cyclosporine for liver transplantation. Acta Derm Venereol 81: 319, 2001.

Openshaw H. Eye movement abnormality associated with ciclosporin. J Neurol Neurosurg Psychiatry 70: 809, 2001.

Openshaw H, Slatkin NE, Smith E. Eye movement disorders in bone marrow transplant patients on cyclosporin and ganciclovir. Bone Marrow Transplant 19(5): 503–505, 1997.

Palmer SL, Bowen A II, Green K. Tear flow in cyclosporine recipients. Ophthalmology 102(1): 118–121, 1995.

Palmer SL, Bowen A II, Green K. Longitudinal tear study after cyclosporine in kidney transplant recipients. Ophthalmology 103(4): 670–673, 1996.

Porges Y, Blumen S, Fireman Z, et al. Cyclosporine-induced optic neuropathy, ophthalmoplegia, and nystagmus in a patient with Crohn's disease. Am J Ophthalmol 126(4): 607–608, 1998.

Rodriguez E, Delucchi A, Cano F. Neurotoxicity caused by cyclosporine A in renal transplantation in children. Rev Med Child 120: 300–303, 1992.

Rubin AM, Kang H. Cerebral blindness and encephalopathy with cyclosporin A toxicity. Neurology 37: 1072, 1987.

Sall K, Stevenson OD, Mundorf TK, et al. Two multicenter, randomized studies of the efficacy and safety of cyclosporine ophthalmic emulsion in moderate to severe dry eye disease. Ophthalmology 107: 631–639, 2000.

Stevenson D, Tauber J, Reis BL, et al. Efficacy and safety of cyclosporine A ophthalmic emulsion in the treatment of moderate-to-severe dry eye disease. Ophthalmology 107: 967–974, 2000.

Stucrenschneider BJ, Meiler WF. Ocular findings following bone marrow transplantation. Ophthalmology 92(suppl): 152, 1992.

Tang-Liu DD, Acheampong A. Ocular pharmacokinetics and safety of ciclosporin, a novel topical treatment for dry eye. Clin Pharmacokinet 44: 247–261, 2005.

Uoshima N, Karasuno T, Yagi T, et al. Late onset cyclosporine-induced cerebral blindness with abnormal SPECT imagings in a patient undergoing unrelated bone marrow transplantation. Bone Marrow Transplant 26: 105–108, 2000.

Walter SH, Bertz H, Gerling J. Bilateral neuropathy after bone marrow transplantation and cyclosporine A therapy. Graefe's Arch Clin Exp Ophthalmol 238: 472–476, 2000.

Weaver SE, et al. Cyclosporin A-induced reversible cortical blindness. J Clin Neuro-Ophthalmol 8: 215–220, 1988.

Generic name: Tacrolimus.

Proprietary names: Prograf, Protopic.

Primary use

Systemic
This potent immunosuppressant is used in the prophylaxis treatment of organ rejection.

Ophthalmic
Used off-label for graft rejection and other conditions helped by immunosuppression.

Ocular side effects

Systemic administration – oral or injection
Certain
1. Decreased vision
2. Visual hallucination
3. Photophobia
4. Eyelids or conjunctiva
   a. Photosensitivity
   b. Increased susceptibility to bacterial, viral or fungal infections

Probable
1. Cortical blindness

Possible
1. Optic nerve
   a. Neuritis
   b. Neuropathy
2. Abnormal visual evoked potential
3. Increase incidence of malignancies (especially lymphoma)
4. Eyelids or conjunctiva
   a. Stevens-Johnson syndrome
   b. Toxic epidermal necrolysis

Conditional/Unclassified
1. Downward gaze deviation
2. Internuclear ophthalmoplegia

Local ophthalmic use of exposure – ointment 0.1–0.3%
Certain
1. Irritation
    a. Burning
    b. Itching

Conditional/Unclassified
1. Mucosal pigmentary changes
2. Hypertrichosis – skin
3. Reactivation of herpes simplex

Clinical significance

This potent agent is often given with ciclosporin. Cortical blindness is consistently associated with tacrolimus from the drug, causing bilateral occipital white matter lesions or a leukoencephalopathy (Shutter et al 1993; Devine et al 1996; Steg et al 1999). Once the drug is stopped, vision usually improves within 1–2 weeks. Devine et al (1996) reported three cases of cortical blindness that followed a pattern similar to ciclosporin-induced cortical blindness, with early onset in the course of therapy, no direct correlation to blood levels of the drug and continued improvement while still on the drug. MRI findings appeared to lag behind the clinical improvements.

Three cases of bilateral optic neuropathy have been attributed to tacrolimus. One was reversible 1 month after discontinuing treatment (Kessler et al 2005), one showed continued deterioration even when the drug was stopped (Brazis et al 2000) and two of the three occurred at the normal or low therapeutic dose range (Brazis et al 2000; Lake and Poole 2003). There are 11 cases of poorly documented optic neuritis in the WHO database. There are isolated reports of downward gaze deviation in tacrolimus-induced mutism (Sokol et al 2003), reversible bilateral internuclear opthalmoplegia (Lai et al 2004) and decreased vision with MRI cerebral abnormalities (Bova et al 2000). Lauzurica et al (2002) reported severe bilateral non-infectious corneal ulcers after oral tacrolimus. The authors postulated either a direct toxic effect or a drug-induced vasculitic response. There are no other cases of corneal ulcers in the National Registry or reported to the manufacturer. Plosker and Foster (2000) pointed out, as with most immunosuppressive therapy, an increased rate of malignancy can happen, especially with lymphomas.

Freeman et al (2004) and Russell (2002), when treating 20 patients with atopic eyelid disease using 0.1% tacrolimus ointment, found that 60–80% reported burning and 25–50% reported itching on application of the ointment, but neither reaction was severe enough to stop the drug. Kang et al (2001), in treating dermatitis in children, found up to an 11% increase in skin infections after topical tacrolimus in the form of herpes simplex, varicella and eczema herpeticum. Joseph et al (2005) reported a patient developing herpes simplex corneal ulcer 1 week after starting topical ocular tacrolimus, but at the time the patient was also on steroids. Russell (2002) felt there was a higher incidence of recurrence of herpes after this drug is applied to or around the eye. Shen and Pedvis-Leftick (2004) reported hyperpigmentation of the oral mucosa after topical tacrolimus. Caelles et al (2005) reported a case and there are an additional five cases in the WHO database of hypertrichosis in the area where tacrolimus ointment was applied. There are reports (Rikker et al 2003) that find no significant adverse ocular events due to tacrolimus ointment applied to the eyelids. The FDA has terminated topical ocular application of this drug in solution form for ocular sicca (Sucampo Pharmaceuticals Inc. 2005).

REFERENCES AND FURTHER READING

Bova D, Shownkeen H, Goldberg K, et al. Delayed transient neurologic toxicity due to tacrolimus: CT and MRI. Neuroradiology 42: 666–668, 2000.
Brazis PW, Spivey JR, Bolling JP, et al. A case of bilateral optic neuropathy in a patient on tacrolimus (FK506) therapy after liver transplantation. Am J Ophthalmol 129: 536–538, 2000.
Caelles IP, Pinto PH, Casado ELD, et al. Focal hypertrichosis during topical tacrolimus therapy for childhood vitiligo. Pediatr Dermatol 22: 86–87, 2005.
Devine SM, Newman NJ, Siegel JL, et al. Tacrolimus (FK506)-induced cerebral blindness following bone marrow transplantation. Bone Marrow Transplant 18: 569–572, 1996.
Freeman AK, Serle J, VanVeldhuisen P, et al. Tacrolimus ointment in the treatment of eyelid sermatitis. Cutis 73: 225–227, 2004.
Joseph MA, Kaufman HE, Insler M. Topical tacrolimus ointment for treatment of refractory anterior segment inflammatory disorders. Cornea 24: 417–420, 2005.
Kang S, Luck AW, Pariser D, et al. Long-term safety and efficacy of tacrolimus ointment for the treatment of atopic dermatitis in children. J Am Acad Dermatol 44(Suppl 1): S58–S64, 2001.
Kessler L, Lucescu C, Pinget M. Tacrolimus-associated optic neuropathy after pancreatic islet transplantation using a sirolimus/tacrolimus immunosuppressive regimen. Tansplantation 81: 636–637, 2005.
Lai MM, Kerrison JB, Miller NR. Reversible bilateral internuclear ophthalmolplegia associated with FK506. J Neurol Neurosurg Psychiatr 75: 776–778, 2004.
Lake DB, Poole TRG. Tacrolimus. Br J Ophthalmol 87: 121–122, 2003.
Lauzurica R, Loscos J, Diaz-Couchod P, et al. Tacrolimus-associated severe bilateral corneal ulcer after renal transplantation. Trans 73: 1006–1007, 2002.
Nakamura M, Fuchinouc S, Sato S, et al. Clinical and radiological features of two cases of tacrolimus-related posterior leukoencephalopathy in living related liver transplantation. Transplant Proc 30: 1477–1478, 1998.
Oliverio PJ, Lucas R, Mitchell SA, et al. Reversible tacrolimus-induced neurotoxicity isolated to the brain stem. Am J Neuroradiol 21: 1251–1254, 2000.
Plosker GL, Foster RH. Tacrolimus: a further update of its pharmacology and therapeutic use in the management of organ transplantation. Drugs 59: 323–389, 2000.
Rikker SM, Holland GN, Drayton GE, et al. Topical tacrolimus treatment of atopic eyelid disease. Am J Ophthalmol 135: 297–302, 2003.
Russell JJ. Topical tacrolimus: a new therapy for atopic dermatitis. Am Fam Physician 66: 1899–1902, 2002.
Shen JT, Pedvis-Leftick A. Mucosal staining after using topical tacrolimus to treat erosive oral lichen planus. J Am Acad Dermatol 50: 326, 2004.
Shutter LA, Green JP, Newman NJ, et al. Cortical blindness and white matter lesions in a patient receiving FK506 after liver transplantation. Neurology 43: 2417–2418, 1993.
Sokol DK, Molleston JP, Filo RS, et al. Tacrolimus (FK560)-induced mutism after liver transplant. Pediatr Neurol 28: 156–158, 2003.
Steg RE, Kessinger A, Wszolek ZK. Cortical blindness and seizures in a patient receiving FK506 after bone marrow transplantation. Bone Marrow Transplant 23: 956–962, 1999.
Sucampo Pharmaceuticals Inc. Sucampo voluntarily halts tacrolimus eye drops development, files complaint against business partner. Media Release, 24 Jun 2005. Available from: http://www.sucampo.com.

CLASS: RETINOIDS

Generic name: Isotretinoin.

Proprietary names: Accutane, Amnesteem, Claravis, Sotret.

Primary use

These retinoids are used in the treatment of psoriasis, cystic acne and various other disorders of the skin.

Ocular side effects

Systemic administration
Certain
1. Eyelids or conjunctiva
    a. Blepharoconjunctivitis
    b. Erythema

   c. Edema
   d. Conjunctivitis – non-specific
   e. Photosensitivity
   f. Angioneurotic edema
   g. Pruritus
2. Decreased or blurred vision
3. Meibomian glands
   a. Meibomitis
   b. Increased viscosity of secretion
   c. Atrophy
   d. Associated increased staphyloccus
4. Lacrimation – variable
5. Tears
   a. Decreased osmolarity
   b. Decreased tear film break-up times
   c. Drug found in tears
   d. Sicca-evaporative form
6. Cornea
   a. Superficial opacities – fine, rough
   b. Superficial punctate keratitis
   c. Ulceration
7. Decreased dark adaptation
   a. Night blindness
   b. Permanent night blindness
8. Myopia – transitory
9. Abnormal ERG (scopic)
10. Decreased tolerance to contact lenses
11. Papilledema secondary to intracranial hypertension

Probable

1. Color vision – decreased

Possible

1. Optic neuritis

Ocular teratogenic effects
Certain

1. Microphthalmia
2. Optic nerve hypoplasia
3. Orbital hypertelorism
4. Cortical blindness

Possible

1. Cataracts
2. Keratoconus

Clinical significance

Ocular side effects are dose related and probably the most frequent adverse drug reactions are blepharoconjunctivitis, subjective complaints of dry eyes and transient blurred vision. Acute refractive changes, especially myopic shifts, are transitory and well documented. The drug is secreted in the tears via the lacrimal gland, which may be the cause of an irritative or drug-induced conjunctivitis. Bozkurt et al (2002) and Mathers et al (1991) believe if given in low doses and not in multiple cycles, the sicca is reversible, but in rare instances it may be permanent (Fraunfelder et al 2001). Some of these signs and symptoms are secondary to isotretinoin's direct effect of decreasing meibomian gland function with resultant increased tear evaporation and tear osmolarity. In some patients, isotretinoin causes keratoconjunctivitis sicca (Fraunfelder et al 2001). This again confirms that drugs that cause oral dryness have the potential to cause ocular sicca as well (Bots et al 2003). Aragona et al (2005) discussed the problems of ocular surface disease in patients on isotretinoin and its management. Miles et al (2006) pointed out the problems of doing laser assisted in situ keratomileusis (LASIK) in patients on isotretinoin and recommend not using this drug for 6 months post surgery. Fine, rounded, subepithelial opacities found in the central and peripheral corneas of patients treated with this medication rarely interfere with vision. They may be of variable sizes, white to gray in color, and disappear within 2–10 months after discontinuation of the drug. This probably occurs partially by changes in tear film along with the drug being secreted in the tears. These factors also affect patients who are contact lens wearers. Some recommend not fitting patients with lenses while on the drug. Approximately 20% of previously successful wearers may need to discontinue their contact lens use, decrease their wearing time or use additional preservative-free lubricating eye drops while on isotretinoin.

There are well-documented cases of decreased ability to see at night in patients after taking this agent (Fraunfelder et al 2001). This may occur as early as after a few weeks or after prolonged drug exposure. This may be irreversible. Retinal dysfunction is probably due to the competition for binding sites between retinoic acid and retinol (vitamin A). The risk of a photosensitizing drug, such as isotretinoin, enhancing the effects of light on the macula and retina is unclear. While there are cases in the National Registry of retinal pigmentary changes, these are few in number and may be unrelated.

Fraunfelder et al (2004) report on 179 cases of intracranial hypertension in patients on isotretinoin. The mean onset was 2.3 months after starting the drug. Six patients in this series had positive rechallenges. Isotretinoin is a synthetic derivative of vitamin A that has well-documented data as being a cause of intracranial hypertension. It is felt this class of drugs alters the lipid concentration of the arachnoid villi, thereby impeding absorption of cerebrospinal fluid (Roytman et al 1988).

The role of isotretinoin as a cataractogenic agent is not yet defined. Although there are a number of reports of cataracts in the National Registry, as well as in a publication by Herman and Dyer (1987), there are little data to prove that isotretinoin is a cataractogenic agent. This drug has been in widespread use for more than two decades and very few cataracts are reported, which suggests that this agent is at worst a very weak cataractogenic agent. Drug exposure is often short-term (i.e. a number of months), indicating the reports are a chance event or consist of a subset of individuals whose lenses are highly sensitive to the drug. Regardless, there is no clear-cut pattern to the cataracts. There are a few cases in the National Registry of a subset of patients in high-light environments who have taken multiple cycles of isotretinoin, developing multiple, small, cortical punctate opacities of various sizes.

Optic neuritis, unilateral and bilateral, has been seen shortly after starting isotretinoin. Since most of these patients are in the multiple sclerosis age group, it is difficult to be confident as to a cause-and-effect relationship. To our knowledge, no case has been rechallenged. However, there are cases that suggest a possible relationship therefore the manufacturer recommends stopping the drug if this occurs.

While keratoconus has been reported with isotretinoin usage, the drug is used in atopic individuals. Keratoconus is seen in 4–6% of atopics. We doubt keratoconus is caused by this agent. Fraunfelder (2001) reviewed 2449 spontaneous isotretinoin ocular side effects and gives the most complete overview.

Offspring of mothers exposed to these drugs during pregnancy may have numerous congenital abnormalities involving the eyes (Guirgis et al 2002).

Recommendations

1. If the patient is below the age of 40 and has not had an eye examination for a few years, or is above age 40 and has not had one within 2 years, it may be prudent to have a baseline dilated ocular examination.
2. Explain risk-benefit ratio to patients with:
   a. retinitis pigmentosa (only theoretical)
   b. severe or chronic blepharoconjunctivitis
   c. significant tear film abnormalities.
3. In selected patients with anterior segment pathology, consider UV blocking lenses since the drug is a photosensitizing agent.
4. Some feel one should consider discontinuing or delaying fitting of contact lenses while on this drug and discontinue the drug during and 6 months post-operatively to LASIK surgery.
5. Patients on long-term isotretinoin should have an annual eye examination.
6. Suggest that patients see you if any significant ocular signs or symptoms occur.
7. Question all patients concerning night blindness, keratitis sicca and decreased color vision. If progressive or persistent, consider discontinuing the drug. Since most cases are transitory, these findings are not necessarily an indication for discontinuing the drug. However, if they persist for a number of weeks consider closer monitoring and further testing. Informed consent should be considered.
8. Consider discontinuing the drug if any of the following occurs until a cause is determined:
   a. intracranial hypertension
   b. optic neuritis
   c. persistent night blindness
   d. decreased color vision.

REFERENCES AND FURTHER READING

Aragona P, Cannavó SP, Borgia F, et al. Utility of studying the ocular surface in patients with acne vulgaris treated with oral isotretinoin: a randomized controlled trial. Br J Dermatol 152: 576–578, 2005.

Bots CP, van Nieuw-Amerongen A, Brand HS. Enduring oral dryness after acne treatment. Ned Tijdschr Tandheelkd 110: 295–297, 2003.

Bozkurt B, Irkec MT, Atakan N, et al. Lacrimal function and ocular complications in patients treated with systemic itotretinoin. Eur J Ophthalmol 12: 173–176, 2002.

Brown RD, Grattan CEH. Visual toxicity of synthetic retinoids. Br J Ophthalmol 73: 286–288, 1989.

Chua WC, Martin PA, Kourt G. Watery eye: a new side-effect of isotretinoin therapy. Eye 15: 115–116, 2001.

Ellies P, Dighiero P, Legeais JM, et al. Persistent corneal opacity after oral isotretinoin therapy for acne. Cornea 19: 238–239, 2000.

Fraunfelder FW. Ocular side effects associated with isotretinoin. Drugs Today 40: 23–27, 2004.

Fraunfelder FT, Fruanfelder FW, Edwards R. Ocular side effects possible associated with isotretinoin usage. Am J Ophthalmol 132: 299–305, 2001.

Fraunfelder FW, Fruanfelder FT, Corbett JJ. Isotretinoin-associated intracranial hypertension. Ophthalmol 111: 1248–1250, 2004.

Gold JA, Shupack JL, Nemec MA. Ocular side effects of the retinoids. Int J Dermatol 28: 218–225, 1989.

Guirgis MF, Wong AMF, Tychsen L, et al. Congenital restrictive external ophthalmoplegia and gustatory epiphora associated with fetal isotretinoin toxicity. Arch Ophthalmol 120: 1094–1095, 2002.

Hazen PG, et al. Corneal effect of isotretinoin: possible exacerbation of corneal neovascularization in a patient with the keratitis, ichthyosis, deafness ('KID') syndrome. J Am Acad Dermatol 14: 141, 1986.

Herman DC, Dyer JA. Anterior subcapsular cataracts as a possible adverse ocular reaction to isotretinoin. Am J Ophthalmol 103: 236, 1987.

Lammer EJ, Chen DT, Hoar RM. Retinoic acid embryopathy. N Engl J Med 313(14): 837–841, 1985.

Mathers WD, Shields WJ, Schdev MS, et al. Meiobomian gland morphology and tear osmolarity: changes with accutane therapy. Cornea 10(4): 286–290, 1991.

Miles S, McGlathery W, Abernathie B. The importance of screening for laser-assisted in situ keratomileusis operation (LASIK) before prescribing isotretinoin. J Am Acad Dermatol 54: 180–181, 2006.

Palestine AJ. Transient acute myopia resulting from isotretinoin (Accutane) therapy. Ann Ophthalmol 16: 661, 1984.

Rismondo V, Ubels JL. Isotretinoin in lacrimal gland fluid and tears. Arch Ophthalmol 105: 416, 1987.

Roytman M, Frumkin A, Bohn TG. Pseudotumor cerebri caused by isotretinoin. Cutis 42: 399–400, 1988.

Saray Y, Seckin D. Angioedema and urticaria due to isotretinoin therapy. J Eur Acad Dermatol Venereol 20: 118–120, 2006.

Weleber RG, et al. Abnormal retinal function associated with isotretinoin therapy for acne. Arch Ophthalmol 104: 831, 1986.

Generic name: Tretinoin (retinoic acid, vitamin A acid, all-trans retinoic acid).

Proprietary names: Avita, Renova, Retin-A, Retin-A-micro, Vesanoid.

Primary use

Systemic
Used in the treatment of various leukemias.

Ophthalmic
Primarily used as a topical ocular medication for xerophthalmia.

Skin
For treatment of various forms of acne vulgaris and aging changes.

Ocular side effects

Systemic administration – oral
Certain
1. Eyelids or conjunctiva
   a. Blepharoconjunctivitis
   b. Erythema
   c. Edema
   d. Conjunctivitis
   e. Photosensitivity
   f. Keratoconjunctivitis
2. Intracranial hypertension – optic nerve edema (Fig. 7.12c)
3. Visual field defect
4. Visual hallucinations
5. Decreased vision

Possible
1. Hypercalcemia

Topical ocular or periocular administration
Certain
1. Cornea
   a. Vascularization
   b. Scarring
   c. Opacities in band or ring pattern
   d. Enhanced epithelial healing
2. Eyelids or conjunctiva – transitory
   a. Irritation
   b. Edema
   c. Hypopigmentation
   d. Hyperpigmentation

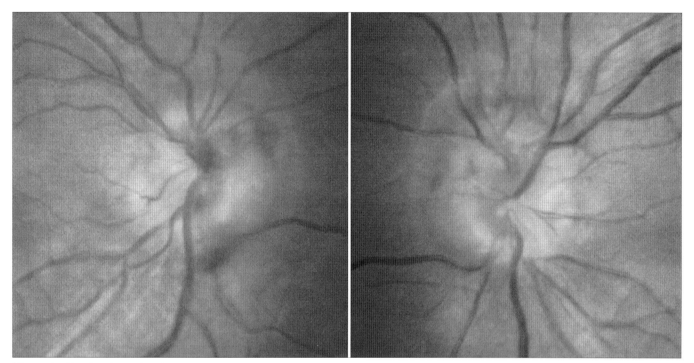

Fig. 7.12c Fundus photo showing optic disc edema and hemorrhage after tretinoin treatment. Photo courtesy of Yu-Chen Y, et al. Pseudotumor cerebri caused by all-trans retinoic acid treatment for acute promyelocytic leukemia. Jpn J Ophthalmol 50: 295–296, 2006.

e. Contact allergy
f. Erythema
g. Peeling
h. Photosensitivity
i. Blister formation
3. May alter some polymers in soft contact lenses
4. May have teratogenic effects

Clinical significance

The oral use of this agent has increased and in high doses the drug is probably secreted in the tears since eyelid and conjunctival findings are similar to topical ocular use of this agent. The most severe ocular side effect is intracranial hypertension with resultant optic nerve edema. There are numerous reports of intracranial hypertension due to tretinoin (Schroeter et al 2000; Tiamkao and Sirijirachi 2000; Colucciello 2003; Guirgis et al 2003; Yeh et al 2006; Yu-Chen et al 2006). Vanier et al (2003) pointed out that various drugs, including fluconazole, may interfere with the metabolism of tretinoin, causing increases in plasma levels and resulting in an increased incidence of intracranial hypertension. The duration and dosage of tretinoin use and the correlation of the onset of intracranial hypertension is variable because of individual variation in the pharmacokinetics of this drug (Lanvers et al 1998). An ophthalmologist seeing a patient with acute promyelocytic leukemia who develops acute papilloedema must consider on the differential diagnosis intracranial hypertension, solid tumor, bacterial meningitis or meningeal leukemic infiltrates. The pathogenesis of intracranial hypertension is felt to be much like an overdose of vitamin A with an impairment of cerebrospinal fluid absorption at the level of the arachnoid villi or granulations (Frankel et al 1994). Increased mucosal and skin dryness is not uncommon with tretinoin use. Hypercalcemia may cause increased corneal deposits. Abu el-Asrar et al (1993) reported a case of bilateral subhyaloid and vitreous hemorrhages that they felt were secondary to this drug.

Topical ocular application of this medication is usually in a vegetable oil or petroleum-based ointment. The amount of ocular irritation is directly proportional to the concentration of the drug and the frequency of application. This product has few side effects if it is used at lower concentrations, and few daily applications. In low dosages, the primary ocular side effects are transient hyperemia, irritation and burning. All other ocular side effects rarely occur except in higher concentrations with five or more applications per day. Avisar et al (1988) noted that with the use of topical ocular tretinoin in sicca patients, calcium-like deposits can appear in the epithelium of the cornea. In one case, the calcium did not resolve after discontinuing the drug; in the other case, the calcium disappeared over a 2-month period. While no human data are available, the manufacturer recently added to the package insert that topical tretinoin might be teratogenic from evidence in animal research.

REFERENCES AND FURTHER READING

Abu el-Asrar AM, al-Momen AK, Harakati MS. Terson's syndrome in a patient with acute promyelocytic leukemia on all-trans retinoic acid treatment. Doc Ophthalmol 84(4): 373–378, 1993.

Avisar R, Deutsch D, Savir H. Corneal calcification in dry eye disorders associated with retinoic acid therapy. Am J Ophthalmol 106: 753–755, 1988.

Colucciello M. Pseudotumor cerebri induced by all-trans retinoic acid treatment of acute promyelocytic leukemia. Arch Ophthalmol 121: 1064–1065, 2003.

Frankel SR, Eardley A, Heller G, et al. All-trans-retinoic acid for acute promyelocytic leukemia: results of the New York study. Ann Intern Med 120: 278–286, 1994.

Gillis JC, Goa KL. Tretinoin: a review of its pharmacodynamic and pharmacokinetic properties and use in the management of acute promyeloctyic leukaemia. Drugs 50(5): 897–923, 1995.

Guirgis MF, Leuder GT. Intracranial hypertension secondary to all-trans retinoic acid treatment for leukemia: diagnosis and management. J AAPOS 7: 432–434, 2003.

Lanvers C, Wagner A, Dubber A, et al. Pharmacokinetics and metabolism of low-dose ATRA in children – first observations. In: Acute Leukemias VII, Hiddemann, et al. (eds), Springer-Verlag, Berlin, pp 565–569, 1998.

Schroeter T, Lanvers C, Herding H, et al. Pseudotumor cerebri induced by all-trans-retinoic acid in a child treated for acute promyelocytic leukemia. Med Pediatr Oncol 34: 284–286, 2000.

Smolin G, Okumoto M. Vitamin A acid and corneal epithelial wound healing. Ann Ophthalmol 13: 563–566, 1981.

Smolin G, Okumoto M, Friedlaender M. Tretinoin and corneal epithelial wound healing. Arch Ophthalmol 97: 545–546, 1979.

Sommer A. Treatment of corneal xerophthalmia with topical retinoic acid. Am J Ophthalmol 95: 349–352, 1983.

Sommer A, Ennran N. Topical retinoic acid in the treatment of corneal xerophthalmia. Am J Ophthalmol 86: 615–617, 1979.

Somsak T, Sirijirachai C. Pseudotumor cerebri caused by all-trans-retinoic acid: a case report. J Med Assoc Thai 83: 1420–1423, 2000.

Soong HK, et al. Topical retinoid therapy for squamous metaplasia of various ocular surface disorders. A multicenter, placebo-controlled double-masked study. Ophthalmology 95(10): 1442–1446, 1988.

Stonecipher KG, et al. Topical application of all-trans-retinoic acid, a look at the cornea and limbus. Graefes Arch Clin Exp Ophthalmol 226: 371–376, 1988.

Tiamkao S, Sirijirachai C. Pesudotumor cerebri caused by all-trans-retinoic acid: a case report. J Med Assoc Thai 83: 1420–1423, 2000.

Vanier KL, Mattiussi AJ, Johnston DL. Interaction of all-trans-retinoic acid with fluconazole in acute promyclocytic leukemia. J Pediatr Hematol Oncol 25: 403–404, 2003.

Wright P. Topical retinoic acid therapy for disorders of the outer eye. Trans Ophthalmol Soc UK 104: 869–874, 1985.

Yeh Y-C, Tang H-F, Fang I-M. Pseudotumor cerebri caused by all-trans-retinoic acid treatment for acute promyelocytic leukemia. Jpn J Ophthalmol 50: 295–296, 2006.

CLASS: SOLVENTS

Generic name: Dimethyl sulfoxide (DMSO).

Proprietary name: Rimso.

Primary use

This is a solvent for various drug deliveries. It is also used in the treatment of musculoskeletal pain, interstitial cystitis and elevated intracranial pressure, and as an anti-inflammatory agent.

Ocular side effects

Systemic administration or absorption from topical application

Certain

1. Potentiates the adverse effects of any drug with which it is combined
2. Problems with color vision – color vision defect (transitory)
3. Photophobia
4. Eyelids or conjunctiva
   a. Allergic reactions
   b. Erythema
   c. Urticaria

Possible

1. Cataracts

Local ophthalmic use or exposure

Certain

1. Irritation
   a. Hyperemia
   b. Burning sensation
2. Eyelids
   a. Erythema
   b. Photosensitivity

Possible

1. Cataracts

Clinical significance

DMSO may enhance the ocular side effects of other drugs by increasing the speed and volume of tissue penetration. Lens opacities and changes in refractive errors have been detected in small animals after systemic DMSO. However, in humans, even with prolonged administration of large amounts of DMSO, no cases of lens changes have been proven due to systemic, topical or local ophthalmic administration. There have recently been scattered reports of lens changes (Rowely and Baer 2001). Using the Scheimpflug camera to follow patients of high dosage DMSO for many years, Saski, Kojima and Fraunfelder (unpublished) could not clearly show an effect of DMSO on the human lens, but did show a change in the refractive index. Metelitsyna (2001) reported that in rabbits DMSO does potentiate lens changes in combination with polychromatic light. Although color vision defects are reported, they are only of a transient nature. Topical ocular DMSO used in high concentrations for its anti-inflammatory properties (i.e. uveitis) commonly causes ocular irritation.

Recommendations

Controversy as to whether or not DMSO causes cataracts requires the package insert to recommend periodical lens examinations. There is no need for these examinations to differ from the routine guidelines of the American Academy of Ophthalmology for regular ophthalmic examination:

- Patients aged 20–29, one examination during this period
- Patients aged 30–39, two examinations during this period
- Patients 40–64, every 2 to 4 years
- Patients aged 65 and over, every 1 to 2 years.

REFERENCES AND FURTHER READING

Dimethyl sulfoxide (DMSO). Med Lett Drugs Ther 22: 94, 1980.

Garcia CA. Ocular toxicology of dimethyl sulfoxide and effects on retinitis pigmentosa. Ann NY Acad Sci 411: 48, 1983.

Hanna C, Fraunfelder FT, Meyer SM. Effects of dimethylsulfoxide on ocular inflammation. Ann Ophthalmol 9: 61, 1977.

Kluxen G, Schultz U. Comparison of human nuclear cataracts with cataracts induced in rabbits by dimethylsulfoxide. Lens Res 3: 161, 1986.

Metelitsyna IP. Potentiation of the cataractogenic effect of light by dimethylsulfoxide and adrenaline. Ukrainskii Biokhimicheskii Zhurnal 73: 114–119, 2001.

Rowley S, Baer R. Lens deposits associated with RIMSO-50 (dimethyl-sulphoxide). Eye 15: 332–333, 2001.

Rubin LF. Toxicologic update of dimethyl sulfoxide. Ann NY Acad Sci 411: 6, 1983.

Use of DMSO for unapproved indications. FDA Drug Bull 10: 20, 1980.

Yellowless P, Greenfield C, McIntyre N. Dimethylsulphoxide-induced toxicity. Lancet 2: 1004, 1980.

CLASS: VACCINES

Generic name: Bacillus Calmette-Guérin (BCG) vaccine.

Proprietary names: Pacis, TherCys, Tice.

Primary use

BCG vaccine is used for active immunization against tuberculosis and in the treatment of various malignant diseases. Intravesical BCG has gained popularity as an adjunctive immunotherapy for superficial carcinomas of the urinary bladder.

Ocular side effects

Systemic administration

Certain

1. Decreased vision
2. Uveitis

3. Conjunctivitis – non-specific

Possible
1. Eyelids or conjunctiva
   a. Urticaria
   b. Purpura
   c. Lupoid syndrome
   d. Erythema multiforme
   e. Eczema
2. Optic neuritis
3. Retinopathy
   a. Focal areas of depigmentation
   b. Choroiditis
   c. Attenuated vascular tree
4. Reiter's syndrome
5. Endophthalmitis
6. Vitritis
7. Subconjunctival or retinal hemorrhages secondary to drug-induced anemia

Local ophthalmic use or exposure
Certain
1. Conjunctiva – follicular conjunctivitis

Clinical significance

Ocular complications following the BCG vaccine are rare, but acute ocular inflammatory or hypersensitivity reactions within the eye, along with a concurrent systemic inflammatory response, have been reported (Lamm et al 1986; Price 1994; Missioux et al 1995; Chevrel et al 1999; Clavel et al 1999; Wertheim and Astbury 2002). While most patients are HLA-B27 positive, Wertheim and Astbury (2002) reported bilateral anterior uveitis presumed secondary to BCG that was HLA-B27 negative. In general, the uveitis is bilateral and anterior, but may also be a panuveitis (Hegde et al 2005). These reactions may occur with or without associated systemic findings such as arthritis, during the first course or after multiple courses of BCG therapy. The uveitis may be granulomatous but is more often non-granulomatous. Clavel et al (1999) reported 26 cases of reactive arthritis secondary to intravesicular BCG. About 8% of these had an associated uveitis and all patients were HLA-B27 positive. Proof of a cause-and-effect relationship is difficult to determine, but the number of reported cases and their similar patterns makes an association almost certain. Donaldson et al (1974) reported two melanoma patients treated with BCG vaccine who developed uveitis associated with vitiligo. Price (1994) reported a patient who, after a second course of BCG therapy for bladder cancer, had his first episode of peripheral arthritis and bilateral iritis with secondary glaucoma. Reports to the National Registry and in the literature suggest that in some patients conjunctivitis may occur, often lasting throughout the injection series. The conjunctivitis is non-specific, but appears to have more chemosis than normally seen. This can be controlled with topical ocular steroids. Hegde et al (2005) as well as Hogarth et al (2000) reported bilateral panuveitis with optic neuritis following BCG vaccination. Han et al (1999) reported a single case of endophthalmitis due to mycobacterium bovis, possibly secondary to BCG therapy. It occurred 14 months after the patient's last treatment (BCG contains live attenuated mycobacteria).

BCG's effect on the retina is not as well established. Cases resembling cancer associated retinopathy (CAR) without a serum reaction to the CAR autoantigen have been reported (Sharon et al 2005). This includes areas of pigmentary disturbances, usually focal, and choroiditis often with narrowed arterioles. Two cases similar to this are in the National Registry. Hodish

et al (2000) reported retinitis syndrome after intravesical BCG. Bilateral cataracts have also been reported in a patient receiving BCG therapy following excision of a cutaneous melanoma.

Pollard and George (1994) described a case of inadvertent direct ocular exposure to BCG vaccine causing follicular conjunctivitis, which was controlled by topical ocular steroids.

REFERENCES AND FURTHER READING

Bouchard R, Bogert M, Tinthoin JF. Eczematides post-BCG. Bull Soc Fr Dermatol Syph 72: 126, 1965.

Chevrel G, Zech C, Miossec P. Severe uveitis followed by reactive arthritis after bacillus Calmette-Guerin therapy. J Rheumatol 26: 1011, 1999.

Clavel G, Grados F, Cayrolle G, et al. Polyarthritis following intravesical BCG immunotherapy. Rev Rheum Engl Ed 66: 115–118, 1999.

Dogliotti M. Erythema multiforme – an unusual reaction to BCG vaccination. S Afr Med J 57: 332, 1980.

Donaldson RC, et al. Uveitis and vitiligo associated with BCG treatment for malignant melanoma. Surgery 76: 771, 1974.

Han DP, Simons KB, Tarkanian CN, et al. Endophthalmitis from mycobacterium bovis-bacille Calmette-Guerin after intravesicular bacilli Calmette-Guering injections for bladder cancer. Am J Ophthalmol 128: 648–650, 1999.

Hegde V, Dean F. Bilateral panuveitis and optic neuritis following bacillus Calmette-Guerin (BCG) vaccination. Acta Paediatr 94: 635–636, 2005.

Hodish I, Ezra D, Gur H, et al. Reiter's syndrome after intravesical bacillus Calmetter-Guerin therapy for bladder cancer. Isr Med Assoc J 2: 240–241, 2000.

Hogarth MB, Thomas S, Seifert MH, et al. Reiter's syndrome following intravesical BCG immunotherapy. Postgrad Med J 76: 791–793, 2000.

Imperia PS, Lazarus HM, Lass JH. Ocular complications of systemic cancer chemotherapy. Surv Ophthalmol 34(3): 20–230, 1989.

Krebs W, Schumann M. Allgenerkrankkung nach BCG.-Impfung. Monatsschr Tuberk-Bekampf 14: 80, 1971.

Lamm DL, Stodgdill VD, Stodgill B, et al. Complications of bacillus Calmette-Guerin immunotherapy in 1278 patients with bladder cancer. J Urol 135: 272–274, 1986.

Missioux D, Hermabessiere J, Sauvezie B. Arthritis and iritis after bacillus Calmetter-Guerin therapy. J Rheumatol 22: 2010, 1995.

Pollard AJ, George RH. Ocular contamination with BCG vaccine (letter). Arch Dis Child 70(1): 71, 1994.

Price GE. Arthritis and iritis after BCG therapy for bladder cancer. J Rheum 21(3): 564–565, 1994.

Sharon S, Thirkill CE, Grigg JR. Autoimmune retinopathy associated with intravesical BCG therapy. Br J Ophthalmol 89: 927–928, 2005.

Vogt D. Tuberkuloseschutz-Impfung. Die Komplikationen der B.C.G.-Impfung. In: Handbuch der Schutzimpfungen, Herrlich A (ed), Springer-Verlag, Berlin, p 345, 1965.

Wertheim M, Astbury N. Bilateral uveitis after intravesical BCG immunotherapy for bladder carcinoma. Br J Ophthalmol 86: 706, 2002.

Generic names: 1. Diphtheria (D) vaccine (adsorbed); 2. diphtheria and tetanus (DT) vaccine (adsorbed); 3. diphtheria and tetanus and pertussis (DPT) vaccine (adsorbed).

Proprietary names: 1. Daptacel, Infanrix, Tripedia.

Primary use

These combinations of diphtheria and tetanus toxoids with pertussis vaccine are the recommended preparations for routine primary immunizations and recall injections in children younger than 7 years of age.

Ocular side effects

Systemic administration
Possible
1. Eyelids or conjunctiva
   a. Allergic reactions
   b. Erythema

c. Conjunctivitis – non-specific (DPT)
d. Angioneurotic edema
e. Urticaria
f. Eczema (DT)
g. Erythema multiforme

Conditional/Unclassified
1. Optic neuritis
2. Extraocular muscles
   a. Paresis or paralysis (D)
   b. Ptosis (DPT)
3. Pupils
   a. Mydriasis (D)
   b. Decreased reaction to light (D)
4. Subconjunctival or retinal hemorrhages secondary to drug-induced anemia (DPT)
5. Corneal graft rejection (tetanus toxoid booster)
6. Papilledema secondary to intracranial hypertension (DPT)
7. Visual field defects (DT)

Clinical significance

For the many millions exposed to these vaccines, there are comparatively exceedingly few ocular complications. Rarely, a partial paralysis of accommodation may occur. This may be unilateral or bilateral, take a few weeks to develop and a few weeks to resolve. The pupils are usually normal or slightly dilated with a normal papillary response to light (Lewin and Guillery 1913). Generalized urticarial reactions have been reported to occur immediately or several hours after injection. Allergic reactions may be due to preservatives or contaminants of the antigens are rarely seen. Conjunctivitis has been seen after DPT shots, but it is transitory and inconsequential. Neurological complications, including papilledema, optic neuritis (McReynolds et al 1953; Hamed et al 1993; Burkhard et al 2001) and decreased vision have been reported as transient adverse effects, sometimes accompanying encephalitis. The National Registry has cases of transitory strabismus post DPT injections, but a cause-and-effect relationship is hard to establish. Steinemann et al (1988) reported a 33-year-old woman with a graft rejection requiring a repeat graft after receiving a tetanus toxoid booster.

REFERENCES AND FURTHER READING

Burkhard C, Choi M, Wilhelm H. Optic neuritis as a complication in preventive tetanus-diphtheria-poliomyelitis vaccination: a case report. Klin Monatsbl Augenheilkd 218: 51–54, 2001.

Dolinova L. Bilateral uveoretinoneuritis after vaccination with Ditepe (diphtheria, tetanus, and pertussis vaccine). Cs Oftal 30: 114, 1974.

Frederiksen MS, Brenoe E, Trier J. Erythema multiforme following vaccination with pediatric vaccines. Scand J Infect Dis 36: 154–155, 2004.

Hamed LM, Silbiger J, Guy J, et al. Parainfectious optic neuritis and encephalomyelitis. A report of two cases with thalamic involvement. J Clin Neuro-Ophthalmol 13(1): 18–23, 1993.

Lewin L, Guillery H. Die wirkungen von arzneimitteln und giften auf das auge, 2nd edn, Berline, August Hirschwald, 1913.

McReynolds WU, Havener WH, Petrohelos MA. Bilateral optic neuritis following smallpox vaccination and diphtheria-tetanus toxoid. Am J Dis Child 86: 601, 1953.

Pembroke AC, Marten RH. Unusual cutaneous reactions following diphtheria and tetanus immunization. Clin Exp Dermatol 4: 345, 1979.

Steinemann TL, Koffler BH, Jennings CD. Corneal allograft rejection following immunization. Am J Ophthalmol 106: 575–578, 1988.

Generic name: Influenza virus vaccine.

Proprietary names: Flumist, Fluvirin, Fluzone.

Primary use

Influenza virus vaccines are used to provide active immunity to influenza virus strains.

Ocular side effects

Systemic administration
Certain
1. Oculo-respiratory syndrome
   a. Conjunctivitis
   b. Lid edema
   c. Photophobia
   d. Blurred vision
   e. Conjunctival discharge
   f. Ocular pain

Probable
1. Corneal graft rejection (Fig. 7.12d)

Possible
1. Decreased vision
2. Eyelids or conjunctiva
   a. Allergic reactions
   b. Erythma
   c. Blepharoconjunctivitis
   d. Urticaria
   e. Purpura
   f. Stevens-Johnson syndrome
   g. Angioneurotic edema
3. Optic nerve
   a. Neuritis
   b. Ischemic optic neuropathy
   c. Edema
4. Extraocular muscles – paresis or paralysis
5. Bell's palsy
6. Problems with color vision – color vision defect, red-green defect

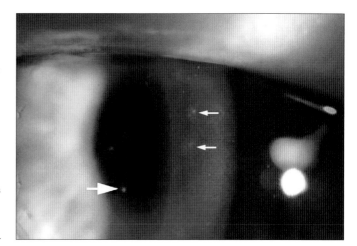

Fig. 7.12d Small arrows showing infiltrates and large arrow showing keratic precipitate of graft rejection. Photo courtesy of Wertheim MS, et al. Corneal transplant rejection following influenza vaccination. Br J Ophthalmol 90: 925–926, 2006.

Conditional/Unclassified
1. Episcleritis
2. Scleritis
3. Orbital myositis
4. Uveitis

Clinical significance

Earlier influenza vaccines were from swine but these have discontinued due to an increased incidence of neurological complications, including optic neuritis, optic atrophy and blindness (Cangemi and Bergen 1980; Macoul 1982). Poser (1982) reported isolated trochlear and 59 facial nerve paresis also using swine vaccine. Manufacturers use various virus strains, which may produce different ocular effects. The best-studied adverse ocular side effect is an influenza-vaccine-induced oculo-respiratory syndrome, which consists of cough, wheeze, chest tightness, difficulty breathing and/or sore throat. The ocular manifestation is bilateral conjunctivitis, which can occur within hours of inoculation. This may or may not include facial edema. Fredette et al (2003) noted photophobia, blurred vision, lid edema, ocular pain and conjunctival concentrates as part of the syndrome. Onset varies between 2 and 24 hours after exposure and resolves within 48 hours. Up to 16% of women between the ages of 50 and 59 had this syndrome, making them the highest risk group (Skowronski et al 2002a). DeSerres et al (2003a) has shown that an earlier onset of this syndrome (less than 2 hours) is more likely in younger patients who have more coughs and sore throats, and a later onset (after 2 hours) is more likely in the older population, who have more ocular symptoms. The frequency of this syndrome substantially decreased with each annual injection over a 4-year follow-up series (DeSerres et al 2005). While the above data are mainly from a specific manufacturer, this vaccine was minimally retrogenic, therefore this syndrome can be associated with influenza vaccines in general (DeSerres et al 2003b; Scheifele et al 2003).

Hull and Bates (1997) reported a case of bilateral optic neuritis developing within 2 weeks of being vaccinated by the newer influenza vaccination. This happened on two separate occasions, 1 year apart. Ray and Dreizin (1996) reported a similar case without rechallenge data. There have been various reports of unilateral and bilateral optic neuritis after vaccination with good recovery, with or without treatment. Kawasaki et al (1998) reported bilateral ischemic optic neuropathy with two cases of permanent visual loss. The authors speculated that an immune complex-mediated vasculopathy following vaccination can cause anterior ischemic optic neuropathy. Knopf (1991) reported a case of complicated cataract surgery with secondary uveitis that had complete recovery. Four months later, following a flu vaccination, the patient had a recurrence of her uveitis with decreased vision and cystoid macular edema. When a rare case of extraocular muscle abnormalities or uveitis occurs, this is usually within 2 to 14 days following inoculation. These may last from a few days to a few weeks.

Patients with corneal grafts who are vaccinated are probably at higher risk for a graft rejection. Most patients who react usually only have mild graft reactions, which can be controlled with topical ocular steroids. However, severe reactions requiring re-grafts have occurred. Steinemann et al (1988), Solomon and Frucht-Pery (1996), Wertheim et al (2006) and the National Registry have a total of eight cases of graft rejection. Thurairajan et al (1997) reported a case of bilateral orbital myositis and posterior scleritis following influenza vaccination. The authors found no other cause for this and felt these ocular side effects, including an associated acute symmetrical polyarthropathy, were due to the vaccine. Mutsch et al (2004) reported 46 cases of Bell's palsy with

an influenza vaccine that was only used in Switzerland. There are cases of episcleritis after inoculation in the National Registry.

REFERENCES AND FURTHER READING

Cangemi FE, Bergen RL. Optic atrophy following swine flu vaccination. Am Ophthalmol 12: 857, 1980.

De Serres G, Boulianne N, Duval B, et al. Oculo-respiratory syndrome following influenza vaccination: evidence for occurrence with more than one influenza vaccine. Vaccine 21: 2346–2353, 2003.

De Serres G, Grenier JL, Toth E, et al. The clinical spectrum of the oculo-respiratory syndrome after influenza vaccination. Vaccine 21: 9726–3732, 2003.

De Serres G, Toth E, Menard S, et al. Oculo-respiratory syndrome after influenza vaccination: trends over four influenza seasons. Vaccine 23: 3732–9726, 2005.

Fredette MJ, De Serres G, Malenfant M. Ophthalmological and biological features of the oculorespiratory syndrome after influenza vaccination. Clin Infect Dis 37: 1136–1138, 2003.

Hull TP, Bates JH. Optic neuritis after influenza vaccination. Am J Ophthalmol 124(5): 703–704, 1997.

Kawasaki A, Purvin VA, Tang R. Bilateral anterior ischemic optic neuropathy following influenza vaccination. J Neuro-Ophthalmol 18(1): 56–59, 1998.

Knopf HL. Recurrent uveitis after influenza vaccination. Ann Ophthalmol 23(6): 213–214, 1991.

Ghosh C. Periorbital and orbital cellulites after H. influenza b vaccination. Ophthalmology 108: 1514–1515, 2001.

Macoul KL. Bilateral optic nerve atrophy and blindness following swine influenza vaccination. Ann Ophthalmol 14: 398, 1982.

Mutsch M, Zhou W, Rhodes P, et al. Use of the inactivated intranasal influenza vaccine and the risk of Bells' palsy in Switzerland. N Engl J Med 350: 896–903, 2004.

Poser CM. Neurological complications of swine influenza vaccination. Acta Neurol Scand 66: 413–431, 1982.

Ray CL, Dreizin IJ. Bilateral optic neuropathy associated with influenza vaccination. J Neuro-Ophthalmol 16(3): 182–184, 1996.

Scheifele DW, Duval B, Russell ML, et al. Ocular and respiratory symptoms attributable to inactivated split influenza vaccine: evidence from a controlled trial involving adults. Clin Infect Dis 36: 850–857, 2003.

Skowronski DM, Bjornson G, Husain E, et al. Oculo-respiratory syndrome after influenza immunization in children. Pediatr Infect Dis J 24: 63–69, 2005.

Skowronski DM, De Serres G, Hebert J, et al. Skin testing to evaluate oculo-respiratory syndrome (ORS) associated with influenza vaccination during the 2000–2001 season. Vaccine 20: 2713–2719, 2002.

Skowronski DM, Lu H, Warrington R, et al. Does antigen-specific cytokine response correlate with the experience of oculorespiratory syndrome after influenza vaccine? J Infect Dis 187: 495–499, 2003a.

Skowronski DM, Strauss B, De Serres G, et al. Oculo-respiratory syndrome: a new influenza vaccine-associated adverse event? Clin Infect Dis 36: 705–713, 2003b.

Skowronski DM, Strauss B, Kendall P, et al. Low risk of recurrence of oculorespiratory syndrome folloing influenza revaccination. CMAJ 167: 853–858, 2002.

Solomon A, Frucht-Pery J. Bilateral simultaneous corneal graft rejection after influenza vaccination. Am J Ophthalmol 121(6): 708–709, 1996.

Steinemann TL, Koffler BH, Jennings CD. Corneal allograft rejection following immunization. Am J Ophthalmol 106: 575–578, 1988.

Thurairajan G, Hope-Ross MW, Situnayake RD, et al. Polyarthropathy, orbital myositis and posterior scleritis: an unusual adverse reaction to influenza vaccine. Br J Rheum 36: 120–123, 1997.

Wetheim MS, Keel M, Cook SD, et al. Corneal transplant rejection following influenza vaccination. Br J Ophthalmol 90: 925–926, 2006.

Generic names: 1. Measles, mumps and rubella virus vaccine live; 2. measles virus vaccine live; 3. mumps virus vaccine live; 4. rubella and mumps virus vaccine live; 5. rubella virus vaccine live.

Proprietary names: 1. MMR II; 2. Attunvax; 3. Mumpsvax; 4. Biavax II; 5. Meruvax II.

Primary use

These vaccines are used to provide active immunity to measles, mumps and rubella.

Ocular side effects

Systemic administration
Possible
1. Optic nerve – optic or retrobulbar neuritis (measles, rubella)
2. Eyelids or conjunctiva
   a. Allergic reactions
   b. Hyperemia
   c. Erythema
   d. Conjunctivitis – non-specific
   e. Ptosis (measles)
   f. Angioneurotic edema
   g. Urticaria
   h. Purpura
   i. Eczema
   j. Stevens-Johnson syndrome
3. Ocular pain

Conditonal/Unclassified
1. Decreased vision
2. Extraocular muscles
   a. Paresis or paralysis
   b. Strabismus
3. Scotomas – centrocecal
4. Retinopathy (rubella)
5. Uveitis

Inadvertent ocular exposure
Certain
1. Keratitis (measles)
2. Conjunctival edema (measles)

Conditional/Unclassified
1. Ocular teratogenic effects (rubella)

Clinical significance
Millions of people have been exposed to these vaccines and there are only a few scattered reports of significant ocular side effects. The most noteworthy ocular side effect reported is optic or retrobulbar neuritis. Onset varies, with Arshi et al (2004) reporting occurrence within a few hours, Kline and Margulie (1982) reporting onset within 1 week and Stevenson et al (1996) and Kazarian and Gager (1982) reporting onset between 2 to 3 weeks. All cases were bilateral and four of the six had a good visual outcome within days to a few weeks. As of 1994, there were five additional reports of optic neuritis with an incidence of 1 in 1 600 000 in the UK (WHO). Based on measles or measles vaccines causing demyelenating disease, most authors felt there was a cause-and-effect relationship between the reports of optic neuritis and the measles vaccination. Regardless, causation has not been proven. In time, some of these patients may develop multiple sclerosis. The risk of neurological complications after natural rubella infections is greater than after rubella vaccines (Krugman 1977).

Islam et al (2000) reported two cases of patients developing anterior uveitis at 4 weeks and at 6 weeks post measles, mumps and rubella vaccinations. Months of conventional therapy were required for management. There are three reports of uveitis in the National Registry. Maspero et al (1984) reported, via a patient survey, a 6% incidence of conjunctivitis after measles vaccine. This is transitory and of no clinical consequence. Marshall et al (1985) reported diffuse retinopathy after rubella vaccination in children, but there are no such reports in the National Registry.

Cases of direct ocular exposure to live measles virus vaccine resulted in keratoconjunctivitis, which resolved within 2 weeks, are in the National Registry.

REFERENCES AND FURTHER READING
Arshi S, Sadeghi-Bazargani H, Ojaghi H, et al. The first rapid onset optic neuritis after measles-rubella vaccination: case report. Vaccine 22: 3240–3242, 2004.
Behan PO. Diffuse myelitis associated with rubella vaccination. BMJ 1: 166, 1977.
Chan CC, Sogg RL, Steinman L. Isolated oculomotor palsy after measles immunization. Am J Ophthalmol 89: 446, 1980.
Hassin H. Ophthalmoplegic migraine wrongly attributed to measles immunization. Am J Ophthalmol 104: 192–193, 1987.
Herman JJ, Radin R, Schneiderman R. Allergic reactions to measles (rubeola) vaccine in patients hypersensitive to egg protein. J Pediatr 102: 196, 1983.
Islam SMM, El-Sheikh HF, Tabbara KF. Anterior uveitis following combined vaccination for measles mumps and rubella (MMR): a report of two cases. Acta Ophthalmol Scand 78: 590–592, 2000.
Kazarian EL, Gager WE. Optic neuritis complicating measles, mumps, and rubella vaccination. Arch Neurol 39: 443, 1982.
Kline L, Margulie SL. Optic neuritis and myelitis following rubella vaccination. Arch Neurol 39: 443–444, 1982.
Krugman S. Present status of measles and rubella immunization in the United States: a medical progress report. Pediatrics 90: 1–12, 1977.
Marshall GS, et al. Diffuse retinopathy following mumps and rubella vaccination. Pediatrics 76: 989, 1985.
Maspero A, Sesana B, Ferrante P. Adverse reactions to measles vaccine. Boll 1st Sieroter Milan 63(2): 125, 1984.
Miller CL. Surveillance after measles vaccination in children. Practitioner 226: 535, 1982.
Morton-Kute L. Rubella vaccine and facial paresthesias. Ann Intern Med 102: 563, 1985.
Preblud SR, et al. Fetal risk associated with rubella vaccine. JAMA 246: 1413, 1981.
Riikonen R. The role of infection and vaccination in the genesis of optic neuritis and multiple sclerosis in children. Acta Neurol Scand 80: 425–431, 1989.
Stevenson VL, Acheson JF, Ball J, et al. Optic neuritis following measles/rubella vaccination in two 13-year-old children. Br J Ophthalmol 80(12): 1110–1111, 1996.
Thomas E, Champagne S. A case of mumps meningitis: a complication of a vaccine? CMAJ 138: 135, 1988.
World Health Organization. Adverse reactions to measles-rubella vaccine. WHO ADR Newslett 4: 10, 1995.

Generic names: 1. Rabies immune globulin; 2. rabies vaccine.

Proprietary names: 1. BayRab, HyperRAB, Imogam Rabies; 2. Imovax Rabies, RabAvert.

Primary use
Rabies immune globulin is used to provide passive immunity to rabies for postexposure prophylaxis of individuals exposed to the disease or virus. Rabies vaccine is used to promote active immunity to rabies in individuals exposed to the disease or virus.

Ocular side effects

Systemic administration
Certain
1. Eyelids or conjunctiva
   a. Allergic reactions
   b. Erythema
   c. Angioneurotic edema
   d. Urticaria
   e. Edema

Possible
1. Optic nerve
   a. Optic neuritis
   b. Retrobulbar neuritis
3. Diplopia

4. Photophobia
5. Scotomas – centrocecal
6. Decreased vision

Conditional/Unclassified
1. Neuroretinitis
   a. Optic disc edema
   b. Macular edema
   c. Hard exudates

Clinical significance

Neurological adverse reactions were much more common with the earlier preparations of rabies vaccine made from infected rabbit brain tissue than from later-generation vaccines. There are reports of optic neuritis (Cormack and Anderson 1934; Srisupan and Konyama 1971; Chayakul et al 1975; Francois and Van Lantschoot 1976; Van de Geijn et al 1994; Dadeya et al 2004). Optic neuritis usually occurs from a few weeks to 3 months post vaccination and is often part of acute disseminated encephalomyelitis (Brain 1962). There are cases (Consul et al 1968; Stratton et al 1994) where the optic neuritis was the only neurological finding. Mostly, patients can recover to good vision, but some permanent damage to the retinal fibers may occur (Consul et al 1968). While neurological complications due to rabies vaccinations are rare, encephalitis, myelitis and encephalomyelitis are well documented. This includes varying degrees of paralysis, including the oculomotor nerves (Walsh 1957). Chayakul et al (1975), along with cases in the National Registry, reported various paresis and paralysis of the ocular motor nerves. This is usually associated with a vaccine-induced encephalomyelitis.

Saxena et al (2005) reported bilateral neuroretinitis using chick embryo cell anti-rabies vaccine. The neuroretinitis was an acute swelling of both the optic discs associated with hard exudates and macular edema.

REFERENCES AND FURTHER READING

Brain WR. Diseases of the Nervous System, 6th edn, Oxford University Press, New York, 1962.

Chayakul V, Ishikawa S, Chotibut S, et al. Convergence insufficiency and optic neuritis due to antirabies inoculation – a case study. Jpn J Ophthalmol 19: 307–314, 1975.

Consul BN, Purohit GK, Chhabra HN. Antirabic vaccine optic neuritis. Indian J Med Sci 22: 630–632, 1968.

Cormack HS, Anderson LAP. Bilateral papillitis following antirabic inoculation: recovery. Br J Ophthalmol 18: 167, 1934.

Cremieux G, Dor JF, Mongin M. Paralysies faciales peripheriques et polyradiculoneurites post-vaccino-rabiques. Acta Neurol Belge 78: 279, 1978.

Dadeya S, Guliani BP, Gupta VS, et al. Retrobulbar neuritis following rabies vaccination. Trop Doct 34: 174–175, 2004.

Francois J, Van Lantschoot G. Optic neuritis and atrophy due to drugs. T Geneesk 32: 151, 1976.

Gupta V, Bandyopadhyay S, Bapuraj JR, et al. Bilateral optic neuritis complicating rabies vaccination. Retina 24: 179–181, 2004.

Saxena R, Sethi HS, Rai HK, et al. Bilateral neuro-retinitis following chick embryo cell anti-rabies vaccination: a case report. BMC Ophthalmol 5: 20, 2005.

Srisupan V, Konyama K. Bilateral retrobulbar optic neuritis following anti-rabies vaccination. Siriraj Hosp Gaz 23: 403, 1971.

Stratton KR, Howe CJ, Johnston RB Jr. Adverse Events Associated with Childhood Vaccines: Evidence Bearing on Causality, Vaccine Safety Committee, Division of Health Promotion and Disease Prevention Institute of Medicine (eds), Washington, DC, National Academy Press, 1994.

Van de Geijn E, Tukkie E, Van Philips L, Punt H. Bilateral optic neuritis with branch retinal artery occlusion associated with vaccination. Doc Ophthalmol 86: 403–408, 1994.

Van der Meyden CH, Van den Ende J, Uys M. Neurological complications of rabies vaccines. S Afr Med J 53: 478, 1978.

Walsh FB. Clinical Neuro-ophthalmology, 2nd edn, Wiliams and Wilkins, Baltimore, p 477, 1957.

Generic name: Smallpox (Vaccinia) vaccine.

Proprietary name: Dryvax.

Primary use

Used as a vaccination against the vaccinia virus.

Ocular side effects

Systemic administration – autoinoculation from vaccination site
Certain
1. Eyelids and conjunctiva
   a. Blepharoconjunctivitis
   b. Vesicles
   c. Pustules
   d. Profound edema
   e. Periorbital erythema (Fig. 7.12e)
   f. Prearicular and submandiublar lymphadenopathy
   g. Scarring
   h. Madrosis
   i. Conjunctivitis
      i. Papillary reaction
      ii. Serous and mucopurulent discharge
      iii. Ulceration
      iv. Symblepharon
   j. Punctal stenosis
2. Cornea
   a. Superficial punctate keratitis
   b. Interstitial and stromal keratitis
   c. Disciform keratitis
   d. Necrosis
   e. Perforation
   f. Subepithelial opacities
   g. Ring infiltrates
3. Iritis
4. Photophobia

Conditional/Unclassified
1. Retina
   a. Cotton wool spots
   b. Branch arteriolar occlusions
   c. Vasculitis

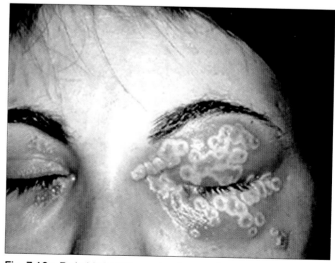

Fig. 7.12e Periorbital edema and erythema after smallpox immunization. Photo courtesy of Pepose JS, et al. Ocular complications of smallpox vaccination. Am J Ophthalmol 136: 343–352, 2003.

2. Optic nerve
   a. Neuropathy
   b. Neuritis

Clinical significance

In the 1980s, the WHO declared smallpox eradicated, but countries not abiding by the promise to destroy the virus have now perpetuated a fear that smallpox may become a biological weapon. This has required mass vaccination in the US military. It is estimated that 10 to 20 per 1 000 000 smallpox immunizations develop ocular complications. The worst complications are in those who are immune compromised, i.e. atopic disease, are allergic to any components of the vaccine or patients with coronary artery disease (Maki and Wis 2003). Ocular complications primarily occur in the very young (age 1–4 years) and occur from autoinoculation from the vaccination site to the eyelid or eye. The most common findings are blepharoconjunctivitis, which occurs between 5 and 11 days after vaccination (Pepose et al 2003). Only rarely does this go on to full-blown cornea involvement, often with significant scarring of the lids and conjunctiva. Uveitis has only been reported with severe corneal involvement. Surprisingly, those with the most severely involved corneal disease rarely have significant visual defects after 5 years (Pepose et al 2003).

There are reports of retinal complications (Redslob 1935; Landa et al 2006) primarily as multiple branch retinal artery occlusions. We know of no other cases. Smallpox and vaccinia have been implicated in encephalopathy and other neurological disorders. Mathur et al (1967) reported a case of bilateral optic nerve inflammation. No other cases were found in the National Registry.

REFERENCES AND FURTHER READING

Fillmore GL, Ward TP, Bower KS, et al. Ocular complications in the department of defense smallpox vaccination program. Ophthalmology 111: 2086–2093, 2004.

Francois J, Molder ED, Gildemyn H. Ocular vaccinia. Acta Ophthalmol 45: 25–31, 1967.

Hu G, Wang MJ, Miller MJ, et al. Ocular vaccinia following exposure to a smallpox vaccine. Am J Ophthalmol 137: 554–556, 2004.

Landa G, Marcovich A, Leiba H, et al. Multiple branch retinal arteriolar occlusions associated with smallpox vaccination. J Infect 52: e7-e9, 2006.

Lee SF, Butler R, Chansue E, et al. Vaccinia keratouveitis manifesting as a masquerade syndrome. Am J Ophthalmol 117: 480–487, 1994.

Maki DG, Wis M. National preparedness for biological warfare and bioterrorism. Arch Ophthalmol 121: 710–711, 2003.

Mathur SP, Makhija JM, Mehta MC. Papillitis with myelitis after revaccination. Indian J Med Sci 21: 469–471, 1967.

McMahon AW, Bryant-Genevier MC, et al. Photophobia following smallpox vaccination. Vaccine 23: 1097–1098, 2005.

Pepose JS, Marcolis TP, LaRussa P, et al. Ocular complications of smallpox vaccination. Am J Ophthalmol 136: 343–352, 2003.

Perera C. Vaccinial disciform keratitis. Arch Ophthalmol 24: 352–356, 1940.

Redslob E. Cecite foudroyanted chez un efant en bas age après vaccination antivariolique. Bull Men Soc Franc Ophtalmol 48: 126–139, 1935.

Rennie A, Cant JS, Foulds WS, et al. Ocular Vaccinia. Lancet 3: 273–275, 1974.

Ruben F, Lane J. Ocular vaccinia: epidemiologic analysis of 348 cases. Arch Ophthalmol 84: 45–48, 1970.

Semba RD. The ocular complications of smallpox and smallpox immunization. Arch Ophthalmol 121: 715–719, 2003.

Generic names: 1. Tetanus immune globulin; 2. tetanus toxoid.

Proprietary names: 1, BayTET, HyperTET; 2. Te Anatxal.

Primary use

Tetanus immune globulin is used prophylactically for wound management in patients not completely immunized. Tetanus toxoid is used for active immunization against tetanus.

Ocular side effects

Systemic side effects
Possible
1. Eyelids or conjunctiva
   a. Allergic reactions
   b. Erythema
   c. Conjunctivitis – non-specific
   d. Angioneurotic edema
   e. Urticaria
   f. Purpura
   g. Stevens-Johnson syndrome
   h. Angioneurotic edema
2. Corneal graft rejection
3. Photophobia

Conditional/Unclassified
1. Decrease or paralysis of accommodation
2. Horizontal nystagmus
3. Visual hallucinations
4. Decreased pupillary response to light
5. Optic neuritis

Clinical significance

Except for local reactions, such as erythema or urticaria, adverse ocular reactions following tetanus immunization are exceedingly rare. Steinemann et al (1988) reported a 33-year-old woman who developed a severe graft rejection within 4 days after receiving a tetanus toxoid booster. This required a repeat graft. Two years later, 6 months after her repeat graft, she received an influenza immunization and she again had a mild graft rejection. A similar case, with a corneal graft reaction after a tetanus immunization, is in the National Registry. Neurological complications probably occur at a rate of 0.4 per 1 million (Immunization Practice Advisory Committee). Nystagmus and accommodative paresis have been reported as adverse ocular symptoms following tetanus vaccine. Optic neuritis and myelitis were reported in an 11-year-old after a tetanus booster (Topaloglu et al 1992).

REFERENCES AND FURTHER READING

Chopra A, Drage LA, Hanson EM, et al. Stevens-Johnson syndrome after immunization with smallpox, anthrax and tetanus vaccines. Mayo Clin Proc 79: 1193–1196, 2004.

Harrer VG, Melnizky U, Wendt H. Akkommodationsparese und Schlucklahmung nach Tetanus-Toxoid-Auffrischungsimpfung. Wien Med Wochenschr 15: 296, 1971.

Immunization Practices Advisory Committee, Centers for Disease Control. Diptheria tetanus and pertussis: guidelines for vaccine prophylaxis and other preventive measures. Ann Intern Med 95: 723–728, 1981.

Jacobs RL, Lowe RS, Lanier BQ. Adverse reactions to tetanus toxoid. JAMA 247: 40, 1982.

McReynolds WU, Havener WH, Petrohelos MA. Bilateral optic neuritis following smallpox vaccination and diphtheria-tetanus toxoid. Am J Dis Child 86: 601, 1953.

Quast U, Hennessen W, Widmark RM. Mono- and polyneuritis after tetanus vaccination. (1970—1977). Dev Biol Stand 43: 25, 1979.

Schlenska GK. Unusual neurological complications following tetanus toxoid administration. J Neurol 215: 299, 1977.

Steinmann TL, Koffler BH, Jennings CD. Corneal allograft rejection following immunization. Am J Ophthalmol 106: 575–578, 1988.

Topaloglu H, Berker M, Kansu T, et al. Optic neuritis and myelitis after booster tetanus toxoid vaccination. Lancet 339: 178–179, 1992.

SECTION 13
DRUGS USED IN OPHTHALMOLOGY

CLASS: AGENTS USED TO TREAT AGE-RELATED MACULAR DEGENERATION

Generic names: 1. Bevacizumab; 2. pegaptanib; 3. ranibizumab.

Proprietary names: 1. Avastin; 2. Macugen; 3. Lucentis.

Primary use

These agents are intended to treat the 'wet' form of age-related macular degeneration (AMD). The aqueous solution of these drugs is injected into the vitreous of the eye and bound with vascular endothelial growth factor (VEGF), inhibiting neovascular formation. Pegaptanib and ranibizumab were developed with the intention of intravitreal injection while bevacizumab was initially approved for intravenous use to treat metastatic colorectal cancer.

Ocular side effects

Local ophthalmic use or exposure (intravitreal injection)
Certain
1. Retina
   a. Pigment epithelial tear (Fig. 7.13a)
   b. Edema
2. Eyelid or conjunctiva
   a. Angioneurotic edema
   b. Allergic reactions
   c. Conjunctival hemorrhage
   d. Blepharitis
   e. Conjunctivitis – non-specific
   f. Conjunctivitis – allergic
   g. Edema
   h. Irritation
3. Anterior eye inflammation
4. Decreased vision
5. Cornea
   a. Edema
   b. Abrasion
6. Irritation
   a. Discharge
   b. Pain
   c. Discomfort
   d. Inflammation
7. Increased intraocular pressure
8. Punctate keratitis
9. Visual disturbance – photopsia
10. Vitreous
    a. Floaters
    b. Opacities
    c. Hemorrhage
11. Endophthalmitis
12. Meibomianitis
13. Periorbital hematoma

Probable
1. Mydriasis

Possible
1. Increased lacrimation
2. Cataract
3. Cornea
   a. Deposits
   b. Epithelium disorder

Clinical significance

These agents act as selective VEGF antagonists through their specific molecular structures. While bevacizumab is a monoclonal antibody that binds VEGF, pegaptanib is an aptamer, which is a pegylated modified oligonucleotide that adopts a three-dimensional conformation, which enables it to bind to extracellular VEGF. Obvious risks exist as these drugs are directly administered into the vitreous of the eye. As with any intraocular surgery there is the risk of bleeding, infection (endophthalmitis), increased eye pressure, iatrogenic cataract, retinal detachment and other eye-related complications. The most frequent adverse ocular events reported during clinical trials were anterior eye inflammation, blurred vision, cataract, conjunctival hemorrhage, corneal edema, eye discharge, eye irritation, eye pain, increased intraocular pressure, ocular discomfort, punctate keratitis, reduced visual acuity, visual disturbance, vitreous floaters and vitreous opacities. These events occurred in 10–40% of patients. The most serious adverse event was endophthalmitis, which occurred in less than 1% of patients. In patients who received pegaptanib, 0.3 mg every 6 weeks intravitreally, 6–10% experienced adverse events, including blepharitis, conjunctivitis, photopsia and vitreous disorders. In 1–5% of patients, adverse events reported included allergic conjunctivitis, conjunctival edema, corneal abrasion, corneal deposits, corneal epithelium disorder, endophthalmitis, eye inflammation, eye swelling, eyelid irritation, meibomianitis, mydriasis, periorbital hematoma, retinal edema and vitreous hemorrhage.

There are potential cardiovascular implications with chronic VEGF inhibition. VEGF plays a vital role in the formation of collateral vessels critical to the viability of ischemic limbs and myocardium. Patients with diabetic retinopathy and AMD may

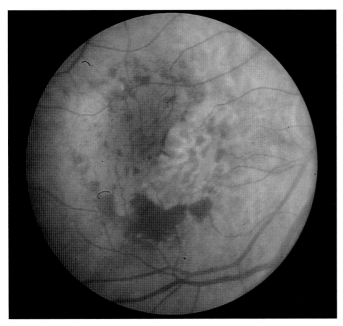

Fig. 7.13a Retinal pigment epithelium tear within the fovea after injection of intravitreal pegaptanib. Photo courtesy of Singh RP, et al. Retinal pigment epithelial tears after pegapanib injections for exudative age-related macular degeneration. Am J Ophthalmol 142: 160–162, 2006.

be at an increased risk of cardiovascular and peripheral vascular disease with chronic inhibition of VEGF. In an editorial by Gillies (2006), the point is made that VEGF inhibitors may eventually cause retinal atrophy by blocking VEGF's neuroprotective actions. Research on the long-term effects of VEGF inhibition are ongoing.

REFERENCES AND FURTHER READING

Asif M, Siddiqui A, Keating GM. Pegatanib: in exudative age-related macular degeneration. Drugs 65: 1571–1577, 2005.

Avery RL, Pearlman J, Pieramici DJ, et al. Intravitreal bevacizumab (avastin) in the treatment of proliferative diabetic retinopathy. Ophthalmology 113: 1695–1705, 2006.

Chun DW, Heier JS, Topping TM, et al. A pilot study of multiple intravitreal injections of ranibizumab in patients with center-involving clinically significant diabetic macular edema. Ophthalmology 113: 1706–1712, 2006.

D'Amico DJ, Masonson HN, Patel M, et al. Pegatanib sodium for neovascular age-related macular degeneration. Ophthalmology 113: 992–1001, 2006.

Dhalla MS, Blinder KJ, Tewari A, et al. Retinal pigment epithelial tear following intravitreal pegatanib sodium. Am J Ophthalmol 141: 752–754, 2006.

Gillies MC. What we don't know about avastin might hurt us. Arch Ophthalmol 123: 1478–1479, 2006.

Hariprasad SM, Shah GK, Blinder KJ. Short-term intraocular pressure trends following intravitreal pegatanib (macugen) injection. Am J Ophthalmol 141: 200–201, 2006.

Manzano RPA, Peyman GA, Khan P, et al. Testing intravitreal toxicity of bevacizumab (avastin). Retina 26: 257–261, 2006.

Singh RP, Sears JE. Retinal pigment epithelial tears after pegatanib injection for exudative age-related macular degeneration. Am J Ophthalmol 142: 160–162, 2006.

Generic name: Verteporfin.

Proprietary name: Visudyne.

Primary use

Administered intravenously, this medication is used during photodynamic therapy (PDT) in the treatment of choroidal neovascularization (CNV). It is photoactivated in the eye by a low-power laser and generates oxygen radicals that damage neovascular endothelial cells and causes thrombus formation, resulting in choroidal vascular occlusion.

Ocular side effects

Systemic administration

Certain

1. Eyelids or conjunctiva
   a. Blepharitis
   b. Conjunctivitis
   c. Conjunctival injection
   d. Photosensitivity (all patients)
   e. Allergic, hypersensitivity reaction
2. Non-specific ocular irritation
   a. Dry eyes
   b. Ocular itching
3. Retina
   a. Subretinal hemorrhage
   b. Detachment (exudative)
   c. Retinal or choroidal vessel non-perfusion
   d. Pigment epithelial detachment
   e. Pigment epithelial tears

4. Vitreous hemorrhage
5. Visual disturbance
6. Blurred vision
7. Visual field defects
8. Diplopia
9. Lacrimation disorder

Probable
1. Abnormal ERG
2. Choroidal infarction
3. Visual hallucination

Possible
1. Non-arteritic anterior ischemic optic neuropathy
2. Cataracts

Clinical significance

Verteporfin, a benzoporphyrin derivative monoacid ring A, is a photosensitizing drug for photodynamic therapy activated by low-intensity, non-heat-generating light of 689 nm wavelength. Activation generates cytotoxic oxygen free radicals, which cause thrombus formation in the target tissues of the choroid. Repeated treatments are usually needed for choroidal neovascularization when instituting photodynamic therapy. PDT has been used to treat CNV from any cause, including ocular histoplasmosis, pathologic myopia, angioid streaks and central serous retinopathy.

The most common side effects from PDT with verteporfin are photosensitivity and back pain. Severe vision decrease, the equivalent of four lines or more, within 7 days after treatment has been reported in 1–5% of patients. Partial recovery of vision was observed in some patients. Photosensitivity reactions usually occurred in the form of a skin sunburn following exposure to sunlight. Blurred vision and visual field defects occur in 10–20% of patients. Conjunctivitis, conjunctival injection, subretinal or vitreous hemorrhage, dry eyes, lacrimation disorder, photosensitivity and possible cataracts occur in 1–10% of patients. There are reports of exudative retinal detachments and significant subretinal hemorrhage soon after PDT using verteporfin. Also reported are retinal pigment epithelial detachments and tears after PDT.

Many of the adverse ocular events listed here are due to the mechanism of action of the drug and not necessarily due to the inherent toxicity of verteporfin. Withdrawal of the drug may be the only treatment in some instances, but many authors feel the benefits of therapy outweigh the risk of the rare event of severe vision loss. Alternative treatments for CNV have emerged which may replace PDT in the future.

Fossarello and Peiretti (2006) describe a case of acute repiratory distress 8 minutes after verteporfin was intravenously injected. They point out the need for the same emergency resources to be available as with fluorescein angiography.

REFERENCES AND FURTHER READING

Beaumont P, Lim CS, Chang A, et al. Acute severe vision decrease immediately after photodynamic therapy. Arch Ophthalmol 122: 1546–1547, 2004.

Colucciello M. Choroidal neovascularization complicating photodynamic therapy for central serous retinopathy. Retina 26: 239–242, 2006.

Do DV, Bressler NM, Bressler SB. Large submacular hemorrhages after verteporfin therapy. Am J Ophthalmol 137(3): 558–560, 2004.

Fossarello M, Peiretti E. Acute repiratory distress due to verteporfin infusion for photodynamic therapy. Arch Ophthalmol 124: 1508–1509, 2006.

Gelisken F, Inhoffen W, Partsch M, et al. Retinal pigment epithelial tear after photodynamic therapy for choroidal neovascularization. Am J Ophthalmol 131: 518–520, 2001.

Gelisken F, Inhoffen W, Karim-Zoda K, et al. Subfoveal hemorrhage after verteporfin photodynamic therapy in treatment of choroidal neovascularization. Graefe's Arch Clin Exp Ophthalmol 243: 198–203, 2005.

Hoz ER, Linare L, Meiler WF, et al. Exudative complications after photodynamic therapy. Arch Ophthalmol 121: 1649–1652, 2003.

Karacorlu M, Karacorlu S, Ozdemir H, et al. Nonarteritic anterior ischemic optic neuropathy after photodynamic therapy for choroidal neovascularization. Jpn J Ophthalmol 48: 418–426, 2004.

Klais CM, Ober MD, Freund KB, et al. Choroidal infarction following photodynamic therapy with verteporfin. Arch Ophthalmol 123: 1149–1153, 2005.

Lai TYY, Chan W-M, Lam DSC. Transient reduction in retinal function revealed by multifocal electroretinogram after photodynamic therapy. Am J Ophthalmol 137: 826–833, 2004.

Mauget-Faysse M, Mimoun G, Ruiz-Moreno JM, et al. Verteporfin photodynamic therapy for choroidal neovascularization associated with toxoplasmic retinochoroiditis. Retina 26: 396–403, 2003.

Mennel S, Meyer CH. Transient visual disturbance after photodynamic therapy. Am J Ophthalmol 139: 748–749, 2005.

Mennel S, Meyer CH, Eggarter F, et al. Transient serous retinal detachment in classic and occult choroidal neovascularization after photodynamic therapy. Am J Ophthalmol 140: 758–760, 2005.

Michels S, Aue A, Simader C, et al. Retinal pigment epithelium tears following verteporfin therapy with intravitreal triamcinolone. Am J Ophthalmol 141: 396–398, 2006.

Noffke AS, Lee J, Weinberg DV, et al. A potentially life-threatening adverse reaction to verteporfin. Arch Ophthalmol 119: 143, 2001.

Ojima Y, Tsujikawa A, Otani A, et al. Recurrent bleeding after photodynamic therapy in polypoidal choroidal vasculopathy. Am J Ophthalmol 141: 958–960, 2006.

Pece A, Introini U, Bottoni F, et al. Acute retinal pigment epithelial tear after photodynamic therapy. Retina 21: 661–665, 2001.

Postelmans L, Pasteels B, Coquelet P, et al. Severe pigment epithelial alterations in the treatment area following photodynamic therapy for classic choroidal neovascularization in young females. Am J Ophthalmol 138: 803–808, 2004.

Ratanasukon M, Wongchaikunakorn N. Exudative retinal detachment after photodynamic therapy: a case report in an Asian patient. Eye 20: 499–502, 2006.

Schnurrbusch UEK, Jochmann C, Einbock W, et al. Complications after photodynamic therapy. Arch Ophthalmol 123: 1347–1350, 2005.

Scott LJ, Goa KL. Verteporfin. Drugs Aging 16: 139–146, 2000.

Srivastava S, Sternberg P Jr.. Retinal pigment epithelial tear weeks following photodynamic therapy with verteporfin for choroidal neovasculization secondary to pathologic myopia. Retina 22: 669–671, 2002.

TAP and VIP Study Groups. Acute severe visual acuity decrease after photodynamic therapy with verteporfin: case reports from randomized clinical trials. TAP and VIP report no. 3. Am J Ophthalmol 137: 683–696, 2004.

Theodossiadis GP, Panagiotidis D, Georgalas IG, et al. Retinal hemorrhage after photodynamic therapy in patients with subfoveal choroidal neovascularization casued by age-related macular degeneration. Graefe's Arch Clin Exp Ophthalmol 241: 13–18, 2003.

Theodossiadis GP, Grigoropoulos VG, Emfietzoglou I, et al. Evolution of retinal pigment epithelium detachment after photodynamic therapy for choroidal neovascularization in age-related macular degeneration. Eur J Ophthalmol 16: 491–494, 2006.

Tzekov R, Lin T, Zhang K-M, et al. Ocular changes after photodynamic therapy. Invest Ophthalmol Vis Sci 47: 377–385, 2006.

CLASS: AGENTS USED TO TREAT ALLERGIES

Generic name: Emedastine difumarate.

Proprietary name: Emadine.

Primary use

Relatively selective H1 receptor antagonist used as a topical ocular agent for the treatment of allergic conjunctivitis.

Ocular side effects

Local ophthalmic use or exposure
Certain
1. Blurred vision
2. Irritation

a. Burning and stinging
b. Foreign body sensation
c. Epiphora
d. Discomfort
e. Photophobia
3. Cornea
a. Infiltrates
b. Superficial punctate keratitis
4. Conjunctival hyperemia

Possible
1. Pruritis
2. Decrease in tear production

Systemic side effects

Local ophthalmic use or exposure
Certain
1. Headaches
2. Drowsiness

Probable
1. Bad taste

Possible
1. Abnormal dreams
2. Asthenia
3. Dermatitis
4. Rhinitis
5. Sinusitis

Clinical significance

This topical ocular antihistamine is one of the stronger agents available, but it is still relatively free of significant side effects. The manufacturer states that many of the reported side effects may be secondary to the underlying disease. The most commonly reported side effects are headache, drowsiness and blurred vision. The reported incidence of headache is 11%. There is a report indicating a significant impairment of the ability to drive due to the sedating effect of emedastine. Some patients complain of unusual dreams or nightmares. Other Systemic side effects appear fairly insignificant and all are reversible.

REFERENCES AND FURTHER READING

AHSF Drug information. Emedastine difumarate. Am Soc Health Syst Pharmacists 1–15, 1998.

Horak F, Stubner P, Zieglmayer R, et al. Clinical study of the therapeutic efficacy and safety of emdastine difumarate versus cetirizine in the treatment of seasonal allergic rhinitis. Arzneimittelforschung 54: 666–672, 2004.

Physicians' Desk Reference for Ophthalmology, 30th edn, Medical Economics Co., Montvale, NJ, p 211, 2002.

Vermeeren A, Ramaekers JG, O'Hanlon JF. Effects of emedastine and cetirizine, alone and with alcohol, on actual driving of males and females. J Psychopharmacol 16: 57–64, 2002.

Generic name: Olopatadine hydrochloride.

Proprietary name: Patanol.

Primary use

Topical ocular histamine H1 receptor antagonist, with a mast cell stabilizing effect, used in the management of ocular allergies.

Ocular side effects

Local ophthalmic use or exposure
Certain
1. Cornea and conjunctiva
   a. Foreign body sensation – stinging
   b. Hyperemia
2. Contact lens use – decreased tolerance

Probable
1. Cornea and conjunctiva
   a. Sicca
   b. Keratitis

Systemic side effects

Local ophthalmic use or exposure
Certain
1. Headache

Probable
1. Nausea
2. Taste perversion

Possible
1. Cold syndrome
2. Pharyngitis
3. Rhinitis
4. Sinusitis

Clinical significance
This antihistamine and mast cell stabilizer is unique due to its longer duration of action, probability of lower ocular irritation and approved use in children 2 years and older. Ocular side effects are minimal and reversible. Since it contains benzalkonium chloride, contact lens use, especially soft lenses, may be a problem. However, the manufacturer and clinicians find that contacts are well tolerated if these drops are given 10–15 minutes before applying the lenses. Headaches are reported at an incidence of 7%. Less than 5% of patients may experience blurred vision, burning or stinging, cold syndrome, dry eye, foreign body sensation, hyperemia, nausea, taste perversion and upper respiratory inflammatory symptoms.

REFERENCES AND FURTHER READING

Anonymous. Olopatadine for allergic conjunctivitis. Med Lett Drugs Ther 39: 108–109, 1997.
Ciprandi G, Buscaglia S, Cerqueti PM, et al. Drug treatment of allergic conjunctivitis: a review of the evidence. Drugs 45: 1005–1008, 1995.
Galindez OA, Kaufman HE. Coping with itchy-burnies: the management of allergic conjunctivitis. Editorial (IDIS 373485). Ophthamology 103: 1335–1336, 1996.
Physicians' Desk Reference for Ophthalmology, 34th edn, Thomson PDR, Montvale, NJ, pp 208–209, 2006.

CLASS: AGENTS USED TO TREAT GLAUCOMA

Generic name: Apraclonidine hydrochloride.

Proprietary name: Iopidine.

Primary use
This topical ocular alpha-adrenergic antagonist is used primarily in the control of elevated ocular pressure. It is also used for acute pressure change post laser or surgical procedures.

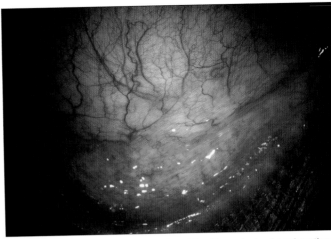

Fig. 7.13b Follicular conjunctivitis involving the palpebral conjunctiva of lower eyelid.

Ocular side effects

Local ophthalmic use or exposure (short exposure, only a few dosages)
Certain
1. Ocular hyperemia
2. Upper lid elevation
3. Conjunctival blanching
4. Mydriasis

Local ophthalmic use or exposure (long-term therapy, not recommended by manufacturer)
Certain
1. Loss of vision
2. Eyelids and conjunctiva
   a. Pruritus
   b. Conjunctivitis – follicular (Fig. 7.13b)
   c. Hyperemia
3. Conjunctival blanching
4. Upper lid elevation
5. Mydriasis

Probable
1. Eyelids or conjunctiva
   a. Contact dermatitis
   b. Blepharitis and dermatitis

Possible
1. Aggravation of ocular sicca
2. Tachyphylaxis
3. Uveitis

Systemic side effects
Certain
1. Dry mouth and nose

Probable
1. Headaches
2. Fatigue
3. Gastrointestinal symptoms
   a. Nausea
   b. Abdominal pain
   c. Diarrhea

4. Cardiovascular episodes
   a. Bradycardia
   b. Palpitations
   c. Orthostatic episodes
5. Taste abnormalities

Clinical significance

With short-term use, apraclonidine has a less than 2% adverse event rate with few adverse events becoming clinically significant. All are reversible and the rare cardiac events may or may not be drug related. The problems with this agent are found in chronic therapy, which is not approved in the USA. Araujo et al (1995) best summarized apraclonidine in a series of patients followed for 35 weeks. Thirty-nine per cent of the patients had side effects occurring as early as after the first drop to as late as the 35th week. Twenty-three per cent of the patients had to stop the drug secondary to adverse drug reactions. The most common side effect was decreased vision. In most cases this was a one line loss on the Snellen chart and was transient. However, a few patients lost two to four lines and in two cases the vision did not return. The allergic reaction was the second most common side effect and the primary reason for stopping the drug. They felt this was either a direct toxic effect or a hypersensitivity reaction. It was unclear if there was an association with a contact dermatitis of the eyelids. In all patients, once the drug was stopped the allergic reaction resolved within 5 days. While ocular adverse effects are transitory and reversible, they may be quite common. Robin et al (1995) noted that 50% get lid retraction, 45% had a small amount (0.4 mm) of mydriasis and between 20 and 50% get the drug-induced allergic reaction. Apraclonidine is a strong vasoconstrictor and conjunctival blanching occurs in 85% of patients (Robin et al 1995). There are a few cases in the National Registry of anterior granulomatous uveitis that promptly resolved when the drug was stopped. A cause-and-effect relationship is not established; however, the referring ophthalmologist considered this as an anterior segment ischemic response.

However in rare patients, systemic adverse drug-related events may occur. The sensation of dry mouth and nose is not unexpected since this group of drugs was initially intended as nasal decongestants. The drug reaches the nasal pharynx through the lacrimal outflow system to cause this effect, and occasionally patients complain of an abnormal taste. Although studies have shown no increase in fatigue compared to controls, many patients would find this hard to believe. This drug has minimal effects on the respiratory, cardiovascular and gastrointestinal systems.

REFERENCES AND FURTHER READING

Araujo SV, Bond BB, Wilson RP, et al. Long term effect of apraclonidine. Br J Ophthalmol 79: 1098–1101, 1995.

Butler P, Mannschreck M, Lin S, et al. Clinical experience with the long-term use of 1% apraclonidine. Arch Ophthalmol 113: 293–296, 1995.

Coleman AL, Robin AL, Pollack IP. Cardiovascular and intraocular pressure effects and plasma concentrations of apraclonidine. Arch Ophthalmol 108: 1264–1267, 1990.

Holdiness MR. Contact dermatitis to topical drugs for glaucoma. Am J Contact Dermatitis 12: 217–219, 2001.

Jampel HD. Hypotony following instillation of apraclonidine for increased intra-ocular pressure after trabeculoplasty. Am J Ophthalmol 108: 191–192, 1989.

Jampel HD. Discussion: Apraclonidine. Ophthalmology 100(9): 1323, 1993

Juzych MS, Robin AL, Novack GD. Alpha-2 Agonists in Glaucoma Therapy. Ocular Pharmacology, Lippincott-Raven, Philadelphia, 1997.

Lin SL, Liang SS. Evaluation of adverse reactions of apraclonidine hydrochloride ophthalmic solution. J Ocul Pharmacol Ther 11(3): 267–278, 1995.

Morrison JC. Side effects of α-adrenergic agonists. J Glaucoma 4(Suppl 1): S36–S38, 1995.

Munden PM, et al. Palpebral fissure responses to topical adrenergic drugs. Am J Ophthalmol 111: 706–710, 1991.

Nagasubramanian S, et al. Comparison of apraclonidine and timolol in chronic open-angle glaucoma. A three-month study. Ophthalmology 100(9): 1318–1323, 1993.

Robin AL, Ritch R, Shin DH, et al. Short-term efficacy of apraclonidine hydrochloride added to maximum-tolerated medical therapy for glaucoma. Apraclonidine maximum-tolerated medical therapy study group. Am J Ophthalmol 120(4): 423–432, 1995.

Silvestre JF, Camero L, Ramon R, et al. Allergic contact dermatitis from apraclonidine in eyedrops. Contact Dermatitis 45: 251, 2001.

Generic names: 1. Betaxolol; 2. levobunolol; 3. timolol.

Proprietary names: 1. Betoptic, Betoptic S, Kerlone; 2. Akbeta, Betagan; 3. Betimol, Blocadren, Istalol, Timoptic, Timoptic-XE.

Primary use

Systemic

Timolol is effective in the management of hypertension and myocardial infarction.

Ophthalmic

These beta-adrenergic blockers are used in the treatment of glaucoma.

Ocular side effects

Systemic administration – timolol
Certain
1. Decreased vision
2. Eyelids or conjunctiva
   a. Allergic reactions
   b. Hyperpigmentation
3. Decreased intraocular pressure
4. Myasthenia gravis
   a. Diplopia
   b. Ptosis
   c. Paresis of extraocular muscles

Probable
1. Eyelids or conjunctiva – loss of eyelashes or eyebrows
2. Visual hallucinations
3. Decreased lacrimation

Local ophthalmic use or exposure
Certain
1. Decreased intraocular pressure
2. Irritation
   a. Hyperemia
   b. Photophobia
   c. Ocular pain
   d. Burning sensation
3. Punctate keratitis
4. Eyelids or conjunctiva
   a. Allergic reactions
   b. Contact dermatitis
   c. Pemphigoid-like lesion with symblepharon
   d. Squamous metaplasia
5. Myasthenia gravis
   a. Ptosis
   b. Diplopia
   c. Paresis of extraocular muscles

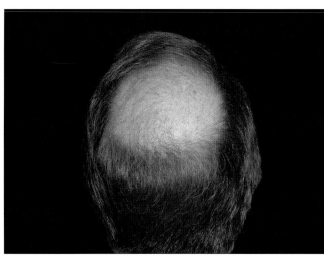

Fig. 7.13c Hair loss from topical ocular timolol.

Probable

1. Myopia
2. Visual hallucinations
3. Corneal anesthesia
4. Contact lens intolerance
5. Tear film break-up time – decreased

Possible

1. Eyelids or conjunctiva
   a. Erythema multiforme
   b. Loss of eyelashes or eyebrows
   c. Blepharoconjunctivitis
   d. Decreased goblet cells
2. Uveitis
3. Recurrent choroidal detachments
4. Iris depigmentation
5. Cystoid macular edema

Systemic side effects

Local ophthalmic use or exposure

Certain

1. Asthma
2. Bradycardia
3. Dyspnea
4. Cardiac arrhythmia
5. Hypotension
6. Impotence
7. Aggravation of chronic obstructive pulmonary disease
8. Nail pigmentation

Probable

1. Dizziness
2. Syncope
3. Bronchospasm
4. Apnea – children
5. Rebound increased blood pressure on beta-blocker withdrawal
6. Increase in high-density lipoprotein
7. Hyperkalemia
8. Respiratory failure
9. Palpitation
10. Hypoglycemia
11. Myasthenia-like syndrome
12. Depression

Possible

1. Headache
2. Congestive heart failure
3. Asthenia
4. Cerebral vascular accident
5. Nausea
6. Rhinitis
7. Nightmares
8. Raynaud's syndrome
9. Arthralgia
10. Alopecia (Fig. 7.13c)
11. Confusion
12. Psoriasis
13. Cardiac arrest
14. Cerebral ischemia

Clinical significance

The above-mentioned potential side effects from the various beta-blockers are all based on timolol. The other beta-blockers should have similar side effect profiles. The more selective beta-blockers, such as betaxolol, in all probability have fewer side effects, especially on the respiratory system. Regardless, any of the beta-blockers seem to have the potential for causing many, if not all, of the above side effects. The topical ocular administration of timolol usually has its peak systemic blood level between 30 and 90 minutes after application. The adverse effects from this drug may occur shortly after application, or may not occur for many weeks, months or even years on therapy. It should be noted that all adverse reactions reported due to systemic beta-blockers have been seen secondary to topical ocular beta blockers. Examples include fingernail and toenail pigmentation, myasthenia gravis neuroblocking effects, psoriasis and impotency. The local ocular effects from ophthalmic use are seldom of major consequence and are rarely an indication to discontinue the drug. Newer formulations and vehicles have decreased some of the initial burning associated with some of these agents. However, if the clinician notices superficial punctate keratitis or erosions, the possibility that this patient is one of a rare group who gets a local anesthetic effect from the medication must be considered. Long-term ocular medications, either due to the drug or its preservative, can cause pemphigoid-like lesions, especially in the inferior cul-de-sac. Many believe beta-blockers can enhance sicca (possibly after long-term use by affecting the microvilli), decrease tear film break-up time and decrease goblet cell density. The suspicion that timolol decreases tear production is real, but in most cases it is of such a mild nature that it is only occasionally of clinical importance. The area in which the beta-blockers cause greatest concern is their Systemic side effects from topical ocular application. Hong et al (2006) showed, as with all chronic topical ocular glaucoma medications, that significant squamous metaplasia occurs with long term use. This may be due to the preservative as well.

The most severe side effects affect the cardiovascular system and the respiratory system. Cardiovascular side effects include bradycardia, which is rarely an indication for stopping the drug. However, for diabetic patients who depend on an increased heart rate (i.e. hypoglycemic attack) as an indication for insulin use, this is of importance because the beta-blocker may mask the increase in heart rate. It is also of importance in exertion because some patients are unable to increase their heart rate. Additional problems include arrhythmia, syncope, congestive heart failure and a possible increase in cerebral vascular accidents, especially in patients with carotid insufficiency with drug-induced decreased blood pressure or pulse rate. In very rare instances, this may be associated with a fatality. Lee et al (2006), in reviewing data from the Blue Mountain Eye Study, suggest a high cardiovascular mortality in glaucoma patients taking topical ocular timolol. Lama's editorial on this article concurs but he feels further studies are necessary (Lama 2006). Since the non-selective beta-blockers decrease heart rate in a different location than the calcium channel blockers, there have been reports of sudden death in patients who are taking both drugs. The combination of these drugs playing a role is only theoretical. The adverse respiratory effects are the most perplexing. It has been well documented that these agents have caused bronchospasm and status asthmaticus with death reported shortly following the use of topical ocular beta-blockers. We have many case reports in the National Registry of status asthmaticus, including death. In approximately two-thirds of patients with a significant bronchospastic attack there was a previous history of asthma. This group of drugs may especially cause problems in patients with chronic obstructive lung disease. Patients recognize that they can breathe more easily after discontinuing these drugs, especially the non-selective beta-blockers. Approximately one-third of patients who develop bronchospasm recognize the problem with the beta-blockers within the first week, and one-quarter within the first day. It seems that patients with chronic pulmonary disease taking these drugs may suffer a decrease in their forced expiratory volume as measurable by spirometry.

There have been reports of apnea in infants who received topical ocular timolol. The central nervous system may also be affected. Clearly, the beta-blockers can cause depression in some patients, and in the younger age group there have been reports of an increased incidence of suicide attempts. The elderly suffer increased emotional liability, vivid dreams and increased anxiety, which may improve after discontinuation of the medication. There have been numerous reports of sexual dysfunction in both men and women while taking timolol. Skin changes from timolol are rare. However, there are well-documented reports of psoriasis, various rashes, increased pigmentation of fingernails and toenails, and male pattern baldness in men and women. This baldness is interesting because it usually does not occur until at least 4 months after the medication is started, although it may take many years for this to occur. Once it is recognized and the drug discontinued, it usually takes 4–8 months for recovery. Myasthenia has been associated with beta-blockers, as has Raynaud's phenomena, arthralgias and one well-documented case with rechallenge of recurrent hyperkalemia. Only with timolol are there data as to interactions between topical ocular medication and oral medication. Timolol and quinine enhance bradycardia. Timolol and halothane also enhance bradycardia and hypotension. Kaiserman et al (2006) feel there is no relationship in the incidence of depression and topical ocular beta-blockers based on data from 250 000 patients.

Recommendations for decreasing systemic effects

1. Have the patient only use 1 drop.
2. Close the lids for 3–5 minutes. You can also lay the head on the side away from the inner canthus with lids closed. Gravity will decrease the amount of drug reaching the lacrimal outflow system.
3. Before and immediately after opening the eyelids, use a tissue to absorb as much of the tears as possible in order to decrease the amount of medication reaching the puncta.
4. Applying pressure over the lacrimal sac during the period of lid closure and while removing excess medication is ideal, but difficult for many patients.

REFERENCES AND FURTHER READING

Akingbehin T, Raj PS. Ophthalmic topical beta blockers: review of ocular and systemic adverse effects. J Toxicol Cut Ocular Toxicol 9: 131–147, 1990.

Ananthanarayan CR, Vaile SJ, Feldman F. Acute episode of asthma following topical administration of betaxolol eyedrops. Can J Ophthalmol 28(2): 80–81, 1993.

Bright RA, Everitt DE. Beta blockers and depression. JAMA 267: 1783–1787, 1992.

Busin M, et al. Overcorrected visual acuity improved by antiglaucoma medication after radial keratotomy. Am J Ophthalmol 101: 374, 1986.

Chun JG, Brodsky MA, Allen BJ. Syncope, bradycardia, and atrioventricular block associated with topical ophthalmic levobunolol. Am Heart J 127(3): 689–690, 1994.

Coleman AL, et al. Topical timolol decreases plasma high-density lipoprotein cholesterol level. Arch Ophthalmol 106: 1260–1263, 1990.

Coppeto JR. Timolol associated myasthenia gravis. Am J Ophthalmol 98: 244–245, 1984.

Doyle E, Liu C. A case of acquired iris depigmentation as a possible complication of levobunolol eye drops. Br J Ophthalmol 83: 1403, 1999.

Duch S, Duch C, Pasto L, et al. Changes in depressive status associated with topical beta blockers. Int Ophthalmol 16(4–5): L331–L335, 1992.

Gorlich W. Experience in clinical research with beta blockers in glaucoma. Glaucoma 9: 21, 1987.

Fraunfelder FT. Ocular beta blockers and systemic effects. Arch Intern Med 146: 1073, 1986.

Fraunfelder FT, Meyer SM. Sexual dysfunction secondary to topical ophthalmic timolol. JAMA 253: 3092, 1985.

Fraunfelder FT, Meyer SM. Systemic side effects from ophthalmic timolol and their prevention. J Ocular Pharmacol 3: 177, 1987.

Geyer O, Neudorfer M, Lazar M. Recurrent choroidal detachment following timolol therapy in previously filtered eye. Choroidal detachment post filtering surgery. Acta Ophthalmol 70(5): 702–703, 1992.

Hannaway PJ, Hopper GDK. Severe anaphylaxis and drug-induced beta-blockade. N Engl J Med 308: 1536, 1983.

Harris LS, Greenstein SH, Bloom AF. Respiratory difficulties with betaxolol. Am J Ophthalmol 102: 274, 1986.

Herreras JM, Pastor JC, Calonge M, et al. Ocular surface alteration after long-term treatment with an antiglaucomatous drug. Ophthalmology 99(7): 1082, 1992.

Hong S, Lee CS, Seo KY, et al. Effects of topical antiglaucoma application on conjunctival impression cytology specimens. Am J Ophthalmol 142: 185–186, 2006.

Jain S. Betaxolol-associated anterior uveitis. Eye 8(Pt. 6): 708–709, 1994.

Kaufman HS. Timolol-induced vasomotor rhinitis: a new iatrogenic syndrome. Arch Ophthalmol 104: 967, 1986.

Kaiserman I, Kaiserman N, Elhayany A, et al. Topical beta blockers are not associated with an increased risk of treatment for depression. Ophthalmology 113: 1077–1080, 2006.

Lama PJ. Topical beta adrenergic blockers and glaucoma: a heart-stopping association?. Ophthalmology 113: 1067–1068, 2006.

Lee AJ, Wang JJ, Kifley A, et al. Open-angle glaucoma and cardiovascular mortality: the Blue Mountains Eye Study. Ophthalmology 113: 1069–1076, 2006.

Mort JR. Nightmare cessation following alteration of ophthalmic administration of a cholinergic and a beta-blocking agent. Ann Pharmacother 26(7–8): 914–916, 1992.

Negi A, Thoung D, Dabbous F. Nightmares with topical beta-blocker. Eye 14(5): 813–814, 2000.

Nelson WL, et al. Adverse respiratory and cardiovascular events attributed to timolol ophthalmic solution, 1978–1985. Am J Ophthalmol 102: 606, 1986.

Nuzzi R, Finazzo C, Cerruti A. Adverse effects of topical antiglaucomatous medications on the conjunctiva and the lachrymal (Brit. Engl) response. Int Ophthalmol 22(1): 31–35, 1998.

Orlando RG. Clinical depression associated with betaxolol. Am J Ophthalmol 102: 275, 1986.

Palmer EA. How safe are ocular drugs in pediatrics? Ophthalmology 93: 1038, 1986.

Schwab IR, et al. Foreshortening of the inferior conjunctival fornix associated with chronic glaucoma medications. Ophthalmology 99: 197–202, 1992.

Sharir M, Nardin GF, Zimmerman TJ. Timolol maleate associated with phalangeal swelling. Arch Ophthalmol 109: 1650, 1991.

Shelley WB, Shelley ED. Chronic erythroderma induced by beta blocker (timolol maleate) eyedrops. J Am Acad Derm 37(5 Pt. 1): 799–800, 1997.

Shore JH, Fraunfelder FT, Meyer SM. Psychiatric side effects from topical ocular timolol, a beta-adrenergic blocker. J Clin Psychopharmacol 7: 264, 1987.

Verkijk A. Worsening of myasthenia gravis with timolol maleate eyedrops. Ann Neurol 17: 211, 1985.

Vogel R. Surface toxicity of timolol (letter). Ophthalmology 100(3): 293–294, 1993.

Vogel R. Topical timolol and serum lipoproteins (letter). Arch Ophthalmol 109: 11341, 1991.

Wilhelmus KR, McCulloch RR, Gross RL. Dendritic keratopathy associated with beta-blocker eyedrops. Cornea 9: 335–337, 1990.

6. Cornea
   a. Edema (travoprost)
   b. Neovascularization
7. Eyelids or conjunctiva
   a. Deepening lid sulcus
   b. Toxic epidermal necrolysis
   c. Poliosis

Probable
1. Cornea – keratitis

Generic names: 1. Bimatoprost; 2. latanoprost; 3. travoprost.

Proprietary names: 1. Lumigan; 2. Xalatan; 3. Travatan.

Primary use
Indicated for the reduction of intraocular pressure in ocular hypertensives and various forms of glaucoma.

Ocular side effects

Local ophthalmic use or exposure
Certain
1. Blurred vision – transitory
2. Irritation
   a. Burning
   b. Stinging
   c. Foreign body sensation
   d. Itching
   e. Pain
   f. Photophobia
3. Conjunctiva
   a. Hyperemia (Fig. 7.13dA)
   b. Hyperkeratosis
   c. Pigmentation
4. Eyelashes
   a. Increased pigmentation
   b. Increased curling
   c. Increased growth – length and thickness
   d. Increased number
5. Iris color change – may be permanent
6. Uvea
   a. Iritis
   b. Uveitis
7. Cystoid macular edema
8. Eyelids
   a. Eyelid pigmentation
   b. Edema
   c. Erythemia
   d. Allergic reactions (Fig. 7.13dB)
   e. Contact dermatitis
   f. Punctal occlusion (Fig. 7.13dC)
9. Activation of herpes simplex
10. Choroidal detachment
11. Iris cysts

Possible
1. Bilateral optic disk edema
2. Uveitis – granulomatous
3. Myopia
4. Bullous keratopathy
5. Angle-closure glaucoma

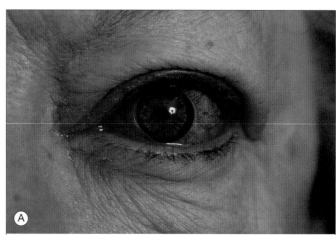

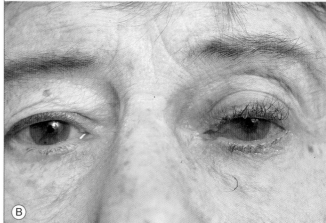

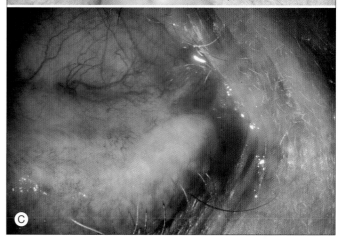

Fig. 7.13d A: Conjunctival hyperemia from topical ocular latanoprost administration. B: Allergic reaction to topical ocular bimatoprost in the left eye only. C: Punctal stenosis from topical ocular latanoprost administration.

Systemic side effects

Local ophthalmic use or exposure
Certain
1. Flu-like symptoms
   a. Abdominal cramps
   b. Malaise
   c. Upper respiratory tract-like infection
2. Muscle, joint and back pain
   a. Aggravation of arthritis
3. Facial burning
4. Facial rash
5. Hypertension

Probable
1. Angina
2. Migraine

Possible
1. Sweating

Clinical significance

These medications are a relatively new class of anti-glaucoma agents. It is somewhat unusual (as with timolol) that so many adverse side effects were missed prior to marketing and were only noted after the drug appeared in the marketplace. The characteristics of different adverse events are still being discovered as more long-term data become available.

The most common adverse ocular events, occurring in 5–15% of subjects, are blurred vision, burning, stinging, conjunctival hyperemia, foreign body sensation, itching, increased pigmentation of the iris and punctate epithelial keratopathy. Conjunctival hyperemia appears to occur more commonly with travoprost and bimatoprost. In 1–4% of subjects, dry eye, excessive tearing, eye pain, lid crusting, lid discomfort/pain, lid edema, lid erythema and photophobia have been reported to occur.

Johnstone (1997) pointed out the rapidity of onset of eyelash changes. For example, curling can occur in less than 5 days, with increased growth and number occurring less than 3 weeks after starting the drug. Iris pigmentation is most evident in patients with mixed color irises, and may be permanent in many subjects. Albert et al (2004) noted that the incidence of iris color changes may occur in more than 50% of patients. It appears there is an increase in melanin content in melanosomes and also an increased number of melanocytes in the iris, but there does not appear to be a predisposition towards malignant transformation. The FDA has not approved latanoprost as a first-line antiglaucoma drug because there are relatively little long-term data on the ocular adverse events reported.

It has become quite apparent that this agent can cause iritis and uveitis, and probably exacerbate old uveitis. In addition, macular edema and cystoid macular edema can occur. Uveitis and macular edema are more common in patients with a prior history of either, or after incisional ocular surgery. These also appear to be more common in aphakic and pseudophakic patients, especially if the posterior capsule is torn or other risk factors are present for macular edema. Miyake et al (1999) have shown that latanoprost therapy enhances disruption of the blood aqueous barrier.

Eyelids may have color changes, usually a darkening in color but there are cases in the National Registry of lightening in color, some in a spotty pattern. Doshi and Edward (2006) reported on 37 Caucasian subjects who developed periocular skin hyperpigmentation that was cosmetically noticeable after 3–6 months of topical ocular bimatoprost. There are multiple reports of herpes simplex keratitis reactivation by this drug. Iris cysts have been reported, which developed within 5 weeks of starting latanoprost. There are now multiple reports of ocular hypotony and choroidal effusions.

The most common systemic side effect is a flu-like syndrome, which occurs in at least 4% of patients. While it is not proven that this drug can exacerbate arthritis symptoms, positive rechallenge data in the National Registry suggest that some patients are convinced and refuse to continue this drug. Facial burning and facial rashes occur, but are rare. An unproven association includes darkening of scalp hair and, in elderly males, increased difficulty urinating. Since prostaglandins cause smooth muscle constriction, this possible latanoprost side effect cannot be ruled out. Increased headaches and increased dreaming or nightmares have also been reported to the National Registry. There are no data to support the case that this drug causes postmenopausal bleeding although the National Registry has a handful of case reports of this nature.

Recommendations for patients

1. Forewarn patients that permanent color changes of iris, eyelids or eyelashes may occur, especially if the drop is not used bilaterally.
2. Use with care in patients who have a past history of uveitis or macular edema.
3. Use with caution or preferably not at all in patients with prior history of herpes simplex keratitis.
4. Contraindicated with contact lens wear because benzalkonium chloride is used as a preservative.
5. Thimerosal will precipitate latanoprost solutions.

REFERENCES AND FURTHER READING

Albert DM, Gangnon RE, Zimbric ML, et al. A study of iridectomy histopathologic features of latanoprost- and non-lantanoprost-treated patients. Arch Ophthalmol 122: 1680–1685, 2004.

Arranz-Marquez E, Teus MA, Saornil MA, et al. Analysis of irises with a latanoprost-induced change in iris color. Am J Ophthalmol 138: 625–630, 2004.

Aslanides IM. Bilateral optic disk oedema associated with latanoprost. Br J Ophthalmol 84: 673, 2000.

Avakian A, Renier SA, Butler PJ. Adverse effects of latanoprost on patients with medically resistant glaucoma. Arch Ophthalmol 116: 679–680, 1998.

Ayyala RS, Cruz DA, Margo CE, et al. Cystoid macular edema associated with latanoprost in aphakic and pseudophakic eyes. Am J Ophthalmol 126: 602–604, 1998.

Callanan D, Fellman RL, Savage JA. Latanoprost-associated cystoid macular edema. Am J Ophthalmol 126: 134–135, 1998.

Doshi M, Edward DP, Osmanovic S. Clinical course of bimatoprost-induced periocular skin changes in Caucasians. Ophthalmology 113: 1961–1967, 2006.

Eisenberg D. CME and anterior uveitis with latanoprost use. Ophthalmology 105: 1978–1983, 1998.

Grierson I, Lee WR, Albert DM. The fine structure of an iridectomy specimen from a patient with latanoprost-induced eye color change. Arch Ophthalmol 117: 394–396, 1999.

Heier JS. Cystoid macular edema associated with latanoprost use. Arch Ophthalmol 116: 680–682, 1998.

Johnstone MA. Hypertrichosis and increased pigmentation of eyelashes and adjacent hair in the region of the ipsilateral eyelids of patients treated with unilateral topical latanoprost. Am J Ophthalmol 124: 544–547, 1997.

Lai IC, Kuo MT, Teng IMC. Iris pigment epithelial cyst induced by topical administration of latanoprost. Br J Ophthalmol 87: 366, 2003.

Miyake K, Ota I, Maekubo K, et al. Latanoprost accelerates disruption of the blood-aqueous barrier and the incidence of angiographic cystoid macular edema in early postoperative pseudophakias. Arch Ophthalmol 117: 34–39, 1999.

Rowe JA, Hattenhauer MG, Herman DC. Adverse side effects associated with latanoprost. Am J Ophthalmol 124: 683–685, 1997.

Stewart WC, Kolker AE, Stewart JA, et al. Conjunctival hyperemia in healthy subjects after short-term dosing with latanoprost, bimatoprost, and travoprost. Am J Ophthalmol 135: 314–320, 2003.

Teus MA, Arranz-Marquez E, Lucea-Suescu P. Incidence of iris colour change in latanoprost treated eyes. Br J Ophthalmol 86: 1085–1088, 2002.

Wand M. Latanoprost and hyperpigmentation of eyelashes. Arch Ophthalmol 115: 1206–1208, 1997.

Wand M, Gilbert CM, Liesegang TJ. Latanoprost and herpes simplex keratitis. Am J Ophthalmol 127(5): 602, 1999.

Wand M, Ritch R, Isbey EK Jr., et al. Latanoprost and periocular skin color changes. Arch Ophthalmol 119: 614–615, 2001.

Warwar RE, Bullock JD, Ballal D. Cystoid macular edema and anterior uveitis associated with latanoprost use. Ophthalmology 105: 263–268, 1998.

Yalvac IS, Tamcelik N, Duman S. Acute angle-closure glaucoma associated with latanoprost. Jpn J Opthalmol 47: 530–531, 2003.

Generic name: Brimonidine tartrate.

Proprietary name: Alphagan.

Primary use

This relatively selective alpha-2 adrenergic agonist is an effective intraocular pressure-lowering agent for open-angle glaucoma and ocular hypertension.

Ocular Side effects

Local ophthalmic use or exposure

Certain

1. Irritation
    a. Allergic reactions (Fig. 7.13eA)
    b. Hyperemia
    c. Pain
    d. Itching
    e. Foreign body sensation
2. Conjunctiva
    a. Blanching
    b. Hyperemia
    c. Edema
    d. Follicles (Fig. 7.13eB)
    e. Hemorrhage
3. Eyelids
    a. Blepharitis
    b. Hyperemia
    c. Edema
4. Blurred vision
5. Ocular pain
6. Cornea – superficial punctate keratitis
7. Photophobia
8. Decreased lacrimations
9. Decreased pupil size

Probable

1. Anterior uveitis

Possible

1. Cornea – erosions
2. Tachyphylaxis – may lose pressure lowering effect

Systemic side effects

Local ophthalmic use or exposure

Certain

1. Headaches
2. Dry nose and mouth

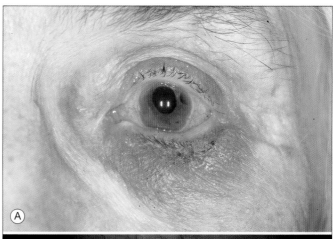

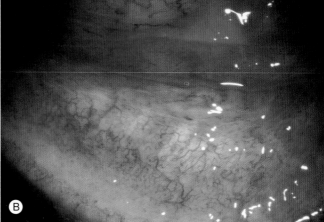

Fig. 7.13e A: Allergic reaction to topical ocular brimonidine in the left eye only. B: Follicular conjunctivitis from topical ocular brimonidine.

3. Drowsiness, fatigue or somnolence
4. Reduction in systolic blood pressure
5. Upper respiratory symptoms
6. Dizziness
7. Gastrointestinal disorders
8. Abnormal taste
9. Infants
    a. Bradycardia
    b. Hypotension
    c. Hypothermia
    d. Hypotonia
10. Contact dermatitis
11. Loss of LASIK flap adherence

Probable

1. Syncope
2. Muscle pain
3. Visual hallucinations

Possible

1. Infants – apnea

Clinical significance

Brimonidine tartrate may need to be discontinued in 5–10% of patients due to ocular or systemic side effects. Side effects may occur within minutes or months and are dose related. It appears that the most common reason for stopping the drug is an allergic reaction consisting of ocular hyperemia, pain, itching, foreign body sensation with a follicular conjunctival response and eyelid swelling. Of critical concern is the brimonidine-induced bradycardia, hypotension, hypothermia, hypotonia and apnea in neonates and infants. There are now multiple reports in the literature and from the National Registry of CNS depression, hypotension, bradycardia, hypersomnolence and even coma secondary to brimonidine eye drops in infants. Fortunately, the child recovers on discontinuation of the medication and supportive care. From the Physicians' Desk Reference, 10–30% of patients may experience oral dryness, ocular hyperemia, burning and stinging, headache, blurring of vision, foreign body sensation, fatigue/drowsiness, conjunctival follicles and ocular allergic reactions. Blurred vision is usually transitory, with vision returning to normal, even if staying on the drug. Schuman (1996) reported that 18% of patients had a clinically significant reduction in tear function. There are multiple reports of uveitis secondary to long-term use of brimonidine. Up to 25% of patients may have a dryness of their nose or mouth. This is not surprising, since this group of drugs was initially developed as nasal decongestants. This is probably due to a direct drug effect via the nasal lacrimal system to the nasal pharynx. LASIK surgeons have noted flap dislocations secondary to a possible lubricant effect from the eye drop preparation. Problems that may require discontinuing the drug include headache, fatigue and somnolence. This drug rarely affects the respiratory or cardiovascular system, however, in rare individuals, clinically significant adverse events may occur. Reports in the National Registry of syncope, which has been reported from 0.5% solution (not commercially available), can also rarely occur in sensitive adults at 0.2% or in the newer 0.15% formulation. We feel this drug is contraindicated in infants.

Recommendation
Do not use in pediatric patients.

REFERENCES AND FURTHER READING

Adkins JC, Balfour JA. Brimonidine. A review of its pharmacological properties and clinical potential in the management of open-angle glaucoma and ocular hypertension. Drugs Aging 12(3): 225–241, 1998.

Becker HI, Walton RC, Diamant JI, Zegans MF. Anterior uveitis and concurrent allergic conjunctivitis associated with long-term use of topical 0.2% brimonidine tartrate. Arch Ophthalmol 122: 1063–1066, 2004.

Berlin RJ, Lee UT, Samples JR, et al. Ophthalmic drops causing coma in an infant. J Pediatr 138: 441–443, 2001.

Byles DB, Frith P, Salmon JF. Anterior uveitis as a side effect of topical brimonidine. Am J Ophthalmol 130: 287–291, 2000.

Carlsen JO, Zabriskie NA, Kwon YH, et al. Apparent central nervous system depression in infants after the use of topical brimonidine. Am J Ophthalmol 128(2): 255–256, 1999.

Derick RJ, Robin AL, Walters TR, et al. Brimonidine tartrate: a one-month dose response study. Ophthalmology 104: 131–136, 1997.

Enyedi LB, Freedman SF. Safety and efficacy of brimonidine in children with glaucoma. J Am Assoc Pediatr Ophthalmol Strabismus 5: 281–284, 2001.

Korsch E, Grote A, Seybold M, Soditt V. Systemic adverse effects of topical treatment with brimonidine in an infant with secondary glaucoma (letter). Eur J Peds 158: 685, 1999.

LeBlanc RP, for Brimonidine Study Group. Twelve-month results of an ongoing randomized trial comparing brimonidine tartrate 0.2% and timolol 0.5% given twice daily in patients with glaucoma or ocular hypertension. Ophthalmology 105: 1960–1967, 1998.

Manlapaz CA, Kharlamb AB, Williams LS, et al. IOP, pulmonary and cardiac effects of anti-glaucoma drugs brimonidine, timolol, and betaxolol. Invest Ophthalmol Vis Sci 38(Suppl): S814, 1997.

McDonald JE II, El-Moatassem Kotb AM, Decker BB. Effect of brimonidine tartrate ophthalmic solution 0.2% on pupil size in normal eyes under different luminance conditions. J Cataract Refract Surg 27: 560–564, 2001.

Mungan NK, Wilson TW, Nischal KK, et al. Hypotension and bradycardia in infants after the use of topical brimonidine and beta-blockers. J Am Assoc Pediatr Ophthalmol Strabismus 7: 69–70, 2003.

Nordlund JR, Pasquale LR, Robin AL, et al. The cardiovascular, pulmonary, and ocular hypotensive effects of 0.2% brimonidine. Arch Ophthalmol 113: 77–83, 1995.

Physicians' Desk Reference, 60th edn, Thomson PDR, Montevale, NJ, pp 563, 2006.

Rosenthal AL, Walters T, Berg E, et al. A comparison of the safety and efficacy of brimonidine 0.2%, BID versus TID, in subjects with elevated intraocular pressure. Invest Ophthalmol Vis Sci 37(3): 1102, 1996.

Schuman JS. Clinical experience with brimonidine 0.2% and timolol 0.5% in glaucoma and ocular hypertension. Surv Ophthalmol 41(Suppl 1): 27–37, 1996.

Schuman JS, Horwitz B, Choplin NT, et al. A 1-year study of brimonidine twice daily in glaucoma and ocular hypertension. Arch Ophthalmol 115: 847–852, 1997.

Serle JB. A comparison of the safety and efficacy of twice daily brimonidine 0.2% versus betaxolol 0.25% in subjects with elevated intraocular pressure. Surv Ophthalmol 41(Suppl 1): S39–S47, 1996.

Sodhi PK, Verma L, Ratan J. Dermatological side effects of brimonidine: a report of three cases. J Dermatol 30: 697–700, 2003.

Tomsak RL, Zaret CR, Weidenthal D. Charles Bonnet syndrome precipitated by brimonidine tartrate eye drops. Br J Ophthalmol 87: 917–929, 2003.

Velasque L, Ducousso F, Pernod L, et al. Anterior uveitis and topical brimonidine: a case report. J Fr Ophthalmol 27: 1150–1152, 2004.

Waldock A, Snape J, Graham CM. Effects of glaucoma medications on the cardiorespiratory and intraocular pressure status of newly diagnosed glaucoma patients. Br J Ophthalmol 84: 710–713, 2000.

Walter KA, Gilbert DD. The adverse effect of perioperative brimonidine tartrate 0.2% on flap adherence and enhancement rates in laser in situ keratomileusis patients. Ophthalmology 108: 1434–1438, 2001.

Walters G, Taylor RH. Severe systemic toxicity caused by brimonidine drops in an infant with presumed juvenile xanthogranuloma (letter). Eye 13: 797–798, 1999.

Generic names: 1. Brinzolamide; 2. dorzolamide.

Proprietary names: 1. Azopt; 2. Trusopt.

Primary use
These topical ocular carbonic anhydrase inhibitors are effective in suppressing aqueous humor production in the management of elevated intraocular pressure.

Ocular side effects

Local ophthalmic use or exposure
Certain
1. Irritation
   a. Burning and foreign body sensation
   b. Stinging
   c. Epiphora
   d. Itching
   e. Allergic reaction
   f. Conjunctivitis
   g. Photophobia
2. Blurred vision
3. Conjunctiva – follicular reaction
4. Eyelids
   a. Irritation
   b. Allergic reaction
   c. Blepharitis
5. Cornea
   a. Superficial punctate keratitis (Fig. 7.13f)
   b. Erosions

Probable
1. Iritis – flare and cell, anterior chamber
2. Hypotony – ciliochoroidal detachment

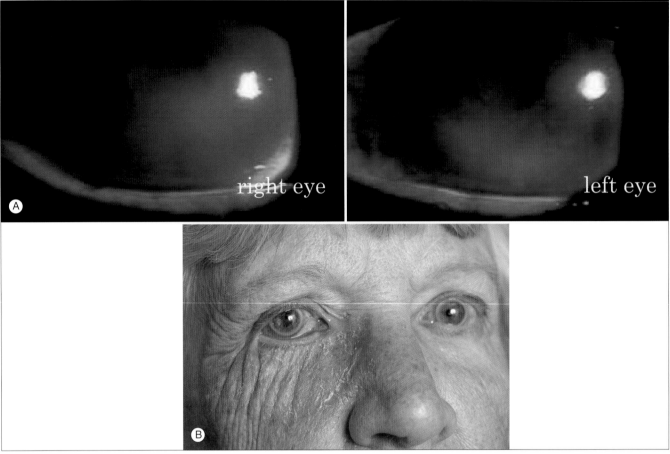

Fig. 7.13f A: Superficial punctuate keratitis with late staining centered on the inferior cornea after treatment with topical ocular brinzolamide. Photo courtesy of Tanimura H, et al. Corneal edema in glaucoma patients after the addition of brinzolamide 1% ophthalmic suspension. Jpn J Ophthalmol 49: 332–333, 2005.

Possible

1. Cornea
   a. Endothelial decompensation
   b. Edema
2. Eyelid or conjunctiva – toxic epidermal necrolysis
3. Choroidal detachment

Systemic side effects

Local ophthalmic use or exposure
Certain

1. Drug in contact with nasopharynx
   a. Taste disturbance
   b. Numbness
   c. Edema
   d. Increased salivation
   e. Nasal congestion
   f. Epistaxis
   g. Dysphonia
   h. Loss of appetite
2. Gastrointestinal disturbances
   a. Gastrointestinal upsets (abdominal cramping)
   b. Nausea
   c. Heartburn
3. CNS effects
   a. Headaches
   b. Asthenia/fatigue
   c. Insomnia

   d. Depression
   e. Paresthesias
4. Eyelids or conjunctiva
   a. Hypersensitivity reactions
   b. Itching
   c. Urticaria
   d. Contact allergy
5. Nephrolithiasis

Possible

1. Eyelids or conjunctiva – Stevens-Johnson syndrome

Clinical significance

The most common side effect in this class (up to one-third of patients) is the bitter metallic-like taste, which may increase salivation. In others, it may be associated with tongue or perioral numbness and edema. The second most common side effects are gastrointestinal complaints, which have occurred in as many as 10% of patients in some series. This may be one of the primary reasons that patients discontinue the drug. The CNS effects are much less common, but striking in some patients (i.e. headaches). Dermatologic conditions may be drug related and can cross-react with other sulfa medications. There are two cases of possible Stevens-Johnson syndrome associated with dorzolamide exposure. There are no proven or suspected blood dyscrasias in the literature or National Registry associated with the topical carbonic anhydrase inhibitors (CAI). There are numerous reports in the National Registry

(50+) of dyspnea, but we cannot determine a positive cause-and-effect relationship. Seizures, as with oral CAI, have also been reported. This association is not proven with topical ocular carbonic anhydrase inhibitors. Carlsen et al (1999) suggest an association with nephrolithiasis and state, 'Perhaps alternative topical glaucoma medication should be considered in patients with a history of renal calculi.' This is also an unproven association.

All topical ocular side effects are transitory and of minimal clinical importance compared to other topical ocular antiglaucomatous medications, except corneal edema. Konowal et al (1999) have shown a subset of patients (usually having had previous ocular surgery, with often borderline endothelial function and disturbed corneal epithelium) who, after starting topical ocular CAI, develop irreversible corneal decompensation. There are pharmacologic and toxicologic data to support a cause-and-effect relationship. These drugs can also cause superficial punctate keratitis and corneal erosions; however, these are seldom an indication to stop the drug. On occasion, the transitory stinging is severe enough that the patient refuses the medication. These effects are probably secondary to the relatively low pH of the eye solution. In rare instances, a low-grade iritis is probably caused by these agents. As with any topical medication, the intended drug effect may not occur (i.e. pressure lowering). However, in individuals hypersensitive to these drugs, ocular hypotony may occur.

Recommendations

1. No need to follow for blood dyscrasias with periodic blood work.
2. We do not feel that informed consent is necessary for systemic side effects since systemic effects appear to be rare and reversible.
3. If bitter taste is a major problem, consider punctal occlusion.
4. It is contraindicated to use oral and systemic CAI concomitantly.
5. Topical ocular sulfonamides may cross-react with other sulfonamides.
6. Use with caution in patients with severe kidney or liver disease.

REFERENCES AND FURTHER READING

Aalto-Korte K. Contact allergy to dorzolamide eyedrops. Contact Dermatitis 39: 206, 1998.
Balfour JA Wilde MI. Dorzolamide – a review of its pharmacology and therapeutic potential in the management of glaucoma and ocular hypertension. Drugs Aging 10: 384–483, 1997.
Callahan C, Ayyala RS, et al. Hypotony and choroidal effusion induced by topical timolol and dorzolamide in patients with previous glaucoma drainage device implantation. Ophthalmic Surg Lasers Imaging 34: 467–469, 2003.
Carlsen J, Durcan J, Zabriskie N, et al. Nephrolithiasis with dorzolamide. Arch Ophthalmol 117: 1087–1088, 1999.
Clineschmidt CM, Williams RD, Snyder E, et al. A randomized trial in patients inadequately controlled with timolol alone comparing the dorzolamide-timolol combination to monotherapy with timolol or dorzolamide. Ophthalmology 105: 1952–1958, 1998.
Epstein RJ, Brown SVL, Konowal A. Endothelial changes associated with topical dorzolamide do appear to be significant. Arch Ophthalmol 122: 1089–1090, 2004.
Fineman MS, Katz LJ, Wilson RP. Topical dorzolamide-induced hypotony and ciliochoroidal detachment in patients with previous filtration surgery (letter). Arch Ophthalmol 114: 1031–1032, 1996.
Florez A, Roson E, Conde A, et al. Toxic epidermal necrolysis secondary to timolol, dorzolamide, and latanoprost eyedrops. J Am Acad Dermatol 53: 909–911, 2005.
Fraunfelder FT, Meyer S, Bagby GC. Hematologic reactions to carbonic anhydrase inhibitors. Reply. Am J Ophthalmol 100: 746, 1985.
Fraunfelder FT, Meyer S, Bagby GC. Hematologic reactions to carbonic anhydrase inhibitors. Letter to the Editor. Am J Ophthalmol 101: 129, 1986.
Goldberg S, Gallily R, Bishara S, et al. Dorzolamide-induced choroidal detachment in surgically untreated eye. Am J Ophthalmol 138: 285–286, 2004.
Gupta R, Vernon SA. An unusual appearance of limbal conjunctival follicles in a patient on brimonidine and dorzolamide. Eye 19: 353–356, 2004.
Harris A, Arend O, Martin B. Effects of topical dorzolamide on retinal and retrobulbar hemodynamics. Acta Ophthalmol Scand 74: 569–572, 1996.
Johnson T, Kass MS. Letter to the editor. Am J Ophthalmol 101: 128–129, 1986.
Konowal A, Morrison JC, Brown SVL, et al. Irreversible corneal decompensation in patients treated with topical dorzolamide. Am J Ophthalmol 127: 403–406, 1999.
Lichter PR. Carbonic anhydrase inhibitors, blood dyscrasias, and standard of care. Ophthalmology 95: 711–712, 1988.
Miller RD. Hematologic reactions to carbonic anhydrase inhibitors. Am J Ophthalmol 100: 745–746. 1985.
Mogk LG, Cyrlin MN. Blood dyscrasias and carbonic anhydrase inhibitors. Letter to the editor. Ophthalmology 95: 768–771, 1988.
Morris S, Geh V, Nischal KK, et al. Topical dorzolamide and metabolic acidosis in a neonate. Br J Ophthalmol 87: 1052–1053, 2003.
Pfeiffer N. Dorzolamide: development and clinical application of a topical carbonic anhydrase inhibitor. Surv Ophthalmol 42: 137–151, 1997.
Schwartzenberg GWS, Trope G. Anorexia, depression and dementia induced by dorzolamide eyedrops (Trusopt). Can J Ophthalmol 34(2): 93–94, 1999.
Sponsel WE, Harrison J, Elliott WR. Dorzolamide hydrochloride and visual function in normal eyes. Am J Ophthalmol 123: 759–766, 1997.
Tanimura H, Minamoto A, Narai A, et al. Corneal edema in glaucoma patients after the addition of brinzolamide 1% ophthalmic suspension. Jpn J Ophthalmol 49: 332–333, 2005.
Wirtitsch MG, Findl O, Kiss B, et al. Short-term effect of dorzolamide hydrochloride on central corneal thickness in humans with cornea guttata. Arch Ophthalmol 121: 621–625, 2003.
Zambarakji HJ, Spencer AF, Vernon SA. An unusual side effect of dorzolamide (letter). Eye 11: 418–419, 1997.
Zhao JC, Chen T, et al. Brinzolamide induced reversible corneal decompensation. Br J Ophthalmol 89: 389–390, 2005.
Zimran A, Beutler E. Can the risk of acetazolamide-induced aplastic anemia be decreased by periodic monitoring of blood cell counts? Am J Ophthalmol 104: 654–658, 1987.

Generic name: Carteolol hydrochloride.

Proprietary names: Ocupress.

Primary use

Ophthalmic
Carteolol is used in the management of glaucoma.

Systemic
Carteolol is a non-selective beta blocker that is used in the management of hypertension and angina pectoris.

Ocular side effects

Local ophthalmic use or exposure
Certain

1. Decreased intraocular pressure
2. Irritation
   a. Ocular pain
   b. Burning sensation
   c. Epiphora
   d. Hyperemia
   e. Photophobia

3. Blurred vision
4. Eyelids or conjunctiva
   a. Allergic reactions
   b. Contact dermatitis
   c. Erythema blepharoconjunctivitis
   d. Chemosis
5. Corneal – variable punctate staining
6. Ptosis

Systemic side effects

Local ophthalmic use or exposure
Certain
1. Asthma
2. Bradycardia
3. Dyspnea
4. Depression
5. Cardiac arrhythmia
6. Headache
7. Asthenia
8. Dizziness
9. Hypotension
10. Syncope
11. Bronchospasm
12. Aggravation of chronic obstructive pulmonary disease
13. Suppression of heart rate and blood pressure elevation
14. Respiratory failure
15. Palpitation

Probable
1. Rhinitis
2. Confusion
3. Taste perversion

Possible
1. Congestive heart failure
2. Cerebral vascular accident
3. Increase in high-density lipoprotein
4. Skin disease
5. Heart block
6. Cerebral ischemia

Clinical significance

Carteolol has not been used as extensively as timolol but, in general, its ocular and systemic side effects are similar to timolol. Clearly, it is better tolerated with regard to stinging and irritation, and most often these symptoms decrease with time. Ocular pain may be a significant side effect, but rarely an indication for discontinuing the drug. To date, the local anesthetic effect of this drug has not been reported in humans. Transient ocular irritation, however, may occur in about 25% of patients. Baudouin and de Lunardo (1998) have shown that using a preservative-free solution enhances the stability of the tear film.

It is apparent from controlled trials that there seem to be fewer systemic side effects with this agent than with timolol. While this agent can reduce the mean heart rate and possibly the mean blood pressure, these have been insignificant clinically. There have been cases in the literature and reports to the National Registry of asthma, decompensated heart failure, headaches, asthenopsia and dizziness, but these are in a much smaller proportion than seen with other non-selective beta blockers. There are two cases in the National Registry, both with challenge and rechallenge, of a bleeding diathesis with nosebleeds and easy bruisability while taking this drug. This has not been reported

with the other beta blockers and, while interesting, this is difficult to understand from a pharmacologic standpoint. Stewart et al (1999) have shown that topical ocular carteolol does not affect serum lipid levels. This is in contrast with timolol maleate, which adversely affects the HDL and TC/HDL ratio in females age 60 and older (see timolol).

REFERENCES AND FURTHER READING

Baudouin C, de Lunardo C. Short-term comparative study of topical 2% carteolol with and without benzalkonium chloride in healthy volunteers. Br J Ophthalmol 82(1): 39–42, 1998.

Brazier DJ, Smith SE. Ocular and cardiovascular response to topical carteolol 2% and timolol 0.5% in healthy volunteers. Br J Ophthalmol 72: 101–103, 1988.

Chrisp P, Sorkin EM. Ocular carteolol – A review of its pharmacological properties, and therapeutic use in glaucoma and ocular hypertension. Drugs Aging 2: 58–77, 1992.

Freedman SF, et al. Effects of ocular carteolol and timolol on plasma highdensity lipoprotein cholesterol level. Am J Ophthalmol 116: 600–611, 1993.

Grunwald JE, Delehanty J. Effect of topical carteolol on the normal human retinal circulation. Inv Ophthalmol Vis Sci 33: 1853–1863, 1992.

Hoh H. Surface anesthetic effect and subjective compatibility of 2% carteolol and 0.6% metipranolol in eye-healthy people. Lens Eye Toxicity Res 7: 347–352, 1990.

Kitazawa Y, Horie T, Shirato S. Efficacy and safety of carteolol hydrochloride: a new beta-blocking agent for the treatment of glaucoma. Int Cong Ophthalmol 1: 683–685, 1983.

Scoville B, et al. Double-masked comparison of carteolol and timolol in ocular hypertension. Am J Ophthalmol 105: 150–154, 1988.

Stewart WC, Dubiner HB, Mundorf TK, et al. Effects of carteolol and timolol on plasma lipid profiles in older women with ocular hypertension or primary open-angle glaucoma. Am J Ophthalmol 127(2): 142–147, 1999.

Generic name: Dipivefrine.

Proprietary names: Akpro, Propine.

Primary use

This sympathomimetic is indicated as initial therapy for the control of intraocular pressure in chronic open-angle glaucoma.

Ocular side effects

Local ophthalmic use or exposure
Certain
1. Decreased intraocular pressure
2. Irritation
   a. Lacrimation
   b. Hyperemia
   c. Ocular pain
   d. Burning sensation
   e. Photophobia
3. Eyelids or conjunctiva
   a. Allergic reactions
   b. Blepharoconjunctivitis
   c. Follicular conjunctivitis
   d. Pemphigoid lesion with symblepharon
4. Mydriasis – may precipitate angle-closure glaucoma
5. Cornea – keratitis

Probable
1. Cornea – intraepithelial vesicles
2. Cystoid macular edema

Systemic side effects

Local ophthalmic use or exposure
Certain
1. Tachycardia
2. Cardiac arrhythmia
3. Hypertension

Probable
1. Headache

Possible
1. Asthma

Clinical significance

Dipivefrine is a prodrug that is biotransformed to epinephrine inside the eye. This topical agent is not used as often in the USA because of the emergence of many alternative anti-glaucoma eye drops. This drug is better tolerated than standard epinephrine preparations, but at concentrations greater than 0.1%, there are increased epinephrine-like systemic side effects. Dipivefrine is a medication surprisingly free of major ocular adverse effects. It rarely shows the epinephrine effects of contact lens discoloration or conjunctival pigment deposits. Upper and lower palpebral conjunctival follicles are common in patients on long-term dipivefrine, with occasional perilimbal, bulbar or plica follicular reactions. Petersen et al (1990) have individually tested each component of commercial preparations and found dipivefrine to be the cause for each of the external ocular findings. Conjunctival shrinkage and symblepharon have also been related to chronic dipivefrine usage. The National Registry has received cases of maculopathy in aphakic eyes and cystoid macular edema in phakic glaucomatous eyes after treatment with dipivefrine. Mehelas et al (1982) and Borrmann and Duzman (1987) have also reported this. This is probably due to the drug, but at a much lower incidence than seen with epinephrine. Single cases of ectropion (Bartley 1991) and central vein occlusion (Fledelius 1990) have also been reported.

The potential for systemic adverse reactions similar to those seen with topical ophthalmic epinephrine also exists for dipivefrine administration, although probably with a lower frequency rate. Clinicians need to be aware of potential sensitivity in patients taking this agent who complain of respiratory difficulties because some of these medications contain sulfites.

REFERENCES AND FURTHER READING

Bartley GB. Reversible lower eyelid ectropion associated with dipivefrin. Am J Ophthalmol 111: 650–651, 1991.

Blanchard DL. Adrenergic-associated symblepharon. Glaucoma 9: 18–20, 1987.

Boerner CF. Dipivefrine. Total punctate keratopathy due to dipivefrin. Arch Ophthalmol 106: 171, 1988.

Borrmann L, Duzman E. Undetected cystoid macular edema in aphakic glaucoma patients treated with dipivefrin. J Toxicol Ocul Toxicol 6: 173–177, 1987.

Cebon L, West RH, Gillies WE. Experience with dipivalyl epinephrine. Its effectiveness, alone or in combination, and its side effects. Aust J Ophthalmol 11: 159, 1983.

Coleiro JA, Sigurdsson H, Lockyer JA. Follicular conjunctivitis on dipivefrin therapy for glaucoma. Eye 2: 440–442, 1988.

Duffey RJ, Ferguson JG Jr. Interaction of dipivefrin and epinephrine with the pilocarpine ocular therapeutic system (Ocusert). Arch Ophthalmol 104: 1135, 1986.

Fledelius HC. Central vein thrombosis and topical dipivalyl epinephrine. Acta Ophthalmol 68: 491–492, 1990.

Kerr CR, et al. Cardiovascular effects of epinephrine and dipivalyl epinephrine applied topically to the eye in patients with glaucoma. Br Ophthalmol 66: 109, 1982.

Liesegang TJ. Bulbar conjunctival follicles associated with dipivefrin therapy. Ophthalmology 92: 228, 1985.

Mehelas TJ, Kollarits CR, Martin WG. Cystoid macular edema presumably induced by dipivefrin hydrochloride (Propine). Am J Ophthalmol 94: 682, 1982.

Petersen PE, et al. Evaluation of ocular hypersensitivity to dipivalyl epinephrine by component eye-drop testing. J Allergy Clin Immunol 85: 954–958, 1990.

Satterfield D, Mannis MJ, Glover AT. Unilateral corneal vesicles secondary to dipivefrin therapy. Am J Ophthalmol 113(3): 339–340, 1992.

Schwab IR, et al. Foreshortening of the inferior conjunctival fornix associated with chronic glaucoma medications. Ophthalmology 99(2): 197–202, 1992.

Schwartz HJ, Sher TH. Bisulfite intolerance manifest as bronchospasm following topical dipivefrin hydrochloride therapy for glaucoma. Arch Ophthalmol 103: 14, 1985.

Wandel T, Spinak M. Toxicity of dipivalyl epinephrine. Ophthalmology 88: 259, 1981.

West RH, Cebon L, Gillies WE. Drop attack in glaucoma. The Melbourne experience with topical miotics, adrenergic and neuronal blocking drops. Aust J Ophthalmol 11: 149, 1983.

Generic name: Metipranolol.

Proprietary name: Optipranolol.

Primary use

Ophthalmic
This non-cardioselective beta blocker is used to reduce intraocular pressure associated with glaucoma.

Systemic
Used in the management of cardiac disorders and hypertension.

Ocular side effects

Local ophthalmic use or exposure
Certain
1. Decreased intraocular pressure
2. Irritation
   a. Hyperemia
   b. Photophobia
   c. Ocular pain
   d. Burning sensation
3. Anterior uveitis
   a. Granulomatous
   b. Non-granulomatous
4. Punctate keratitis
5. Eyelids or conjunctiva
   a. Allergic reactions
   b. Erythema
   c. Blepharoconjunctivitis
6. Corneal anesthesia
7. Contact lens intolerance
   a. Corneal erosion
   b. Unable to wear
8. Tear film break-up time – decreased
9. Conjunctival keratinization

Probable
1. Blurred vision

Systemic side effects
Similar to timolol.

Clinical significance

This non-selective beta blocker has been popular because of its lower cost, lower concentration of preservatives, fewer CNS side effects and, possibly, less corneal anesthesia than seen with other beta blockers. This agent has the potential to cause any of the systemic side effects seen with other non-selective beta blockers (see timolol). All non-selective beta blockers have been reported to cause anterior uveitis in rare instances. Possibly due to the radiation sterilization techniques, large keratic precipitates, flare and cells, and elevated intraocular pressures were first reported in Germany and Great Britain as a fairly common side effect. The current preparation appears to make granulomatous uveitis rare. The uveitis does recur on rechallenge, with common signs and symptoms disappearing on drug withdrawal and the uveitis incidence increasing with increased drug concentration. The uveitis may be granulomatous with large mutton fat keratic precipitates or it can be a low-grade non-granulomatous reaction (Patel et al 1997). The incidence of this side effect, as per Melles and Wong (1994), is about 0.49%. They also suggest that argon laser trabeculoplasty may play a role in sensitizing patients to metipranolol. Watanabe and Hodes (1997) reported a case with bilateral granulomatous uveitis due to metipranolol (without argon treatment). Beck et al (1996) found no cases of uveitis in retrospective studies of 1928 patients on 0.3% metipranolol or in 3903 patients on other topical ocular beta blockers. On topical ocular steroids, the uveitis usually subsides within 4–6 weeks. In some cases, a marked elevation of intraocular pressure, blepharoconjunctivitis and periorbital dermatitis is associated with uveitis. De Groot et al (1998) describe three cases of contact allergies secondary to this drug. Wolf et al (1998) show that both systemic and topical ocular metipranolol lead to increased retinal blood flow velocity. The authors state that the implications of these results for treatment with beta blockers are not clear.

REFERENCES AND FURTHER READING

Akingbehin T, Villada JR. Metripranolol-associated granulomatous anterior uveitis. Br J Ophthalmol 75: 519, 1991.

Beck RW, Moke P, Blair RC, et al. Uveitis associated with topical beta blockers. Arch Ophthalmol 114(10): 1181–1182, 1996.

Cervantes R, Hernandez HH, Frati A. Pulmonary and heart rate changes associated with nonselective beta-blocker glaucoma therapy. J Toxicol Cut Ocular Toxicol 5: 185–193, 1986.

De Groot AC, Van Ginkel CJ, Bruynzeel DP, et al. Contact allergy to eyedrops containing beta blockers. Nederlands Tijdschrift voor Geneeskunde 142(18): 1034–1036, 1998.

Derous D, et al. Conjunctival keratinization, an abnormal reaction to an ocular beta blocker. Acta Ophthalmol 67: 333–338, 1989.

Drager J, Winter R. Corneal sensitivity and intraocular pressure. In: Glaucoma Update II, Krieglstein, Leydhecker (eds), Springer-Verlag, Berlin, pp 63–70 1983.

Flaxel C, Samples JR. Metipranolol. J Toxicol Cut Ocular Toxicol 10: 171–174, 1991.

Hoh H. Surface anesthetic effect and subjective compatibility of 2% carteolol and 0.6% metipranolol in eye-healthy people. Lens Eye Toxic Res 7: 347–352, 1990.

Kessler C, Christ T. Incidence of uveitis in glaucoma patients using metipranolol. J Glaucoma 2: 166–170, 1993.

Melles RB, Wong IG. Metipranolol-associated granulomatous iritis. Am J Ophthalmol 118: 712–715, 1994.

Patel NP, Patel KH, Moster MR, et al. Metipranolol-associated nongranulomatous anterior uveitis. Am J Ophthalmol 123(6): 843–846, 1997.

Schultz JS, Hoenig JA, Charles H. Possible bilateral anterior uveitis secondary to metipranolol (OptiPranolol) therapy. Arch Ophthalmol 111: 1607, 1993.

Serle JB, Lustgarten JS, Podos SM. A clinical trial of metipranolol, a non-cardioselective beta-adrenergic antagonist, in ocular hypertension. Am J Ophthalmol 112: 302–307, 1991.

Stempel I. Different beta blockers and their short-time effect on break-up time. Ophthalmologica 192: 11, 1986.

Watanabe TM, Hodes BL. Bilateral anterior uveitis associated with a brand of metipranolol. Arch Ophthalmol 115: 421–422, 1997.

Wolf S, Werner E, Schulte K, et al. Acute effect of metipranolol on the retinal circulation. Br J Ophthalmol 82: 892–896, 1998.

Generic name: Unoprostone isopropyl.

Proprietary name: Rescula.

Primary use

A prostanoid derivative used to treat glaucoma and ocular hypertension.

Ocular side effects

Local ophthalmic use or exposure
Certain
1. Conjunctiva – hyperemia
2. Iris – increased pigmentation
3. Eyelashes – changes similar to latanoprost

Probable
1. Conjunctiva – follicles
2. Cornea – superficial punctate keratitis

Possible
1. Conjunctiva – edema
2. Cornea
   a. Epithelial erosions
   b. Persistent epithelial defects
3. Cystoid macular edema

Systemic side effects

Local ophthalmic use or exposure
Probable
1. Headaches
2. Numbness (tip of tongue)
3. Oral dryness
4. Nasal congestion
5. Nausea and vomiting
6. Bradycardia

This medication is a prostaglandin F2-alpha analogue and exhibits some of the same adverse ocular and systemic reactions this class of medication is known for, i.e. changes in eyelashes and iris color. The ocular side effects are transient and seldom of clinical significance. The most common adverse ocular event is conjunctival hyperemia, which resolves in most patients even if the drug is continued. Corneal changes can be an indication to stop the drug if epithelial defects persist. Iris and eyelash changes similar to those seen with latanoprost have been reported with isopropyl unoprostone, although the incidence is less than other topical eye drops in the same class. Systemic side effects are mild, transient and usually disappear while the patient is still on therapy.

REFERENCES AND FURTHER READING

Haria M, Spencer CM. Unoprostone (Isopropyl Unoprostone). Drugs Aging 9(3): 213–218, 1996.

Kokawa N, Yokoi N, Matsumoto Y, et al. Seven cases of severe ocular surface disorders following topical antiglaucoma agents. Jpn J Clin Ophthalmol 50: 1105–1108, 1996.

McCarey BE, Kapik BM, Kane FE. Unoprostone monotherapy study group. Low incidence of iris pigmentation and eyelash changes in 2 randomized clinical trials with unoprostone isopropyl 0.15%. Ophthalmology 111: 1480–1488, 2004.

Nordmann J-P, Mertz B, Yannoulis NC, et al. Unoprostone monotherapy study group. A double-masked randomized comparison of the efficacy and safety of unoprostone with timolol and betaxolol in patients with primary open-angle glaucoma including pseudoexfoliation glaucoma or ocular hypertension. 6 month data. Am J Ophthalmol 133: 1–10, 2002.

Sakamoto Y, Iwasaki N, Maeda N, et al. Corneal epithelial lesion induced by prostaglandin F2a ophthalmic solution. Jpn J Clin Ophthalmol 49: 1845–1848, 1995.

Wand M, Gaudio AR. Cystoid macular edema associated with ocular hypotensive lipids. Am J Ophthalmol 133: 403–405, 2002.

CLASS: ANTIVIRAL AGENTS

Generic name: Aciclovir (Acyclovir).

Proprietary name: Zovirax.

Primary use

This purine nucleoside is used in the treatment and management of herpes simplex infections.

Ocular side effects

Systemic administration
Certain
1. Visual hallucinations
2. Eyelids
   a. Erythema
   b. Urticaria
   c. Edema
3. Keratoconjunctivitis sicca – aggravates
4. Phospholipidosis
   a. Corneal epithelial vacuoles
   b. Conjunctival hyperemia

Probable
1. Decreased vision
2. Perioral numbness

Possible
1. Eyelids or conjunctiva
   a. Erythema multiforme
   b. Stevens-Johnson syndrome
   c. Toxic epidermal necroylsis
2. Subconjunctival or retinal hemorrhages secondary to drug-induced anemia

Local ophthalmic use or exposure
Certain
1. Irritation
   a. Lacrimation
   b. Hyperemia
   c. Ocular pain
   d. Edema
   e. Burning sensation
   f. Sicca
2. Superficial punctate keratitis
3. Eyelids or conjunctiva
   a. Allergic reaction
   b. Blepharitis
   c. Conjunctivis – follicular
4. Narrowing or occlusion of lacrimal puncta

Clinical significance

Oral aciclovir has very few ocular side effects. The most common is probably periocular edema with or without perioral numbness. Common systemic adverse reactions are gastrointestinal disturbances such as nausea, vomiting and diarrhea. Renal failure has occurred in rare instances. Since the drug is secreted in human tears, ocular sicca can be aggravated. Visual hallucinations have been reported secondary to systemic aciclovir therapy.

Topical ophthalmic aciclovir is commonly prescribed for herpes keratitis according to guidelines recommended by the Herpes Eye Disease Study and it is generally well tolerated. A mild transient burning or a stinging sensation has been reported immediately following application of the drug. Punctate epithelial staining of the inferior bulbar conjunctiva and limbus is reversible with discontinuation of the agent. Punctal stenosis or occlusion, follicular conjunctivitis, contact blepharoconjunctivitis, palpebral allergy or other signs of hypersensitivity have also occurred occasionally. Aciclovir does not appear to interfere significantly with the healing of stromal wounds. Colin et al (1997) felt that healing rates were better with ganciclovir than with acyclovir gel, but these data were not statistically significant. Ohashi (1997) reviewed herpes simplex keratitis treated with topical ocular aciclovir. He suggests that a more persistent superficial punctate keratitis can occur with emergence of an acyclovir-resistant strain of the virus, and an increase in progressive corneal endotheliitis. Wilhelmus et al (1995) felt that drug-induced phospholipidosis is a cause of punctate epitheliopathy seen in AIDS patients, but it is not clear if this is due to aciclovir and/or ganciclovir given systemically.

REFERENCES AND FURTHER READING

Auwerx J, Knockaert D, Hofkens P. Acyclovir and neurologic manifestations. Ann Intern Med 99: 882, 1983.

Colin J, Hoh HB, Easty DL, et al. Ganciclovir ophthalmic gel (Virgan; 0.15%) in the treatment of herpes simplex keratitis. Cornea 16(4): 393–399, 1997.

Collum LMT, Logan P, Ravenscroft T. Acyclovir (Zovirax) in herpetic disciform keratitis. Br J Ophthalmol 67: 115, 1983.

de Koning EWJ, van Bijsterveld OP, Cantell K. Combination therapy for dendritic keratitis with acyclovir and α-interferon. Arch Ophthalmol 101: 1983, 1866.

Jones PG, Beier-Hanratty SA. Acyclovir: neurologic and renal toxicity. Ann Intern Med 104: 892, 1986.

Koliopoulos J. Acyclovir – a promising antiviral agent: a review of the preclinical and clinical data in ocular herpes simplex management. Ann Ophthalmol 16: 19, 1984.

Ohashi Y. Treatment of herpetic keratitis with acyclovir: benefits and problems. Ophthalmologica 221(Suppl 1): 29–32, 1997.

Richards DM, et al. Acyclovir. A review of its pharmacodynamic properties and therapeutic efficacy. Drugs 26: 378, 1983.

Wilhelmus KR, Keener MJ, Jones DB, et al. Corneal lipidosis in patients with the acquired immunodeficiency syndrome. Am J Ophthalmol 119: 14–19, 1995

Generic name: Cidofovir.

Proprietary name: Vistide.

Primary use

A nucleotide analogue used in the treatment of cytomegalovirus retinitis in patients with AIDS.

Ocular side effects

Topical administration
1. Toxicity to skin and conjunctiva

Intravenous or intravitreal administration
Certain
1. Anterior uveitis
2. Intraocular pressure
   a. Decreased
   b. Hypotony
3. Decreased vision
4. Vitritis (intravitreal injections)
5. Ciliary body
   a. Non-pigment epithelial alterations
   b. Choroidal detachment

Systemic side effects

Ophthalmic use or exposure
Certain
1. Renal failure

Clinical significance

Cidofovir is an antiviral drug used intravenously or injected into the vitreous in HIV infected patients with cytomegalovirus retinitis (CMV). The most serious systemic adverse event, nephrotoxicity, can be minimized with intravitreal injection. Topical application of cidofovir 1% eye drops has been attempted without success due to local toxicity. Ocular side effects are dose and time dependent. While the drug may need to be discontinued due to severe uveitis with synechiae and cataracts, this is unusual. Acute anterior uveitis occurs in up to 44% in one series with up to 12% of patients developing hypotony. Taskintuna et al (1997) reported a 3% incidence of chronic hypotony with intravitreal injections. It is not unusual to lose more than two lines on the Snellen chart, but fortunately most patients recover most of this vision. Some visual loss may be permanent. How much loss is drug related versus CMV related is unclear. Many of the side effects are tolerable with lower dosages, and in most cases the iritis is controlled with topical ocular steroids and cycloplegics. While retinal detachments have been reported, it is unclear whether this is drug related or associated with the intraocular injection. Chavez de la Paz et al (1997) felt concomitant use of probenecid will decrease the incidence and severity of iritis. Pretreatment with topical ocular steroids was ineffective in decreasing the severity or incidence of the iritis. Davis et al (1997) pointed out that reduction of the dosage is effective in decreasing the severity of the ocular adverse reaction; however, if severe inflammation or hypotony persists, other medication should be considered. They also pointed out that it is unclear whether the drug and its ocular side effects are cumulative, although they have one case that suggests this. They have three cases of positive rechallenge.

REFERENCES AND FURTHER READING

Akler ME, Johnson DW, Burman WJ, Johnson SC. Anterior uveitis and hypotony after intravenous cidofovir for the treatment of cytomegalovirus retinitis. Ophthalmology 105(4): 651–657, 1998.

Barrier JH, Bani-Sadr F, Gaillard F, Raffi F. Recurrent iritis after intravenous administration of cidofovir. CID 25: 337, 1997.

Chavez de la Paz E, Arevalo JF, Kirsch LS, et al. Anterior nongranulomatous uveitis after intravitreal HPMPC (cidofovir) for the treatment of cytomegalovirus retinitis. Analysis and prevention. Ophthalmology 104(3): 539–544, 1997.

Davis JL, Taskintuna I, Freeman WR, et al. Iritis and hypotony after treatment with intravenous cidofovir for cytomegalovirus retinitis. Arch Ophthalmol 115(6): 733–736, 1997.

Fraunfelder FW, Rosenbaum T. Drug-induced uveitis – incidences, prevention and treatment. Drug Safety 17(3): 197–207, 1997.

Friedberg DN. Hypotony and visual loss with intravenous cidofovir treatment of cytomegalovirus retinitis. Arch Ophthalmol 115: 801–802, 1997.

Hillenkamp J, Reinhard T, Rudolf RS, et al. The effects of cidofovir 1% with and without cyclosporin A 1% as a topical treatment of acute adenoviral keratoconjunctivitis. A controlled clinical pilot study. Ophthalmology 109: 845–850, 2002.

Jabs DA. Cidofovir. Arch Ophthalmol 115: 785–786, 1997.

Kirsch LS, Arevalo JF, Chavez de la Paz E, et al. Intravitreal cidofovir (HPMPC) treatment of cytomegalovirus retinitis in patients with acquired immune deficiency syndrome. Ophthalmology 102(4): 533–542, 1995.

Kirsch LS, Arevalo JF, De Clercq E. Phase I/II study of intravitreal cidofovir for the treatment of cytomegalovirus retinitis in patients with the acquired immunodeficiency syndrome. Am J Ophthalmol 119(4): 466–476, 1995.

Labetoulle M, Goujard C, Frau E, et al. Cidofovir ocular toxicity is related to previous ocular history. AIDS 14: 622–623, 2000.

Lin AP, Holland GN, Engstrom RE Jr. Vitrectomy and silicone oil tamponade for cidofovir-associated hypotony with ciliary body detachment. Retina 19(1): 75–76, 1999.

Scott RAH, Pavesio C. Ocular side-effects from systemic HPMPC (cidofovir) for a non-ocular cytomegalovirus infection. Am J Ophthalmol 130: 126–127, 2000.

Taskintuna I, Rahhal FM, Rao NA, et al. Adverse events and autopsy findings after intravitreous cidofovir (HPMPC) therapy in patients with acquired immune deficiency sydrome (AIDS). Ophthalmology 104(11): 1827–1836, 1997.

Generic names: 1. Idoxuridine (IDU); 2. trifluridine (F3T, trifluorothymidine).

Proprietary names: 1. Dendrid, Herplex; 2. Viroptic.

Primary use
Idoxuridine and trifluridine are used in the treatment of herpes simplex keratitis.

Ocular side effects

Local ophthalmic use or exposure
Certain
1. Irritation
   a. Lacrimation
   b. Hyperemia
   c. Photophobia
   d. Ocular pain
   e. Edema
2. Cornea
   a. Superficial punctate keratitis
   b. Edema
   c. Filaments
   d. Delayed wound healing
   e. Erosions or indolent ulceration
   f. Stromal opacities
   g. Superficial vascularization (late)
3. Eyelids or conjunctiva
   a. Allergic reactions
   b. Hyperemia
   c. Blepharitis
   d. Conjunctivitis – follicular
   e. Edema
   f. Pemphigoid-like lesion with symblepharon
   g. Perilimbal filaments
   h. Conjunctival punctate staining
   i. Conjunctival scarring
   j. Conjunctival squamous metaplasia (Fig. 7.13g)

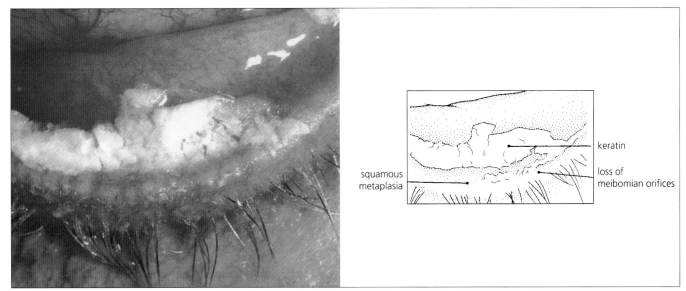

Fig. 7.13g Conjunctiva squamous metaplasia from topical idoxuridine. Photo courtesy of Spalton DJ, Hitchings RA, Hunter PA. Atlas of Clinical Ophthalmology, 3rd edn, Mosby Elsevier, London, 2005.

4. Lacrimal system
   a. Canaliculitis
   b. Stenosis
   c. Occlusion
5. Ptosis

Probable

1. Cornea – epithelial dysplasia (chronic therapy)

Possible

1. Eyelids or conjunciva – ischemia (trifluridine)

Clinical significance

Adverse ocular reactions to topical ophthalmic antivirals are often overlooked and frequently assumed to be a worsening of the clinical disease. Ocular side effects seem to occur most frequently in eyes with decreased tear production and on long-term therapy. Idoxuridine causes the highest degree of local irritation and toxicity, followed by trifluridine. There is evidence of cross-reactivity with the other pyrimidine analogues, not only ocular but cutaneous as well. The occasional appearance of corneal clouding, stippling and small punctate defects in the corneal epithelium is common. These corneal changes can be painful, even in partially anesthetic corneas, but resolve after the drug has been discontinued. Ocular side effects secondary to these agents are confusing, in large part due to the normal sequelae of the disease and already compromised tissue being exposed frequently to the drug and its preservatives. However, probably the most clinically important side effect is when the epithelial viral disease is in check, but the antiviral medication plus the preservatives will not allow the epithelium to heal. Topical rose bengal stain of the epithelial edges will be ragged (fiord pattern), meaning the virus is still active, while a smooth, often slightly elevated edge means the viral process is inactive. While most of the above Ocular side effects are reversible once the drug is stopped, some are quite indolent or irreversible. Ptosis, either from habit, chronic edema or possibly drug enhanced, may never completely recover. Occlusion of the lacrimal outflow system may be permanent. Some of the stromal scarring may be enhanced by the delay in wound healing by these agents. Ischemic changes have been reported in the conjunctiva and anterior segment, possibly secondary to trifluridine (Falcon et al 1981; Shearer and Bourne 1990). These changes were described as irreversible, including iris atrophy.

Jayamanne et al (1997) described a case of reversible anterior ischemia possibly due to trifluridine.

Although several instances of premalignant changes have occurred after application of topical antivirals, the causal relationship has not been proven, in part since herpes type II has been associated with malignant changes. These agents are best not used during pregnancy. While they have teratogenic effects in animals in high dosages, at the dosages used in ophthalmology, with punctal occlusion, they may be safe. However, every effort should be made not to use them during pregnancy, and if you do, a signed informed consent seems prudent. The agents should be safe in nursing mothers, since the dosages are low; however, again, it is prudent not to use these agents, even though they are probably safe.

REFERENCES AND FURTHER READING

Falcon MG, Jones BR, Williams HP, et al. Adverse reactions in the eye from topical therapy with idoxuridine, adenine arabinoside and trifluorothymidine. In: Herpetische Augenerkrankungen, Sundmacher R (ed), JF Bergmann, Munich, pp 263–268, 1981.

Jayamanne DGR, Vize C, Ellerton CR, et al. Severe reversible ocular anterior segment ischaemia following topical trifluorothymidine (F3T) treatment for herpes simplex keratouveitis (letter). Eye 11(Pt 5): 757–759, 1997.

Kaufman HE. Chemical blepharitis following drug treatment. Am J Ophthalmol 95: 703, 1983.

Kremer I, Rozenbaum D, Aviel E. Immunofluorescence findings in pseudo-pemphigoid induced by short-term idoxuridine administration. Am J Ophthalmol 111(3): 375–377, 1991.

Lass JH, Troft RA, Dohlman CH. Idoxuridine-induced conjunctival cicatrization. Arch Ophthalmol 101: 747, 1983.

Maudgal PC, Van Damme B, Missotten L. Corneal epithelial dysplasia after trifluridine use. Graefes Arch Clin Exp Ophthalmol 220: 6, 1983.

Patten JT, Cavanagh HD, Allansmith MR. Induced ocular pseudopemphigoid. Am J Ophthalmol 82: 272, 1976.

Shearer DR, Bourne WM. Severe ocular anterior segment ischemia after long-term trifluridine treatment for presumed herpetic keratitis. Am J Ophthalmol 109: 346–347, 1990.

Udell IJ. Trifluridine-associated conjunctival cicatrization. Am J Ophthalmol 99: 363, 1985.

CLASS: CARBONIC ANHYDRASE INHIBITORS

Generic names: 1. Acetazolamide; 2. methazolamide.

Proprietary names: 1. Diamox; 2. generic only.

Primary use

These enzyme inhibitors are effective in the treatment of all types of glaucomas. Acetazolamide is also effective in edema due to congestive heart failure, drug-induced edema and centrencephalic epilepsies.

Ocular side effects

Systemic administration
Certain
1. Decreased vision
2. Myopia
3. Lens
   a. Hydration
   b. Forward displacement
   c. Posterior displacement
4. Eyelids or conjunctiva
   a. Allergic reactions
   b. Erythema
   c. Photosensitivity
   d. Urticaria
   e. Purpura
   f. Loss of eyelashes or eyebrows
5. Problems with color vision (methazolamide)
   a. Color vision defect
   b. Objects have yellow tinge
6. Ocular signs of gout
7. Subconjunctival or retinal hemorrhages secondary to drug-induced anemia
8. Retinal or macular edema (hypotony)
9. Iritis

Probable
1. ERG changes

Possible
1. Eyelids or conjunctiva
   a. Erythema multiforme
   b. Stevens-Johnson syndrome
   c. Lyell's syndrome

Systemic side effects

Systemic administration
Certain
1. Malaise syndrome
   a. Acidosis
   b. Asthenia
   c. Anorexia
   d. Weight loss
   e. Depression
   f. Somnolence
   g. Confusion
   h. Impotence
2. Paresthesia
3. Taste disoders
4. Gastrointestinal disorder
   a. Nausea
   b. Vomiting
   c. Gastrointestinal irritation
5. Renal disorder (usually in persons with pre-existing renal disease)
   a. Urolithiasis
   b. Polyuria
   c. Hematuria
   d. Glycosuria
   e. Calculi
   f. Tubular acidosis
6. Eyelids or conjunctiva
   a. Allergic reactions
   b. Erythema
   c. Photosensitivity
   d. Urticaria
   e. Purpura
   f. Hair loss or new growth
7. Respiratory problems
   a. Acidosis
   b. Aggravation of severe chronic lung disease
8. Increased aspirin-induced CNS toxicity
9. Blood dyscrasia
   a. Aplastic anemia
   b. Pancytopenia
   c. Thrombocytopenia
   d. Agranulocytosis
   e. Hypochromic anemia
   f. Eosinophilia
10. Gout
   a. Increased serum uric acid
   b. Gouty arthritis
11. Ammonia intoxication
12. Teratogenicity – contraindicated in pregnancy (in animal studies)

Probable
1. Osteomalacia – primarily with dilantin use

Possible
1. Anaphylactic shock or death
2. Eyelids or conjunctiva
   a. Erythema multiforme
   b. Stevens-Johnson syndrome
   c. Lyell's syndrome

Clinical significance

Ocular side effects secondary to carbonic anhydrase inhibitors are transient and usually insignificant. Acute reversible myopia, ranging from 1 to 8 diopters, usually occurs within hours to days after starting the drug. This can occur especially in the last months of pregnancy when the drug is given for water retention without toxemia. There are also numerous reports of deepening or shallowing of the anterior chamber with or without alterations in the hydration of the lens. One of the more unusual side effects, however, is reported by Vela and Campbell (1985), in which the drug induced a ciliochoroidal detachment after glaucoma surgery. Other ocular side effects are usually of minimal importance and do not appear to be dose related.

Systemic side effects from oral or intravenous CAI are common. Patients may be unaware of how poorly they tolerate these drugs until they are discontinued. The quality of life in some patients is profoundly affected. One of the most bothersome side effects is the overall malaise and weakness that these drugs may cause. This syndrome may include marked changes in perception of taste, anorexia, generalized malaise, severe depression, decreased libido and impotence. This overall syndrome is the primary cause of patients discontinuing the drug. Paresthesia is one of the most common initial side effects, with numbness and tingling around the mouth, face and extremities. This side effect usually gets better with time. Gastrointestinal disturbances are common and characterized by generalized stomach and gastrointestinal irritation. Delayed release forms of this medicine have markedly improved this side effect. Renal problems are more common in those patients with a prior history of renal disease and stone producers. Uric acid retention with elevation of serum uric acid occasionally with gouty arthritis can be seen secondary to oral CAI.

Numerous skin problems have been reported. Most are those typically seen with sulfa drugs and are usually transitory if the medication is stopped. However, recent reports by Flach et al (1995) pointed out a possible increased incidence of Stevens-Johnson syndrome in Japanese Americans exposed to CAI. In patients with severe chronic obstructive lung disease, CAI may cause significant CO_2 retention with respiratory acidosis and respiratory failure. In the elderly, severely diabetic and those with severe renal disease, metabolic acidosis may also occur. This may be enhanced in patients simultaneously receiving medication that causes frank hypokalemia. The need to watch for potassium depletion is well recognized. Tabbara et al (1998) recently reported that CAIs, when used in a uveitis patient on cyclosporine, may have a marked elevation in blood levels of cyclosporine.

In severe liver disease, including cirrhosis, CAIs are contraindicated since ammonia intoxication can result. In patients on high oral dosages of salicylates, CAI may increase salicylate concentration in the CNS, causing salicylate toxicity, including convulsions.

While there are few reports of CAI-associated teratogenic effects (Worshan-sacrococcygeal teratoma) there is a host of animal work showing that these agents are highly suspect therefore most feel these agents are contraindicated in pregnancy.

As with all pure sulfa preparations, drug-induced blood dyscrasias can occur. However, few sulfas are used for as long a period as those for glaucoma patients. Keisu et al (1990) provided an estimate of the frequency of CAI-associated aplastic anemia. Their data for Sweden show that exposure to acetazolamide has an incidence 25 times higher in males and 10 times higher in females than the control group. They calculate one case of aplastic anemia for 18 000 patient years of exposure, which is significantly higher than with oral chloramphenicol. In their study, as also in the almost 400 cases of possible CAI-related blood dyscrasis in the National Registry, between 35 and 45% are aplastic anemia, with the remainder leukopenia, agranulocytosis, pancytopenia, thrombocytopenia, hypochromic anemia or eosinophilia. New methods of treatment may salvage one-third of aplastic anemia cases and a majority of the rest of the dyscrasias. Early discovery, stopping the inciting agent, finding this with blood tests prior to symptoms, and earlier treatment have increased the cure rate.

Recommendations for following patients on carbonic anhydrase inhibitors

To date, we have not had any blood dyscrasias associated with topical ocular CAIs nor do we have any reports of blood dyscrasia in the National Registry from oral CAI exposure of less than 2 weeks. We consider short-term CAI therapy to be safe. Our current recommendations for following patients on oral CAIs include:

1. Before starting the drug, obtain a complete blood count, which should be repeated every 2 months during the first 6 months, and then every 6 to 12 months.
2. Have the patient call you if any of the following develop:

   persistent sore throat   pallor
   fever   fatigue
   easy bruising   jaundice
   nosebleeds   red blotches

3. A drop in any level of formed blood element calls for stopping the drug and seeking hematologic consultation.

Since the majority of the ophthalmic community has not accepted the above recommendations, as long as informed consent has been explained to the patient, this should not be considered at this point in time to be the standard of ophthalmic practice.

REFERENCES AND FURTHER READING

Aminlari A. Falling scalp hairs. Glaucoma 6: 41–42, 1984.

Barbey F, Nseir G, Ferrier C, et al. Carbonic anhydrase inhibitors and calcium phosphate stones. Nephrologie 25: 169–172, 2004.

Elinav E, Ackerman Z, Gotteherer NP, et al. Recurrent life-threatening acidosis induced by acetazolamide in a patient with diabetic type IV renal tubular acidosis. Ann Emerg Med 40: 259–260, 2002.

Epstein RJ, Allen RC, Lunde MW. Organic impotence associated with carbonic anhydrase inhibitor therapy for glaucoma. Ann Ophthalmol 19: 48, 1987.

Flach AJ, Smith RE, Fraunfelder FT. Stevens-Johnson syndrome associated with methazolamide treatment reported in two Japanese-American women. Ophthalmology 102: 1677–1680, 1995.

Fraunfelder FT, et al. Hematologic reactions to carbonic anhydrase inhibitors. Am J Ophthalmol 100: 79, 1985.

Gallerani M, Manzoli N, Fellin R, et al. Anaphylactic shock and acute pulmonary edema after a single oral dose of acetazolamide. Am J Emerg Med 20: 371–372, 2002.

Keisu M, Wiholm BE, Ost A, Mortimer O. Acetazolamide-associated aplastic anemia. J Int Med 228: 627–632, 1990.

Kodjikian L, Duran B, Burillon C, et al. Acetazolamide-induced thrombocytopenia. Arch Ophthalmol 122: 1543–1544, 2004.

Lichter PR. Reducing side effects of carbonic anhydrase inhibitors. Ophthalmology 88: 266, 1981.

Margo CE. Acetazolamide and advanced liver disease. Am J Ophthalmol 100: 611, 1986.

Niven BI, Manoharan A. Acetazolamide-induced anaemia. Med J Aust 142: 120, 1985.

Shirato S, Kagaya F, Suzuki Y, et al. Stevens-Johnson syndrome induced by methazolamide treatment. Arch Ophthalmol 115: 550–553, 1997.

Shuster JN. Side effects of commonly used glaucoma medications. Geriatr Ophthalmol 2: 30, 1986.

Tabbara KF, Al-Faisal Z, Al-Rashed W. Interaction between acetazolamide and cyclosporine. Arch Ophthalmol 116: 832–833, 1998.

Vela MA, Campbell DG. Hypotony and ciliochoroidal detachment following pharmacologic aqueous suppressant therapy in previously filtered patients. Ophthalmology 92: 50–57, 1985.

White GL, Pribble JP, Murdock RT. Acetazolamide and the sulfonamide-sensitive patient. Ophthalmol Times 10: 15, 1985.

CLASS: DECONGESTANTS

Generic names: 1. Naphazoline; 2. tetryzoline hydrochloride.

Proprietary names: 1. Albalon, Clear eyes, Nafazair, Vasocon; 2. Tyzine, Visine.

Primary use

These sympathomimetic amines are effective in the symptomatic relief of ophthalmic congestion of allergic or inflammatory origin.

Ocular side effects

Local ophthalmic use or exposure
Certain
1. Conjunctival vasoconstriction
2. Irritation
   a. Lacrimation
   b. Reactive hyperemia
   c. Ocular pain
   d. Burning sensation

3. Mydriasis – may precipitate angle-closure glaucoma
4. Increased intraocular pressure
5. Decreased vision
6. Punctate keratitis
7. Allergic reactions
   a. Conjunctivitis
   b. Blepharoconjunctivitis

Probable
1. Increased pigment granules in anterior chamber
2. Decreased tolerance to contact lenses
3. Increased width of palpebral fissures

Systemic side effects

Local ophthalmic use or exposure
Certain
1. Headache
2. Hypertension
3. Nervousness
4. Nausea
5. Dizziness
6. Asthenia
7. Somnolence

Possible
1. Stroke
2. Cardiac arrhythmia
3. Hyperglycemia
4. Hypothermia
5. Anaphylaxis

Clinical significance

Ocular side effects due to these ocular decongestants are seldom significant, except with frequent or long-term use. The conjunctival vasculature may fail to respond to the vasoconstrictive properties when these agents are used excessively or for prolonged periods. Abelson et al (1980) have shown that if these drugs are given nasally, no rebound vasodilatation occurs, even with frequent and prolonged exposure. They postulate that if the clinician sees this, it is due to 1) the tissue returning to baseline which is already hyperemic from another cause, 2) a hypersensitivity reaction to a component of the ophthalmic solution or toxicity from overuse, or 3) tachyphylaxis. Naphazoline and tetryzoline are over-the-counter preparations. There are over 400 spontaneous reports of mydriasis associated with these agents (especially with naphazoline) that have been given to the FDA. A warning about angle-closure glaucoma has now been included. Cases of bilateral acute angle-closure glaucoma secondary to tetryzoline use have been reported to the National Registry and are in the literature. Soparkar et al (1997) did a landmark study of these over-the-counter vasoconstrictors, used from 8 hours to 20 years. Clinical patterns included conjunctival hyperemia, follicular conjunctivitis and eczematoid blepharoconjunctivitis. The most interesting part of this study was the length of time off medication before these adverse effects resolved. This ranged from 1 to 24 weeks with a mean of 4 weeks. Any preparation used this long, especially those containing benzalkonium chloride (which most of these do), has the potential for conjunctival scarring, including epithelial changes with occlusion of the lacrimal outflow system. Adverse ocular reactions secondary to these drugs are almost always reversible with discontinuation of the drug; however, keratitis requiring months to resolve has been reported.

In addition, the National Registry has received reports of a possible association of acute central retinal artery occlusion related to topical ocular naphazoline. Major systemic adverse reactions following use of ocular decongestants are rare and occur primarily when ocular decongestants are used more frequently than recommended by the manufacturer.

REFERENCES AND FURTHER READING

Abelson MB, Allansmith MR, Friedlaender MH. Effects of topically applied ocular decongestant and antihistamine. Am J Ophthalmol 90: 254, 1980.

Abelson MB, Yamamoto GK, Allansmith MR. Effects of ocular decongestants. Arch Ophthalmol 98: 856, 1980.

Abelson MB, et al. Tolerance and absence of rebound vasodilation following topical ocular decongestant usage. Ophthalmology 91: 1364–1367, 1984.

Cook BE Jr., Holtan SB. Mydriasis from inadvertent topical application of naphazoline hydrochloride. Contact Lens Assoc Ophthalmol 24(2): 72, 1998.

Gandolfi C. Therapeutic ocular application of sympathomimetic substances. Boll Oculist 26: 397–400, 1947.

Grossmann EE, Lehman RH. Ophthalmic use of Tyzine. Am J Ophthalmol 42: 121, 1956.

Khan MAJ, Watt LL, Hugkulstone CE. Bilateral acute angle-closure glaucoma after use of Fenox nasal drops. Eye 16: 662–663, 2002.

Lisch K. Conjunctival alterations by sympathomimetic drugs. Klin Mbl Augenheilk 173: 404–406, 1973.

Menger HC. New ophthalmic decongestant, tetrahydrozoline hydrochloride. JAMA 170: 178, 1959.

Rich LF. Toxic drug effects on the cornea. J Toxicol Cut Ocular Toxicol 1: 267, 1982–1983.

Skilling FC Jr, Weaver TA, Kato KP, et al. Effects of two eye drop products on computer users with subjective ocular discomfort. Optometry 76: 47–54, 2005.

Soparkar CN, Wilhelmus KR, Koch DD, et al. Acute and chronic conjunctivitis due to over-the-counter ophthalmic decongestants. Arch Ophthalmol 115(1): 34–38, 1997.

Stamer UM, Buderus S, Wetegrove S, et al. Prolonged awakening and pulmonary edema after general anesthesia and naphazoline application in an infant. Anesth Analg 93: 1162–1164, 2001.

Williams TL, Williams AJ, Enzenauer RW. Case report: unilateral mydriasis from topical Opcon-A and soft contact lens. Aviat Space Environ Med 68(11): 1035–1037, 1997.

CLASS: MIOTICS

Generic name: Acetylcholine.

Proprietary names: Miochol, Miochol-E.

Primary use

This intraocular quaternary ammonium parasympathomimetic agent is used to produce prompt, short-term miosis.

Ocular side effects

Local ophthalmic use or exposure – subconjunctival or intracameral injection
Certain
1. Miosis
2. Decreased intraocular pressure
3. Conjunctival hyperemia
4. Accommodative spasm
6. Lacrimation
7. Decreased anterior chamber depth
8. Cataract – transient

Probable
1. Paradoxical mydriasis – rare
2. Blepharoclonus

Systemic side effects

Local ophthalmic use or exposure – subconjunctival or intracameral injection

Certain
1. Bradycardia
2. Hypotension
3. Vasodilation
4. Dyspnea
5. Perspiration

Clinical significance

Few ocular side effects due to acetylcholine are seen. Although miosis is the primary ophthalmic effect, mydriasis may occur on rare occasions. Ocular side effects are rarely of clinical significance. A few cases of corneal edema have been reported to the National Registry, but it is difficult to distinguish the drug's effects from surgical trauma. Once a new buffering system was added to the formulation, the incidence of corneal clouding almost disappeared. Most of the endothelial damage is possibly secondary to the 'fire hose' effect of forcing fluid through a small bore needle, which then causes fluid to come out at a high velocity and damages endothelial cells. The current products have been shown to be non-toxic to the endothelium. Transient lens opacities have been reported, probably on the basis of an osmotic effect. To date, no long-term effect on the lens has been seen due to this drug. If acetylcholine is administered intraocularly, it may cause lacrimation. Bradycardia and hypotension have been seen following irrigation of the anterior chamber with acetylcholine.

REFERENCES AND FURTHER READING

Brinkley JR Jr., Henrick A. Vascular hypotension and bradycardia following intraocular injection of acetylcholine during cataract surgery. Am J Ophthalmol 97: 40, 1984.

Fraunfelder FT. Corneal edema after use of carbachol. Arch Ophthalmol 97: 975, 1979.

Fraunfelder FT. Recent advances in ocular toxicology. In: Ocular Therapeutics, Srinivasan BD (ed), Masson, New York, pp 123–126, 1980.

Gombos GM. Systemic reactions following intraocular acetylcholine instillation. Ann Ophthalmol 11: 529, 1982.

Grimmett MR, Williams KK, Broocker G, et al. Corneal edema after miochol (letter). Am J Ophthalmol 116(2): 236–238, 1993.

Hagan J. Severe bradycardia and hypotension following intraocular acetylcholine in patients who previously tolerated the medication. Missouri Med 87: 4, 1990.

Hollands RH, Drance SM, Schulzer M. The effect of acetylcholine on early postoperative intraocular pressure. Am J Ophthalmol 103: 749–753, 1987.

Lazar M, Rosen N, Nemet P. Miochol-induced transient cataract. Ann Ophthalmol 9: 1142, 1977.

Leopold IH. The use and side effects of cholinergic agents in the management of intraocular pressure. In: Glaucoma: Applied Pharmacology in Medical Treatment, Drance SM, Neufeld AH (eds), Grune & Stratton, New York, p 357–393, 1984.

Rasch D, et al. Bronchospasm following intraocular injection of acetylcholine in a patient taking metoprolol. Anesthesiology 59: 583, 1983.

Yee RW, Meenakshi S, Yu HS, et al. Effects of acetylcholine and carbachol on bovine corneal endothelial cells in vitro. J Cataract Refract Surg 22(5): 591–596, 1996.

Generic name: Dapiprazole hydrochloride.

Proprietary name: Rev-eyes.

Primary use

This agent is an alpha-adrenergic receptor blocker that is used topically on the eye to reverse mydriasis after pharmacologic dilation. It is also used to treat pigmentary glaucoma and to decrease night haloes after excimer keratectomy. Some clinicians may prescribe this medication for photic phonomena following refractive surgery.

Ocular side effects

Local ophthalmic use or exposure

Certain
1. Burning/stinging
2. Conjunctiva
   a. Bulbar injection
   b. Palpebral injection
   c. Chemosis
3. Conjunctiva
   a. Superficial punctate keratitis
   b. Edema
4. Eyelids
   a. Edema
   b. Ptosis
   c. Erythema
   d. Allergic or irritative reactions
5. Dryness
6. Browache
7. Photophobia
8. Epiphora
9. Blurred vision
10. Ocular pain

Systemic side effects

Local ophthalmic use or exposure

Certain
1. Headaches
2. Allergic or anaphylactic reactions – rare

Clinical significance

Dapiprazole blocks the alpha-adrenergic receptor in smooth muscle and produces miosis through an effect on the dilator muscle of the iris. Many of the adverse drug effects are due to the pharmacologic alpha-adrenergic properties of the drug, such as dilatation of the conjunctival blood vessels therefore close to 100% of eyes will show hyperemia. In rare instances this can be severe, but mostly it resolves within 20–30 minutes or, at worst, within 24 hours. Ocular stinging and burning occur 20–30% of the time with lid edema and ptosis in the 10% range. All side effects are transitory and reversible. Corneal changes may occur, but are also transitory. Theoretically, this agent should be used with care in patients with disturbed epithelium since the drug can be toxic to the corneal endothelium. Unlike pilocarpine, dapiprazole has little effect on accommodation, anterior chamber depth or lens thickness.

There have been reports to the National Registry of urinary incontinence, but this is hard to prove as drug related. The only major systemic findings are occasional headaches. The manufacturer suggests two drops per eye, repeated in 5 minutes. Wilcox et al (1995) suggest giving only one drop once, not twice, as being efficacious with fewer side effects.

REFERENCES AND FURTHER READING

Bonomi L, Marchinni G, De Gregorio M. Ultrasonographic study of the ocular effects of topical dorzolamide. Glaucoma 8: 30–31, 1986.

Cheeks L, Chapman JM, Green K. Corneal endothelial toxicity of dapiprazole hydrochloride. Lens Eye Toxicity Res 9: 79–84, 1992.

Dudley DF, et al. Counteracting the effects of pharmacologic mydriasis with dapiprazole. Investi Ophthalmol Vis Sci 35(4): 32, 1994.

Iuglio N. Ocular effects of topical application of dapiprazole in man. Glaucoma 6: 110–116, 1984.

Marx-Gross S, Krummenauer F, Dick HB, et al. Brimonidine versus dapiprazole: influence on pupil size at various illumination levels. J Cataract Refract Surg 31: 1372–1376, 2005.

Wilcox CS, et al. Comparison of the effects on pupil size and accommodation of three regimens of topical dapiprazole. Br J Ophthalmol 79: 544–548, 1995.

Generic name: Ecothiopate iodide.

Proprietary name: Phospholine iodide.

Primary use

This topical anticholinesterase is used in the management of open-angle glaucoma, conditions in which movement or constriction of the pupil is desired, and in accommodative esotropia.

Ocular side effects

Local ophthalmic use or exposure
Certain
1. Miosis
2. Decreased vision
3. Accommodative spasm
4. Irritation
   a. Lacrimation
   b. Hyperemia
   c. Photophobia
   d. Ocular pain
   e. Edema
   f. Burning sensation
5. Cataracts
   a. Anterior or posterior subcapsular
6. Eyelids or conjunctiva
   a. Allergic reactions
   b. Conjunctivitis – follicular
   c. Chemosis
   d. Depigmentation (isoflurophate)
7. Myopia
8. Iris or ciliary body cysts – especially in children
9. Intraocular pressure
   a. Increased – initial
   b. Decreased
10. Iritis
    a. Occasional fine keratitic precipitates (KP)
    b. Activation of latent iritis or uveitis
    c. Formation of anterior or posterior synechiae
11. Decreased scleral rigidity
12. Occlusion of lacrimal canaliculi
13. Decreased anterior chamber depth
14. Retinal detachment
15. May aggravate myasthenia gravis

Probable
1. Eyelids or conjunctiva
   a. Pemphigoid lesion with symblepharon
2. Decreased size of filtering bleb

Possible
1. Blepharoclonus
2. Hyphema – during surgery
3. Vitreous hemorrhages
4. Cystoid macular edema

Systemic side effects

Local ophthalmic use or exposure
Certain
1. Gastrointestinal disorders
   a. Nausea
   b. Vomiting
   c. Abdominal pain
   d. Diarrhea
2. Urinary incontinence
3. Increased saliva
4. Dyspnea
5. Bradycardia
6. Cardiac arrhythmia
7. Perspiration
8. Asthenia

Clinical significance

Visual complaints with or without accommodative spasm are the most frequent adverse ocular reactions. Drug-induced lens changes are well documented and are primarily seen in the older age group. In shallow anterior chamber angles, these agents are contraindicated because they may precipitate angle-closure glaucoma. This is probably due to peripheral vascular congestion of the iris and a possible forward shift of the lens-iris diaphragm, which may further aggravate an already compromised angle. While irritative conjunctival changes are common with long-term use, allergic reactions are rare. This strong miotic, primarily in diseased retinas, may cause retinal detachments by exerting traction on the peripheral retina. (See Pilocarpine for a more detailed explanation of possible cause.) Halperin and Goldman (1993) report a case of cystoid macular edema after echothiophate iodide. We do not know of any other cases. Cases of irreversible miosis due to long-term therapy have been reported. An atypical band-shaped keratopathy has been said to be due to long-term miotic therapy; however, others suggest that this is due to long-term elevation of intraocular pressure and is not drug-induced. A slowly progressive drug-related cicatricial process of the conjunctiva may be clinically indistinguishable from ocular cicatricial pemphigoid and may occur with this drug. Patients receiving topical ocular anticholinesterases and those being treated for myasthenia may have increased systemic and ocular side effect risks if exposed to organic phosphorus insecticides. In addition, anesthetic deaths have been reported in patients on topical ocular anticholinesterases after receiving suxamethonium. This effect is due to the lowered blood cholinesterase from the topical ocular anticholinesterase agents. Mezer et al (1996) described a case of hyper- and hypothyroidism induced by echothiophate iodide eye drops. They felt that the thyroid dysfunction was secondary to excessive iodide intake found in the eye drops. Ellenberg et al (1992) and Flach and Donahue (1994) pointed out that animal flea products contain anticholinesterase agents, which can get into the eyes by finger-to-eye contact or the insertion of contaminated contact lenses. This can cause a transitory miosis. Without this knowledge, a cascade of tests could occur if the patient entered an emergency room. Flach and Donahue (1994) pointed out that these agents are rapidly hydrolyzed by water and simply washing one's hands prevents this ocular contamination.

REFERENCES AND FURTHER READING

Adams SL, Mathews J, Grammer LC. Drugs that may exacerbate myasthenia gravis. Ann Emerg Med 13: 532, 1984.

Adler AG, et al. Systemic effects of eye drops. Arch Intern Med 142: 2293, 1982.

Eggers NM. Toxicity of drugs used in diagnosis and treatment of strabismus. In: Ocular Therapeutics, Srinivasan D (ed), Masson, New York, pp 115–122, 1980.

Ellenberg DJ, Spector LD, Lee A. Flea collar pupil. Ann Emerg Med 21: 1170, 1992.

Eshagian J. Human posterior subcapsular cataracts. Trans Ophthalmol Soc UK 102: 364, 1982.

Flach AJ, Donahue ME. Pet flea and tick collar-induced anisocoria. Arch Ophthalmol 112: 586, 1994.

Halperin LS, Goldman HB. Cystoid macular edema associated with topical echothiophate iodide. Ann Ophthalmol 25(12): 457–458, 1993.

Hirst LW, et al. Drug-induced cicatrizing conjunctivitis simulating ocular pemphigoid. Cornea 1: 121, 1982.

Mezer E, Krivoy N, Scharf J, et al. Echothiophate iodide induced transient hyper- and hypothyroidism. J Glaucoma 5(3): 191–192, 1996.

Tseng SCG, et al. Topical retinoid treatment for various dry-eye disorders. Ophthalmology 92: 717, 1985.

West RH, Cebon L, Gillies WE. Drop attack in glaucoma. The Melbourne experience with topical miotics, adrenergic and neuronal blocking drops. Aust J Ophthalmol 11: 149, 1983.

Wood JR, Anderson RL, Edwards JJ. Phospholine iodide toxicity and Jones' tubes. Ophthalmology 87: 346, 1980.

Generic name: Pilocarpine.

Proprietary names: Pilopine HS, Salagen.

Primary use

This topical ocular parasympathomimetic agent is used in the management of glaucoma and in conditions in which constriction of the pupil is desired.

Ocular side effects

Local ophthalmic use or exposure
Certain
1. Pupils
   a. Miosis
   b. Mydriasis – rare
2. Decreased vision (light hunger)
3. Paralysis or spasm of accommodation
4. Intraocular pressure
   a. Increased – initial
   b. Decreased
5. Anterior chamber
   a. Decreases depth
   b. Increases angle width in narrow angles
6. Eyelids or conjunctiva
   a. Allergic reactions
   b. Hyperemia
   c. Conjunctivitis – follicular
   d. Muscle spasms
7. Irritation
   a. Lacrimation
   b. Burning sensation
   c. Decreased tear production
8. Myopia – transient
9. Retina
   a. Bleeds (vitreous hemorrhage)
   b. Detachment
10. Cornea
    a. Punctate keratitis
    b. Edema
    c. Epithelial microcysts
    d. Atypical band keratopathy
11. Decreased dark adaptation
12. Iris cysts
13. Increased axial lens diameter
14. Decreased scleral rigidity
15. Malignant glaucoma

Probable
1. Eyelids or conjunctiva
   a. Angioneurotic edema
   b. Pseudomembrane
   c. Pseudo-ocular pemphigoid
   d. Cicatricial shortening of fornices
   e. Conjunctival dysplasia or epithelial proliferation (Fig. 7.13h)
   f. Conjunctival hemorrhage
2. Cornea – dysplasia or epithelial proliferation
3. Blepharoclonus
4. Cataracts
5. Iritis
6. Punctal or canalicular stenosis
7. Increases corneal transplant rejection

Possible
1. Retina – macular hole
2. Problems with color vision – color vision defect

Systemic side effects

Local ophthalmic use or exposure
Certain
1. Headache, browache
2. Perspiration
3. Gastrointestinal disorder
   a. Nausea
   b. Vomiting
   c. Diarrhea
   d. Spasms
4. Saliva increased
5. Tremor

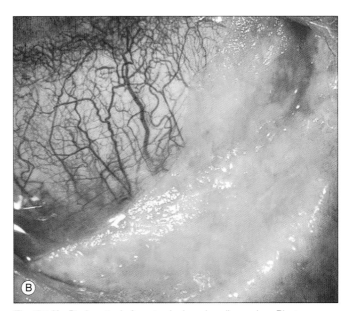

Fig. 7.13h Dsykeratosis from topical ocular pilocarpine. Photo courtesy of Spalton DJ, Hitchings RA, Hunter PA. Atlas of Clinical Ophthalmology, 3rd edn, Mosby Elsevier, London, 2005.

6. Bradycardia
7. Hypotension
8. Bronchospasm
9. Pulmonary edema
10. Mental status changes
    a. Confusion
    b. Short-term memory loss
    c. Depression
    d. Aggravation of Alzheimer's syndrome
    e. Aggravation of Parkinson's syndrome
11. Rhinorrhea

Probable

1. Epistaxis
2. Voice changes, including hoarseness

Possible

1. Tenesmus

Clinical significance

Side effects from pilocarpine can be divided by those that are primarily seen within minutes to hours and those that may take weeks, months or years to develop. The most frequent immediate effects are these that affect the pupil, including miosis that causes 'light hunger', effects on accommodation, transient myopia and periocular muscle spasms. Acute toxic or allergic reactions of the anterior segment are infrequent. The most bothersome effects are superficial punctate keratitis and, rarely, corneal edema. Cases of edema are primarily seen with a poor corneal epithelium, possibly allowing a direct drug or preservative effect on the corneal endothelium. The most serious side effects, however, are retinal detachment and malignant glaucoma. Retinal detachments or macular holes may be aggravated by drug-induced accommodation with forward displacement of the posterior lens surface and elongation of the eye. This causes a more anterior position of the vitreous face and body. This forward movement may cause traction in areas where the vitreous is attached to the retina. A partial macular hole (Stage 1-A) that resolved on discontinuation of the miotic has also been reported (Benedict and Shami 1992). Animal data show that a miotic can cause a pull on the peripheral retina by constriction of the ciliary body. Either of these mechanisms (i.e. forward vitreous displacement or accommodation in already diseased retinas) may precipitate a retinal hole or tear in an already compromised area of the retina. Vitreous hemorrhages have been reported secondary to this process involving a retinal vessel. Pilocarpine's ability to increase the A-P diameter of the lens and decrease the depth of the anterior chamber may also play a prominent role in some forms of malignant glaucoma. Massry and Assil (1995) and cases in the National Registry support the fact that pilocarpine does diminish corneal allograft immune privilege and enhances graft rejection. Kobayashi et al (1999) have shown that pilocarpine increases angular width in angle-closure eyes, and this is the reason that it is of value in the management of angle-closure glaucoma. Nuzzi et al (1998) described decreased tear secretion compared to controls after topical ocular pilocarpine. Fraunfelder and Morgan (1994) reported bizarre behavior after topical ocular pilocarpine was administered in elderly patients. This is possibly due to miosis causing 'light hunger', thereby causing a decrease in sensory input that may be enough to cause confusion in some patients. Reyes et al (1987) believe that this is most common in subclinical Alzheimer's syndrome patients. They postulated that this may be a direct pilocarpine effect on the CNS and noted an increase of symptomatology in patients with Parkinson's disease after taking topical ocular pilocarpine.

Ocular changes secondary to the long-term use of pilocarpine may be divided into those specifically due to the drug itself or due to various combinations of the drug, preservatives or vehicles. Iris cysts are due to the miosis induced by this drug. Pilocarpine may be a weak cataractogenic agent, but this is unproven. It is likely that most of the other side effects are due to repeated exposure of the drug and its preservatives over a period of months to years. This includes conjunctival, corneal and lacrimal outflow system changes. Epithelial microcysts similar in appearance to Cogan's microcystic dystrophy, but often smaller and usually clear, can be seen after long-term pilocarpine therapy. Corneal and conjunctival dysplasia or hyperplasia occur most often on the inferior nasal limbus. Chronic topical ocular drug exposure has been implicated in changes in the conjunctiva and Tenon's capsule to the extent that they may adversely influence the success of filtration procedures for glaucoma. Baudouin et al (1999), as well as Nuzzi et al (1998), have shown that these effects in the conjunctiva and trabecular meshwork are mainly due to benzalkonium chloride, but chronic exposure to the drug itself can also play a minor role. The above can also cause cicatricial shortening in the fornices, lacrimal outflow system and even pseudo-ocular pemphigoid.

The most frequent finding in the spontaneous reporting systems includes literally hundreds of reports of pilocarpine, of various concentrations, having no effect on intraocular pressure. Even today, with improved manufacturing, there are still occasional reports of pilocarpine causing mydriasis and cycloplegia. This is due to an impurity of the stereoisomer of pilocarpine, jaborine, an atropinelike drug. There have been numerous reports in the past of an atypical band keratopathy caused by phenylmercuric nitrate, a preservative no longer in use with pilocarpine. However, rare reports are still received by the National Registry of peripheral, white, subepithelial deposits occurring with pilocarpine use. This seems to occur more frequently in eyes with pre-existing band keratopathy. Iritis has been reported secondary to pilocarpine use. Human data support the fact that pilocarpine increases the blood-aqueous barrier permeability to plasma protein in a dose-dependent manner. In some individuals this will give cells and flare on slit lamp examination. Mothers on topical ocular pilocarpine giving birth may have infants with signs mimicking neonatal meningitis – hyperthermia, restlessness, convulsions and diaphoresis. Pediatricians should be made aware of this syndrome so unnecessary tests and manipulations are avoided. It is not known whether pilocarpine is excreted in human milk, but caution should be advised when miotics are administered to nursing mothers. Recently, pilocarpine has been found to cause a counter-productive backward shift in accommodating intraocular lenses.

REFERENCES AND FURTHER READING

Abramson DH, MacKay C, Coleman J. Pilocarpine-induced retinal tear: an ultrasonic evaluation of lens movements. Glaucoma 3: 9, 1981.

Ancelin ML, Artero S, Portet F, et al. Non-degenerative mild cognitive impairment in elderly people and use of anticholinergic drugs: longitudinal cohort study. BMJ [online]. http://www.bmj.com, 2006.

Baudouin C, Pisella PJ, Fillacier K, et al. Ocular surface inflammatory changes induced by topical antiglaucoma drugs: Human and animal studies. Ophthalmology 106(3): 556–563, 1999.

Beasley H, Fraunfelder FT. Retinal detachments and topical ocular miotics. Ophthalmology 86(1): 95–98, 1979.

Benedict WL, Shami M. Impending macular hole associated with topical pilocarpine. Am J Ophthalmol 114(6): 765–766, 1992.

Crandall AS, et al. Characterization of subtle corneal deposits. J Toxicol Cut Ocular Toxicol 3: 263, 1984.

Flore PM, Jacobs IH, Goldberg DB. Drug-induced pemphigoid. Arch Ophthalmol 105: 1660–1663, 1987.

Fraunfelder FT, Morgan R. The aggravation of dementia by pilocarpine. JAMA 271(22): 1742–1743, 1994.

Kastl PR. Inadvertent systemic injection of pilocarpine. Arch Ophthalmol 105: 28, 1987.

Kobayashi H, Kobayashi K, Kiryu J, et al. Pilocarpine induces an increase in the anterior chamber angular width in eyes with narrow angles. Br J Ophthalmol 83: 553–558, 1999.

Koeppl C, Findl O, Menapace R. Pilocarpine-induced shift of an accommodating intraocular lens: AT-45 Crystalens. J Cataract Refract Surg 31: 1290–1297, 2005.

Levine RZ. Uniocular miotic therapy. Trans Am Acad Ophthmol Otolaryngol 79: 376–380, 1975.

Littman L, et al. Severe symptomatic atrioventricular block induced by pilocarpine eye drops. Arch Intern Med 147: 586, 1987.

Massry GG, Assil KK. Pilocarpine-associated allograft rejection in post-keratoplasty patients. Cornea 14(2): 202–205, 1995.

Merritt JC. Malignant glaucoma induced by miotics postoperatively in open-angle glaucoma. Arch Ophthalmol 95: 1988–1989, 1977.

Mishra P, et al. Intraoperative bradycardia and hypotension associated with timolol and pilocarpine eye drops. Br J Anaesth 55: 897, 1983.

Mori M, Araie M, Sakurai M, Oshika T. Effects of pilocarpine and tropicamide on blood-aqueous barrier permeability in man. Invest Ophthalmol Vis Sci 33(2): 416–423, 1992.

Naveh-Floman N, Stahl V, Korczyn AD. Effect of pilocarpine on intraocular pressure in ocular hypertensive subjects. Ophthalmic Res 18: 34, 1986.

Nuzzi R, Finazzo C, Cerruti A. Adverse effects of topical antiglaucomatous medications on the conjuncitva and the lachrymal response. Intern Ophthalmol 22(1): 31–35, 1998.

Pouliquen Y, Patey A, Foster CS, et al. Druginduced cicatricial pemphigoid affecting the conjunctiva. Ophthalmology 93(6): 775–783, 1986.

Reyes PF, et al. Mental status changes induced by eye drops in dementia of the Alzheimer type. J Neurol Neurosurg Psychiatry 50: 113, 1987.

Samples JR, Meyer SM. Use of ophthalmic medications in pregnant and nursing women. Am J Ophthalmol 106(5): 616–623, 1988.

Schuman JS, Hersh P, Kylstra J. Vitreous hemorrhage associated with pilocarpine. Am J Ophthalmol 108(3): 333–334, 1989.

Schwab IR, Linberg JV, Gioia VM, Benson WH, Chao GM. Foreshortening of the inferior conjunctival fornix associated with chronic glaucoma medications. Ophthalmology 99(2): 197–202, 1992.

Sherwood MB, Grierson I, Millar L, Hitchings RA. Long-term morphologic effects of antiglaucoma drugs on the conjunctiva and Tenon's capsule in glaucomatous patients. Ophthalmology 96(3): 327–335, 1989.

CLASS: MYDRIATICS AND CYCLOPLEGICS

Generic names: 1. Cyclopentolate hydrochloride;
2. tropicamide.

Proprietary names: 1. Akpentolate, Cyclogyl, Pentolair;
2. Topicacyl, Mydriacyl.

Primary use
These topical ocular short-acting anticholinergic mydriatic and cycloplegic agents are used in refractions and fundus examination.

Ocular side effects

Local ophthalmic use or exposure
Certain
1. Decreased vision
2. Mydriasis – may precipitate angle-closure glaucoma
3. Irritation
   a. Hyperemia
   b. Photophobia
   c. Ocular pain
   d. Burning sensation
4. Decrease or paralysis of accommodation
5. Increased intraocular pressure
6. Eyelids or conjunctiva
   a. Allergic reactions
   b. Blepharoconjunctivitis
   c. Urticaria

7. Keratitis
8. Ambloypia (patients 3 months or younger)

Systemic side effects

Local ophthalmic use or exposure
Certain
1. CNS effects
   a. Personality disorders
   b. Psychosis
   c. Ataxia
   d. Speech disorder
   e. Agitation
   f. Hallucinations
   g. Confusion
   h. Convulsion
   i. Emotional changes
   j. Loss of equilibrium
   k. Seizures
2. Tachycardia
3. Fever
4. Vasodilation
5. Urinary retention
6. Nausea
7. Dry mouth
8. Paresthesia
9. Generalized urticaria
10. Myasthenia-like syndrome
11. Weakness

Probable
1. Gastrointestinal disorder
2. Paralytic ileus

Clinical significance
Significant ocular side effects due to these drugs are quite rare. Topical ocular cyclopentolate and tropicamide can elevate intraocular pressure in open-angle glaucoma and precipitate angle-closure glaucoma. Cycloplegics have been shown to decrease the coefficient outflow. Some have suggested that the use of these agents may cause an instability of vitreous face, which could aggravate cystoid macular edema. Visual hallucinations or psychotic reactions after topical applications are primarily seen with cyclopentolate.

Systemic adverse reactions from these agents are not uncommon, especially in children. Disorientation, somnolence, hyperactivity, vasomotor collapse, tachycardia and even death have been reported. Kellner and Esser (1989) have the most complete review of cyclopentolate-induced acute psychosis. The pattern is one of onset between 20 and 60 minutes after ocular exposure. This is followed by disorientation, dysarthria, ataxia, various types of hallucinations and retrograde amnesia. Recovery is between 30 minutes and 7 hours. There are cases in the literature and in the National Registry of dilation (with decreased sensory input) aggravating patients who are elderly or those with Alzheimer's. There have also been cases of addiction to topical ocular application of these drugs, since some patients get a CNS 'high' from their use. Sato et al (1992) reaffirmed this in two patients. Mori et al (1992) showed that tropicamide reduces aqueous barrier permeability. McCormack (1990) showed reduced mydriasis from both of these drugs with repeat dosage. He recommended that they not be used the day before surgery if one wants to achieve maximum dilation at surgery. Hermansen and Sullivan (1985) and Isenberg et al (1985) warned against the use of 0.5%

cyclopentolate in preterm infants since there appears to be a risk of developing necrotizing enterocolitis. They performed studies that showed that 0.25% cyclopentolate has no effect on gastric functions; however, case reports from Sarici et al (2001) and Lim et al (2003) describe bowel obstruction in neonates requiring cyclopentolate. Newman and Jordan (1996) reported a case of generalized urticaria secondary to topical ocular cyclopentolate. Meyer et al (1992) reported a case with rechallenge of a myasthenia-like syndrome induced by 1.0% tropicamide.

REFERENCES AND FURTHER READING

Brooks AMV, West RH, Gillies WE. The risks of precipitating acute angle-closure glaucoma with the clinical use of mydriatic agents. Med J Aust 145: 34, 1986.

Demayo AP, Reidenberg MM. Grand mal seizure in a child 30 minutes after cyclogyl (cyclopentolate hydrochloride) and 10% Neo-Synephrine (phenylephrine hydrochloride) eye drops were instilled. Pediatrics 113: e499–e500, 2004.

Eggers MN. Toxicity of drugs used in diagnosis and treatment of strabismus. In: Ocular Therapeutics, Srinivasan D (ed), Masson, New York, p 115–122, 1980.

Fitzgerald DA, et al. Seizures associated with 1% cyclopentolate eyedrops. J Paediatr Child Health 26: 106–107, 1990.

Hermansen MC, Sullivan LS. Feeding intolerance following ophthalmologic examination. Am J Dis Child 139: 367, 1985.

Isenberg SJ, Abrams C, Hyman PE. Effects of cyclopentolate eyedrops on gastric secretory function in pre-term infants. Ophthalmology 92: 698, 1985.

Jones LWJ, Hodes DT. Cyclopentolate. First report of hypersensitivity in children: 2 case reports. Ophthalmic Physiol Opt 11: 16–20, 1991.

Kellner U, Esser J. Acute psychosis caused by cyclopentolate. Klin Mbl Augenheilk 194: 458–461, 1989.

Lim DL, Batilando M, Rajadurai VS. Transient paralytic ileus following the use of cyclopentolate-phenylephrine eye drops during screening for retinopathy of prematurity. J Paediatr Child Health 39: 318–320, 2003.

Marti J, Anton E, Ezcurra I. An unexpected cause of delirium in an old patient. J Am Geriatr Soc 52: 545, 2005.

McCormack DL. Reduced mydriasis from repeated doses of tropicamide and cyclopentolate. Ophthal Surg 21(7): 508–512, 1990.

Meyer D, Hamilton RC, Gimbel HV. Myasthenia gravis-like syndrome induced by topical ophthalmic preparations. A case report. J Clin Neuro-Ophthalmol 12(3): 210–212, 1992.

Mirshahi A, Kohnen T. Acute psychotic reaction caused by topical cyclopentolate use for cycloplegic refraction before refractive surgery. J Cataract Refract Surg 29: 1026–1030, 2003.

Mori M, et al. Effects of pilocarpine and tropicamide on blood-aqueous permeability in man. Invest Ophthalmol Vis Sci 33(2): 416–423, 1992.

Newman DK, Jordan K. Generalized urticaria induced by topical cyclopentolate. Eye 10(Pt 6): 750–751, 1996.

Rosales T, et al. Systemic effects of mydriatrics in low weight infants. Pediatr Ophthalmol 18: 42, 1981.

Rush R, Rush S, Nicolau J, et al. systemic manifestations in response to mydriasis and physical examination during screening for retinopathy of rematurity. Retina 24: 242–245, 2004.

Sarici SU, Yurdakok M, Unal S. Acute gastric dilatation complicating the use of mydriatics in a preterm newborn. Pediatr Radiol 31: 581–583, 2001.

Sato EH, de Freitas D, Foster CS. Abuse of cyclopentolate hydrochloride (Cyclogyl) drops. N Engl J Med 326: 1363–1364, 1992.

Shihab ZM. Psychotic reaction in an adult after topical cyclopentolate. Ophthalmologica 181: 228, 1980.

Generic name: Hydroxyamfetamine hydrobromide.

Proprietary names: Multi-ingredient preparations only.

Primary use

Ophthalmic
This topical sympathomimetic amine is used as a mydriatic.

Ocular side effects

Local ophthalmic use or exposure
Certain
1. Mydriasis – may precipitate angle–closure glaucoma
2. Decreased vision
3. Irritation
   a. Lacrimation
   b. Photophobia
   c. Ocular pain
4. Palpebral fissure – increase in vertical width
5. Paradoxical pressure elevation in open-angle glaucoma
6. Eyelids or conjunctiva – allergic reactions
7. Paralysis of accommodation – minimal

Probable
1. Problems with color vision – objects have a blue tinge

Clinical significance
Other than precipitating angle-closure glaucoma, Ocular side effects from topical ocular administration of hydroxyamfetamine are insignificant and reversible. An increase in vertical palpebral fissure width reaches a maximum 30 minutes after topical ocular application. This is secondary to stimulation of Mueller's muscle. Some feel this may be the safest mydriatic to use with a shallow anterior chamber since it is slow acting and possibly more easily counteracted by miotics. Administration of 1% hydroxyamfetamine eye drops causes a more pronounced mydriasis in patients with Down's syndrome. A letter to ophthalmologists from the manufacturer described three cases of significant cardiac events following the use of a topical ocular hydroxyamfetamine/tropicamide ophthalmic solution (1%/0.25%).

REFERENCES AND FURTHER READING

Burde RM, Thompson HS. Hydroxyamphetamine. A good drug lost? Am J Ophthalmol 111(1): 100–102, 1991.

Gartner S, Billet E. Mydriatic glaucoma. Am J Ophthalmol 43: 975, 1957.

Grant WM. Toxicology of the Eye, 2nd edn, Charles C Thomas, Springfield, IL, 567–568, 1974.

Kronfeld PC, McGarry HI, Smith HE. The effect of mydriatics upon the intraocular pressure in so-called primary wide-angle glaucoma. Am J Ophthalmol 26: 245, 1943.

Munden PM, et al. Palpebral fissure responses to topical adrenergic drugs. Am J Ophthalmol 111: 706–710, 1991.

Priest JH. Atropine response of the eyes in mongolism. Am J Dis Child 100: 869, 1960.

CLASS: NEUROTOXINS

Generic name: Botulinum A or B toxin.

Proprietary names: Botox, Myobloc.

Primary use
This neurotoxin is used primarily to treat blepharospasm, hemifacial spasms and Meige's syndrome. It has also been used in selected strabismus and various neuromuscular disorders of the head and neck. Retrobulbar injections for acquired nystagmus have been advocated.

Ocular side effects

Periocular injection
Certain
1. Ptosis

2. Sicca
3. Extraocular muscles
   a. Paresis (in muscles other than those intended)
   b. Hemorrhage
   c. Diplopia
   d. Hyperdeviation
4. Eyelids
   a. Hemorrhage (associated with injection)
   b. Lagophthalmos
   c. Edema
   d. Pruritis
   e. Paralytic ectropion
   f. Paralytic entropion
   g. Allergic reaction
5. Cornea – exposure keratitis (associated with eyelid paresis)
6. Facial weakness or numbness
7. Blurred vision
8. Brow droop
9. Epiphora (associated with dry eye reflex tearing)

Probable
1. Photophobia

Possible
1. Eyelids
   a. Permanent cutaneous depigmentation
   b. Erythema multiforme
2. Pupil
   a. Mydriasis
   b. Acute glaucoma
   c. Inverse Argyll Robertson pupil
3. Myasthenia gravis (exacerbation)
   a. Ptosis
   b. Diplopia
   c. Paresis of extraocular muscles

Retrobulbar injection
Certain
1. Diplopia
2. Ptosis
3. Ophthalmoplegia
4. Filamentary keratitis (associated with dry eyes)

Clinical significance
There have been no proven systemic side effects from periocular injections of botulinum toxin. Ocular side effects are transitory and are usually gone by 2 weeks, but can last up to 6 weeks. The most frequently encountered side effect is ptosis with or without lagophthalmos and decreased blink rate. Sicca is the second most commonly seen adverse effect, but it is unclear if this is due to increased ocular exposure or a decrease in tear production. The incidence of both ptosis and dry eyes is roughly between 6 and 8%. The next most common side effect is diplopia, which occurs in approximately 3% of patients. Wutthiphan et al (1997) reported these same side effects in children, but at a lower incidence. The inferior oblique is the most commonly involved extraocular muscle. This side effect is surprisingly well tolerated by most patients. Scott (1997) suggests injections of human botulinum immune globulin following injections of the toxin to avoid ptosis. It also been suggested that diplopia will be decreased by avoiding treatment of the medial two-thirds of the lower eyelids and keeping the injection superficial when treating blepharospasm. There have been reports of injection around eyelids for blepharospasm in which mydriasis with

secondary acute glaucoma occurred. Keech et al (1990) reported possible enhancement of anterior segment ischemia following vertical muscle transposition after botulinum injection. They recommend injections of botulinum toxin several days after strabismus surgery rather than intraoperatively. Sanders et al (1986) reported a questionable case of the toxin causing transitory paresis of an arm after periocular injection. Roehm et al (1999) treated 26 African Americans without any alteration of skin pigmentation, although Friedland and Burde (1996) reported three white patients with permanent periocular cutaneous depigmentation. Nussgens and Roggenkamper (1997) compared the incidence of side effects of Dysport with Botox. Statistical significance included fewer cases of ptosis with Botox (1.4% versus 6.6%) and fewer side effects with Botox (17.0% versus 24.1%). Attempts to find antibody production secondary to botulinum toxin have been negative. Histologic features have shown no persistent toxic changes to the muscle, although there were some changes in the nerve fiber endings.

REFERENCES AND FURTHER READING

Averbuch-Heller L, von Maydell RD, Poonyathalang A, et al. Inverse Argyll Robertson pupil in botulism: Late central manifestation. Ophthal Lit 50(2): 132, 1997.

Biglan AW, et al. Absence of antibody production in patients treated with botulinum A toxin. Am J Ophthalmol 101: 232–235, 1986.

Burns CL, Gammon A, Gemmill MC. Ptosis associated with botulinum toxin treatment of strabismus and blepharospasm. Ophthalmology 93(12): 1621–1627, 1986.

Corridan P, et al. Acute angle-closure glaucoma following botulinum toxin injection for blepharospasm. Br J Ophthalmol 74: 309–310, 1990.

Dunlop D, Pittar G, Dunlop C. Botulinum toxin in ophthalmology. Aust N Z J Ophthalmol 16: 15–20, 1988.

Dutton JJ, Buckley EG. Long-term results and complications of botulinum A toxin in the treatment of blepharospasm. Ophthalmology 95(11): 1529–1534, 1988.

Engstrom PF, et al. Effectiveness of botulinum toxin therapy for essential blepharospasm. Ophthalmology 94(8): 971–975, 1987.

Friedland S, Burde RM. Porcealinizing discoloration of the periocular skin following botulinum A toxin injections. J Neuroophthalmol 16: 70–71, 1996.

Frueh BR, et al. The effect of omitting botulinum toxin from the lower eyelid in blepharospasm treatment. Am J Ophthalmol 106: 45–47, 765–766, 1988.

Harris CP, et al. Histologic features of human orbicularis oculi treated with botulinum A toxin. Arch Ophthalmol 109: 393–395, 1991.

Huges AJ. Botulinum toxin in clinical practice. Practical therapeutics. Drugs 48(6): 888–893, 1994.

Kalra HK, Magoon EH. Side effects of the use of botulinum toxin for treatment of benign essential blepharospasm and hemifacial spasm. Ophthal Surg 21(5): 335–338, 1990.

Keech RV, et al. Anterior segment ischemia following vertical muscle transposition and botulinum toxin injection. Arch Ophthalmol 108: 176, 1990.

Magoon EH. Chemodenervation of strabismic children. Ophthalmology 96(7): 931–934, 1989.

Mauriello JA, Coniaris H, Haupt EJ. Use of botulinum toxin in the treatment of one hundred patients with facial dyskinesias. Ophthalmology 94(8): 976–979, 1987.

Nussgens Z, Roggenkamper P. Comparison of two botulinum-toxin preparations in the treatment of essential blepharospasm. Graefes Arch Clin Exp Ophthalmol 235(4): 197–199, 1997.

Repka MX, Savino PJ, Reinecke RD. Treatment of acquired nystagmus with botulinum neurotoxin A. Arch Ophthalmol 112: 1320–1324, 1994.

Roehm PC, Perry JD, Girkin CA, et al. Prevalence of periocular depigmentation after repeated botulinum toxin A injections in African American patients. J Neuro-Ophthalmol 19(1): 7–9, 1999.

Sanders DB, Massey EW, Buckley EG. Botulinum toxin for blepharospasm. Neurology 36: 545–547, 1986.

Scott AB. Preventing ptosis after botulinum treatment. Ophthalmic Plast Reconstr Surg 13(2): 81–83, 1997.

Tomsak RL, Remler BF, Averbuch-Heller L, et al. Unsatisfactory treatment of acquired nystagmus with retrobulbar injection of botulinum toxin. Am J Ophthalmol 119(4): 489–496, 1995.

Wutthiphan S, Kowal L, O'Day J, et al. Diplopia following subcutaneous injections of botulinum A toxin for facial spasms. J Pediatr Ophthalmol Strabismus 34(4): 229–234, 1997.

CLASS: OPHTHALMIC DYES

Generic names: 1. Indocyanine green; 2. lissamine green; 3. rose bengal; 4. trypan blue.

Proprietary names: 1. IC-Green; 2. Generic only; 3. Rosets; 4. Visionblue.

Primary use
These dyes are used in various ocular diagnostic tests.

Ocular side effects

Local ophthalmic use or exposure
Certain
1. Staining
   a. Mucus
   b. Devitalized epithelium
   c. Epithelium not adequately covered by periocular tear film (rose bengal)
   d. Degenerated epithelial cells (trypan blue)
   e. Connective tissue
   f. Posterior capsule (trypan blue)
   g. Internal limiting membrane (trypan blue)
   h. Soft contact lens
2. Irritation
   a. Ocular pain
   b. Burning sensation
3. Eyelids or conjunctivitis
   a. Blue discoloration (trypan blue)
   b. Red discoloration (rose bengal)
   c. Green discoloration (lissamine green)
   d. Photosensitizer (rose bengal)
4. Visual field defect (indocyanine green)
5. Rentinal pigment epithelium toxicity (indocyanine green)
6. Nerve fiber layer toxicity (indocyanine green)
7. Retained subretinal dye (indocyanine green)

Probable
1. Inhibit PCR detection of herpes simplex virus (rose bengal, lissamine green)

Possible
1. Cystoid macular edema (trypan blue)
2. Reduced efficacy of infrared laser treatment (indocyanine green)
3. Enhanced photothermal effect with infrared laser treatment (indocyanine green)

Systemic side effects

Local ophthalmic use or exposure (indocyanine green)
Certain
1. Nausea and vomiting
2. Urticaria
3. Vasovagal episodes
4. Cardiorespiratory arrest
5. Hypotension
6. Urge to defecate
7. Anaphylactic shock

Clinical significance
Rose bengal, especially in concentrations above 1%, may occasionally cause significant ocular irritation after topical ocular instillation. It was thought that rose bengal was a vital dye, but it has recently been shown to stain primarily epithelium not adequately covered by periocular tear film. If the corneal or conjunctival epithelium is not intact, the topical application of rose bengal may cause long-term or even permanent stromal deposits of the dye. Lee et al (1996) reaffirmed that light augmentation can enhance the toxic effects of rose bengal. Manning et al (1995) showed that lissamine green had similar staining properties to rose bengal with much better patient acceptance with the duration of ocular discomfort significantly less with lissamine green. Rose bengal and lissamine green may inhibit detection of herpes simplex virus by PCR.

Gale et al (2004) showed that indocyanine green (ICG) dye demonstrated more toxicity than trypan blue to the human retinal pigment epithelium in cell cultures and Balayre et al (2005) showed that 0.15% trypan blue facilitated ERM peeling without any retinal toxicity. Still, trypan blue has been reported to cause significant retina pigment abnormalities from prolonged exposure, usually when the dye migrates to the subretinal space.

Trypan blue has also been reported to inadvertently stain the posterior capsule during phacoemulsification in a previously vitrectomized eye and is known to stain the internal limiting membrane of the retina. It does not appear to damage endothelial cells but can stain hydrogel intraocular lenses if used intraoperatively. Cystoid macular edema associated with trypan blue use during phacoemulsification has also been reported.

ICG dye has been used for more than 30 years in other areas of medicine and has gained popularity in ophthalmology more recently. The side effects of this drug are less frequent than with fluorescein. Mild adverse reactions to fluorescein were between 1 and 10%, while mild adverse reactions to this dye were approximately 0.15%. The rate of moderate reactions to fluorescein was 1.6% compared with 0.2% for ICG. Severe reactions were 0.05% with ICG, which was similar to that with fluorescein (Hope-Ross et al 1994). ICG dye may absorb infrared laser light and could produce a photothermal effect, leading to unwanted damage to the inner retinal layers during retinal laser surgery. There are multiple reports of ICG dye toxicity of the outer retina and retinal pigment epithelium after macular hole surgery, although this is rare. Cheng et al (2005) reported that ocular toxicity caused by ICG dye used in macular hole surgery may present as pigment epithelial atrophy, which is characteristically larger than the previous area of the macular hole and surrounding cuff. Disc atrophy, retinal toxicity and ocular hypotony were also observed in some instances. To prevent toxicity, residual ICG and ICG-stained internal limiting membrane must be removed as completely as possible.

Indocyanine green dye is an established iodine allergen, is metabolized in the liver and will cross the placental barrier therefore its use is contraindicated in patients with iodine allergies, who are pregnant or who have liver or kidney disease. Patients with uremia have a higher incidence of significant adverse systemic reactions to indocyanine green than normal. The reason for this is unknown but may be due to an allergic hypersensitivity reaction. Deaths have been reported with this agent, and are probably due to an anaphylactic reaction and cardiorespiratory arrest. There may be an increased incidence of reactions with repeat administration, but this has not been proven.

REFERENCES AND FURTHER READING

Ang GS, Ang AJS, Burton RL. Iatrogenic macula hole and consequent macular detachment caused by intravitreal trypan blue injection. Eye 18: 759–760, 2004.

Aydin P, Tayanc E, Dursun D, et al. Anterior segment indocyanine green angiography in pterygium surgery with conjunctival autograft transplantation. Am J Ophthamol 135: 71–75, 2003.

Balayre S, Boissonnot M, Paquereau J, et al. Evaluation of trypan blue toxicity in idiopathic epiretinal membrane surgery with macular function test using multifocal electroretinography: seven prospective case studies. J Fr Opthalmol 28: 169–176, 2005.

Benya R, Quintana J, Brundage B. Adverse reactions to indocyanine green: a case report and a review of the literature. Cathet Cardiovasc Diagn 17: 231–233, 1989.

Blem RI, Huynh PD, Thall EH. Altered uptake of infrared diode laser by retina after intravitreal indocyanine green dye and internal limiting membrane peeling. Am J Ophthalmol 134: 285–286, 2002.

Birchall W, Matthew R, Turner G. Inadvertent staining of the posterior lens capsule with trypan blue dye during phacoemulsification. Arch Ophthalmol 119: 1082, 2001.

Bisol T, Rezende RA, Guedes J, et al. Effect of blue staining of expendable hydrophilic intraocular lenses on contrast sensitivity and glare vision. J Cataract Refract Surg 30: 1732–1735, 2004.

Bonte CA, Ceuppens J, Leys AM. Hypotensive shock as a complication of infracyanine green injection. Retina 18(5): 476–477, 1998.

Cheng S-N, Yang T-C, Ho J-D, et al. Ocular toxicity of intravitreal indocyanine green. J Ocul Pharmacol Ther 21: 85–93, 2005.

Chodosh J, Banks MC, Stroop WG. Rose bengal inhibits herpes simplex virus replication in vero and human corneal epithelial cells in vitro. Invest Ophthalmol Vis Sci 33(8): 2520–2527, 1992.

Chowdhury PK, Raj SM, Vasavada AR. Inadvertent staining of the vitreous with trypan blue. J Cataract Refract Surg 30: 274–276, 2004.

Ciardella AP, Schiff W, Barile G, et al. Persistent indocyanine green fluorescence after vitrectomy for macular hole. Am J Ophthalmol 136: 174–177, 2003.

Doughty MJ, Naase T, Donald C, et al. Visualization of 'Marx's line' along the marginal eyelid conjunctiva of human subjects with lissamine green dye. Ophthalmic Physiol Opt 24: 1–7, 2004.

Feensra RPG, Tseng, SCG. What is actually stained by rose bengal? Arch Ophthalmol 110: 984–993, 1992.

Gale JS, Proulx AA, Gonder JR, et al. Comparison of the in vitro toxicity of indocyanine green to that of trypan blue in human retinal pigment epithelium cell cultures. Am J Ophthalmol 138: 64–69, 2004.

Gaur A, Kayarkar VV. Inadvertent vitreous staining. J Cataract Refract Surg 31: 649, 2005.

Gouws P, Merriman M, Goethals S, et al. Cystoid macular oedema with trypan blue use. Br J Ophthalmol 88: 1348–1349, 2004.

Guyer DR, et al. Digital indocyanine-green angiography in chorioretinal disorders. Ophthalmology 99: 287–291, 1992.

Ho J-D, Tsai RJ, Chen S-N, et al. Toxic effect of indocyanine green on retinal pigment epithelium related to osmotic effects of the solvent. Am J Ophthalmol 135: 258–259, 2003.

Ho J-D, Tsai RJ, Chen S-N, et al. Cytotoxicity of indocyanine green on retinal pigment epithelium. Arch Ophthalmol 121: 1423–1429, 2003.

Hope-Ross M, et al. Adverse reactions due to indocyanine green. Ophthalmology 101(3): 529–533, 1994.

Iriyama A, Yanagi Y, Uchida S, et al. Retinal nerve fibre layer damage after indocyanine green assisted vitrectomy. Br J Ophthalmol 88: 1606–1607, 2004.

Kampik A, Sternberg P. Indocyanine green in vitreomacular surgery – (why) it is a problem? Am J Opthalmol 136: 527–529, 2003.

Kanda S, Uemura A, Yamashita T, et al. Visual field defects after intra-vitreous administration of indocyanine green in macular hole surgery. Arch Ophthalmol 122: 1447–1451, 2004.

Kogure K, et al. Infrared absorption angiography of the fundus circulation. Arch Ophthalmol 83: 209–214, 1970.

Lee YC, Park CK, Kim MS, et al. In vitro study for staining and toxicity of rose bengal on cultured bovine corneal endothelial cells. Cornea 15(4): 376–385, 1996.

Lee JE, Yoon TJ, Oum BS, et al. Toxicity of indocyanine green injected into the subretinal space. Retina 23: 675–681, 2003.

Manning FJ, Wehrly SR, Foulks GN. Patient tolerance and ocular surface staining characteristics of lissamine green versus rose bengal. Ophthalmology 102(12): 1953–1957, 1995.

Menon IA, et al. Reactive oxygen species in the photosensitization of retinal pigment epithelial cells by rose bengal. J Toxicol Cut Ocular Toxicol 11(4): 269–283, 1992.

Nanikawa R, et al. A case of fatal shock induced by indocyanine green (ICG) test. Jpn Leg Med 32: 209–214, 1978.

Obana A, et al. Survey of complications of indocyanine green angiography in Japan. Am J Ophthalmol 118: 749–753, 1994.

Olsen TW, Lim JI, Capone A Jr, et al. Anaphylactic shock following indocyanine green angiography (letter). Arch Ophthalmol 114(1): 97, 1996.

Rezai KA, Farrokh-Siar L, Ernest JT, et al. Indocyanine green induced apoptosis in human retinal pigment epithelial cells. Am J Ophthalmol 93: 931–933, 2004.

Rezai KA, Farrokh-Siar L, Gasyna EM, et al. Trypan blue induces apoptosis in human retinal pigment epithelial cells. Am J Ophthalmol 138: 492–495, 2004.

Schatz H. Sloughing of skin following fluorescein extravasation. Ann Ophthalmol 10: 625, 1978.

Seitzman GD, Cevallos V, Margoli TP. Rose bengal and lissamine green inhibit detection of herpes simplex virus by PCR. Am J Ophthalmol 141: 756–758, 2006.

Speich R, et al. Anaphylactoid reactions after indocyanine green administration. Ann Intern Med 109: 345–346, 1988.

Uemura A, Kanda S, Sakamoto Y, et al. Visual field defects after uneventful vitrectomy for epiretinal membrane with indocyanine green-assisted internal limiting membrane peeling. Am J Ophthalmol 136: 252–257, 2003.

Uemoto R, Yamamoto S, Takeuchi S. Changes in retinal pigment epithelium after indocyanine green-assisted internal limiting lacmina peeling during macular hole surgery. Am J Ophthalmol 140: 752–755, 2005.

Uno F, Malerbi F, Maia M, et al. Subretinal trypan blue migration during epiretinal membrane peeling. Retina 26: 237–239, 2006.

van Dooren BTH, DeWaard PWT, Nouhuys HPV, et al. Corneal endothelial cell density after trypan blue capsule staining in cataract surgery. J Cataract Refract Surg 28: 574–575, 2002.

Werner L, Apple DJ, Crema AS, et al. Permanent blue discoloration of a hydrogel intraocular lens by intraoperative trypan blue. J Cataract Refract Surg 28: 1279–1286, 2002.

Yannuzzi LA, et al. Fluorescein angiography complication survey. Ophthalmology 93: 611–617, 1986.

Yannuzzi LA, et al. Digital indocyanine green videoangiography and choroidal neovascularization. Retina 12: 191–223, 1992.

Yuen HKL, Lam RF, Lam DSC, et al. Cystoid macular oedema with trypan blue use. Br J Ophthalmol 89: 644–645, 2005.

Generic name: Fluorescein.

Proprietary names: Fluorescite, Fluor-I-Strip.

Primary use

Intravenous fluorescein is used to study various ocular and systemic vascular perfusions. Topical ocular fluorescein is used as a diagnostic test.

Ocular side effects

Systemic administration – intravenous
Certain
1. Stains ocular fluids and tissues yellow-green
2. Eyelids or conjunctiva
    a. Allergic reactions
    b. Hyperemia
    c. Yellow-orange discoloration
    d. Angioneurotic edema
    e. Urticaria
    f. Eczema
3. Blurred vision (transient)

Local ophthalmic use or exposure
Certain
1. Stains ocular fluids and tissues yellow-green
2. Eyelids or conjunctiva
    a. Yellow-orange discoloration
    b. Chemosis
3. Tears and/or contact lenses stained yellow-green

4. Phototoxicity
5. Irritation

Possible
1. Iritis (radial keratotomy)

Systemic side effects

Systemic administration
Certain
1. Nausea
2. Vomiting
3. Urine discoloration
4. Headache
5. Dizziness
6. Fever
7. Syncope
8. Hypotension
9. Dyspnea
10. Shock
11. Thrombophlebitis – injection site
12. Skin necrosis – injection site
13. Cardiac arrest
14. Myocardial infarction
15. Anaphylaxis
16. Generalized seizure
17. Phototoxic reactions

Intrathecal injection
Certain
1. Lower extremity weakness
2. Numbness
3. Generalized seizures
4. Opisthotonos
5. Cranial nerve paralysis
6. Paralysis lower extremities

Clinical significance

Hundreds of thousands of intravenous fluorescein angiographies are done annually. While widely perceived as a safe drug, significant adverse events do occur. The most common systemic reactions are nausea and vomiting, which occur between 3 and 9% of the time, and pruritus and urticaria from a Type 1 reaction about 0.5 to 1.5% of the time. The most serious and occasionally fatal reactions include laryngeal edema or anaphylactic reactions. Butrus et al (1999) reported the first case of elevated levels of beta-tryptase in serum, which indicates a systemic reaction to fluorescein that was mast cell dependent. This test can be done several hours after the reaction to confirm an anaphylactic reaction. Danis and Stephens (1997) reported three patients who experienced marked cutaneous erythema, edema and pain in the sun-exposed areas 1 hour after sunlight exposure after an ocular fluorescein angiogram. Fluorescein is a photosensitive agent and patients have complained even after an ocular fluorescein angiogram that their vision became worse. Since these were persons with diseased maculae, it is difficult to prove a cause-and-effect relationship. Johnson et al (1998) reported a delayed allergic reaction which resulted in a rash, chills and fever 2 hours after an intravenous injection. Hara et al (1998) reported 1787 patients who had oral fluorescein for ocular angiography and stated that the side effects were significantly less than intravenous injections. Local reactions from infiltration of fluorescein in the area of the injection site range from pain and tenderness to tissue necrosis.

Ocular side effects due to topical ocular fluorescein are rare and transient. Brodsky et al (1987) reported that if microperforations occur following radial keratotomy incisions, topical ocular fluorescein may cause acute iritis with an inflammatory membrane. Corneal transplant surgeries commonly use topical ocular fluorescein and have not reported this problem. Solutions of fluorescein can become contaminated with Pseudomonas because fluorescein inactivates the preservatives found in most ophthalmic solutions. Valvano and Martin (1998) reported a case of periorbital urticaria after topical ocular fluorescein.

REFERENCES AND FURTHER READING

Antoszyk AN, et al. Subretinal hemorrhages during fluorescein angiography. Am J Ophthalmal 103: 111, 1987.

Brodsky ME, Bauerberg JM, Sterzovsky A. Case report: probably flourescein-induced uveitis following radial keratotomy. J Refract Surg 3(1): 29, 1987.

Butrus SI, Negvesky GJ, Rivera-Velazques PM, et al. Serum tryptase: an indicator of anaphylaxis following fluorescein angiography. Graefes Arch Clin Exp Ophthalmol 237(5): 433–434, 1999.

Chishti MI. Adverse reactions to intravenous fluorescein. Pak J Ophthalmol 2: 19, 1986.

Danis RP, Stephens T. Phototoxic reactions caused by sodium fluorescein. Am J Ophthalmol 123(5): 694–696, 1997.

Danis RP, Wolverton S, Steffens T. Phototoxicity from systemic sodium fluorescein. Retina 20: 370–373, 2000.

Duffner LR, Pflugfelder SC, Mandelbaum S, et al. Potential bacterial contamination in fluorescein-anesthetic solutions. Am J Ophthalmol 110: 199–202, 1990.

Foster RE, Kode R, Ross D, et al. Unusual reaction to fluorescein dye in patients with inflammatory eye disease. Retina 24: 263–266, 2004.

Hara T, Inami M, Hara T. Efficacy and safety of fluorescein angiography with orally administered sodium fluorescein. Am J Ophthalmol 126(4): 560–564, 1998.

Hitosugi M, Omura K, Yokoyama T, et al. An autopsy case of fatal anaphylactic shock following fluorescein angiography: a case report. Med Sci Law 44: 264–265, 2004.

Johnson RN, McDonald HR, Schatz H. Rash, fever, chills after intravenous fluorescein angiography. Am J Ophthalmol 126(6): 837–838, 1998.

Karhunen U, Raitta C, Kala R. Adverse reactions to fluorescein angiography. Acta Ophthalmol 64: 282, 1986.

Kratz RP, Davidson B. A case report of skin necrosis following infiltration with IV fluorescein. Ophthalmology 12: 654–656, 1980.

Kurli M, Hollingworth K, Kumar V, et al. Fluorescein angiography and patchy skin discoloration: a case report. Eye 17: 422–424, 2003.

Kwiterovich KA, Maguire MG, Murphy RP, et al. Frequency of adverse systemic reactions after fluorescein angiography; results of a prospective study. Surv Ophthalmol 98(7): 1139–1142, 1991.

Spaeth GL, Nelson LB, Beaudoin AR. Ocular teratology. In: Ocular Anatomy, Embryology and Teratology, Jakobiec FA (ed), JB Lippincott, Philadelphia, pp 955–975, 1982.

Valvano MN, Martin TP. Periorbital urticaria and topical fluorescein. Am J Emerg Med 16(5): 525–526, 1998.

Yannuzzi LA, et al. Fluorescein angiography complication survey. Ophthalmology 93: 611, 1986.

CLASS: OPHTHALMIC IMPLANTS

Generic name: Silicone.

Proprietary names: None.

Primary use
Various silicone polymers of various viscosities or solids are used in ophthalmology as lubricants, implants and volume expanders.

Ocular side effects

Local ophthalmic use or exposure
Certain
1. Conjunctiva
   a. Irritation
   b. Burning sensation

Intraocular – oil
Certain
1. Cornea
   a. Edema
   b. Opacity
   c. Vascularization
   d. Thinning
   e. Vacuoles (silicone)
   f. Keratopathy – bullous and/or band
2. Chamber angle
   a. Glaucoma
   b. Vacuoles (silicone)
3. Iris – vacuoles (silicone)
4. Retina – vacuoles (silicone)
5. Optic nerve – vacuoles (silicone)

Probable
1. Lens – intravitreal silicone may attach to silicone lenses
2. Eyelid
   a. Vacuoles (silicone)
   b. Ptosis
3. Migration of silicone into brain
4. Visual field defect

Possible
1. Optic nerve – atrophy
2. Cornea – perforation
3. Cataract
4. Sympathetic ophthalmia
5. Vitreoretinopathy

Implants – ocular, eyelid or lacrimal system
Certain
1. Granulomatous reactions

Probable
1. Increase in infections

Clinical significance
Silicone solutions or solids rarely cause adverse ocular reactions, but significant side effects may occur under certain circumstances. Silicone plugs are used frequently in the management of keratitis sicca. Like any foreign body buried within tissue, the implant, even if inert, may be encased by scar tissue or granulomatous tissue. Rapoza and Ruddat (1992) first reported pyogenic granulomas caused by these devices. Most granulomas resolved after the plugs were removed. Granulomas may also form after retinal surgery and when silicone is used in augmentation of the eyelids. Amemiya and Dake (1994) have shown that this latter procedure may also cause degeneration of the orbicularis muscle.

As with silicone liquids placed in other areas of the body, the silicone liquid within the eye may migrate to new locations with time. Since the usual site of injection is intravitreal, occasionally the solution may come in contact with the lens or enter the anterior chamber, with the potential to affect the outflow channels, lens or cornea. Apple et al (1996) reported three cases of intravitreal silicone oil injection migrating forward to come into contact with a silicone intraocular lens. The silicone oil coated the intraocular lens as droplet formations. These adherences could not be removed with instrumentation or viscoelastics. They caused decreased vision and aberrations such as halos or rainbow patterns. Shields et al (1989) have also shown that silicone liquids have the potential to migrate posteriorly to affect glaucomatous optic nerves and enhance atrophy, probably on a mechanical basis.

Multiple authors have now reported on the potential for migration of silicone oil from the vitreous, through the optic nerve, and into the brain. This appears to be a rare but potential complication of silicone oil retinal tamponade. Eckle et al (2005) have shown visual field defects in association with chiasmal migration of intraocular silicone oil and Fangtian et al (2005) reported a case of migration of intraocular silicone oil into the cerebral ventricles. There are also rare reports of eyelid swelling and blepharoptosis from migration into the eyelid from silicone oil instilled into the eye during vitreoretinal surgery. Corneal changes are probably not a toxic process, but rather, as pointed out by Norman et al (1990), act as a nutritional barrier. Silicone oils may increase permeability by dissolving substances such as cholesterol and other lipophilic substances out of membranes in the corneal endothelium and retina. Hutton et al (1994) have shown that silicone oil removal after anatomically successful retinal surgery has significance in improving visual acuity with some slight increase of redetachment.

REFERENCES AND FURTHER READING

Al-Jazzaf AM, Netlan PA, Charles S. Incidence and management of elevated intraocular pressure after silicon oil injection. J Glaucoma 14: 40–46, 2005.

Amemiya T, Dake Y. Granuloma after augmentation of the eyelids with liquid silicone: An electron microscope study. Ophthalmic Plast Reconstr Surg 10(1): 51–56, 1994.

Ando F. Intraocular hypertension resulting from pupillary block by silicone oil. Am J Ophthalmol 99: 87, 1985.

Apple DJ, Federman JL, Krolicki TJ, et al. Irreversible silicone oil adhesion to silicone intraocular lenses. Ophthalmology 103(10): 1555–1562, 1996.

Beekhuis WN, van Rij G, Zivojnovic R. Silicone oil keratopathy: Indication for keratoplasty. Br J Ophthalmol 69: 247, 1985.

Bennett SR, Abrams GW. Band keratopathy from emulsified silicone oil. Arch Ophthalmol 108: 1387, 1990.

Chuo N, et al. Intravitreous silicone injection. Histopathologic findings in a human eye after 12 years. Arch Ophthalmol 101: 1399, 1983.

Donker DLT, Paridaens D, Mooy CM, et al. Blepharoptosis and upper eyelid swelling due to lipogranulomatous inflammation caused by silicone oil. Am J Ophthalmol 140: 934–936, 2005.

Eckle D, Kampik A, Hintschich C, et al. Visual field defect in association with chiasmal migration of intraocular silicone oil. Br J Ophthalmol 89: 918–920, 2005.

Eller AW, Frieberg TR, Mah F. Migration of silicone oil into the brain: a complication of intraocular silicone for retinal tamponade. Am J Ophthalmol 129: 685–688, 2000.

Fangtian D, Rongping D, Lin Z, et al. Migration of intraocular silicone into the cerebral ventricles. Am J Ophthalmol 140: 156–158, 2005.

Foulks GN, et al. Histopathology of silicone oil keratopathy in humans. Cornea 10: 29–37, 1991.

Friberg TR, Verstraeten TC, Wilcox DK. Effects of emulsification, purity, and fluorination of silicone oil on human retinal pigment epithelial cells. Invest Ophthalmol Vis Sci 32: 2030–2034, 1991.

Hotta K, Sugitani A. Refractice changes in silicone oil-filled pseudophakic eyes. Retina 25: 167–170, 2005.

Hutton WL, Azen SP, Blumenkranz MS, et al. The effects of silicone oil removal. Arch Ophthalmol 112: 778–785, 1994.

Jackson TL, Thiagarajan M, Murthy R, et al. Pupil block glaucoma in phakic and pseudophakic patients after vitrectomy with silicone oil injection. Am J Ophthalmol 132: 414–416, 2001.

Jalkh AE, et al. Silicone oil retinopathy. Arch Ophthalmol 104: 178, 1986.

Laroche L, et al. Ocular findings following intravitreal silicone injection. Arch Ophthalmol 101: 1422, 1983.

Norman BC, et al. Corneal endothelial permeability after anterior chamber silicone oil. Ophthalmology 97(12): 1671–1677, 1990.

Parmley VC, et al. Foreign-body giant cell reaction to liquid silicone. Am J Ophthalmol 101: 680, 1986.

Quintyn J, Genevois O, Ranty M, et al. Silicone oil migration in the eyelid after vitrectomy for retinal detachment. Am J Ophthalmol 136: 540–542, 2003.

Rapoza PA, Ruddat MS. Pyogenic granuloma as a complication of silicone punctal plugs. Am J Ophthalmol 113(4): 454–455, 1992.

Shields CL, et al. Silicone oil. Optic atrophy: case report. Arch Ophthalmol 107: 683–686, 1989.

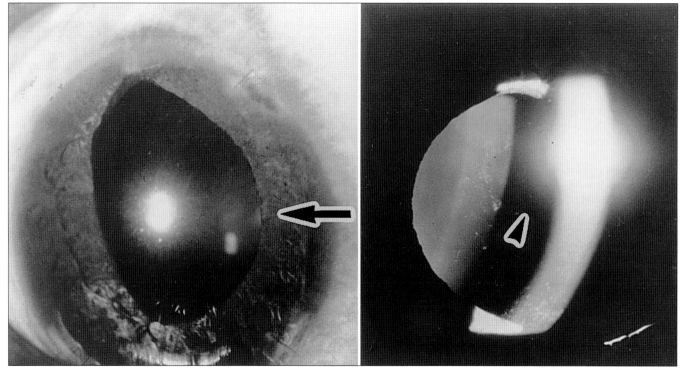

Fig. 7.13i Left: Anterior segment photoshowing iridocorneal contact nasally (arrow) due to silicone oil between iris and lens. Right: Deep anterior chamber of same eye (arrowhead). Photo courtesy of Jackson TL, et al: Pupil block glaucoma in phakic and pseudophakic patients after vitrectomy with silicone oil injection. Am J Ophthalmol 132: 414-416, 2001.

Vankatesh P, Chawla R, Tewari HK. Spontaneous perforation of the cornea following silicon oil keratopathy. Cornea 24: 347–348, 2005.

Wang LC, Wang TJ, Yang CM. Entrapped preretinal oil bubble: report of two cases. Jpn J Ophthalmol 50: 277–279, 2006.

CLASS: OPHTHALMIC PRESERVATIVES AND ANTISEPTICS

Generic name: Benzalkonium chloride.

Proprietary names: Benza, Zephiran.

Primary use

This topical ocular quaternary ammonium agent is used as a preservative in ophthalmic solutions and as a germicidal cleaning solution for contact lenses.

Ocular side effects

Local ophthalmic use or exposure
Certain
1. Irritation
   a. Lacrimation
   b. Hyperemia
   c. Photophobia
   d. Ocular pain
   e. Burning sensation
2. Eyelids or conjunctiva
   a. Allergic reactions
   b. Hyperemia
   c. Erythema
   d. Blepharitis
   e. Conjunctivitis
   f. Edema
   g. Contact allergies
3. Cornea
   a. Punctate keratitis
   b. Edema
   c. Pseudomembrane formation
   d. Decreased epithelial microvilli
   e. Vascularization
   f. Scarring
   g. Delayed wound healing
   h. Increased transcorneal permeability
   i. Decreased stability of tear film
4. May aggravate keratoconjunctivitis sicca

Probable
1. Eyelids or conjunctiva – pemphigoid lesion with symblepharon (Fig. 7.13jA)
2. Cystoid macular edema
3. Corneal endothelial cell damage
4. Leukoplakia (Fig. 7.13jB)

Possible
1. Decreased lacrimation
2. Cataract

Clinical significance

This bactericide is a popular preservative because its antimicrobial effects cover a broad pH range of formulations. In fact, the antibacterial properties are almost as good as the currently available topical ocular antibiotics even in human clinical trials. Adverse ocular reactions to benzalkonium are not uncommon, even at exceedingly low concentrations, and may cause cell damage by emulsification of the lipids in the cell wall. De Saint Jean et al (1999) reported that this chemical can cause cell growth

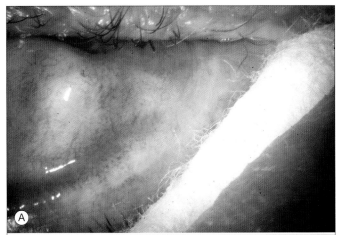

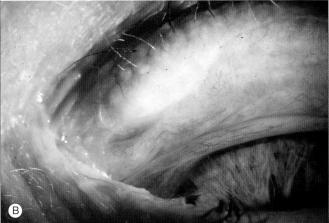

Fig. 7.13j A: Cicatricial changes associated with topical ocular application of eyedrops containing benzalkonium chloride. B: Lekoplakia from topical ocular application of eyedrops containing benzalkonium chloride.

arrest and death at concentrations as low as 0.0001%. Most adverse effects, with short-term use in healthy corneas, are inconsequential after this agent is discontinued since the damage is fairly superficial. However, long-term use has caused extensive corneal damage requiring corneal transplantation. Benzalkonium may destroy the corneal epithelial microvilli, and thereby possibly prevent adherence of the mucoid layer of the tear film to the cornea. This drug also allows for increased penetration of some drugs through the corneal epithelium, and is added to some commercial ophthalmic preparations for this reason.

Topical epithelial cell sensitization to benzalkonium chloride has been postulated to cause increased fibrosis and inflammation, decreasing the success of glaucoma filtration procedures.

Benzalkonium binds to soft contact lenses, and the use of preservatives has been said to concentrate in the contact lens, possibly causing increased epithelial breakdown. Baudouin (Baudouin 1996; Baudouin and Lunardo 1998; Baudouin et al 1994, 1999) has written a series of articles on immune and inflammatory infiltrates in glaucoma filtering procedures that are probably factors for filter failures. Benzalkonium chloride along with other factors may be involved in this process. The Baudoin group also showed that the above process affects not only the epithelial cells of the conjunctiva and cornea, but also the endothelial cells of the trabecular meshwork. Means et al (1994) clearly showed the toxicity of benzalkonium chloride from irrigating solutions on the endothelial cells of the cornea. A case report to the National Registry showed irreversible corneal damage

with vascularization when 1:1000 benzalkonium was inadvertently placed in both eyes and irrigated out 20 minutes later. This agent, as pointed out by Lemp and Zimmerman (1988), is toxic to the corneal endothelium. Even in the small amounts used in ophthalmic solutions, it may cause problems in diseased denuded corneas that receive multiple topical ocular applications daily. Benzalkonium used in solutions introduced within the eye is equally damaging to the corneal endothelium.

Relatively recent reports indicate that chronic anti-glaucoma therapy can damage the cornea, lens and retina. These changes are presumably from benzalkonium but could also be from the antiglaucoma agent itself. An editorial by Brandt (2003) explores the possibility of cataracts. Goto et al (2003) and others describe the possible mechanism behind how this could occur. It is 'possible' but undetermined if cataracts form after chronic therapy with benzalkonium-containing products. Maculopathy has been postulated to occur by Miyake et al (2003) and 'pseudophakic preservative maculopathy' is poorly understood at this time and we feel it is only 'possible'.

REFERENCES AND FURTHER READING

Baudouin C. Mechanisms of failure in glaucoma filtering surgery: A consequence of antiglaucoma drugs? Int J Clin Pharm Res 16(1): 29–41, 1996.

Baudouin C, de Lunardo C. Short-term comparative study of topical 2% carteolol with and without benzalkonium chloride in healthy volunteers. Br J Ophthalmol 82(1): 9–42, 1998.

Baudouin C, et al. Expression of inflammatory membrane markers by conjunctival cells in chronically treated patients with glaucoma. Ophthalmology 101(3): 454–460, 1994.

Baudouin C, Pisella PJ, Fillacier K, et al. Ocular surface inflammatory changes induced by topical antiglaucoma drugs: human and animal studies. Ophthalmology 106(3): 556–563, 1999.

Bernal DL, Ubels JL. Quantitative evaluation of the corneal epithelial barrier: effect of artificial tears and preservatives. Curr Eye Res 10: 645–656, 1991.

Brandt JD. Does benzalkonium chloride cause cataract? Arch Ophthalmol 121: 892–893, 2003.

Burstein NL. Corneal cytotoxicity of topically applied drugs, vehicles and preservatives. Surv Ophthalmol 25: 15, 1980.

Chapman JM, Cheeks L, Green K. Interactions of benzalkonium chloride with soft and hard contact lenses. Arch Ophthalmol 108: 244–246, 1990.

De Saint Jean M, Brignole F, Bringuier AF, et al. Effects of benzalkonium chloride on growth and survival of change conjunctival cells. Invest Ophthalmol Vis Sci 40: 619–630, 1999.

Gibran SK. Unilateral drug-induced ocular pseudopemphigoid. Eye 18: 1270–1278, 2004.

Goto Y, Ibaraki N, Miyake K. Human lens epithelial cell damage and stimulation of their secretion of chemical mediators by benzalkonium chloride rather than latanoprost and timolol. Arch Ophthalmol 121: 835–839, 2003.

Ishibashi T, Yokoi N, Kinoshita S. Comparison of the short-term effects on the human corneal surface of topical timolol maleate with and without benzalkonium chloride. J Glaucoma 12: 486–490, 2003.

Keller N, et al. Increased corneal permeability induced by the dual effects of transient tear film acidification and exposure to benzalkonium chloride. Exp Eye Res 30: 203, 1980.

Lavine JB, Binder PS, Wickham MG. Antimicrobials and the corneal endothelium. Ann Ophthalmol 11: 1517, 1979.

Lemp MA, Zimmerman LE. Toxic endothelial degeneration in ocular surface disease treated with topical medications containing benzalkonium chloride. Am J Ophthalmol 105: 670–673, 1988.

Means TL, et al. Corneal edema from an intraocular irrigating solution containing benzalkonium chloride. J Toxicol Cut Ocular Toxicol 13(1): 67–81, 1994.

Miyake K, Ibaraki N, Goto Y, et al. ESCRS Binkhorts Lecture 2002: pseudophakic preservative maculopathy. J Cataract Refract Surg 29: 1800–1810, 2003.

Samples JR, Binder PS, Nayak S. The effect of epinephrine and benzalkonium chloride on cultured corneal endothelial and trabecular meshwork cells. Exp Eye Res 49: 1–12, 1989.

Generic name: Chlorhexidine.

Proprietary names: Betasept, Dyna-Hex, Exidine, Hibiclens, Hibistat, Peridex, Periochip, Periogard.

Primary use

Topical

This disinfectant is used as an antiseptic wound and general skin cleanser for preoperative preparation of the patient, as a surgical scrub and as a handwash for health care personnel.

Ophthalmic

Chlorhexidine is a topical antiseptic and surfactant commonly used in contact lens solutions and in the treatment of *Acanthamoeba* infection.

Ocular side effects

Inadvertent ocular exposure (4.0%)
Certain
1. Corneal
   a. Decreased endothelial counts
   b. Punctate keratitis
   c. Edema (including bullous)
   d. Opacification (all layers)
   e. Vascularization (all layers)
   f. Decreased sensation
2. Conjunctiva
   a. Hyperemia
   b. Lacrimation
   c. Photophobia
   d. Ocular pain
   e. Burning sensation

Topical ocular exposure (0.02–0.04% for Acanthamoeba)
Certain
1. Keratitis – transitory
2. Corneal edema – transitory
3. Cataracts – higher concentrations
4. Iris atrophy – higher concentrations
5. Loss of endothelial cells – higher concentrations
6. Conjunctiva
   a. Hyperemia
   b. Lacrimation
   c. Photophobia
   d. Ocular pain
   e. Burning sensation

Clinical significance

Serious and permanent eye injury may occur during inadvertent ocular exposure of 4.0% chlorhexidine, mainly from preoperative scrub of the head with accidental ocular exposure. Most severe injuries in the National Registry's experience are cases of head surgeries where this agent was used as a disinfectant. The head is usually turned and gravity allows the chemical to be exposed to the dependent eye. The head drape covers this area therefore a significant delay occurs before recognition of the problem and irrigation of the eye. Almost total destruction of the corneal endothelium can occur, with only variable success gained from conventional corneal grafting. In general, with immediate irrigation, only superficial punctate keratitis and mild corneal edema with conjunctivitis lasting 7 to 10 plus days occurs. The role of the detergent with this chemical is unclear, but it has been suggested that this enhances the penetration of chlorhexidine, allowing for great stromal and anterior chamber concentration with toxicity to the corneal endothelium.

Chlorhexidine and propamidine in combination is commonly used for the treatment of *Acanthamoeba*. Propamidine may cause epithelial cyst, but chlorhexidine may cause conjunctival irritation and keratitis, especially at high dosage and prolonged therapy. Ehler and Hjortal (2004) suggested that on rare instances in prolonged treatment and with already damaged corneas, chlorhexidine may more easily enter the anterior chamber. This chemical can destroy the membrane of the *Acanthamoeba* cyst wall, keratocytes, and even fibrocytes as well as the iris and lens membranes. We have no other reports of iris, lens or corneal endothelial damage from topical 0.02–0.04% chlorhexidine in the National Registry. Wright has shown in animals that 0.02% chlorhexidine within the anterior chamber irrigation is cytotoxic to rabbit endothelial.

Concentrations of 0.002–0.005% chlorhexidine used as a chemical disinfectant of soft contact lenses may rarely present problems of toxic anterior segment irritation. Transitory corneal edema and 'chlorhexidine conjunctivitis' can occur. Okuda et al (1994) reported a case of anaphylactic shock secondary to an ophthalmic wash containing chlorhexidine.

REFERENCES AND FURTHER READING

Apt L, Isenberg SJ. Hibiclens keratitis. Am J Ophthalmol 104: 670, 1987.

Ehlers E, Hjortdal J. Are cataract and iris atrophy toxic complications of medial treatment of acanthamoeba keratitis? Acta Ophthalmol Scand 82: 228–231, 2004.

Hamed LM, et al. Hibiclens keratitis. Am J Ophthalmol 104: 50, 1987.

Khurana AK, Ahluwalie BK, Sood S. Savlon keratopathy, a clinical profile. Acta Ophthalmol 67: 465–466, 1989.

MacRae SM, Brown B, Edelhauser HF. The corneal toxicity of presurgical skin antiseptics. Am J Ophthalmol 97: 221, 1984.

Morgan JF. Complications associated with contact lens solutions. Ophthalmology 86: 1107, 1979.

Murthy S, Hawksworth NR, Cree I. Progressive ulcerative keratitis related to the use of topical chlorhexidine gluconate (0.02%). Cornea 21(2): 237–239, 2002.

Nasser RE. The ocular danger of Hibiclens. Plast Reconstr Surg 89(1): 164–165, 1992.

Okuda T, Funasaka M, Arimitsu M, et al. Anaphylactic shock by ophthalmic wash solution containing chlorhexidine. Jpn J Anesthesiol 43(9): 1352–1355, 1994.

Paugh JR, Caywood TG, Peterson SD. Toxic reactions associated with chemical disinfection of soft contact lenses. Int Contact Lens Clin 11: 680, 1984.

Phinney RB, Mondino BJ, et al. Corneal edema related to accidental Hibiclens exposure. Am J Ophthalmol 106: 210–215, 1988.

Shore JW. Hibiclens keratitis. Am J Ophthalmol 104: 670–671, 1987.

Scott WG. Antiseptic (Hibiclens) and eye injuries. Med J Aust 2: 456, 1980.

Tabor E, Bostwick DC, Evans CC. Corneal damage due to eye contact with chlorhexidine gluconate. JAMA 261: 557–558, 1989.

Generic names: 1. Thiomersal; 2. yellow mercuric oxide (hydrargyric oxide flavum).

Proprietary names: 1. Aeroaid, Mersol; 2. Stye.

Primary use

These topical ocular organomercurials are used as antiseptics, preservatives and antibacterial or antifungal agents in ophthalmic solutions and ointments.

Ocular side effects

Local ophthalmic use or exposure
Certain
1. Irritation
   a. Lacrimation
   b. Hyperemia
   c. Photophobia
   d. Ocular pain
   e. Burning sensation
2. Eyelids or conjunctiva
   a. Allergic reactions
   b. Hyperemia
   c. Erythema
   d. Blepharitis
   e. Conjunctivitis – follicular
   f. Edema
   g. Urticaria
   h. Eczema
3. Bluish-gray mercury deposits
   a. Eyelids
   b. Conjunctiva
   c. Cornea
   d. Lens
4. Cornea (thiomersal)
   a. Punctate keratitis
   b. Opacities
   c. Edema
   d. Subepithelial infiltrates
   e. Vascularization
   f. Band keratopathy
   g. Hypersensitivity reactions
5. Decreased tolerance to contact lenses (thiomersal)

Clinical significance

Adverse ocular side effects due to these organomercurials are rare and seldom of significance. The most striking side effect is mercurial deposits in various ocular and periocular tissues. This is an apparently harmless side effect since it is asymptomatic and no related visual impairments have been reported. Conjunctival mercurial deposits can be seen around blood vessels near the cornea. Corneal deposits are in the peripheral Descemet's membrane and lens deposits are mainly in the visual axis. No deposits have been reported in any other ocular tissues with the topical ocular use of thiomersal. Thiomersal is now a commonly used preservative in many ophthalmic contact lens solutions. Mercurialentis has not been seen with thiomersal at concentrations of 0.005%, the concentration used as a preservative in some ophthalmic solutions. There are a surprisingly large number of people allergic to thiomersal. In a Japanese series, up to 50% of eye patients became hypersensitive, while in the USA this rate was about 10%. To evaluate this agent as a factor for ocular intolerance, thiomersal skin testing can be performed. Soft contact lenses cleaned and stored in thiomersal-containing solution may produce an ocular inflammatory process similar to superior limbic keratoconjunctivitis. The corneal changes are transient and range from faint epithelial opacities to a coarse, punctate epithelial keratopathy.

REFERENCES AND FURTHER READING

Binder PS, Rasmussen DM, Gordon M. Keratoconjunctivitis and soft contact lens solutions. Arch Ophthalmol 99: 87, 1981.
Brazier DJ, Hitchings RA. Atypical band keratopathy following longterm pilocarpine treatment. Br J Ophthalmol 73: 294–296, 1989.
De la Cuadra J, Pujol C, Aliagia A. Clinical evidence of cross-sensitivity between thiosalicyclic acid, a contact allergen, and piroxicam, a photo-allergen. Cont Dermatol 21: 349–351, 1989.
Gero G. Superficial punctuate keratitis with CSI contact lenses dispensed with the Allergan Hydrocare cold kit. Int Contact Lens Clin 11: 674, 1984.
Mondino BJ, Salamon SM, Zaidman GW. Allergic and toxic reactions in soft contact lens wearers. Surv Ophthalmol 26: 337, 1982.
Rietschel RL, Wilson LA. Ocular inflammation in patients using soft contact lenses. Arch Dermatol 118: 147, 1982.
Wilson LA, McNatt J, Reitschel R. Delayed hypersensitivity to thimerosal in sort contact lens wearers. Ophthalmology 88: 804, 1981.
Wilsonholt N, Dart JKG. Thiomersal keratoconjunctivitis, frequency, clinical spectrum and diagnosis. Eye 3: 581–587, 1989.
Wright P, Mackie I. Preservative-related problems in soft contact lens wearers. Trans Ophthalmol Soc UK 102: 3, 1982.

CLASS: PROTEOLYTIC ENZYMES

Generic name: Urokinase.

Proprietary name: Abbokinase.

Primary use

This proteolytic enzyme is injected into the anterior chamber or vitreous to possibly aid in the removal of blood.

Ocular side effects

Local ophthalmic use or exposure
Certain
1. Hypopyon (sterile)
2. Uveitis
3. Intraocular pressure
   a. Increased
   b. Decreased
4. Abnormal ERG
5. Cornea
   a. Edema
   b. Fold in Descemet's membrane

Clinical significance

After intravitreal injections of urokinase an incidence of sterile hypopyon as high as 50% has occurred. This is thought to be cellular debris in the anterior chamber that usually absorbs within 5 days. Uveitis is usually mild, although severe cases have been reported. A transient decrease in the b-wave of the ERG, corneal edema and folds in the Descemet's membrane have been reported following intravitreal injection of urokinase for treatment of vitreous hemorrhage. In addition, one patient developed a discrete posterior subcapsular opacity 2 months after the third injection of 15 000 units of urokinase. Fourteen months after discontinuing treatment, the posterior lens capsule ruptured.

REFERENCES AND FURTHER READING

Berman M, et al. Plasminogen activator (urokinase) causes vascularization of the cornea. Invest Ophthalmol Vis Sci 22: 191, 1982.
Bramsen T. The effect of urokinase on central corneal thickness and vitreous hemorrhage. Acta Ophthalmol 56: 1006, 1978.
Higuchi M, Hinokuma R. The effect of intravitreal injection of urokinase on longstanding vitreous hemorrhage. Folia Ophthalmol Jpn 32: 316, 1981.
Hull DS, Green K. Effect of urokinase on corneal endothelium. Arch Ophthalmol 98: 1285, 1980.
Koch H-R. Experimental approaches to elucidate clinical cataract problems. In: Symposium on the Lens, Regnault F (ed), Elsevier, Amsterdam, pp 5–12, 1981.
Textorius O, Stenkula S. Toxic ocular effects of two fibrinolytic drugs. An experimental electroretinographic study on albino rabbits. Acta Ophthalmol 61: 322, 1983.

CLASS: TOPICAL LOCAL ANESTHETICS

Generic name: Cocaine.

Proprietary name: Generic only.

Street name: Nasal, oral: base, bernice, bernies, blow, C, coke, crack, flake, freebase, girl, gold dust, happy dust, heaven dust, pearl, rock, snow, toot.

Primary use

Injection
Intravenous cocaine may be used by drug abusers.

Nasal, oral
Cocaine is a potent CNS stimulant that is commonly available on the illicit drug market.

Ophthalmic
This topical local anesthetic is used in diagnostic and surgical procedures.

Ocular side effects

Systemic administration – nasal or oral
Certain
1. Decreased vision
2. Visual hallucinations
3. Photosensitivity
4. Pupils
   a. Mydriasis
   b. Absence of reaction to light – toxic states
5. Paralysis of accommodation
6. Secondary optic nerve involvement (sinusitis)
   a. Optic neuritis
   b. Optic atrophy

Possible
1. Exophthalmos
2. Madarosis
3. Iritis

Local ophthalmic use or exposure
Certain
1. Mydriasis – may precipitate angle-closure glaucoma
2. Corneal epithelium
   a. Punctate keratitis
   b. Gray, ground glass appearance
   c. Edema
   d. Softening, erosions and sloughing
   e. Filaments
   f. Ulceration
   g. Anesthesia
3. Corneal stroma
   a. Yellow-white opacities (Fig. 7.13k)
   b. Vascularization
   c. Scarring
4. Irritation
   a. Lacrimation
   b. Hyperemia
   c. Ocular pain
   d. Burning sensation

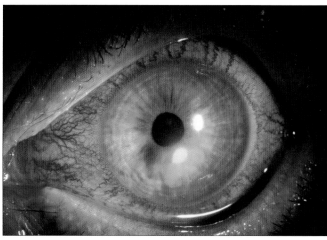

Fig. 7.13k Corneal opacities from cocaine exposure to the eye.

5. Eyelids or conjunctiva
   a. Allergic reactions
   b. Blepharoconjunctivitis
   c. Widening of palpebral aperture
6. Decreased stability of corneal tear film
7. Subconjunctival hemorrhages
8. Decreased blink reflex
9. Hypopyon
10. Decreased vision
11. Conjunctival vasoconstriction
12. Paralysis of accommodation
13. Visual hallucinations – especially Lilliputian
14. Abnormal ERG (reduced blue cone responses)
15. Delayed corneal wound healing

Possible
1. Iritis

Systemic side effects

Local ophthalmic use or exposure
Certain
1. Nervousness
2. Tremors
3. Convulsion
4. Bradycardia
5. Asthma
6. Apnea

Clinical significance

Topical ocular cocaine can cause all the side effects that one sees from the topical abuse of local anesthetics. It differs, however, from other local anesthetics in that it causes conjunctival vasoconstriction. It also causes mydriasis, which may affect accommodation, and only rarely precipitates angle-closure glaucoma. Visual hallucinations, especially Lilliputian, may occur. A potential problem is that a detectable level of cocaine may be present in the urine for 72 hours after the application of topical ocular cocaine by ophthalmologists. There has been a marked increase in the illicit use of cocaine with new and more potent drugs available. One of the most common methods of using this drug systemically is by applying it to the nasal mucosa. There have been a number of cases of optic neuropathies associated with chronic sinusitis and orbital inflammation secondary to chronic cocaine-induced nasal pathology. These have included optic neuritis, optic atrophy and blindness. Intracranial hemorrhages have occurred secondary to cocaine use, including bilateral and unilateral intranuclear ophthalmoplegia secondary to micro-infarcts in the medial longitudinal vesicles. Vascular infarcts with secondary visual field changes and extraocular muscle dysfunction have been reported. There have been reports of precipitation of angle-closure glaucoma secondary to the mydriatic effect of the drug. Ocular teratogenic effects secondary to cocaine administration probably occur. Dominguez et al (1991) reported that nine infants had ophthalmic abnormalities, including strabismus, nystagmus and hypoplastic optic discs. Good et al (1992) reported 13 cocaine-exposed infants who had optic nerve abnormalities, delayed visual maturation and prolonged eyelid edema. There have also been reports of abnormal visual evoked potentials in 11 of 12 neonates with cocaine present in their urine. Stafford et al (1994), however, showed no significant effects of prenatal cocaine exposure on the infant eye, with axial lengths consistent with the statistical norm, along with other parameters that were normal for fetal growth. Nucci and Brancato (1994) reported a 24% incidence of congenital esotropia in infants who were cocaine-exposed newborns. It is apparent, however, that many of the infants who have cocaine in their urine at birth may show increased congestion, engorgement and bleeding of their retinal and iris vessels.

Another form of cocaine use is crack cocaine, in which the fumes from the cocaine cause significant ocular irritation, dryness and loss of eyebrows. It has become advisable to consider crack cocaine on the differential diagnosis if a young patient comes in with corneal ulcers or epithelial defects and no related medical or traumatic cause. Various bacterial and fungal organisms have been identified in these ulcers. McHenry et al (1993) reported central retinal artery occlusions, unilateral mydriasis, cranial nerve palsies and optic neuropathies with crack cocaine use. They also believe that crack cocaine babies have an increased incidence of strabismus and nystagmus.

REFERENCES AND FURTHER READING

Block SS, Moore BD, Scharre JE. Visual anomalies in young children exposed to cocaine. Optom Vis Sci 74(1): 28–36, 1997.
Cruz OA, et al. Urine drug screening for cocaine after lacrimal surgery. Am J Ophthalmol 111: 703–705, 1991.
Dominguez AA, et al. Brain and ocular abnormalities in infants with in utero exposure to cocaine and other street drugs. Am J Dis Child 145: 688–695, 1991.
Goldberg RA, et al. Orbital inflammation and optic neuropathies associated with chronic sinusitis of intranasal cocaine abuse. Arch Ophthalmol 107: 831–835, 1989.
Good WV, et al. Abnormalities of the visual system in infants exposed to cocaine. Ophthalmology 99(3): 341–346, 1992.
Jacobson DM, Berg R, Grinstead GF, et al. Duration of positive urine for cocaine metabolite after ophthalmic administration: implications for testing patients with suspected horner syndrome using ophthalmic cocaine. Am J Ophthalmol 131: 742–747, 2001.
McHenry JG, et al. Ophthalmic complications of crack cocaine (letter). Ophthalmology 100(12): 1747, 1993.
Mitchell JD, Schwartz AL. Acute angle-closure glaucoma associated with intranasal cocaine abuse. Am J Ophthalmol 122(3): 425–426, 1996.
Munden PM, et al. Palpebral fissure responses to topical adrenergic drugs. Am J Ophthalmol 111: 706–710, 1991.
Nucci P, Brancato R. Ocular effects of prenatal cocaine exposure (letter). Ophthalmology 101(8): 1321–1324, 1994.
Perinatal toxicity of cocaine. Med Newslett 30: 59–60, June 1988.
Sachs R, Zagelbaum BM, Hersh PS. Corneal complications associated with the use of crack cocaine. Ophthalmology 100(2): 187–191, 1993.
Silva-Araujo AL, Tavares MA, Patacao MH, et al. Retinal hemorrhages associated with in utero exposure to cocaine. Retina 16: 411–418, 1996.
Stafford JR Jr, et al. Prenatal cocaine exposure and the development of the human eye. Ophthalmology 101(2): 301–308, 1994.
Steinkamp PN, Watzke RC, Solomon JD, et al. An unusual case of solar retinopathy. Arch Ophthalmol 121: 1798, 2003.
Stominger MB, Sachs R, Hersh PS. Microbial keratitis with crack cocaine. Arch Ophthalmol 108: 1672, 1990.
Tames SM, Goldenring JM. Madarosis from cocaine use. N Engl J Med May 15: 1324, 1986.
Zagelbaum BM, Tannenbaum MH, Hersh PS. Candida albicans corneal ulcer associated with crack cocaine. Am J Ophthalmol 111(2): 248–249, 1991.
Zeiter JH, McHenry JG, McDermott ML. Unilateral pharmacologic mydriasis secondary to crack cocaine (letter). Am J Emerg Med 8: 568, 1990.
Zeiter JH, et al. Sudden retinal manifestations of intranasal cocaine and methamphetamine abuse (letter). Am J Ophthalmol 114: 780–781, 1992.

Generic names: 1. Proxymetacaine hydrochloride (proparacaine); 2. tetracaine.

Proprietary names: 1. Alcaine, Ophthetic, Paracaine; 2. Pontocaine.

Primary use

Ophthalmic
These topical local anesthetics are used in diagnostic and surgical procedures.

Ocular side effects

Local ophthalmic use or exposure
Certain
1. Corneal epithelium
   a. Punctate keratitis
   b. Gray, ground glass appearance
   c. Edema
   d. Softening, erosions and sloughing
   e. Filaments
   f. Ulceration
2. Corneal stroma
   a. Yellow-white opacities
   b. Vascularization
   c. Scarring
   d. Ulceration
   e. Crystalline keratopathy
   f. Perforation
   g. Increased incidence of *Acanthamoeba keratitis*
   h. Increased incidence of *Candida keratitis*
   i. Melting (Fig. 7.13l)
3. Corneal endothelium
   a. Loss of cells
   b. Variation in cell size
4. Uveitis
   a. Fibrinous
   b. Hypopyon
5. Irritation
   a. Lacrimation
   b. Hyperemia
   c. Ocular pain
   d. Burning sensation
6. Delayed wound healing
7. Eyelids or conjunctiva
   a. Allergic reactions
   b. Blepharoconjunctivitis
   c. Puritis
   d. Erythema
   e. Contact dermatitis
8. Decreased stability of corneal tear film

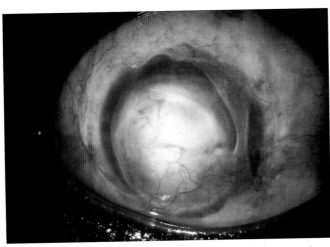

Fig. 7.13l Corneal melt and vascularization from topical proxymetacaine hydrochloride abuse.

9. Subconjunctival hemorrhages
10. Decreased blink reflex
11. Inhibits fluorescence of fluorescein
12. Decreased vision
13. Atonic pupil

Possible

1. Eyelids or conjunctiva – Stevens-Johnson syndrome (proparacaine)

Systemic side effects

Local ophthalmic use or exposure
Probable

1. Nervousness
2. Tremors
3. Convulsion
4. Bradycardia
5. Asthma
6. Apnea

Clinical significance

Few significant ocular side effects are seen with these agents if they are given topically for short periods of time, but prolonged use will inevitably cause severe and permanent corneal damage, including visual loss. Local anesthetics inhibit the rate of corneal epithelial cell migration by disruption of cytoplasmic action in filaments and destruction of superficial corneal epithelial microvilli. This allows for permanent epithelial defects and disruption of the corneal tear film with continued drug use. Chronic use of local anesthetics causes denuding of corneal epithelium, which may cause dense yellow-white rings in the corneal stroma. This may occur as early as the sixth or as late as the 60th day after initial use. The corneal ring resembles a Wessely ring and often resolves once the local anesthetic is discontinued. Moreira et al (1999) have shown a direct toxic effect of local anesthetics on stromal keratocytes. Secondary infection is common, and an increase in the frequency of *Acanthamoeba* may be seen. Chern et al (1996) described four patients who, after local anesthetic abuse, developed *Candida* keratitis. Infectious crystalline keratopathy has been reported due to topical local anesthetic abuse (Kinter et al 1990). Risco and Millar (1992) have shown irreversible destruction of the endothelial cells secondary to topical ocular local anesthetic abuse. With prolonged use, from one-third to two-thirds of the endothelial loss may occur. Various degrees of uveitis have been reported, including plastic and fibrinous forms. Rosenwasser et al (1990) have an excellent review of this subject, including cases of ocular perforation requiring enucleation.

Numerous systemic reactions from topical ocular applications of local anesthetics have been reported. Many are probably not drug-induced if they occur immediately after the eye drop is administered, but may be emotionally mediated. They may occur, in part, from fear of the impending procedure or possibly an oculocardiac reflex. Side effects include syncope, convulsions and anaphylactic shock. Liesegang and Perniciaro (1999) described an ophthalmologist with fingertip dermatitis secondary to exposure to proparacaine on a daily basis. Taddio et al (2006) reported a pre-term infant developing bradycardia and contact dermatitis on 4% tetracaine gel.

REFERENCES AND FURTHER READING

Burns RP, Gipson I. Toxic effects of local anesthetics. JAMA 240: 347, 1978.

Chern KC, Meisler DM, Wilhelmus KR, et al. Corneal anesthetic abuse and *Candida keratitis*. Ophthalmology 103: 37–40, 1996.

Dannaker CJ, Maibach HI, Austin E. Allergic contact dermatitis to proparacaine with subsequent cross sensitization to tetracaine from ophthalmic preparations. Am J Contact Dermatitis 12: 177–179, 2001.

Duffin RM, Olson RJ. Tetracaine toxicity. Ann Ophthamol 16: 836, 1984.

Fraunfelder FT, Sharp JD, Silver BE. Possible adverse effects from topical ocular anesthetics. Doc Ophthalmol 18: 341, 1979.

Gild WM, et al. Eye injuries associated with anesthesia. Anesthesiology 76: 24–208, 1992.

Grant WM, Schuman JS. Toxicology of the Eye. 4th edn. Charles C Thomas, Springfield, IL, 144–157, 1993.

Haddad R. Fibrinous iritis due to oxybuprocaine. Br J Ophthalmol 73: 76–77, 1989.

Hodkin MJ, Cartwright MJ, Kurumety UR. In vitro alteration of Schirmer's tear strip wetting by commonly instilled anesthetic agents. Cornea 13(2): 141–147, 1994.

Kinter JC, et al. Infectious crystalline keratopathy associated with topical anesthetic abuse. Cornea 9(1): 77–80, 1990.

Lemagne JM, et al. Purtscher-like retinopathy after retrobulbar anesthesia. Ophthalmology 97(7): 859–861, 1990.

Liesegang TJ, Perniciaro C. Fingertip dermatitis in an ophthalmologist caused by proparacaine. Am J Ophthalmol 127(2): 240–241, 1999.

Moreira LB, Kasetsuwan N, Sanchez D, et al. Toxicity of topical anesthetic agents to human keratocytes in vivo. J Cataract Refract Surg 25: 975–980, 1999.

Risco JM, Millar LC. Ultrastructural alterations in the endothelium in a patient with topical anesthetic abuse keratopathy. Ophthalmology 99(4): 628–633, 1992.

Roche G, Brunette I, Le Francois M. Severe toxic keratopathy secondary to topical anesthetic abuse. Can J Ophthalmol 30(4): 198–202, 1995.

Rosenwasser GOD, et al. Topical anesthetic abuse. Ophthalmology 97(8): 967–972, 1990.

Taddio A, Lee CM, Parvez B, et al. Contact dermatitis and bradycardia in a pre-term infant given tetracaine 4% gel. Ther Drug Monit 28: 291–294, 2006.

CLASS: TOPICAL OCULAR NONSTEROIDAL ANTI-INFLAMMATORY DRUGS

Generic names: 1. Bromfenac sodium; 2. diclofenac; 3. ketorolac trometamol (tromethamine); 4. nepafenac.

Proprietary names: 1. Xibrom; 2. Solaraze, Voltaren, Voltaren XR; 3. Acular, Acular LS, Toradol; 4. Nevanac.

Primary use

These topical ocular non-steroidal anti-inflammatory agents are used in the management of inflammation associated with cataract surgery (diclofenac, bromfenac, nepafenac) and for relief of ocular itching due to seasonal allergies (ketorolac tromethamine).

Ocular side effects

Local ophthalmic use or application
Certain
1. Irritation
    a. Burning
    b. Stinging
    c. Lacrimation
2. Eyelids or conjunctiva
    a. Allergic reactions
    b. Angioneurotic edema
3. Cornea
    a. Superficial punctate keratitis
    b. Anesthesia
    c. Delayed epithelial healing
    d. Persistent epithelial defects
    e. Melting
    f. Perforation (Fig. 7.13m)
    g. Edema
4. Conjunctiva
    a. Conjunctivitis
    b. Erosions
    c. Perforation
    d. Hyperemia
5. Scleral
    a. Melting
    b. Perforation
6. Pupil
    a. Inhibits surgical-induced miosis
    b. Postsurgical atonic mydriasis
7. Potentiates ocular bleeding
8. Iritis

Probable
1. Dry eye

Possible
1. Increased intraocular pressure
2. Eyelids or conjunctiva
    a. Toxic epidermal necrolysis
    b. Stevens-Johnson syndrome

Systemic side effects

Local ophthalmic use or exposure
Certain
1. Nausea and vomiting
2. Exacerbation of asthma
3. Abdominal pain
4. Asthenia
5. Chills
6. Dizziness
7. Facial edema
8. Headaches
9. Insomnia

Clinical significance
These topical non-steroidal anti-inflammatory agents rarely cause serious ocular side effects if used according to guidelines in the Physicians' Desk Reference. The most common ocular side effect is transitory irritation, which may be present in up to 40% of patients. This is seldom an indication for not using the drug. Szerenyi et al (1994) documented that diclofenac can cause a significant decrease in corneal sensitivity. Superficial keratitis can be found with this class of medicine but this resolves once the drug is discontinued. There are convincing data that persistent epithelial defects occur in 42% of post-operative penetrating keratoplasty cases when diclofenac eye drops are used. It is postulated that denervated tissue or vulnerable corneal epithelium may be more susceptible to diclofenac toxicity. Multiple reports implicate all of the topical ocular NSAIDs with causing corneal melting in rare instances. It is probable that all NSAIDs, when used in excess both pre and post operatively, can on occasion cause severe superficial punctate keratitis, delayed wound healing, corneal erosion, corneal ulcers and perforations. These processes can occur in the conjunctiva as well as the sclera. These agents have not caused elevation in intraocular pressure. They have, however, caused cross-sensitivity with other non-steroidal antiinflammatory agents, including acetylsalicylic acid, and have the potential to increase bleeding time. This is especially true if they are used in conjunction with other systemic drugs that also cause this side effect. It is believed that this is probably due to inhibition of platelet aggregation. Because of this, there may be a higher incidence of postoperative hyphemas if these drugs are used. Sharir (1997) reported a patient with exacerbation of asthma after topical ocular diclofenac. This has also been reported from the other NSAIDs. Other systemic findings include nausea and vomiting in approximately 1% of patients.

Recommendations
1. Use with caution in patients with predisposing conditions for conjunctival, corneal or scleral melting.
2. Take care in using topical ocular NSAIDs in patients on concurrent steroids.
3. May cause ocular irritation in contact lens wearers.
4. Not recommended, especially surgically, when taking oral NSAIDs for fear of increased bleeding tendencies.
5. Potential for cross-sensitivity to acetylsalicylic acid, phenylacetic acid derivatives and other NSAIDs.
6. Denervated tissue (post-operative penetrating keratoplasty) or damaged corneal epithelium may be more vulnerable to secondary topical ocular NSAIDs toxicity.
7. Do not use in patients with aspirin allergies or those with a combination of asthma and nasal polyps.

REFERENCES AND FURTHER READING

Appiotti A, Gualdi L, Alberti M, et al. Comparative study of the analgesic efficacy of flurbiprofen and diclofenac in patients following excimer laser photorefractive keratectomy. Clin Ther 20: 913–920, 1998.

Asai T, Nakagami T, Mochizuki M, et al. Three cases of corneal melting after instillation of new nonsteroidal anti-inflammatory drug. Cornea 25: 224–224, 2006.

Buckley MMT, Brogden RN. Ketorolac: A review of its pharmacodynamic and pharmacokinetic properties, and therapeutic potential. Drugs 39: 86–109, 1990.

Eiferman RA, Hoffman RS, Sher NA. Topical diclofenac reduces pain following photorefractive keratectomy. Arch Ophthalmol 111: 1022, 1993.

Flach AJ. Cyclo-oxygenase inhibitors in ophthalmology. Surv Ophthalmol 36: 259–285, 1992.

Flach AJ. Topically applied nonsteroidal anti-inflammatory drugs and corneal problems: an interim review and comment. Ophthalmology 107: 1224–1226, 2000.

Flach AJ. Corneal melts associated with topically applied nonsteroidal anti-inflammatory drugs. Trans Am Ophth Soc 99: 205–212, 2001.

Flach AJ, et al. Quantitative assessment of postsurgical breakdown of the blood aqueous barrier following administration of 0.5% ketorolac tromethamine solution. Arch Ophthalmol 106: 344–347, 1988.

Gabison EE, Chastang P, Menashi S, et al. Late corneal perforation after photorefractive keratectomy associated with topical diclofenac. Ophthalmology 11: 1626–1631, 2003.

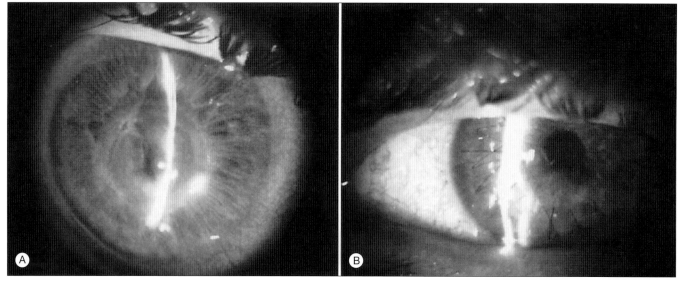

Fig. 7.13m A: Central corneal perforation from topical ocular diclofenac. B: Corneal transplant to repair (1 week post-op). Photo courtesy of Gabison EE, et al: Late corneal perforation after photorefractive keratectomy associated with topical diclofenac. Ophthalmology 110: 1626-1631, 2003.

Goes F, Richard C, Trinquand C. Comparative study of two nonsteroidal anti-inflammatory eyedrops, 0.1% indomethacin versus 0.1% diclofenac in pain control postphotorefractive keratectomy. Bull Soc Belge Ophtalmol 267: 11–19, 1997.

Guidera AC, Luchs JI, Udell IJ. Keratitis, ulceration, and perforation associated with topical nonsteroidal anti-inflammatory drugs. Ophthalmology 108: 936–944, 2001.

Hersh PS, et al. Topical nonsteroidal agents and corneal wound healing. Arch Ophthalmol 108: 577–583, 1990.

Hettinger ME, Gill DJ, Robin JB, et al. Evaluation of diclofenac sodium 0.1% ophthalmic solution in the treatment of ocular symptoms after bilateral radial keratectomy. Cornea 16: 406–413, 1997.

Jampol LM, et al. Nonsteroidal anti-inflammatory drugs and cataract surgery. Arch Ophthalmol 112: 891–893, 1994.

Koch DD. Corneal complications and NSAIDs. Ophthalmology 108: 1519–1520, 2001.

Lin JC, Rapauano CJ, Laibson PR, et al. Corneal melting associated with use of topical nonsteroidal anti-inflammatory drugs after ocular surgery. Arch Ophthalmol 118: 1129–1132, 2000.

Reid ALA, Henderson R. Diclofenac and dry, irritable eyes. Med J Aust 160: 308, 1994.

Seitz B, Sorken K, LaBfree LD, et al. Corneal sensitivity and burning sensation. Comparing topical ketorolac and diclofenac. Arch Ophthalmol 114: 921–924, 1996.

Sharir M. Exacerbation of asthma by topical diclofenac. Arch Ophthalmol 115: 294–295, 1997.

Sitenga GL, Ing EB, Van Dellen RG, et al. Asthma caused by topical application of ketorolac. Ophthalmology 103: 890–892, 1996.

Solomon KD, Turkalj JW, Whiteside SB, et al. Topical 0.5% ketorolac vs 0.03% flurbiprofen for inhibition of miosis during cataract surgery. Arch Ophthalmol 115: 1119–1122, 1997.

Strelow SA, Sherwood MB, Broncata LJ, et al. The effect of diclofenac sodium ophthalmic solution on intraocular pressure following cataract extraction. Ophthalmic Surg 23: 170–175, 1992.

Szerenyi K, et al. Decrease in normal human corneal sensitivity with topical diclofenac sodium. Am J Ophthalmol 118(3): 312–315, 1994.

Yee RW, the Ketorolac Radial Keratotomy Study Group. Analgesic efficacy and safety of nonpreserved ketorolac tromethamine ophthalmic solution following radial keratotomy. Am J Ophthalmol 125: 472–480, 1998.

Zaidman GW. Diclofenac and its effect on corneal sensation. Arch Ophthalmol 113: 262, 1995.

Zanini M, Savini G, Barboni P. Corneal melting associated with topical diclofenac use after laser-assisted subepithelial keratectomy. J Cataract Refract Surg 32: 1570–1572, 2006.

CLASS: TOPICAL OSMOTIC AGENTS

Generic name: Sodium chloride.

Proprietary name: Muro 128.

Primary use

This topical ocular hypertonic salt solution is used to reduce corneal edema.

Ocular side effects

Local ophthalmic use or exposure – topical application
Certain
1. Irritation
   a. Hyperemia
   b. Ocular pain
   c. Burning sensation
2. Corneal dehydration
3. Subconjunctival hemorrhages
4. Nose bleeds

Local ophthalmic use or exposure – subconjunctival injection
Certain
1. Conjunctival hyperemia
2. Increased intraocular pressure

Clinical significance

Few significant adverse ocular reactions are seen with commercial topical sodium chloride solutions. The most frequent ocular side effects are irritation and discomfort, which are primarily related to the frequency of application. At suggested dosages, all ocular side effects are reversible and transient. Kushner (1987) reported that nosebleeds may occur after use of topical ocular hypertonic salt solutions or ointment; cases in the National Registry support this. This is not unexpected because conjunctival hemorrhages are seen as well. Numerous patients experience ocular irritation and keratitis induced by preserved saline solution used in soft contact lens wear but the symptoms are usually alleviated with the use of preservative-free saline.

REFERENCES AND FURTHER READING

Barabino S, Rolando M, Camicione P, et al. Effects of a 0.9% sodium chloride. ophthalmic solution on the ocular surface of symptomatic contact lens wearers. Can J Ophthalmol 40: 45–50, 2005.

Kushner FH. Sodium chloride eye drops as a cause of epistaxis. Arch Ophthalmol 105: 1643, 1987.

Shapiro A, et al. The effect of salt loading diet on the intraocular pressure. Acta Ophthalmol 60: 35, 1982.

Shaw EL. Allergies induced by contact lens solution. Contact Lens 6: 273, 1980.

Spizziri LJ. Stromal corneal changes due to preserved saline solution used in soft contact lens wear: report of a case. Ann Ophthalmol 13: 1277, 1981.

CLASS: VISCOELASTICS

Generic name: Sodium hyaluronate.

Proprietary names: AMO Vitrax, Amvisc, Coease, Euflexxa, Healon, Hyalgan, Orthovisc, Provisc, Restylane, Shellgel, Supartz, Synvisc, Viscoat.

Primary use

These are primarily used as viscoelastic materials in ophthalmic surgery.

Ocular side effects

Local ophthalmic use of exposure – intraocular
Certain
1. Elevated intraocular pressure
2. Opacities (corneal injection)
3. Crystalline deposition on intraocular lenses (high molecular weight)
4. Myopia
5. Ciliary block glaucoma

Possible
1. Uveitis – transient

Clinical significance

Improvements have been made in the manufacture of viscoelastics since the 1970s, and many of the initial adverse events, such as uveitis or precipitation of calcium salts due to excessive phosphate in the buffer, have now been eliminated. Floren (1998) showed that since autoclaving degrades high molecular weight hyaluronic acid molecules, it may still be a problem to keep these products free of endotoxins. The sodium salt of hyaluronic acid is sodium hyaluronate, which is one of the more commonly used viscoelastics. All of the viscoelastics can cause transitory elevations in pressure, usually peaking between 6 and 12 hours and returning to normal within 24 hours. This pressure elevation seems to be more acute and lasting in patients with glaucoma. There is some evidence that lower molecular weight viscoelastics do not produce as great a pressure elevation as those with higher molecular weights. Tanaka et al (1997) have shown that viscosity is important as well. It is recommended that washout times of at least 10 seconds are necessary to help prevent intraocular pressure elevations. Shammas (1995), Holtz (1992) and Reck et al (1998) describe entrapment of a viscoelastic in the capsular bag. This material is very slow to absorb and may require a surgical procedure, as it did in these three cases,

to prevent myopia, shallow anterior chamber and a distended capsular bag. Berger et al (1999) described a case of suspected ciliary block glaucoma caused by the viscoelastic agent being misdirected into the vitreous through an unsuspected small zonular dialysis. This required a vitrectomy and peripheral iridectomy to resolve. Since postoperative uveitis is common, it is difficult to determine a true incidence of inflammation attributed directly to these agents. However, this was more of a problem initially than it is currently. Studies by Storr-Paulsen and Larsen (1991) show little difference in the severity of iritis among the various viscoelastics. In general, these products seldom cause a significant inflammatory response. Jensen et al (1994) described a series of patients with visually significant deposition of a high molecular weight sodium hyaluronate (Healon GV®). These deposits may remain up to 6 months and decrease vision to 20/40 or worse. Isolated cases have been reported of corneal opacities occurring after inadvertent corneal injection of viscoelastics but they seem to absorb and resolve in a matter of months. There is little evidence that the viscoelastics bind with drugs to inhibit their action in the eye.

REFERENCES AND FURTHER READING

Alpar JJ. Comparison of healon and amvisc. Ann Ophthalmol 17: 647–651, 1985.

Berger RR, Kenyeres AM, Powell DA. Suspected ciliary block associated with Viscoat use. J Cataract Refract Surg 25(4): 594–596, 1999.

Daily L. Caution on sodium hyaluronate (Healon) syringe. Am J Ophthalmol 94(4): 59, 1982.

Floren I. Viscoelastic purity. J Cataract Refract Surg 24(2): 145–146, 1998.

Glasser DB, Matsuda M, Edelhauser HF. A comparison of the efficacy and toxicity of and intraocular pressure response to viscous solutions in the anterior chamber. Arch Ophthalmol 104: 1819–1824, 1986.

Goa KL, Benfield P. Hyaluronic acid: A review of its pharmacology and use as a surgical aid in ophthalmology, and its therapeutic potential in joint disease and wound healing. Drugs 47(3): 536–566, 1994.

Holtz SJ. Postoperative capsular bag distension. J Cataract Refract Surg 18: 310–317, 1992.

Hoover DL, Giangiacomo J, Benson RL. Descemet's membrane detachment by sodium hyaluronate. Arch Ophthalmol 103: 805–808, 1985.

Jensen MK, et al. Crystallization on intraocular lens surfaces associated with the use of Healon GV. Arch Ophthalmol 112: 1037–1042, 1994.

MacRae SM, et al. The effects of sodium hyaluronate, chondroitin sulfate, and methylcellulose on the corneal endothelium and intraocular pressure. Am J Ophthalmol 95: 332–341, 1983.

McDermott ML, Edelhauser HF. Drug binding of ophthalmic viscoelastic agents. Arch Ophthalmol 107: 261–263, 1989.

Pape LG, Balazs EA. The use of sodium hyaluronate (Healon®) in human anterior segment surgery. Ophthalmology 87(7): 699–705, 1980.

Passo MS, Ernest JT, Goldstick TK. Hyaluronate increases intraocular pressure when used in cataract extraction. Br J Ophthalmol 69(8): 572–575, 1985.

Reck AC, Pathmanathan T, Butler RE. Post-operative myopic shift due to trapped intracapsular Healon (letter). Eye 12(Pt 5): 900–901, 1998.

Shammas HJ. Relaxing the fibrosis capsulorhexis rim to correct induced hyperopia after phacoemulsification. J Cataract Refract Surg 21: 228–229, 1995.

Sholohov G, Levartovsky S. Retained ophthalmic viscosurgical device material in the capsular bag 6 months after phacoemulsification. J Cataract Refract Surg 31: 627–629, 2005.

Storr-Paulsen A. Analysis of the short-term effect of two viscoelastic agents on the intraocular pressure after extracapsular cataract extraction. Acta Ophthalmol 71: 173–176, 1993.

Storr-Paulsen A, Larsen M. Long-term results of extracapsular cataract extraction with posterior chamber lens implantation. Acta Ophthalmol 69: 766–769, 1991.

Tanaka T, Inoue H, Kudo S, et al. Relationship between postoperative intraocular pressure elevation and residual sodium hyaluronate following phacoemulsification and aspiration. J Cataract Refract Surg 23(2): 284–288, 1997.

8

Chemical-induced ocular side effects

Devin Gattey, MD

CLASS: ACIDS

Generic name: 1. Hydrofluoric acid; 2. hydrochloric acid; 3. sulfuric acid.

Synonyms: 1. Fluoric acid, fluohydric acid, hydrofluoride, fluorine monohydride; 2. hydrogen chloride, muriatic acid; 3. battery acid, sulfuric acid, hydrogen sulfate, sulfine acid.

Proprietary names/products containing: 1. Eagle One Chrome and Wire Cleaner, Ultradent Porcelain Etch, FPPF Acid Enhanced Trailer Brightener, Whink Rust Remover, Arrobrite Aluminum Brightener, Briter 601 Glass Cleaner; 2. Lysol Brand Toilet Bowl Cleaner, Humidifier Plastic Cleaner, Febreze Laundry Odor Eliminator, Lime A Way Toilet Bowl Cleaner, Zep Grout Cleaner and Whitener, Zep Calcium, Lime, and Rust Stain Remover, C Flux (Lead Free) maintenance paste, Kem Tek Calcium & Metal Eliminator, Kem Tek Tile & Spa Cleaner, Parks Muriatic Acid 20%.; 3. Rain Away Rain Repellent, Naval Jelly Rust Dissolver, Loctite Sink Jelly, Goddards Silver Dip, Instant Power Liquid Drain Opener, Duro Aluminum Jelly Corrosion Remover, pH Down, pH Adjust

Primary use

Hydrofluoric acid
This compound is used to clean and etch glass and metal in the manufacture of silicone wafers and in the synthesis of many fluorine-containing organic compounds, including teflon and refrigerants such as freon. It is also used in many household rust removers.

Hydrochloric acid
Sold as muriatic acid, this is used for a variety of household, scientific research and construction purposes. Hydrochloric acid is also used to clean and electroplate metal, and to tan leather. It is used to adjust pH in many products.

Sulfuric acid
A principal component in the manufacture of batteries, this is also used in the fertilizer, petroleum refining and printing industries as well as in metal cleaning and electroplating and in the paper industry.

Ocular side effects

Direct ocular exposure
Certain
1. Ocular irritation
   a. Eye pain
2. Lacrimation
3. Non-specific blepharospasm
4. Conjunctiva
   a. Hyperemia
   b. Edema
   c. Blanching of vascular bed
   d. Symblepharon
5. Cornea
   a. Edema
   b. Scarring
   c. Ulceration
   d. Vascularization
   e. Perforation
   f. Fibrovascular pannus
6. Entropion
7. Iritis

Possible
1. Cataracts
2. Increased intraocular pressure

Clinical significance
In general, acids are less injurious to the eye than alkalis. As is the case for alkalis, concentration, time and surface area of exposure, and pH are the factors which most influence the extent of the injury. Once the pH drops to 2.5 or below the extent of injury is likely to be much more severe. Hydrofluoric, hydrochloric and sulfuric acids can all cause extensive corrosive damage, initially from the high concentration of hydrogen ions. However, hydrofluoric acid is considered the acid most likely to cause severe ocular and skin injuries.

Most acids cause a coagulative necrosis of the corneal epithelium, which helps to prevent penetration of the acid into the deeper layers of the cornea or the anterior chamber. With hydrofluoric acid, the fluoride ion itself can penetrate the cornea and cause severe damage. In fact, the ability of the free fluoride ion to penetrate tissue and combine with internal body calcium stores makes splash exposures potentially fatal. Hypocalcemia may ensue in cases where less than 10% of the body surface area has been exposed to hydrofluoric acid, causing cardiac arrhythmia and bone damage.

The ocular injury pattern for hydrofluoric and other concentrated acids is very similar to that for alkalis. A higher concentration and longer exposure time may be needed to achieve the same degree of injury, but the same types of injury are possible, including corneal and conjunctival scarring, and symblepharon formation.

Recommendations
The most important intervention in ocular exposure to concentrated acids is immediate irrigation. Many studies have been done to identify the optimal irrigating solution for various types of chemical exposure, but the subtle advantages of one solution

over another are far less important than the rapidity of applying irrigation. In an industrial setting, eyewash stations are often prevalent. If an ocular exposure to a strong acid occurs away from such resources, rescuers should immediately apply whatever non-toxic aqueous solution is at hand.

Once a victim is in a medical care center, extensive irrigation must be started immediately using normal saline or sterile water. This is aided by the use of topical anesthetic and a lid speculum. One liter of fluid should be used to flush the eye surface over a period of 10 minutes. A few minutes should be allowed to pass following this first liter for accurate testing of the pH of the conjunctival cul-de-sac using litmus paper accurate in the neutral range. If the pH does not rise above 7, cycles of irrigation should be continued for 15 minutes followed by a check of the pH. One study suggested that repeating cycles of irrigation could prolong corneal epithelial healing time with acid injuries. After the initial round of irrigation, a brief ocular examination should take place, checking vision and intraocular pressure, and examining the conjunctival fornices for foreign bodies, which may act as a reservoir for acid. At this point, the necrotic corneal epithelium should be removed.

Following irrigation and neutrality of pH, medical therapy should ensue. Topical cycloplegic eye drops, antibiotic ointment and corticosteroid eye drops should be instituted for the first week. After this time, corticosteroids may inhibit wound healing. The surgical care of the late sequelae of severe ocular burns from acids is a complicated subject and beyond the scope of this text.

Calcium gluconate gel, 2.5%, is often applied in first-aid settings for hydrofluoric acid burns of the skin. There are reports of using this chemical in subcutaneous, intra-arterial and inhaled forms following hydrofluoric acid exposures. Unfortunately, it has not proven as effective in the treatment of ocular injuries, and it is not currently considered to be the standard of care.

REFERENCES AND FURTHER READING

Beiran I, Miller B, Bentur Y. The efficacy of calcium gluconate in ocular hydrofluoric acid burns. Hum Exp Toxicol 16(4): 223–228, 1997.

Blomet J, Hall AH, Mathieu L, Nehles J. Efficacy of hexafluorine for emergent decontamination of hydrofluoric acid eye and skin splashes. Vet Hum Toxicol 43(5): 263–265, 2001.

Fung JF, Kenneally CZ, Sengelmann RD. Chemical injury to the eye from trichloroacetic acid. Dermatol Surg 28(7): 609–610, 2002.

Grant WM, Schuman JS. Toxicology of the Eye. Effects on the eyes and visual system from chemicals, drugs, metals and minerals, plants, toxins and venoms; also, systemic side effects from eye medications, 4th edn, Charles C. Thomas, Springfield, IL, 1993.

Lauberm SE, McCulley JP, Petitt MG, Whiting DW. Hydrofluoric acid burns of the eye. J Occup Med 25(6): 447–450, 1983.

McCulley JP. Ocular hydrofluoric acid burns: animal model, mechanism of injury and therapy. Trans Am Ophthalmol Soc 88: 649–684, 1990.

Rubinfeld RS, Silbert DI, Arentsen JJ, Laibson PR. Ocular hydrofluoric acid burns. Am J Ophthalmol 114: 420–423, 1992.

Wagoner MD, Kenyon KR. Chemical injuries of the eye. In: Principles and Practice of Opthalmology, 2nd edn. Albert DM, Jacobiec FA (eds), Philadelphia, WB Saunders, 2000.

CLASS: AEROSOLS

Generic names: 1. Ortho-chlorobenzalmalononitrile (CS); 2. Chloracetophenone; 3. Oleoresin capsicum (OC).

Synonyms: Tear gas; 1. CS gas; 2. CN gas, mace; 3. OC-pepper spray.

Primary use

Used as 'chemical batons' for control of individuals or crowds, primarily in law enforcement. CS and CN gas are white crystals with low vapor pressures and are not gases. OC is an extract from chilli peppers and is a reddish-orange oily liquid that is dispersed as an aerosol.

Ocular side effects

Direct ocular exposure
Certain
1. Profuse lacrimation
2. Eyelids
   a. Blepharospasm
   b. Erythema
   c. Blisters (high concentrations)
3. Severe ocular pain – burning
4. Decreased corneal sensitivity (OC)
5. Cornea
   a. Superficial punctate keratitis (OC)
   b. Erosions (OC)
6. Blurred vision
7. Conjunctiva
   a. Erythema
   b. Chemosis

Probable
1. Allergic reactions

Defective or improper delivery – powder form of CS and CN
Certain
1. Conjunctiva and/or cornea
   a. Erosions
   b. Scarring
   c. Vascularization

Systemic side effects

Topical ocular exposure
Certain
1. Coughing (CS, CN)
2. Increase mucus secretion (CS, CN)
3. Severe headaches (CS, CN)
4. Dizziness (CS, CN)
5. Dyspnea (CS, CN)
6. Tightness of chest (CS, CN)
7. Difficulty breathing (CS, CN)
8. Excessive salivation (CS, CN)

Possible
1. Bradycardia (OC)
2. Hypotension (OC)

Clinical significance

CS is one of the most commonly used tear gases in the world. CS and CN are effective because when released, they are dispersed as a microscopic powder, which acts as a 'powdered barb'. This powder attaches to moist mucus membranes and skin, where it becomes a liquid and a potent sensory irritant. OC is an irritant causing neurogenic inflammation with the same ocular finding as CS and CN.

CS causes symptoms within 20–60 seconds after exposure and if the recipient seeks fresh air, these findings generally cease within 10–30 minutes with currently used forms of CS delivery. OC effects last up to 40 minutes after irrigation, with some minor irritation up to a few hours. The medical literature, in the main, supports the safety of CS gas (Ballantyne 1977/1978; Beswick 1983; Danto 1987), however, significant reactions have been reported (Hu et al 1989; Parneix-Spake et al 1993; Scott 1995). In over 30 plus years of use of 1% CS tear gas, no lawsuits for bodily damages have been awarded in the USA. In the UK, however, 5% CS tear gas is used and there appears to be some concern on its use (Ro and Lee 1991).

Chloracetophenone (mace) is a more caustic agent and if the eye is exposed to high concentrations (non-standard use) or defective delivery this can cause cicatrisation, corneal and conjunctival erosions, and scarring with vascularization.

These sprays may aggravate asthma, chronic obstructive airway disease, hypertension, cardiovascular disease and possibly those on neuroleptic drugs. Based on our current knowledge, if properly trained law personnel use these agents, and if the combatant leaves the gas area rapidly, significant long-term effects should not occur.

Recommendations

The current recommendations in the UK for treatment of CS ocular exposure are to 'blow dry air directly onto the eye' (Yih 1995). The recommendation of the manufacturers in the USA suggests copious ocular irrigation to dislodge, dilute and wash away the irritant. Liquids initially may increase the pain secondary to CS, therefore an ocular anesthetic might first be applied to facilitate irrigation. If ocular exposure does occur, take the following steps:
1. Remove contact lenses.
2. Use copious amounts of water for irrigation (cold isotonic saline is ideal).
3. Move to an environment free of the gas.
4. Wash skin twice with soap and do not rub.
5. Do not apply oily lotions or oily soaps.
6. Remove contaminated clothing.
7. Pain can be reduced by over-the-counter medication such as ibuprofen.
8. Over-the-counter antihistamines may alleviate some of the effects of pepper spray, especially if used before exposure.
9. Slit lamp examination may be required to remove any corneal or conjunctival particulate matter.

REFERENCES AND FURTHER READING

Ballantyne B. Riot control agents. Med Annu 7–41, 1977/1978.
Beswick FW. Chemical agents used in riot control and warfare. Human Toxicol 2: 247–256, 1983.
Danto BL. Medical problems and criteria regarding the used of tear gas by police. Am J Forensic Med Pathol 8: 317–322, 1987.
Fraunfelder FT. Is CS gas dangerous?. BMJ 320: 458–459, 2000.
Gray PJ. Treating CS gas injuries to the eye: exposure at close range is particularly dangerous [letter] 311: 871, 1995.
Hu H, Fine J, Epstein P, et al. Tear gas – harassing agent or toxic chemical weapon? JAMA 262: 660–663, 1989.
Parneix-Spake A, Theisen A, Roujean JC, et al. Severe cutaneous reactions to self-defense sprays. Arch Dermatol 129: 913, 1993.
'Safety' of chemical batons. Editorial. Lancet 352: 159, 1998.
Ro YS, Lee CW. Tear gas dermatitis: allergic contact sensitization due to CS. J Dermatol 30: 576–577, 1991.
Scott RAH. Treating CS gas injuries to the eye: illegal 'mace' contains more toxic CN particles [letter]. BMJ 311: 871, 1995.
Treudler R, Tebbe B, Blume-Peytavi U, et al. Occupational contact dermatitis due to 2-chloroacetophenone tear gas. Br J Dermatol 140: 531–534, 1999.
Wheeler H, Murray V. Treating CS gas injuries to the eye: exposure at close range is particularly dangerous [letter]. BMJ 311: 871, 1995.
Willoughby CF, Ilango B, Hughes A. CS gas ocular injury [comment]. Eye 12: 164, 1998.
Yih JP: CS gas injury to the eye. Blowing dry air on to the eye is preferable to irrigation. BMJ 311: 276, 1995.
Zollman TM, Bragg RM, Harrison DA. Clinical effects of oleoresin capsicum (pepper spray) on the human cornea and conjunctiva. Ophthalmology 107: 2186–2189, 2000.

CLASS: ALCOHOLS

Generic name: Alcohol (ethanol, ethyl alcohol)

Proprietary name: None

Primary use

This colorless liquid is used as a solvent, an antiseptic, a beverage and as a nerve block in the management of certain types of intractable pain.

Ocular side effects

Systemic administration – acute intoxication
Certain
1. Extraocular muscles
   a. Phoria
   b. Diplopia
   c. Nystagmus – various types, including downbeat nystagmus
   d. Esophoria or exophoria
   e. Convergent strabismus
   f. Decreased convergence
   g. Jerky pursuit movements
   h. Decreased spontaneous movements
2. Pupils
   a. Mydriasis
   b. Decreased reaction to light
   c. Anisocoria
3. Decreased vision
4. Decreased accommodation
5. Problems with color vision
   a. Color vision defect, blue-yellow or red-green defect
   b. Objects have blue tinge
6. Decreased dark adaptation
7. Decreased intraocular pressure – transitory
8. Constriction of visual fields
9. Decreased depth perception
10. Decreased optokinetic and peripheral gaze nystagmus
11. Visual hallucinations
12. Prolonged glare recovery
13. Ptosis (unilateral or bilateral)
14. Impaired oculomotor coordination
15. Toxic amblyopia
16. Abnormal ERG, VEP or critical flicker fusion

Systemic administration – chronic intoxication
Certain
1. Extraocular muscles
   a. Paralysis
   b. Jerky pursuit movements
2. Downbeat nystagmus
3. Paralysis of accommodation
4. Pupils
   a. Miosis
   b. Decreased or absent reaction to light

5. Decreased vision
6. Visual fields
   a. Papillomacular scotomas
   b. Abnormal static perimetry
   c. Abnormal kinetic perimetry
7. Problems with color vision – color vision defect, red-green defect
8. Oscillopsia
9. Lacrimation increased
10. Decreased intraocular pressure – transitory
11. Visual hallucinations

Probable
1. Cataracts
   a. Posterior subcapsular
   b. Nuclear

Possible
1. Optic nerve
   a. Neuritis
   b. Temporal pallor
2. Corneal deposits (arcus senilis)
3. Toxic amblyopia

Ocular teratogenic effects (fetal alcohol syndrome)
Certain
1. Retinal blood vessels – increased tortuosity
2. Decreased vision
3. Optic nerve – hypoplasia
4. Palpebral fissure – horizontal shortening
5. Ptosis
6. Strabismus (convergent or divergent)
7. Abnormalities of anterior chamber angles
8. Secondary glaucoma
9. Duane's retraction syndrome
10. Cornea
    a. Decreased polymegathism
    b. Decreased hexagonality

Local ophthalmic use or exposure – retrobulbar injection
Certain
1. Irritation
   a. Hyperemia
   b. Ocular pain (acute)
   c. Edema
2. Keratitis
3. Paralysis of extraocular muscles
4. Nystagmus
5. Ptosis
6. Corneal ulceration
7. Decreased vision
8. Eyelids – depigmentation
9. Ocular anesthesia

Inadvertent ocular exposure
Certain
1. Irritation
   a. Lacrimation
   b. Hyperemia
   c. Ocular pain
   d. Edema
   e. Burning sensation
2. Keratitis
3. Corneal necrosis or opacities (prolonged exposure)

Clinical significance

Inadvertent splashes of alcoholic beverage onto the eye surface are a frequent occurrence and result in irritation of the conjunctiva and cornea, but there are no reports of permanent damage. Most distilled alcoholic beverages are 40% alcohol by volume, but concentrations up to 75% are available commercially in the USA. In the photorefractive keratectomy procedure, ophthalmic surgeons use concentrations of less than 40% alcohol to remove corneal epithelium. It has been shown that the duration of application of 20% alcohol is important to corneal epithelial cell survival. A 30-second or less application allows cell survival, while a 60-second application may lead to cell death. There is a report of an adverse event in which alcohol was placed in the anterior chamber during cataract surgery, resulting in permanent endothelial damage.

Consumption of alcoholic beverages leads to a host of well-known ocular side effects. Acute intoxication may result in nystagmus, a finding used by law enforcement personnel to screen for inebriated motor vehicle operators. Pupil abnormalities, ptosis and strabismus are also well known effects of inebriation. Also reported are temporary corneal clouding, and a methanol-like loss of vision associated with alcohol-induced metabolic acidosis. Alcoholism also leads to malnutrition in severe cases, which may lead to xerophthalmia or toxic amblyopia. Various types of cataracts have been reported to be more common in heavy users of ethanol, but large population-based studies have shown that nuclear sclerosis is more common in people who smoke and drink heavily. It is suspected that alcoholics are also more prone to infectious keratitis. Children born with fetal alcohol syndrome have multiple orbital and ocular structural abnormalities.

Recommendations

1. Inadvertent ocular splashes of high concentrations of ethanol should be treated with routine irrigation, and patients should be followed for the development of corneal abrasion or ulceration.
2. The ocular side effects of retrobulbar alcohol injections are many, and thus its use in cases of blind and painful eyes should be considered if evisceration or enucleation are not possible.
3. The neuroophthalmic side effects of acute ethanol intoxication usually reverse within 24 hours. Chronic use of alcohol will have less untoward ocular effects if the diets are supplemented with vitamins.

REFERENCES AND FURTHER READING

Al-Faran MF, Al-Omar OM. Retrobulbar alcohol injection in blind painful eyes. Ann Ophthalmol 22: 460–462, 1990.

Dreiss AK, Winkler von Mohrenfels C, Gabler B, et al. Laser epithelial keratomileusis (LASEK): histological investigation for vitality of corneal epithelial cells after alcohol exposure. Klin Monatsbl Augenheilkd 219: 365–369, 2002.

Garber JM. Steep corneal curvature: a fetal alcohol syndrome landmark. J Am Optom Assoc 55: 595–598, 1984.

Hsu HY, Piva A, Sadun AA. Devastating complication from alcohol cauterization of recurrent Rathke cleft cyst. Case report. J Neurosurg 100: 1087–1090, 2004.

Kondo M, Ogino N. An accidental irrigation of the anterior chamber with ethanol during cataract surgery. Jpn J Clin Ophthalmol 43: 1851–1853, 1989.

Leibowitz HM, Ryan W, Kupferman A, Vitale JJ. The effect of alcohol intoxication on inflammation of the cornea. Arch Ophthalmol 103: 723–725, 1985.

Reisin I, Reisin LH, Aviel E. Corneal melting in a chronic contact lens wearer. CLAO J 22: 146–147, 1996.

Roncone DP. Xerophthalmia secondary to alcohol-induced malnutrition. Optometry 77: 124–133, 2006.

Shiono T, Asano Y, Hashimoto T, Mizuno K. Temporary corneal edema after acute intake of alcohol. Br J Ophthalmol 71: 462–465, 1987.

Stein HA, Stein RM, Price C, Salim GA. Alcohol removal of the epithelium for excimer laser ablation: outcomes analysis. J Cataract Refract Surg. 23: 1160–1163, 1997.

Yanagawa Y, Kiyozumi T, Hatanaka K, et al. Reversible blindness associated with alcoholic ketoacidosis. Am J Ophthalmol 137: 775–777, 2004.

Generic name: Ethylene glycol.

Synonyms: 1,2-dihydroxyethane; 1,2-ethandiol; ethane-1,2-diol; ethylene alcohol; ethylene dihydrate; glycol; 2-hydroxyethanol; meg; monoethylene glycol.

Proprietary names/products containing: Fridex; Tescol; Lutrol-9; Macrogol; Snap Fix A Flat Tire Sealant; Wagner Premium Brake Fluid; Rally Cream Car Wax; Snap Windshield Spray De Icer; Prestone Antifreeze/Coolant; Epson Ink Cartridges; Red Devil EZ Caulk; Behr Premium Plus Interior Flat.

Primary use

Ethylene glycol is principally used as antifreeze. It is also used in hydraulic brake fluid, as a solvent in the paint and plastics industries, and in inks, fire extinguishing agents, and synthetic waxes. There are longer-chain glycol ethers such as diethylene glycol, triethylene glycol and polyethylene glycol that have similar uses, and they may be combined in various products.

Ocular side effects

Direct ocular exposure
Certain
1. Irritation
   a. Burning sensation
2. Conjunctiva
   a. Hyperemia

Systemic exposure
Certain
1. Nystagmus
2. Pupils
   a. Poorly reactive
   b. Dilated (comatose)
3. Strabismus
4. Blurred vision
5. Optic disc edema

Possible
1. Optic atrophy
2. Retinal edema

Clinical significance

Ocular splash injuries with ethylene glycol are quite common as it is the main component of automobile antifreeze and hydraulic fluids. At room temperature, this substance is known to be fairly innocuous, causing minor to moderate irritation. A data pull from the American Association of Poison Control Centers Toxic Exposure Surveillance System database revealed 601 exposures to ethylene glycol and brake fluid. Of these, four cases were judged to have an outcome severity graded as 'major' (indicating some type of significant residual disability). The data do not indicate the nature of the injury, and it is possible that ethylene glycol of high temperature or pressure was involved in these cases.

Systemic poisoning with ethylene glycol is unfortunately not uncommon. It leads to a metabolic acidosis similar to that which occurs with methanol. Although blurred vision has been reported, vision damage is not the hallmark of this toxin. Severe cases usually lead to renal damage and cardiopulmonary failure. Neurotoxicity is often present in these severe (and frequently fatal) cases, including multiple cranial nerve dysfunction, cerebral edema and coma. These patients may experience strabismus, optic disc edema and pupil abnormalities as part of the neurotoxicity.

Longer chain glycol ethers are typically less toxic, although diethylene glycol can cause a similar toxic syndrome when taken orally. Polyethylene glycols are generally harmless topically and systemically, and are found in many medications and cosmetics.

Recommendations

Ocular splash injury should be treated with brief rinsing unless an accompanying thermal burn is suspected, in which case urgent ophthalmic consultation should be sought. Systemic poisoning with ethylene glycol leads to a complex toxic syndrome and should be managed in an intensive care setting. Treatment is similar to that for methanol and often includes competitive inhibition of metabolic enzymes with ethanol or fomepizole, reversal of metabolic acidosis and dialysis.

REFERENCES AND FURTHER READING

Ahmed MM. Ocular effects of antifreeze poisoning. Br J Ophthalmol 55(12): 854–855, 1971.

American Association of Poison Control Centers Toxic Exposure Surveillance System database, 2002–2005, human ocular exposures by substance. Data pull 8/23/06.

Berger JR, Ayyar DR. Neurological complications of ethylene glycol intoxication. Report of a case. Arch Neurol 38(11):724–726, 1981.

Brent J. Current management of ethylene glycol poisoning. Drugs 61(7): 979–988, 2001.

DaRoza R, Henning RJ, Sunshine I, Sutheimer C. Acute ethylene glycol poisoning. Crit Care Med 12(11): 1003–1005, 1984.

Fruijtier-Polloth C. Safety assessment on polyethylene glycols (PEGS) and their derivatives as used in cosmetic products. Toxicology 214(1–2): 1–38, 2005.

Jacobsen D, McMartin KE. Methanol and ethylene glycol poisonings. Mechanism of toxicity, clinical course, diagnosis and treatment. Med Toxicol 1(5): 309–334, 1986.

McDonald TO, Kasten K, Hervey R, et al. Acute ocular toxicity for normal and irritated rabbit eyes and subacute ocular toxicity for ethylene oxide, ethylene glycol. Bull Parenter Drug Assoc 31(1): 25–32, 1977.

Morgan BW, Ford MD, Follmer R. Ethylene glycol ingestion resulting in brainstem and midbrain dysfunction. J Toxicol Clin Toxicol 38(4): 445–451, 2000.

Generic name: Isopropyl alcohol.

Synonyms: Rubbing alcohol, isopropanol, methylethanol, 2-hydroxypropane, 2-propanol, 2-propyl alcohol, dimethylcarbinol, dimethyl carbinol, sec-propyl alcohol, persprit, propan-2-ol.

Proprietary names/products containing: Found in household cleaners, adhesives and antifog or rain formulations.

Primary use

Isopropyl alcohol is used in antifreeze products, as a solvent for gums, shellac and essential oils, and in quick-drying inks and oils. It can also be found in body rubs, hand lotions, after-shave lotions, cosmetics and pharmaceuticals. It is used in the manufacture of acetone, glycerol and isopropyl acetate. In medicine, it receives widespread use as an antiseptic for skin and instrumentation, including the antisepsis of applanation tonometer tips.

Ocular side effects

Direct ocular exposure
Certain
1. Irritation – burning
2. Conjunctiva – hyperemia
3. Cornea
   a. Abrasion
   b. Punctate keratitis

Clinical significance

Isopropyl alcohol is well known to cause ocular surface irritation, epithelial keratitis and occasional corneal abrasion. Most commonly, isopropyl alcohol comes into contact with the eye surface during Goldmann applanation tonometry. Tonometer tips are frequently cleaned with a wipe saturated in 70% isopropyl alcohol or soaked for at least 5 minutes in a 70% solution (the method recommended by the US Center for Disease Control) and applied to the corneal surface. If this is done before the alcohol has completely dried, a familiar round epithelial defect, a burning sensation or frank eye pain may ensue. Another potential route of ocular injury includes pre-surgical preparation of the peri-ocular skin with alcohol wipes. Occupational exposures to isopropyl alcohol vapors have been reported to cause eye irritation but no significant injury.

Recommendations

As with most chemical eye injuries, rapid irrigation with isotonic saline or sterile water is the best first aid. Unlike methanol, drinking isopropyl alcohol, although potentially fatal, does not cause loss of vision.

REFERENCES AND FURTHER READING

Griffith JF, Nixon GA, Bruce RD, et al. Dose-response studies with chemical irritants in the albino rabbit eye as a basis for selecting optimum testing conditions for predicting hazard to the human eye. Toxicol Appl Pharmacol 55(3): 501–513, 1980.

Mac Rae SM, Brown B, Edelhauser HF. The corneal toxicity of presurgical skin antiseptics. Am J Ophthalmol 97(2): 221–232, 1984.

Roseman MJ, Hill RM. Aerobic responses of the cornea to isopropyl alcohol, measured in vivo. Acta Ophthalmol (Copenh) 65(3): 306–312, 1987.

Segal WA, Pirnazar JR, Arens M, Pepose JS. Disinfection of Goldmann tonometers after contamination with hepatitis C virus. Am J Ophthalmol 131(2): 184–187, 2001.

Smeets MA, Maute C, Dalton PH. Acute sensory irritation from exposure to iso propanol (2-propanol) at TLV in workers and controls: objective versus subjective effects. Ann Occup Hyg 46(4): 359–373, 2002.

Smith CA, Pepose JS. Disinfection of tonometers and contact lenses in the office lenses in the office setting: are current techniques adequate? Am J Ophthalmol 127(1): 77–84, 1999.

Soukiasian SH, Asdourian GK, Weiss JS, Kachadoorian HA. A complication from alcohol-swabbed tonometer tips. Am J Ophthalmol 105(4): 424–425, 1988.

Generic name: Methanol.

Synonyms: Methyl alcohol, wood alcohol, wood spirits.

Proprietary names/products containing: Found in automobile engine cleaners, antifreeze, de-icers and paint/stain removers.

Primary use

Known as wood alcohol, methanol was once produced by the distillation of wood. It is now produced synthetically. Methanol is the simplest alkyl alcohol. It is used primarily as a solvent and as an antifreeze. It is also found in several cleaners and is used to denature ethanol. Methanol occurs in small amounts naturally in the environment.

Ocular side effects

Topical ocular exposure
Possible
1. Irritation

Systemic exposure
Certain
1. Blindness
2. Blurred vision
3. Optic atrophy
4. Optic disc hyperemia
5. Visual field defects
6. Decreased pupil reactions.
7. Death

Clinical significance

Many unfortunate accidents involving the consumption of methanol have been recorded in the literature. Methanol is often used to denature ethanol for industrial uses, and as its odor is milder and sweeter than ethanol, so its presence in denatured alcohol is difficult to detect. People may accidentally consume methanol while consuming what they believe to be unadulterated ethanol. A report of multiple victims of methanol toxicity in Port Moresby, Papua New Guinea showed that a dose-related response exists with ocular effects ranging from none to blindness. With consumption of higher volumes, vision loss often precedes death. Rarely, significant systemic toxicity may occur via percutaneous or inhalational exposure.

Temporary reactions to systemic methanol exposure include peripapillary edema, optic disc hyperemia, diminished pupillary reactions and central scotomata. Permanent ocular abnormalities include decreased visual acuity, blindness, optic disc pallor, attenuation or sheathing of arterioles, diminished pupillary reaction to light and visual field defects. MRI studies have shown one location of neurological damage from methanol to be in the putamen. Pathologic studies reveal that methanol probably damages mitochondria in the photoreceptors.

Recommendations

People who are suspected to have ingested methanol need immediate care, preferably in an intensive care unit setting. Treatment of systemic methanol poisoning consists of trying to prevent the metabolism of methanol to formaldehyde, which then is converted to formic acid. Formic acid inhibits cytochrome oxidase, a key protein in the production of ATP within mitochondria, and its formation is thought to precipitate the neurological side effects of methanol consumption. Peak concentrations of methanol occur within an hour of ingestion. A latent period occurs while the methanol is converted to formic acid, and a metabolic acidosis ensues. Visual loss often precedes the potentially fatal side effects of the formic acidosis. To block the metabolism towards formic acid, competitive inhibition of alcohol dehydrogenase may be achieved by giving the patient ethanol or fomepizole (which does not cause inebriation). Hemodialysis may enhance the elimination of methanol and its metabolic byproducts, allowing improved chances of recovery.

REFERENCES AND FURTHER READING

Barceloux DG, Bond GR, Krenzelok EP, et al. American Academy of Clinical Toxicology practice guidelines on the treatment of methanol poisoning. J Toxicol Clin Toxicol 40(4): 415–416, 2002.

Brent J, McMartin K, Phillips S, et al. Fomepizole for the treatment of methanol poisoning. N Engl J Med 344(6): 424–429, 2001.

Dethlefs R, Naragi S. Ocular manifestations and complications of acute methyl alcohol intoxication. Med J Aust 4:2(10)): 483–485, 1978.

Eells JT, Henry MM, Summerfelt P, et al. Therapeutic photobiomodulation for methanol-induced retinal toxicity. Proc Natl Acad Sci USA 100(6): 3439–3444, 2003.

Onder F, Ilker S, Kansu T, et al. Acute blindness and putaminal necrosis in methanol intoxication. Int Ophthalmol 22(2): 81–84, 1998–1999.

Seme MT, Summerfelt P, Neitz J, et al. Differential recovery of retinal function after mitochondrial inhibition by methanol intoxication. Invest Ophthalmol Vis Sci 42(3): 834–841, 2001.

Generic name: Phenol (hydroxybenzene).

Synonyms: Carbolic acid, fenol, phenic acid, phenylic acid, phenolum, phenyl hydrate, phenylic alcohol, phenyl hydroxide, benzaphenol.

Proprietary names/products containing: Noxema Shaving Cream, Campho-Phenique, Chloraseptic Sore Throat Spray, Ulcer Ease Mouth Wash.

Primary use

Phenols are a class of organic compounds containing a hydroxyl group and a benzene ring, the simplest of which is referred to as phenol. Commonly used in organic synthesis, phenol is a precursor in the production of resins and nylons. It is used in the manufacture of many products, including insulation materials, adhesives, lacquers, paint, solvents, rubber, ink, dyes, illuminating gases, perfumes, soaps and toys. Also used in embalming and research laboratories, it is found in commercial disinfectants, antiseptics, lotions and ointments. Phenol is also used as a topical anesthetic, in ear drops and as a sclerosing agent. Other medical applications of phenol include use as a neurolytic agent and in dermatology for chemical face peeling.

Ocular side effects

Direct ocular exposure
Certain
1. Eyelid
   a. Scarring
   b. Entropion
2. Cornea
   a. Opacification
   b. Hypesthesia
3. Conjunctiva – chemosis

Systemic exposure
Certain
1. Sclera – discoloration (carbolochronosis) – blue-gray and brown

Clinical significance

Phenol is well known to be caustic and may cause severe chemical burns of the skin or eyes in higher concentrations. Use of this agent in lower concentrations for cosmetic 'skin-peeling' has become widespread. In most consumer products, the concentration of phenol is quite low. Although ocular damage from concentrated phenol is well documented in the literature prior to 1950, there have been no recent reports. This may indicate a substantial improvement in industrial hygiene practices over the last century. Phenol is used by percutaneous retrogasserian injection in the treatment of trigeminal neuralgia, and there is a single report of unilateral blindness following such a procedure.

Recommendations

In dermal burns from phenol, first-aid treatment with isopropyl alcohol or polyethylene glycol has been recommended. Isopropyl alcohol is toxic to the corneal epithelium and should be avoided. Polyethylene glycol is well tolerated by the eye, but there is not substantial evidence that this treatment improves visual outcomes. Standard immediate irrigation practices with water or isotonic saline should be pursued.

REFERENCES AND FURTHER READING

Aydemir O, Yilmaz T, Onal SA, et al. Acute unilateral total visual loss after retrogasserian phenol injection for the treatment of trigeminal neuralgia: a case report. Orbit 25(1): 23–26, 2006.

Kligman AM, Baker TJ, Gordon HL. Long-term histologic follow-up of phenol face peels. Plast Reconstr Surg. 75(5): 652–659, 1985.

Monteiro-Riviere NA, Inman AO, Jackson H, et al. Efficacy of topical phenol decontamination strategies on severity of acute phenol chemical burns and dermal absorption: in vitro and in vivo studies in pig skin. Toxicol Ind Health 17(4): 95–104, 2001.

Todorovic V. Acute phenol poisoning [in Serbian]. Med Pregl 56 Suppl 1: 37–41, 2003.

CLASS: ALKALI

Generic name: Ammonia.

Synonyms: Hydrogen nitride, ammonium hydroxide.

Proprietary names/products containing: Found in a variety of cleaners and polishes.

Primary use

Pure ammonia is present as a gas at room temperature, but it is dissolvable in water and readily forms ammonium salts. Its primary use is in the production of fertilizers. It is also used to produce explosives. In household products 5–10% solutions are used in many glass cleaners and polishes.

Ocular side effects

Topical Ocular Exposure
Certain
1. Irritation – eye pain
2. Cornea (Fig. 8.1)
   a. Ulceration
   b. Scarring
3. Conjunctiva – hyperemia
4. Glaucoma
5. Cataract
6. Iris
   a. Degeneration
   b. Pupillary abnormality

Clinical significance

Exposure to ammonia gas is clearly irritating to the eyes. Significant eye injuries from ammonia gas typically occur only with high pressure or in conjunction with severe systemic injury. When

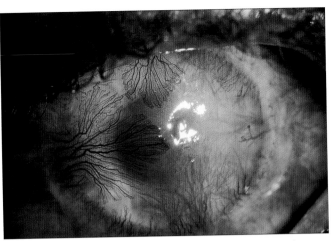

Fig. 8.1 Massive neovascularization of the cornea and stromal scarring after direct eye exposure to ammonia. Photo courtesy of Spalton DJ, Hitchings RA, Hunter PA. Atlas of Clinical Ophthalmology, 3rd edn, London, Mosby Elsevier, 2005.

dissolved in water ammonia forms ammonium hydroxide, a moderately strong base. When dissolved in water in the concentrations found in household cleaning supplies (5–10%), ammonia is unlikely to cause severe eye injury with a liquid splash into the eye, although corneal abrasion is possible. In concentrations higher than 10%, significant tissue injury has frequently been reported, including corneal scarring, glaucoma, cataracts and iris degeneration. Ammonium hydroxide seems to penetrate the anterior chamber more easily than other alkalis, leading to severe intraocular damage. Although most severe ammonia injuries occur in the agriculture industry, there are reports of ocular damage occurring during the illicit production of methamphetamine.

Recommendations

Exposure to ammonia gas in higher concentrations may result in an injury pattern common to alkalis. Emergent medical evaluation is required as the risk of severe pulmonary injury is high.

1. Ocular splashes from household cleaners containing less than 10% ammonia should be treated with routine irrigation using isotonic saline, and patients should receive a consultation with an ophthalmologist to follow possible corneal or anterior chamber injuries.
2. If liquid or solid industrial preparations of higher concentration ammonia-containing products are involved in ocular injuries, then the irrigation strategy should follow the guidelines for the treatment of alkali burns (see section on lye), with prompt referral to an ophthalmologist.

REFERENCES AND FURTHER READING

Charukamnoetkanok P, Wagoner MD. Facial and ocular injuries associated with methamphetamine production accidents. Am J Ophthalmol Nov; 138(5): 875-876, 2004.

Lee JH, Farley CL, Brodrick CD, et al. Anhydrous ammonia eye injuries associated with illicit methamphetamine production. Ann Emerg Med 41: 157, 2003.

McGuiness R. Ammonia in the eye. BMJ 1: 575, 1969.

Wrong O. Ammonia burns of the eye. BMJ (Clin Res Ed) 296(6631): 1263, 1988.

Generic name: Lime.

Synonyms: Calcium oxide, calcium hydroxide, burnt lime, pebble lime, quicklime, slaked lime, hydrated lime.

Proprietary names/products containing: DAP All Purpose Stucco Patch; QuikCrete Concrete Mix; Custom Tile Grout; Custom LevelQuik Self Leveling Underlayment; Thoro Super Quickseal; QuickRete Polyutherane Construction Adhesive; Bonide Hydrated Lime.

Primary use

Lime, or calcium oxide, is a principle ingredient in the production of Portland cement, the basis for most mortars and concrete. Hydrated or 'slaked' lime is the chemical calcium hydroxide. This chemical is also used in mortars. Both types of lime are strong bases and are also used in food production (calcium hydroxide is commonly used in making corn tortillas), petroleum refining and sewage treatment. In the household it is used by aquarium hobbyists to add bioavailable calcium to fish tanks. It is also found in hair relaxers.

Ocular side effects

See section on lye.

Clinical significance

Lime has the properties of a strong alkali and thus carries similar risks to those presented in the section on lye. In addition, since lime is often present in the form of mortar pastes, ocular injuries are more likely to involve solid particles lodged on the ocular surface. Although lime may penetrate the anterior chamber less well than lye or ammonia, it has the capacity to cause severe ocular injury, especially if the solid particles are not removed and instead are allowed to act a reservoir of alkaline material.

Recommendations

See the recommendations for lye. In addition, particular attention must be paid to removing adherent foreign bodies. Mortar and cement debris may be difficult to remove with forceps or cotton-tipped applicators. Some authors have advocated the use of EDTA solutions such as those used to remove band keratopathy. Unfortunately, these solutions are not readily available in most first-aid settings.

REFERENCES AND FURTHER READING

See references for lye.

Generic name: Lye.

Synonyms: Sodium hydroxide (soda lye, caustic soda); potassium hydroxide (potash lye, caustic potash, potassium hydrate).

Proprietary names/products containing: Available in a variety of household, outdoor and industrial cleaners.

Primary use

Lye refers to both sodium and potassium hydroxide. Soap-making via saponification is the most traditional chemical process using sodium hydroxide. It is also used in the manufacture of biodiesel and in food production. Sodium hydroxide is used most commonly in the home in products that unblock drains, and it is also found in many strong household cleaners. In research and industrial applications, sodium and potassium hydroxide are used to control the pH of various products.

Ocular side effects

Direct ocular exposure
Certain
1. Ocular irritation
   a. Eye pain
2. Lacrimation
3. Non-specific blepharospasm
4. Conjunctiva
   a. Hyperemia
   b. Edema
   c. Blanching of vascular bed
   d. Symblepharon
5. Cornea
   a. Edema
   b. Scarring
   c. Ulceration
   d. Vascularization
   e. Perforation
   f. Fibrovascular pannus
6. Cataracts
7. Increased or decreased intraocular pressure
   a. Glaucoma
   b. Hypotony
   c. Phthisis bulbi
8. Entropion
9. Iritis

Clinical significance

Many severe ocular injuries occur every year from exposure to alkalis. A data pull covering the years 2002–2005 from the American Association of Poison Control Centers Toxic Exposure Surveillance System database revealed 34 ocular injuries from alkalis that were rated as 'major' (indicating some type of significant residual disability). This number did not include injuries due to ammonia, detergents or other products with an alkaline pH. The total number of emergency visits for ocular exposure to alkalis was greater than 3000, a number rivaled only by gasoline and bleach exposures. Some automobile airbags release minor amounts of sodium hydroxide, which may complicate ocular injuries received via direct trauma during motor vehicle accidents.

Alkalis owe their toxicity to their ability to penetrate the eye surface more readily than other chemicals, including acids. The corneal epithelium and its mucoid coating are effective barriers to many substances, but they are quickly distorted in the presence of strong alkalis. The concentration of hydroxyl ion and the nature of its associated cation play a role in the ocular injury pattern caused by the different alkalis, but the pH of the substance seems to correlate most closely to the extent of the damage. As the pH of a substance rises above 11, there is a large increase in its potential for ocular damage. Of the three most common alkalis, ammonium hydroxide (see section on ammonia) penetrates the eye most rapidly, followed by sodium hydroxide and then calcium hydroxide (see section on lime). Magnesium hydroxide is another alkali known to cause ocular injury, and is a common ingredient in fireworks so chemical injury with this compound is often accompanied by thermal injury.

If the eye is exposed to concentrated lye, the initial response is one of pain, lacrimation and blepharospasm. The latter makes immediate irrigation of the eye more difficult. Conjunctival injuries may include ischemic necrosis of the limbal tissue and loss of the vascular bed. Later, severe dry eye may ensue along with the development of symblepharon and entropion. Severe ocular burns from alkalis can injure sensory nerves and lead to ocular anesthesia, a bad prognostic sign. As the lye causes corneal epithelial necrosis and disruption of the surface barriers, it immediately begins to penetrate to the deeper layers of the cornea, potentially arriving in the anterior chamber within a minute. The presence of lye in the stroma may lead to permanent corneal opacification, corneal vascularization, stromal thinning, and perforation. Lye in the anterior chamber raises the pH, causing damage to the trabecular meshwork and elevated intraocular pressure. Although some patients eventually develop chronic intraocular pressure elevation, damage to the ciliary body may occur, leading to hypotony and phthisis bulbi. The lens may be permanently injured by the elevated intraocular pH, leading to cataract. There are also case reports of retinal toxicity from alkali injury.

The true severity of an ocular injury from lye may not be known for a few days. Healing may be retarded by chronic inflammation, an imbalance in collagen synthesis/degradation and death of limbal stem cells. Sterile ulcers may form and eventually a fibrovascular pannus may cover the cornea.

Recommendations

The most important intervention in ocular exposure to lye or other alkalis is immediate irrigation. Many studies have been done to identify the optimal irrigating solution for various types of chemical exposure, but the subtle advantages of one solution over another are far less important than the rapidity of applying irrigation. In an industrial setting, eyewash stations are often prevalent. If an ocular exposure to a strong alkali occurs away from such resources, rescuers should immediately apply whatever non-toxic aqueous solution is at hand.

Once a victim is in a medical care center, extensive irrigation must be started immediately using normal saline or sterile water. This is aided by the use of topical anesthetic and a lid speculum. One liter of fluid should be used to flush the eye surface over a period of 10 minutes. A few minutes should be allowed to pass following this first liter for accurate testing of the pH of the conjunctival cul-de-sac using litmus paper accurate in the neutral range. If the pH does not drop below 8, one should continue cycles of irrigation for 15 minutes followed by a check of the pH. Some experts advocate irrigation for at least 2 hours to help neutralize the anterior chamber pH while others have advocated anterior chamber paracentesis and washout. After the initial round of irrigation, a brief ocular exam should take place, checking vision and intraocular pressure and examining the conjunctival fornices for foreign bodies, which may be acting as a reservoir for the alkali. At this point, the necrotic corneal epithelium should be removed.

Following irrigation and neutrality of pH, medical therapy should ensue. Topical cycloplegic eye drops, antibiotic ointment and corticosteroid eye drops should be instituted for the first week. After this time, corticosteroids may inhibit wound healing. Antiglaucoma therapy should be started if necessary. High dose oral ascorbate is possibly helpful and of low toxicity. Many other substances have been advocated via both oral and topical routes to aid in healing from these injuries, but none have become the standard of care. The surgical care of the late sequelae of severe ocular burns from alkalis is a complicated subject and beyond the scope of this text.

REFERENCES AND FURTHER READING

American Association of Poison Control Centers Toxic Exposure
  Surveillance System database, 2002–2005, Human ocular exposures
  by substance. Data pull 8/23/06.
Brahma AK, Inkster C. Alkaline chemical ocular injury from Emla cream.
  Eye 9(Pt 5): 658–659, 1995.
Brodovsky SC, McCarty CA, Snibson G, et al. Management of alkali
  burns: an 11-year retrospective review. Ophthalmology 107:
  1829–1835, 2000.
Corazza M, Trincone S, Virgili A. Effects of airbag deployment: lesions,
  epidemiology, and management. Am J Clin Dermatol 5: 295–300,
  2004.
Davis AR, Ali QK, Aclimnados WA, Hunter PA. Topical steroid use in
  the treatment of ocular alkali burns. Br J Ophthalmol 81: 732–734,
  1997.
He J, Bazan NG, Bazan HE. Alkali-induced corneal stromal melting
  prevention by a novel platelet-activating factor receptor antagonist.
  Arch Ophthalmol 124: 70–78, 2006.
Ikeda N, Hayasaka S, Hayasaka Y, Watanabe K. Alkali burns of the eye:
  effect of immediate copious irrigation with tap water on their severity.
  Ophthalmologica 220: 225–228, 2006.
Kompa S, Schareck B, Tympner J, et al. Comparison of emergency eye-wash
  products in burned porcine eyes. Graefes Arch Clin Exp Ophthalmol
  240: 308–313, 2002.
Kuckelkorn R, Schrage N, Keller G, Redbrake C. Emergency treatment of
  chemical and thermal eye burns. Acta Ophthalmol Scand 80: 4–10,
  2002.
Laria C, Alio JL, Ruiz-Moreno JM. Combined non-steroidal therapy in
  experimental corneal injury. Ophthalmic Res 29: 145–153, 1997.
Merle H, Donnio A, Ayeboua L, et al. Alkali ocular burns in Martinique
  (French West Indies). Evaluation of the use of an amphoteric solution as
  the rinsing product. Burns 31: 205–211, 2005.
Schrage NF, Kompa S, Haller W, Langefeld S. Use of an amphoteric lavage
  solution for emergency treatment of eye burns. First animal type
  experimental clinical considerations. Burns 28: 782–786, 2002.
Sekundo W, Augustin AJ, Strempel I. Topical allopurinol or corticosteroids
  and acetylcysteine in the early treatment of experimental corneal alkali
  burns: a pilot study. Eur J Ophthalmol 12: 366–372, 2002.
Wagoner MD. Chemical injuries of the eye: current concepts in
  pathophysiology and therapy. Surv Ophthalmol 41: 275–313, 1997.
Wagoner MD, Kenyon KR. Chemical injuries of the eye. In: Albert DM,
  Jacobiec FA, eds Principles and Practice of Ophthalmology, 2nd edn.
  WB Saunders, Philadelphia, 2000.

CLASS: BLEACHES

Generic name: Boric acid.

Synonyms: Orthoboric acid; boracic acid.

Proprietary names/products containing: In a variety of household laundry detergents, hand soaps and lotions.

Primary use

Borax (or sodium tetraborate) is a naturally occurring alkaline compound that is a precursor in the manufacture of boric acid. Used as a preservative, buffer, antiseptic and fungicide, boric acid is also used to manufacture glazes and enamels, and to fireproof textiles and wood. In the household, boric acid and borates as tablets or powder are used to kill insects. It is a frequent ingredient in soaps and detergents. It is used in conjunction with borax to buffer and preserve certain eye drops.

Ocular side effects

Topical ocular exposure
Certain
1. Irritation

Clinical significance

Boric acid dust has been reported as an ocular irritant in industrial exposures although it is generally considered non-toxic to the eyes. In low concentrations, it has historically been used as an eye wash. In a private data pull, the American Association of Poison Control Centers Toxic Exposure Surveillance System database recorded a low incidence of ocular injury from 2001–2005, but there were two reports of ocular injury rated as 'major' (indicating some type of significant residual disability) and 10 reports of injury rated as 'moderate' (indicating an injury with prolonged symptoms requiring treatment but not resulting in permanent injury). However, this data does not detail the nature of the injuries reported or their treatment.

Recommendations

Standard irrigation with sterile water or isotonic saline is recommended for ocular exposure to boric acid dust. As boric acid and borax are usually present in the form of soaps and cleansers, most exposures to these substances will coincide with exposures to surfactants. See the section on surfactants for how to treat these injuries.

REFERENCES AND FURTHER READING

American Association of Poison Control Centers Toxic Exposure
  Surveillance System database, 2002–2005, human ocular exposures
  by substance. Data pull 8/23/06.
Garabrant DH, Bernstein L, Peters JM, Smith TJ. Respiratory and eye irritation
  from boron oxide and boric acid dusts. J Occup Med 26: 585–6. 1984.

Generic name: Chlorine

Synonyms: Bleach, chlorine gas, sodium hypochlorite, calcium hypochlorite; hypochlorous acid, chloramines, chlorinated isocyanurates, chlorinated hydantoins, chlorinated lime, chlorine dioxide, tosylchloramide sodium, sodium oxychloride.

Proprietary names/products containing: Found in a variety of household and commercial cleaners.

Primary use

A halogen gas, chlorine is also available as a pressurized solution. There are many more stable compounds that release chlorine in the form of hypochlorous acid and hypochlorite ion when exposed to water. When otherwise stable chlorine-releasing compounds are combined with acids, chlorine gas may be liberated, and when combined with ammonia, poisonous chloramines may be released.

The ability of chlorine gas or the non-ionized hypochlorous acid molecule to chlorinate proteins yields its extreme effectiveness in disinfection. Chlorine gas is used to sanitize public water supplies. Various chlorine compounds are used to disinfect swimming pools. In medical clinics, bleach (sodium hypochlorite 5-10%) is commonly used as a surface disinfectant, including the disinfection of applanation tonometer tips.

Ocular side effects

Topical ocular exposure
Certain
1. Irritation
2. Cornea
   a. Edema
   b. Punctate epithelial erosions
3. Conjunctiva – hyperemia

Clinical significance

Industrial exposure to chlorine gas is irritating to mucous membranes, including the conjunctiva, although reports of severe pathology are few. If concentrations are high enough or if duration of exposure is lengthy, fatal outcomes are possible from pulmonary damage. Severe ocular damage in these patients may be masked by the systemic pathology.

The American Association of Poison Control Centers Toxic Exposure Surveillance System database recorded that from 2001–2005 there were over 6000 ocular exposures to hypochlorite-containing bleach products. Of these, there were four 'major' (indicating some type of significant residual disability) and 522 'moderate' (indicating more prolonged symptoms requiring some type of treatment but resulting in no permanent injury) outcomes in their ratings of severity. Unfortunately, this data pull did not detail the specific injuries or define the final outcome in terms of visual acuity or other measure. Typically, ocular splashes from household cleaners containing chlorinated compounds do not result in serious injury. Some chlorinated compounds are made more stable by the addition of alkaline substances and some of the more serious injuries may occur as a result of the elevated pH. Household bleach is usually 5–10% sodium hypochlorite and has a pH near 11.

It is well known that extended ocular exposure to chlorine products in swimming pools will lead to corneal edema and punctate erosions. Higher concentrations of available chlorine in the pool water, the pH and the concentration of chloramines (products of reaction between chlorine and nitrogen-containing compounds such as urea) all affect the degree of irritation.

Chlorine crystals have been reported to form on tonometer tips chronically soaked in bleach solution for anti-sepsis and, despite rinsing of the tips, such crystals may cause minor corneal injury. Although chlorine bleach is an excellent disinfectant, alcohol wiping may be a less problematic method of cleaning tonometer tips. It is important to remind patients to use appropriate eye protection to guard against splash-type injuries while using concentrated cleaning products, including bleach. These products can be corrosive to mucous membranes and substantial irrigation should ensue, and as they are usually quite alkaline, pH testing of the conjunctival cul-de-sac should be tested during irrigation.

Recommendations

1. Industrial ocular exposures to chlorine gas should be treated with copious irrigation, but it is extremely important to immediately assess possible pulmonary injury as this can lead to fatal outcomes.
2. Typical ocular splash exposures to bleach should be treated with copious irrigation using sterile water or saline as the pH is typically near 11.

REFERENCES AND FURTHER READING

American Association of Poison Control Centers Toxic Exposure Surveillance System database, 2002–2005, Human ocular exposures by substance. Data pull 8/23/06.

Hery M, Hecht G, Gerber JM, et al. Exposure to chloramines in the atmosphere of indoor swimming pools. Ann Occup Hygiene 39(4): 427–439, 1995.

Hery M, Gerber JM, Hecht G, et al. Exposure to chloramines in a green salad processing plant. Ann Occup Hygiene 42: 437–451, 1998.

Horton DK, Berkowitz Z, Kaye WE. The public health consequences from acute chlorine releases, 1993–2000. J Occup Environ Med 44(10): 906–913, 2002.

LoVecchio F, Blackwell S, Stevens D. Outcomes of chlorine exposure: a 5 year poison center experience in 598 patients. Eur J Emerg Med 12: 109–110, 2005.

Martinez TT, Long C. Explosion risk from swimming pool chlorinators and review of chlorine toxicity. J Toxicol Clin Toxicol 33(4): 349–354, 1995.

Mauger TF, Laxson LC. Effect of hydrogen peroxide and sodium hypochlorite on the corneal oxygen uptake rate. J Toxicol Cutaneous Ocul Toxicol 11: 369–374, 1992.

Maurer JK, Molai A, Parker RD, et al. Pathology of ocular irritation with bleaching agents in the rabbit low-volume eye test. Toxicol Pathol 29(3): 308–319, 2001.

Racioppi F, Daskaleros PA, Besbelli N, et al. Household bleaches based on sodium hypochlorite: Review of Acute Toxicology and Poison Control Center Experience. Food Chem Toxicol 32(9): 845–861, 1994.

Saunders SK, Kempainen R, Blanc PD. Outcomes of ocular exposures reported to a regional poison control center. J Toxicol Cutaneous Ocul Toxicol 15(3): 249–259, 1996.

Generic name: Hydrogen peroxide.

Synonyms: Hydrogen dioxide hydroperoxide, peroxide, albone, dihydrogen dioxide, hioxyl, inhibine, interox, kastone, oxydol, perhydrol, perone, peroxan.

Proprietary names/products containing: Available as a generic name product in a variety of laundry bleaches, cleaners and hair dyes.

Primary use

This molecule has many applications in medicine and industry. It is used as an antiseptic, disinfectant and deodorant. It is a strong oxidizing agent that is frequently used to catalyze chemical reactions. Some disinfectant solutions for contact lenses contain 3% hydrogen peroxide. Hydrogen peroxide is used as a 6% solution for wound cleansing, disinfecting equipment, including tonometer tips, and for bleaching hair and fabrics. Some household fabric stain removers and bleaches contain 5–15% hydrogen peroxide. Hydrogen peroxide used for industrial purposes is made in concentrations as high as 90%. Solutions of 90% hydrogen peroxide are also used as rocket fuel.

Ocular side effects

Topical ocular exposure
Certain
1. Irritation – eye pain
2. Cornea – punctate keratitis
3. Conjunctiva – hyperemia

Probable
1. Cornea
   a. Haze
   b. Edema
   c. Ulceration

Possible
1. Cornea
   a. Descemet's membrane detachment
   b. Recurrent erosion

Clinical significance

Historically, hydrogen peroxide has been used in eye drops at concentrations up to 20% for the treatment of corneal ulcers without reports of long-term corneal damage. Inadvertent ocular application of 3% solution occurs frequently when contact lens disinfectant solution is mistaken for re-wetting drops. This causes moderate to severe pain and conjunctival hyperemia but no long-term ocular damage. Reports of ocular exposure to high concentrations of hydrogen peroxide (greater than 25%) show that permanent injury is possible, including corneal ulceration, scarring and detachment of Descemet's membrane. There is a report detailing a patient who repeatedly applied high concentrations of hydrogen peroxide to the eye surface as a home remedy, resulting in a cicatricial pemphigoid-type injury.

Experiments in rabbit corneas show that long-term exposure or exposure to higher concentrations result in corneal cell death. Hydrogen peroxide exists normally in human tissue with especially high concentration in the anterior chamber. Intact cornea seems to protect against penetration of exogenous hydrogen peroxide from the eye surface into the anterior chamber.

Hydrogen peroxide is used to sterilize Goldmann applanation tips. Ocular injury has occurred when the tips are not rinsed with sterile water prior to contact with the cornea. The hydrogen peroxide is typically kept in a reservoir in which the tips are soaked. Concentration of the hydrogen peroxide via evaporation may occur if the solution is not replaced frequently. If allowed to dry completely without rinsing, the tip may accumulate a residue that acts as a highly concentrated solution on application to the cornea, and this has resulted in injuries causing long-term corneal haze.

Recommendations

1. Patients who have inadvertent ocular exposure to contact lens disinfectant solution need only observation, analgesia and lubrication as these patients nearly always recover from this injury within a few days. Patients should also be reminded that the neutralizing case, which contains a platinum-coated disk, should be replaced according to the manufacturer's instructions as they lose effectiveness with time. The eye could therefore be exposed to a higher concentration of hydrogen peroxide over time with contact lens insertion. Rinsing the lenses in sterile saline prior to their insertion should also reduce the concentration of any residual hydrogen peroxide on the contact lens surface. The disinfectant solution itself should be replaced regularly as the concentration may change with time.
2. When used in the clinic to disinfect tonometer tips, hydrogen peroxide solution in reservoirs should be changed daily and tips should be rinsed in sterile water prior to application to the cornea.
3. If a cornea is exposed to a higher concentration of hydrogen peroxide, copious irrigation should follow. The patient should be followed carefully for the development of ulceration, Descemet's membrane damage and scarring of the anterior cornea. Topical steroids and antibiotic drops have been employed successfully to aid in the healing of such injuries.

REFERENCES AND FURTHER READING

Kaplan EN, Gundel RE, Sosale A, Sack R. Residual hydrogen peroxide as a function of platinum disc age. CLAO J 18(3): 149–154, 1992.
Knopf HL. Reaction to hydrogen peroxide in a contact-lens wearer. Am J Ophthalmol 97(6): 796, 1984.
Maurer JK, Molai A, Parker RD, et al. Pathology of ocular irritation with bleaching agents in the rabbit low-volume eye test. Toxicol Pathol 29(3): 308–319, 2001.
Memarzadeh F, Shamie N, Gaster RN, Chuck RS. Corneal and conjunctival toxicity from hydrogen peroxide: a patient with chronic self-induced injury. Ophthalmology 111(8): 1546–1549, 2004.
Pandit RT, Farjo AA, Sutphin JE, et al. Iatrogenic corneal and conjunctival toxic reaction from hydrogen peroxide disinfection [letter]. Arch Ophthalmol 121: 904–906, 2003.
Paugh JR, Brennan NA, Efron N. Ocular response to hydrogen peroxide. Am J Optom Physiol Opt 65(2): 91–98, 1988.
Riley MV, Wilson G. Topical hydrogen peroxide and the safety of ocular tissues. CLAO J 19(3): 186–190, 1993.
Tripathi BJ, Tripathi RC, Millard CB, Borisuth NS. Cytotoxicity of hydrogen peroxide to human corneal epithelium in vitro and its clinical implications. Lens Eye Toxic Res 7(3–4): 385–401, 1990.
Wilson G, Riley MV. Does topical hydrogen peroxide penetrate the cornea? Invest Ophthalmol Vis Sci 34: 2752–2760, 1993.
Yuen HK, Yeung BY, Wong TH, et al. Descemet membrane detachment caused by hydrogen peroxide injury. Cornea 23(4): 409–411, 2004.

CLASS: DETERGENTS

Generic name: 1. Cationic surfactant; 2. anionic surfactant; 3. zwitterionic surfactant; 4. non-ionic surfactant.

Synonyms: Surface active agent, detergent, soap, wetting agent.

Proprietary names/products containing: 1. Cationic – cetyl trimethylammonium bromide, cetylpyridinium chloride, polyethoxylated tallow amine, benzalkonium chloride, benzethonium chloride; 2. Anionic – sodium dodecyl sulfate, ammonium lauryl sulfate, sodium laureth sulfate, alkyl benzene sulfonate, Ivory soap, Triton X-200, cholic acid. 3. Zwitterionic (amphoteric) – dodecyl betaine, dodecyl dimethylamine oxide, cocamidopropyl betaine, CHAPS, dodecyl dimethyl ammonio propane sulfonate; 4. Non-ionic – polyethylene glycol ether W-1, Span 20, Polysorbate 80, Tergitol, Type 15-S-12, Triton X-15, Tween 20, Tyloxapol.

Primary use

These compounds have a multitude of uses in many industries, including food and agriculture, cosmetics and medicine. Products containing surfactants include shampoo, dishwashing detergent, emulsifiers, foaming, wetting and dispersing agents, creams, lotions, toothpaste, foods and pharmaceuticals. They are used in laboratories for preparing samples, especially in gel electrophoresis.

Ocular side effects

Topical ocular exposure
Certain
1. Irritation
   a. Burning
   b. Hyperemia
2. Cornea
   a. Punctate keratitis
   b. Abrasion (Fig. 8.2)
   c. Edema – intraocular exposure

Clinical significance

Surfactants frequently gain access to the ocular surface in the form of shampoos and soaps, and are generally well tolerated. Stinging and burning sensations are common and resolve relatively quickly with brief rinsing. Those surfactants that are frequently used in detergents and shampoos have received substantial animal testing and have proved themselves as being safe after years in the marketplace.

In general, cationic surfactants are the most irritating and most destructive to the conjunctival and corneal epithelium. Exposure to industrial concentrations of certain detergents may cause more significant injury, with corneal edema and opacification. There are

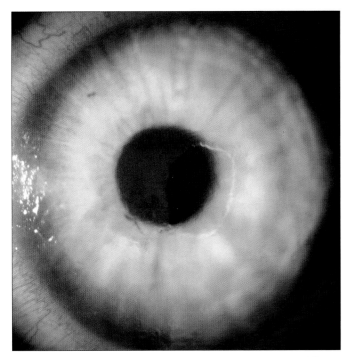

Fig. 8.2 Corneal abrasion from ocular exposure to detergents. Photo courtesy of the Krachmer JH, Palay DA. Cornea Atlas, 2nd edn, Mosby Elsevier, London, 2006.

no recent reports of serious eye injury with topical surfactant exposure, but animal studies show that high concentrations of certain detergents cause corneal scarring. There are recent reports of alkali liquid detergent packets causing moderate conjunctival and corneal injury in children without scarring. The surfactant in this product may have contributed to the injuries but the alkaline formulation (pH 9) probably exacerbated the toxicity. Benzalkonium chloride is a cationic surfactant that is commonly used as a preservative in eye drops. Several studies suggest that chronic use of eye drops containing this preservative may alter the tear film-epithelial interface on the ocular surface. Some pharmaceutical companies have recently brought to the market eye drops with alternative preservatives.

Although surfactants are not thought to penetrate through the cornea into the anterior chamber, there is considerable concern regarding the role of surfactants in the toxic anterior segment syndrome. Although this syndrome may have multiple etiologies, some cases have been tied to inadequate cleaning of intraocular instruments such as cannulas. It is suspected that residue from the detergents used to clean these instruments may not get fully rinsed off, making its way into the anterior chamber during subsequent cataract surgery and causing irreversible endothelial damage and corneal edema.

Recommendations

1. Detergent splashes into the eye are generally well tolerated and require brief rinsing with water. However, certain automatic dishwasher and laundry detergents are significantly alkaline and, in these cases, alkali burn protocols should be followed (see the section on alkalis).
2. If a surgery center suspects a series of cases of toxic anterior segment syndrome has occurred, efforts should be made to review the instrument cleaning protocol of the institution. The use of disposable cannulas may reduce the likelihood of inadvertent inoculation of surfactant into the anterior chamber during intraocular surgery.

REFERENCES AND FURTHER READING

Baradaran-Dilmaghani R, Ergun E, Krepler K. Keratoconjunctivitis after exposure to party foam. Br J Ophthalmol 81(6): 515, 1997.

Cater KC, Harbell JW. Prediction of eye irritation potential of surfactant-based rinse off personal care formulations by the bovine corneal opacity and permeability (BCOP) assay. Cutan Ocul Toxicol 25(3): 217–233, 2006.

Debbasch C, Brignole F, Pisella PJ, et al. Quarternary ammoniums and other preservatives' contribution in oxidative stress and apoptosis on Chang conjunctival cells. Invest Ophthalmol Vis Sci 42(3): 642–652, 2001.

De Saint Jean M, Brignole F, Bringuier AF, et al. Effects of benzalkonium chloride on growth and survival of Chang conjunctival cells. Invest Ophthalmol Vis Sci 40(3): 619–630, 1999.

Eleftheriadis H, Cheong M, Sandeman S, et al. Corneal toxicity secondary to inadvertent use of benzalkonium chloride preserved viscoelastic material in cataract surgery. Br J Ophthalmol 86(3): 299–305, 2002.

Fayers T, Munneke R, Strouthidis NG. Detergent capsules causing ocular injuries in children. J Pediatr Ophthalmol Strabismus 43(4): 250–251, 2006.

Gettings SD, Lordo RA, Feder PI, Hintze KL. A comparison of low volume, Draize and in vitro irritation test data. III. Surfactant-based formulations. Food Chem Toxicol 36(3): 209–231, 1998.

Jester JV, Maurer JK, Petroll WM, et al. Application of in vivo confocal microscopy to the understanding of surfactant-induced ocular irritation. Toxicol Pathol 24(4): 509–510, 1996.

Maudgal PC. Ocular burn caused by soft brown soap. Bull Soc Belge Ophthalmol 263:81–84, 1996.

Maurer JK, Parker RD. Light microscopic comparison of surfactant-induced eye irritation in rabbits and rats at three hours and recovery/day 35. Toxicol Pathol 24(4): 403–411, 1996.

Parikh C, Sippy BD, Martin DF, Edelhauser HF. Effects of enzymatic sterilization detergents on the corneal endothelium. Arch Ophthalmol 120(2): 165–172, 2002.

CLASS: GLUES

Generic name: Cyanoacrylate adhesives.

Synonyms: Bucrilate, enbucrilate, mecrilate, ocrilate.

Proprietary names: Commonly known as 'superglue', available under many proprietary names.

Primary use
Household glue, artificial fingernail adhesive, surgical tissue adhesive (skin, cornea, mucous membrane).

Ocular side effects

Topical Ocular Exposure
Certain
1. Irritation
2. Eyelids – inadvertent adhesion of lid margins (Fig. 8.3)
3. Cornea – abrasion
4. Conjunctiva
   a. Giant papillary conjunctivitis
   b. Symblepharon and scarring

Probable
1. Lacrimal outflow system (as surgical plug) – dacryocystitis
2. Cornea (as surgical adhesive)
   a. Infectious and inflammatory keratitis
   b. Endothelial toxicity
3. Anterior chamber (as surgical adhesive)
   a. Pupillary block
   b. Irido-lenticular and irido-corneal adhesions

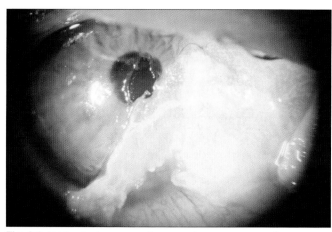

Fig. 8.3 Inadvertent exposure to superglue on cornea surface.

Clinical significance

Ocular toxicity from cyanoacrylate adhesives most often occurs from the inadvertent application of household glue preparations into the eye (Fig. 8.1). Most of these accidental exposures result in no long-term tissue damage. Placement of the glue in the conjunctival fornices may occur when the patient mistakes the glue container for an eye drop container. This type of application may cause adherence of the upper and lower lids to each other via lashes or eyelid margin. The glue polymerizes in the presence of water on the ocular surface and may form a foreign body capable of abrading the cornea and conjunctiva.

Cyanoacrylate tissue adhesives utilize longer side-chain esters than the household preparations because of the more toxic nature of adhesives containing shorter methyl or ethyl side chains. These preparations have a long history in ophthalmology with applications including closing blepharoplasty incisions, occluding the lacrimal puncta, creating temporary tarsorrhaphies and sealing small corneal perforations. A few reports exist of inadvertent spillage of adhesive into the anterior chamber with resultant iritis, iridocorneal and iridolenticular adhesions, and even one case of pupillary block. When used to seal corneal perforations, glue plugs are often left in place for several weeks, typically under a bandage contact lens. Infectious keratitis under the glue plug may occur in these patients despite evidence showing that cyanoacrylate adhesives have anti-microbial properties, especially against gram-positive organisms.

Recommendations

1. In cases of accidental tarsorrhaphy, the glue may be protruding posteriorly, causing corneal or conjunctival erosions. Use of scissors or manual lid separation is appropriate. Typically, focal lash loss or lid margin abrasions result. Some clinicians have advocated the use of cotton-tip applicators soaked in acetone to dissolve the glue, but extreme care should be taken as the acetone can be toxic to the ocular surface.
2. Glue plugs in the conjunctival cul-de-sac should probably be removed upon presentation as household cyanoacrylate preparations are composed of shorter side-chain esters, which are more tissue toxic. Others advocate awaiting spontaneous glue rejection as long-term ocular surface damage from these exposures is rare in any event.
3. Intraocular exposure occurs during the clinical application of tissue glue to corneal perforations. Any spillage into the anterior chamber should be surgically removed. There are several published application techniques that assist in avoidance of this complication.

REFERENCES AND FURTHER READING

Cavanaugh TB, Gottsch JD. Infectious keratitis and cyanoacrylate adhesive. Am J Ophthalmol 111(4): 466–472, 1991.

Chan SM, Boisjoly H. Advances in the use of adhesives in ophthalmology. Curr Opin Ophthalmol Aug 15(4): 305–310, 2004.

de Almeida Manzano RP, Naufal SC, Hida RY, et al. Antibacterial analysis in vitro of ethyl-cyanoacrylate against ocular pathogens. Cornea 25(3): 350–351, 2006.

Markowitz GD, Orlin SE, Frayer WC, et al. Corneal endothelial polymerization of histoacryl adhesive: a report of a new intraocular complication. Ophthal Surg 26(3): 256–258, 1995.

Ritterband DC, Meskin SW, Shapiro DE, et al. Laboratory model of tissue adhesive (2-octyl cyanoacrylate) in sealing clear corneal cataract wounds. Am J Ophthalmol 140(6): 1039–43, 2005.

Strempel I. Complications by liquid plastics in ophthalmic surgery. Histopathologic study. Dev Ophthalmol 13: 137–146, 1987.

Vote BJ, Elder MJ. Cyanoacrylate glue for corneal perforations: a description of a surgical technique and a review of the literature. Clin Exp Ophthalmol 28: 437–442, 2000.

CLASS: HERBICIDES AND INSECTICIDES

Generic name: Diethyltoluamide.

Synonyms: DEET.

Proprietary names/products containing: Cutter Insect Repellant; Off! Deep Woods For Sportsmen Insect Repellent; Bonide Mosquito Beater; Champion Sprayon Insect Repellent; Repel Insect Repellent; Cutter Family All Insect Repellent; Cutter All Family Mosquito Wipes (and most other Cutter products); Macchar Insect Repellent; PreStrike Mosquito Repellent; Cutter Tick Defense.

Primary use

Insect repellant.

Ocular side effects

Topical ocular exposure
Certain
1. Irritation
2. Eyelids – urticaria

Clinical significance

This chemical has been in use as an insect repellant for over five decades. It is formulated in various concentrations, often with alcohol as a base. In the USA alone there are estimated to be over 90 million exposures to this product per year. A private data pull indicated that from 2001 to 2005, the American Association of Poison Control Centers recorded 931 cases of ocular exposure to DEET. Of these, 23 were categorized to have a severity outcome rated as 'moderate' (indicating more prolonged symptoms requiring some type of treatment but resulting in no permanent injury) and there were none rated as 'major' (indicating some type of significant residual disability). Exposure to this toxin appears to cause minimal harm to ocular health. There are several reports of urticaria of the face after even a single exposure. No reports of scarring in the periocular area were found.

Recommendations

Inadvertent ocular exposure of DEET is probably frequent and generally of low toxicity. Patients should be treated with copious irrigation using sterile water or isotonic saline.

REFERENCES AND FURTHER READING

American Association of Poison Control Centers Toxic Exposure
Surveillance System database, 2002–2005, Human ocular exposures
by substance. Data pull 8/23/06.
Bell JW, Veltri JC, Page BC. Human exposures to N,N-diethyl-m-toluamide
insect repellents reported to the American Association of Poison
Control Centers 1993–1997. Int J Toxicol 21(5): 341–352, 2002.
MacRae SM, Brown BA, Ubels JL, et al. Ocular toxicity of diethyltoluamide
(DEET). J Toxicol Cut Ocular Toxicol 3: 17–30, 1984.
Sudakin DL, Trevathan WR. DEET: a review and update of safety and risk in
the general population. J Toxicol Clin Toxicol 41(6): 831–839, 2003.

Generic names: 1. Glyphosate; 2. N-(phosphonomethyl) glycine.

Synonyms: Phosphonomethyliminoacetic acid.

Proprietary names/products containing: Roundup, Polado, Fozzate, Gly-Flo, Glygran, Glyphogan, Kleeraway Systemic Weed & Grass Killer 2, Kull Tgai, Recoil Broad Spectrum Herbicide, Standout Herbicide, Touchdown Herbicide.

Primary use

Used as a herbicide to control post-emergent weed growth, glyphosate is usually formulated as an isopropylamine salt in an aqueous solution with surfactants added and has a pH of 4.4–7.5. It comes in a variety of concentrations and in a dry form. It is one of the best-selling herbicides worldwide.

Ocular side effects

Topical ocular exposure
Certain
1. Lacrimation
2. Irritation – eye pain
3. Blurred vision
4. Cornea – abrasion

Possible
1. Conjunctiva
   a. conjunctivitis
   b. pseudomembranes

Clinical significance

Amongst herbicides and pesticides, glyphosate is the most commonly reported to cause ocular injury in calls to poison centers. The vast majority are of the 'minor' classification (indicating rapid resolution of symptoms without permanent injury). Most reports are of lacrimation, blurred vision, and eye pain. Most of the reports in the 'moderate' category involve corneal abrasions. Since glyphosate is usually formulated with surfactants, these injuries may be a result of surfactant injury rather than of the active ingredient itself.

There was a single report of pseudomembranous conjunctivitis in a contact-lens wearer which resulted in no permanent ocular damage. Studies in which rabbits were exposed to high concentrations over long duration demonstrated that permanent corneal scarring is possible, but the most commonly available concentrations to the consumer caused no serious injuries in animal studies.

Recommendations

Standard irrigation technique with sterile water or isotonic saline is all that is indicated in most cases. Patients with injuries from herbicides containing glyphosate should be assessed for corneal abrasion.

REFERENCES AND FURTHER READING

Acquavella JF, Weber JA, Cullen MR, et al. Human ocular effects from
self-reported exposures to Roundup herbicides. Hum Exp Toxicol
18: 479–486, 1999.
American Association of Poison Control Centers Toxic Exposure
Surveillance System database, 2002–2005, Human ocular exposures
by substance. Data pull 8/23/06.
Goldstein DA, Acquavella JF, Mannion RM, et al. An analysis of glyphosate
data from the California Environmental Protection Agency Pesticide
Illness Surveillance Program. J Toxicol Clin Toxicol 40(7): 885–892,
2002.
Smith EA, Oehme FW. The biological activity of glyphosate to plants and
animals: a literature review. Vet Hum Toxicol 34(6): 531–543, 1992.

Generic name: Organophosphate insecticides.

Synonyms: OPs, organophosphorus pesticides, organophosphate cholinesterase inhibitors.

Proprietary names/products containing: Azinphosmethyl, chlorpyrifos, diazinon, disulfoton, fonofos, malathion, methyl parathion, parathion, phosmet, physostigmine, pyridostigmine.

Primary use

Organophosphates are a class of chemicals that block cholinesterase in humans, animals and insects, inhibiting the breakdown of acetylcholine, an important neurotransmitter, in the nerve terminal. This makes them effective insecticides. Physostigmine and pyridostigmine are organophosphates used in treating myasthenia gravis.

Ocular side effects

Systemic exposure – acute effects
Certain
1. Pupils – miosis
2. Accommodative spasm
3. Blurred vision
4. Eye pain
5. Conjunctiva – hyperemia

Probable
1. Nystagmus
   a. Upbeat nystagmus
   b. Opsoclonus
   c. Ocular bobbing

Systemic exposure – chronic effects
Possible
1. Smooth pursuit – delayed
2. Visual field defects
3. Retina – pigmentary degeneration
4. Myopia – pathologic
5. Color vision deficit
6. Contrast sensitivity – decreased

Clinical significance

Systemic exposure to these compounds mostly occurs in the agriculture industry. Suicide attempts using organophosphates are another means of intoxication. Young children may receive accidental systemic exposure to these toxins from lawn and garden applications. Toxicity from organophosphates leads to a build-up of acetylcholine in nerve synapses, which can cause myriad neurological dysfunctions. In humans poisoning with these agents may cause acute excess secretory activity, including involuntary salivation, lacrimation, urination, emesis, defecation, muscle weakness and seizures.

As with muscarinic compounds such as pilocarpine, miosis and accommodative spasm are part of the symptom complex. Ocular bobbing, opsoclonus and upbeat nystagmus have all been reported as transient effects from toxicity due to organophosphates.

Chronic effects from exposure to organophosphates may include eye findings but these are more controversial. In the 1970s, Japanese researchers identified a symptom complex including myopia, visual field defects, difficulty with ocular pursuit movements and pigmentary changes to the retina occurring in people living in agricultural areas that received heavy organophosphate use. They coined the term 'Saku disease' after the name of the region in which a high proportion of the affected patients resided, and they presumed the cause to be chronic exposure to organophosphates. Other work has suggested subclinical effects from chronic exposure to these compounds, including changes in color vision, contrast sensitivity and pupil contractility. There is a well-accepted non-ocular syndrome of peripheral neuropathy resulting from chronic exposure to certain organophosphates. The mechanism of this distal axonal dysfunction seems to be related not to decreased cholinesterase activity but to phosphorylation of a receptor protein, neurotoxic esterase. In any case, there is no consensus on whether long-term systemic exposure to organophosphates causes any type of chronic eye toxicity.

Recommendations

Patients suspected to have acute organophosphate poisoning need emergent evaluation. Care may be best provided in an intensive care setting as seizures and cardiopulmonary arrest are possible. Treatment involves anticholinergic drugs such as atropine and pralidoxime chloride. Ocular symptoms require no special treatment as systemic therapy will reverse the eye findings as well.

REFERENCES AND FURTHER READING

Dementi B. Ocular effects of organophosphates: a historical perspective of Saku disease. J Appl Toxicol 14(2): 119–129, 1994.

Dick RB, Steenland K, Krieg EF, Hines CJ. Evaluation of acute sensory-motor effects and test sensitivity using termiticide workers exposed to chlorpyrifos. Neurotoxicol Teratol 23(4): 381–393, 2001.

Dyro FM. Organophosphates. The Emedicine from WebMD page. Available at: http://www.emedicine.com/neuro/topic286.htm. Accessed November 25, 2006.

Geller AM, Sutton LD, Marshall RS, et al. Repeated spike exposure to the insecticide chlorpyrifos interferes with the recovery of visual sensitivity in rats. Doc Ophthalmol 110(1): 79–90, 2005.

Hata S, Bernstein E, Davis LE. Atypical ocular bobbing in acute organophosphate poisoning. Arch Neurol 43(2): 185–186, 1986.

Ishikawa S. Ophthalmology due to environmental toxic substances especially intoxication by organophosphorus pesticides. Nippon Ganka Gakkai Zasshi 100(6): 417–432, 1996.

Jay WM, Marcus RW, Jay MS. Primary position upbeat nystagmus with organophosphate poisoning. J Pediatr Ophthalmol Strabismus 19(6): 318–319, 1982.

Liang TW, Balcer LJ, Messe SR, Galetta SL. Supranuclear gaze palsy and opsoclonus after Diazinon poisoning. J Neurol Neurosurg Psychiatry 74(5): 677–679, 2003.

Paraoanu LE, Mocko JB, Becker-Roeck M, et al. Exposure to diazinon alters in vitro retinogenesis: retinospheroid morphology, development of chicken retinal cell types, and gene expression. Toxicol Sci 89(1): 314–324, 2006.

Pullicino P, Aquilina J. Opsoclonus in organophosphate poisoning. Arch Neurol 46(6): 704–705, 1989.

Rosenstock L, Keifer M, Daniell WE, et al. Chronic central nervous system effects of acute organophosphate pesticide intoxication. The Pesticide Health Effects Study Group. Lancet 338(8761): 223–227, 1991.

CLASS: HYDROCARBONS

Generic name: Gasoline.

Synonyms: Petrol, motor fuel, benzene, motor spirits.

Proprietary names/products containing: There are many brands of gasoline and gasoline/ethanol blends.

Primary use

Primarily used as fuel in internal combustion engines, gasoline is a complex mixture of hundreds of hydrocarbons. The hydrocarbons vary by class (paraffins, olefins, naphthenes and aromatics) and by the number of carbon atoms in the molecule. Gasoline typically contains dozens of additives to enhance performance, cleanliness, etc., including oxidation inhibitors (aromatic amines and hindered phenols), corrosion inhibitors (carboxylic acids and carboxylates), antiknock compounds (tetraethyl lead, tetramethyl lead, methylcyclopentadienyl manganese tricarbonyl, and ferrocene), anti-icing additives (surfactants, alcohols, and glycols), dyes and drag reducers (high-molecular-weight polymers).

Ocular side effects

Topical ocular exposure
Certain
1. Irritation
   a. Hyperemia
   b. Burning
   c. Lacrimation

Systemic exposure
Possible
1. Visual hallucination (leaded gasoline)
2. Visually evoked potential abnormalities (leaded gasoline)
3. Corneal anesthesia

Clinical significance

Gasoline splashes in the eye are ubiquitous. A data mining from the American Association of Poison Control Centers Toxic Exposure Surveillance System database revealed 6119 ocular exposures to gasoline and related hydrocarbons over a recent 5-year period. Of these exposures, only 318 had an outcome severity rated as 'moderate' (indicating more prolonged symptoms requiring some type of treatment but resulting in no permanent injury) and only five were rated 'major' (indicating some type of significant residual disability). The nature of the injuries was not available. There are no recent reports detailing ocular injuries from direct ocular exposure.

Systemic absorption of gasoline by workers in the petroleum industry or by persons seeking psychotropic effects by 'huffing' gasoline fumes may cause some visual side effects, including hallucinations and abnormalities in the visually evoked potential. The reports detailing these findings are older and reflect gasoline that was formulated with lead, which is no longer in use in the USA and most developed countries.

Recommendations

Ocular splashes with gasoline should be treated with routine irrigation techniques using water or isotonic saline. Ophthalmic follow-up should focus on the development of ocular surface-disease.

REFERENCES AND FURTHER READING

American Association of Poison Control Centers Toxic Exposure Surveillance System database, 2002–2005, Human ocular exposures by substance. Data pull 8/23/06.
Nelson JD, Kopietz LA. Chemical injuries to the eyes. Emergency, intermediate, and long-term care. Postgrad Med 81(4): 62–75, 1987.
Reese E, Kimbrough RD: Acute toxicity of gasoline and some additives. Environ Health Perspec 101: 115–131, 1993.

in regards to ocular injury. The fluorescent dyes used in these compounds are not known to be toxic.

Recommendations

No detailed study has been done exploring exposure to this compound, so it is difficult to recommend any particular treatment aside from copious irrigation. As hydrogen peroxide may be the irritating ingredient in the chemiluminescent compound, similar treatment strategies may be indicated.

REFERENCES AND FURTHER READING

American Association of Poison Control Centers Toxic Exposure Surveillance System database, 2002–2005, Human ocular exposures by substance. Data pull 8/23/06.
Hoffman RJ, Nelson LS, Hoffman RS. Pediatric and young adult exposure to chemiluminescent glow sticks. Arch Pediatr Adolesc Med 156: 901–904, 2002.
Vettese T, Hurwitz JJ. Toxicity of the chemiluminescent material Cyalume in anatomic assessment of the nasolacrimal system. Can J Ophthalmol 18: 131–135, 1983.

CLASS: MISCELLANEOUS

Generic name: Chemiluminescent liquid compound.

Synonyms: Glow Stick Compound (phenyl oxylate ester, hydrogen peroxide, fluorescent dyes).

Proprietary names/products containing: Cyalume, Glow Sticks and Jewelry.

Primary use

This compound is found primarily in glow sticks and related products, which have applications in sporting, scuba diving and military activities, and glow-in-the-dark jewelry and toys. Once the dye is activated by crushing an ampoule of hydrogen peroxide inside the flexible plastic wall of the glow stick, the dye will emit fluorescent light of various colors until the chemical reaction has extinguished itself.

Ocular side effects

Topical ocular exposure
Probable
1. Irritation

Clinical significance

Multiple ocular exposures to this compound are reported by poison centers annually, mostly in the pediatric and young adult populations. Glow sticks and jewelry are popular for use at dance clubs and during certain holidays. There have been no detailed reports of ocular pathology in response to these exposures. The American Association of Poison Control Centers Toxic Exposure Surveillance System database reported 21 ocular injuries of 'moderate' severity due to the chemiluminescent compound during the period 2001–2005. Hydrogen peroxide, a known ocular irritant and an ingredient in the chemiluminescent compound, is the possible source of these injuries. Dibutyl phthalate, a phenyl oxylate ester found in some chemiluminescent compounds in small quantities is known to cause anaphylaxis or death when ingested in large quantities, but it is probably insignificant

Generic name: Methyl ethyl ketone peroxide.

Synonyms: 2-butanone peroxide, MEKP.

Proprietary names: Butanox, Chaloxyd, Esperfoam, FR 222, Hi-point, Kayamek, Lucidol, Lupersol, Permek, Quickset, Sprayset MEKP, Superox, Trigonox M.

Primary use

Commonly used as a curing agent for thermosetting polyester resins and a cross-linking agent and catalyst in the production of other polymers. It is a lipophilic peroxide used in the automobile, airline, boating, fabric and paint industries. It is a catalyst for most polyester resins.

Ocular side effects

Topical ocular exposure
Certain
1. Pain
   a. Ocular
   b. Periorbital
   c. Orbital
2. Lacrimation
3. Photophobia
4. Eyelids – erythema
5. Conjunctiva – bulbar and palpebral
   a. Hyperemia
   b. Chemosis
6. Vision loss
   a. All grades
   b. Total blindness
7. Cornea
   a. Demyelination of nerves
   b. Edema – superficial to full thickness
   c. Epithelial erosions
   d. Endothelial cell death
   e. Pannus
   f. Interstitial keratitis
   g. Abnormal tear film break-up time

h. Thinning
i. Necrosis
8. Anterior uveitis
9. Increased intraocular pressure
10. Phthisis

Clinical significance

The usual concentration of commercial MEKP is 40–60%. Animal research shows that concentrations of less than 10%, while irritating, seldom cause permanent damage. Clinically the main factor as to severity of prognosis is speed of getting the eye irrigated (especially with a local anesthetic so adequate irrigation can occur). This needs to be performed in a manner of seconds rather than minutes. No severe cases, even with marked exposure, have been reported if immediate irrigation occurred.

Mild exposure occurs with hand to eye contact with MEKP, vapor exposure, minimal inadvertent contact with MEKP solutions or with immediate irrigation. Even with mild exposure, lid erythema resolved in 3–7 days and conjunctiva hyperemia without corneal findings after a few weeks. However, symptoms of ocular discomfort may persist for many months.

Moderate to extensive exposure is due to a rupture of a container by dropping or an object falling on the container, explosion of a canister or tubing containing MEKP or confusing a bottle with MEKP and an eyedropper, resulting in directly dropping MEKP onto the eye. The classic syndrome of moderate exposure is reoccurring corneal and conjunctival abnormalities, which are triggered by external ocular stimulus (wind, dust and light). This pattern of multiple reoccurrences, lasting for 6 months, is the sign of a moderate injury. If signs and symptoms are severe or last for more than 6 months there is usually progression or persistence of corneal edema, pannus or interstitial keratitis, and the prognosis is poor. A cyclic course of reoccurrences may extend over a 20-year plus period. In cases when irrigation was delayed for over 1 hour the eye sustains complete corneal endothelial cell death and chronic corneal edema and possible phthsis.

The long-term course of MEKP ocular injury mimics nitrogen mustard gas injury in many ways, with a slow progression of multiple exacerbations and remission over decades. It differs in lack of eyelid changes, conjunctival ischemia, scleral disease, tortuous corneal blood vessels and corneal lipoidal-cholesterol deposit degeneration. MEKP may act by causing molecular alteration of tissue macromolecules such as DNA. This creates an autoimmune response primarily in the limbus and cornea. Surprisingly, the rest of the eye and eyelid are generally not affected in the long-term, unless damaged at the time of the original exposure.

Recommendations

1. Main effort should be on prevention with:
   a. Safety goggles
   b. Local anesthetic drops available – pain from the chemical is so severe one cannot adequately perform immediate irrigation without an anesthetic. Make sure to single and double evert lids while using copious amounts of saline irrigation.
2. Use of topical ocular steroids over the first few weeks should be avoided. Treat frequently with preservative-free lubricants, reduction of external stimulant (light, fumes, etc.), protection of the eyes with goggles or patching, and use of as few irritating topical ocular medications as possible. Avoid preservatives in all topical ocular medications.
3. Cases with delayed irrigation are universally the most difficult to treat. There is no effective treatment for serious MEKP injury. The primary goal is to attempt to decrease or impede corneal neovascularization to maintain the immune privilege. The use of topical ocular steroids, limiting external stimuli, oral or injectable vitamin E (alpha-tocopherol) or topical ocular sulphydryl agents (n-acetylcysteine) should be considered after the first month. We have found liquid nitrogen application to the limbus impedes and destroys limbal blood vessels as shown by regrafts of corneal transplants, which have a high success rate (Fraunfelder et al 1990). This may be considered in severe cases, although no one has treated any MEKP injuries in this way. Once extensive corneal pannus or interstitial keratitis occurs the prognosis is universally poor.

REFERENCES AND FURTHER READING

Ando M, Tappel AL. Effect of dietary vitamin E on methyl ethyl ketone peroxide damage to microsomal cytochrome P-450 peroxidase. Chem Biol Interact 55:317, 1985.

Chaudiere J, Clement M, Gerard D, et al. Brain alterations induced by vitamin E deficiency and intoxication with methyl ethyl ketone peroxide. Neurotoxicology 2:173, 1988.

Floyd EP, Stokinger HE. Toxicity studies of certain organic peroxides and hydroperoxides. Am Ind Hyg Assoc J 19:205, 1958.

Fraunfelder FT, Coster DJ, Drew R, et al. Ocular injury induced by methyl ethyl ketone peroxide. Am J Ophthalmol 110:635–640, 1990.

Litov RE, Mathews LC, Tappel AL. Vitamin E protection against in vivo lipid peroxidation initiated in rats by methyl ethyl ketone peroxide as monitored by pentane. Toxicol Appl Pharmacol 59:96, 1981.

Slansky HH, Berman MB, Dohlman CH, et al. Cysteine and acetylcysteine in the prevention of corneal ulcerations. Ann Ophthalmol 2:488, 1970.

Summerfield FW, Tappel AL. Vitamin E protects against methyl ethyl ketone peroxide-induced peroxidative damage to rate brain DNA. Mutat Res 126:113, 1984.

Herbal medicine and dietary supplement induced ocular side effects

Frederick W. Fraunfelder, MD

Herbal or supplement name: Canthaxanthine.

Primary use

This agent is used in cosmetics, as a food coloring and to produce an artificial suntan when administered orally. It is naturally occurring and is found in crustaceans and chanterelle mushrooms.

Ocular side effects

Systemic administration
Certain
1. Retina
    a. Extracellular yellow or gold-like particles (Fig. 9.1)
    b. Predisposed to macular area
    c. Decreased retinal sensitivity
2. Blurred vision
3. Decreased dark adaptation
4. ERG
    a. Hypernormal scotopic amplitudes (low doses)
    b. Increased scotopic latencies (higher doses)
    c. Depressed photopic activity

Clinical significance

For over two decades canthaxanthine has been known to cause deposition of a crystalline form of it in all layers of the retina, primarily the superficial layers. These may cover retinal blood vessels. There is a predisposition for deposition in the macular area, areas of prior trauma or areas of retinal pathology. The deposits are dose related, and may be more common in the elderly and patients with pre-existing ocular disease (i.e. glaucoma or pigmentary retinopathies). Chang et al (1995) described a case in which deposits significantly increased around a branch vein occlusion. The deposits will absorb with time if the supplement is discontinued, but this may take many years. In general, these crystals cause no visual problems, although in rare cases some visual complaints are seen. Static threshold perimetry. (Harnois et al 1988), dark adaptation, (Philipp 1985), and electroretinography (Weber et al 1987) can show abnormalities, which are reversible. If 37 g of canthaxanthine are given over time to enhance skin tanning, 50% of individuals will have retinal deposition, and at the 60-g level 100% will show retinal deposits (Harnois et al 1988). Harnois' paper, along with Sharkey (1993) and cases in the National Registry, suggest that in sensitive individuals dietary intake may rarely show mild cases similar to those described here. There has also been canthaxanthine retinopathy without direct intake of canthaxanthine due to deposits from food coloring (Oosterhuis et al 1989). This naturally occurring carotenoid is a commonly used food color and can be found in crustaceans, chanterelle mushrooms and in some pink-colored fish flesh. The most complete review of this subject is by Arden and Barker (1991).

REFERENCES AND FURTHER READING

Arden GB, Barker FM. Canthaxanthin and the eye: A critical ocular toxicologic assessment. J Toxicol Cut Ocul Toxicol 10(1&2): 115–155, 1991.

Arden GB, et al. Monitoring of patients taking canthaxanthin and carotene: An electroretinographic and ophthalmological survey. Hum Toxicol 8: 439–450, 1989.

Barker FM. Canthaxanthin retinopathy. J Toxicol Cut Ocul Toxicol 7: 223–236, 1988.

Bluhm R, et al. Aplastic anemia associated with canthaxanthin ingested for 'tanning' purposes. JAMA 264: 1141–1142, 1990.

Chan A, Ko TH, Duker JS. Ultrahigh-resolution optical coherence tomography of canthaxanthine retinal crystals. Ophthalmic Surg Lasers Imaging 37: 138–139, 2006.

Chang TS, Aylward W, Clarkson JG, et al. Asymmetric canthaxanthin retinopathy. Am J Ophthalmol 119(6): 801–802, 1995.

Cortin P, et al. Gold sequin maculopathy. Can J Ophthalmol 17: 103–106, 1982 (French).

Espaillat A, Aiello LP, Arrigg PG, et al. Canthaxanthine retinopathy. Arch Ophthalmol 113: 412–413, 1999.

Harnois C. Canthaxathine retinopathy. Anatomic and functional reversibility. Arch Ophthalmol 107: 538–540, 1989.

Harnois C, et al. Static perimetry in canthaxanthin maculopathy. Arch Ophthalmol 106: 58–60, 1988.

Leyon H, et al. Reversibility of canthaxanthin within the retina. Acta Ophthalmol 68: 607–611, 1990.

Lonn LI. Canthaxanthin retinopathy. Arch Ophthalmol 105: 1590, 1987.

Oosterhuis JA, et al. Canthaxanthin retinopathy without intake of canthaxanthin. Klin Monatsbl Augenheilkd 194: 110–116, 1989.

Philipp W. Carotinoid deposits in the retina. Klin Mbl Augenheilk 187: 439–440, 1985.

Sharkey JA. Idiopathic canthaxanthine retinopathy. Eur J Ophthalmol 3(4): 226–228, 1993.

Weber U, Goerz G. Carotinoid-Retinopathie. III. Reversibilitat. Klin Mbl Augnheilk 188: 20–22, 1986.

Weber U, Kern W, et al. Experimental cartenoid retinopathy. I. Functional and morphological alterations of the rabbit retina after 11 months dietary carotenoid application. Graefes Arch Clin Exp Ophthalmol 225: 198–205, 1987.

Herbal or supplement name: Chamomile *(Matricariae chamomilla)*.

Primary use

Chamomile is used to treat inflammation of the eye as well as insomnia, indigestion, migraine headaches, bronchitis, fevers, colds, inflammation and burns. The indications for the eye include eye irritation, styes, epiphora and inflammation.

Ocular side effects

Local ophthalmic use or exposure
Certain
1. Allergic conjunctivitis (severe)
2. Angioedema

Clinical significance

Chamomile tea, which is a common drink worldwide, is made from the dried flower heads of the German or common chamomile plant. There is strong evidence that this tea, when applied topically in or around the eye, can cause a severe conjunctivitis. Subiza et al (1990) described seven patients who rinsed their eyes with chamomile tea to treat styes and runny, irritated eyes. All subjects developed severe conjunctivitis, with angioedema occurring in two patients. All seven subjects had a history of seasonal allergic rhinitis.

A possible mechanism for these patients' conjunctivitis could be sensitivity to the allergens present in *Matricaria chamomilla* pollen. Cross-reactivity with other allergenic pollens to which the patient is already sensitive could lead to the severe conjunctivitis observed in Subiza's study. Because patients are using chamomile to treat their eyes, clinicians should recognize the possibility of *Matricaria chamomilla* sensitivity in cases of what appears to be allergic conjunctivitis, especially in patients who already have an atopic history.

REFERENCES AND FURTHER READING

Subiza J et al. Allergic conjunctivitis to chamomile tea. Ann Allergy 65: 127–132, 1990.

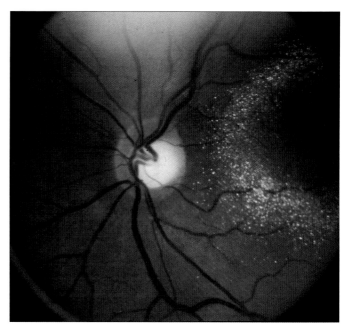
Fig. 9.1 Canthaxanthine crystalline retinopathy.

Herbal or supplement name: Chrysanthemum (lice shampoo). (Fig. 9.2)

Primary use

Pyrethrum (*Chrysanthemum cinerarifolium*) is used as an insecticide for scabies, head lice, crab lice and their nits. Not Nice to Lice® (NNTL) shampoo is used to kill head lice and their nits. The ingredients of the latter, according to the product label, include purified water, anionic/non-ionic surfactant blend, glycerin, enzymes and peppermint oil.

Ocular side effects

Local ophthalmic use or exposure
Certain
1. Keratitis
2. Irritative conjunctivitis
3. Allergic conjunctivitis (severe)
4. Corneal abrasions

Clinical significance

From the WHO and the National Registry, there are 54 reports of keratitis and 19 reports of irritative conjunctivitis from topical use of pyrethrum, which presumably got into the eye of the patients inadvertently. In addition, there are 15 case reports of severe surface ocular reactions from Not Nice to Lice (Ginesis, Nashville, Tennessee, USA) which got into the eyes of the user. Seven of these cases were corneal abrasions. It may not be unusual for eye irritation to occur when a topical solution is used around the eyes (i.e. lice shampoo on the head) but it is unusual for the reaction to cause more than transient eye irritation or red eye. Specifically, reports of corneal abrasions are worrisome, as patients will need to seek emergency treatment due to severe ocular pain and the risk of a bacterial infection superimposed on the corneal epithelial defect. Corneal abrasions may be due to the proteolytic enzymes present in the shampoo preparation.

From the available data, all adverse reactions were immediate and resolved after 1–2 days after discontinuation of the product. The dosage in all patients was per manufacturer instructions for use of Not Nice to Lice®; however, the concentration of pyrethrum is unknown in products such at NNTL and others.

REFERENCES AND FURTHER READING

Fraunfelder FW, Fraunfelder FT, Goetsch RA. Adverse ocular effects from over-the-counter lice shampoo. Arch Ophthalmol 121: 1790-1791, 2003.

Herbal or supplement name: *Datura*.

Primary use

The dried leaves of this flower are used to treat inflammation of the eye as well as asthma, bronchitis, influenza and coughs. The leaves contain alkaloids that are anticholinergic and parasympatholytic in extremely varying concentrations. Jimson weed (*Datura stramonium*) is the main member of this genus utilized for its potential therapeutic value.

Ocular side effects

Systemic administration
Certain
1. Pupils – mydriasis

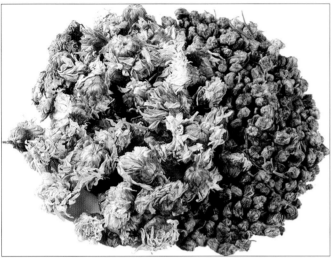

Fig. 9.2 Chrysanthemum From: Ayurvedic Medicine: The Principles of Traditional Practice. London, Elsevier, 2006.

Clinical significance

Hayman reported *Datura wrightii* induced mydriasis in a 4-year-old girl as she was picking flowers in her garden. Thin-layer chromatography showed large quantities of scopolamine, the highest concentration being in the seed pod. There were also trace amounts of hyoscyamine and atropine in all the samples. There are seven more cases of dilated pupils reported in young adults who used this flower for its hallucinogenic properties in Europe (Reader 1977).

Clinicians should remain aware of this ocular side effect from this wild flower, especially in the southwest USA, where it is most prevalent.

REFERENCES AND FURTHER READING

Hayman J. Datura poisoning – the angel's trumpet. Pathology 17: 465-466, 1985.
Reader AL. Mydriasis from *Datura wrightii*. Am J Ophthalmol 82: 263-264, 1977.

Herbal or supplement name: *Echinacea purpurea* (Fig. 9.3).

Primary use

This plant's roots, leaves or the whole plant in various stages of development are used to treat the common cold, cough, fevers, urinary tract infections, burns and influenza.

Ocular side effects

Systemic administration
Certain
1. Irritative conjunctivitis
2. Allergic conjunctivitis

Clinical significance

The evidence of efficacy for *Echinacea* has been studied through randomized placebo-controlled, double-blind studies and the results are mixed, especially for upper respiratory infections.

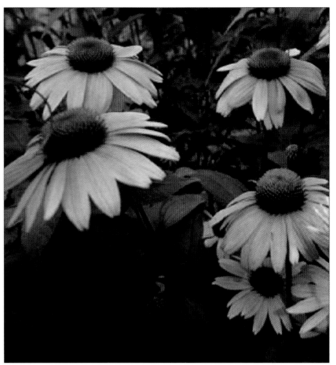

Fig. 9.3 Echinacea purpurea From: Ayurvedic Medicine: The Principles of Traditional Practice. London, Elsevier, 2006.

There are seven reports to the National Registry of eye irritation and conjunctivitis secondary to *Echinacea*. All reports were in adults and in all cases the ocular symptoms resolved within at least a day after stopping this agent.

The conjunctivitis may be due to an anaphylactic reaction. There is evidence that *Echinacea* may activate the autoimmune response and the Physicians' Desk Reference suggests it be avoided in patients with autoimmune diseases.

REFERENCES AND FURTHER READING

Grimm W, Muller H. A randomized controlled trial of the effect of fluid extract of *Echinacea purpurea* on the incidence and severity of colds and respiratory infection. Am J Med 106: 138–143, 1999.
Mullins RJ. Echinacea-associated anaphylaxis. Med J Aust 168: 170–171, 1998.

Herbal or supplement name: *Ginkgo biloba.*

Primary use

The flower and seeds separated from their fleshy outer layer provide medicinal effects, not limited to a mechanism similar to aspirin, in that it inhibits platelet aggregation. The therapeutic benefits have been studied for dementia, peripheral occlusive arterial disease and equilibrium disorders. It is also used to treat tinnitus, asthma (inhibits bronchoconstriction), hypertonia, angina pectoris and tonsillitis.

Ocular side effects

Systemic administration
Certain
1. Spontaneous hyphema

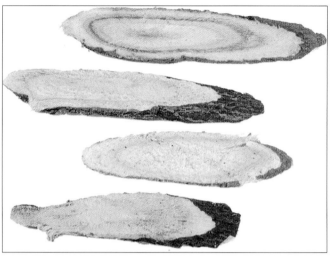

Fig. 9.4 Licorice. From: Ayurvedic Medicine: The Principles of Traditional Practice. London, Elsevier, 2006.

2. Retinal hemorrhage
3. Increased bleeding time

Clinical significance

Ginkgo biloba is one of the best selling and most popular herbal medicines in the USA and worldwide. There are numerous manufacturers who produce this product alone or in combination with other herbal medicines.

There are numerous case reports of bleeding tendencies in patients taking *Ginkgo biloba*. From 27 spontaneous reports to the National Registry, there are two cases of spontaneous hyphema and seven reports of retinal hemorrhages in patients taking this agent. The literature reveals a well-documented case of spontaneous hyphema in a 70-year-old man and a retrobulbar hemorrhage in a 65-year-old woman after retrobulbar injection for cataract surgery. The blood thinning properties and propensity to bleed in patients taking *Ginkgo biloba* appear to be real and this agent should be used with caution in patients who are also taking coumadin or aspirin, as the effects could be additive.

REFERENCES AND FURTHER READING

Benjamin JT, Muir T, Briggs K. A case of cerebral haemorrhage: can ginkgo biloba be implicated? Postgrad Med J 77: 112–113, 2001.
Fong KCS, Kinnear PE. Retrobulbar haemorrhage associated with chronic gingko biloba ingestion. Postgrad Med J 79: 532–533, 2003.
Rosenblatt M. Spontaneous hyphema associated with ingestion of ginkgo biloba extract. N Engl J Med 336: 1108, 1997.

Herbal or supplement name: Licorice.

Primary use

Used to treat patients with gastric ulcers, peptic ulcers and hepatitis C. Indian medicine sometimes uses licorice for eye diseases, and it is frequently used by some patients to treat upper respiratory tract infections, ulcers of the gastrointestinal tract, appendicitis, constipation and other conditions.

Ocular side effects

Systemic administration
Certain
1. Transient visual loss similar to the visual symptoms associated with migraine headaches

Clinical significance

Licorice (*Glycyrrhiza glabra*) root derives some of its medicinal properties from the isoflavonoid glabridin. Glabridin inhibits cyclooxygenase activity and has an anti-inflammatory effect and an anti-platelet effect. Dobbins and Saul (2000) reported five cases of transient visual loss after licorice ingestion. The visual symptoms were similar to what one might see with an ocular migraine without headache. The authors postulate that vasospasm of the brain, retinal and/or optic nerve blood vessels play a role in the visual symptoms as there is strong evidence licorice, through its glucocorticoid and noradrenaline effects, can cause vasospasm throughout the body. Clinically, it appears subjects need to consume large amounts of licorice for the ocular side effects to occur. One should use caution, however, if patients have a history of migraine headaches as the effects could be additive.

REFERENCES AND FURTHER READING

Dobbins KR, Saul RF. Transient visual loss after licorice ingestion. J Neuroophthalmol 20: 38-41, 2000.

Herbal or supplement name: 1. Aluminum nicotinate; 2. niacin (nicotinic acid); 3. niacinamide (nicotinamide); 4. nicotinyl alcohol.

Primary use

Nicotinic acid and its derivatives are used as peripheral vasodilators, as vitamins and as a first-line drug in the treatment of hyperlipidemia.

Ocular side effects

Systemic administration
Certain
1. Decreased vision
2. Macula
   a. Edema
   b. Cystoid macular edema

Probable
1. Sicca sensation
2. Eyelids or conjunctiva
   a. Allergic reactions
   b. Hyperpigmentation
   c. Edema

Possible
1. Diplopia
2. Proptosis (minimal)
3. Decreased risk of cataracts
4. Eyelids or conjunctiva
   a. Angioneurotic edema
   b. Urticaria

c. Loss of eyelashes or eyebrows
d. Edema

Clinical significance

All of the above signs and symptoms are dose related to niacin (nicotinic acid) although the other agents may cause these symptoms as well. These drugs cause macular edema with resultant blurred vision. This may occur from even one dose and last for 1 to 2 hours; however, with prolonged use, some can develop cystoid macular edema. If this goes unrecognized, permanent damage to the macula may occur. Spirn et al (2003) have shown that these cystoid spaces are in the inner nuclear and outer plexiform layers of the retina. Macular edema occurs primarily in patients who are taking at least 3 g per day, although it has been seen in patients taking as little as 1.5 g per day. Macular edema is 10 times more common in men than women, especially in the third to fifth decades of life. The edema usually disappears on discontinuation of the drug. In all probability this drug is also secreted in the tears and will aggravate patients who already have a sicca-type problem. It is debatable if it can induce sicca. There is also a group of patients who will develop some lid or periorbital edema with or without minimal proptosis while on this drug. Occasionally, a transitory, grayish discoloration of the eyelids occurs as well. There are a few cases in the National Registry of superficial punctate keratitis and two cases of eyelash or eyebrow loss. A retrospective survey (Fraunfelder et al 1995) showed that 7% of patients had to discontinue niacin in dosages above 3 g per day secondary to adverse ocular effects. All of the above side effects seem to be dose related, so if the patient prefers to continue therapy, he or she may consider titrating the drug. If decreased vision occurs, one needs to consider macular edema in the differential diagnosis. Although this agent decreases lipids, and other lipid-lowering agents have been linked to cataract formation, no relationship with niacin and cataracts has been established. In fact, a case-control study (Leske 1991) suggests that the antioxidant potential of niacin is inhibitory in the formation of cortical, nuclear or mixed cataracts.

REFERENCES AND FURTHER READING

Callanan D, Blodi BA, Martin DF. Macular edema associated with nicotinic acid. JAMA 279(21): 1702, 1998.
Chazin BJ. Effect of nicotinic acid on blood cholesterol. Geriatrics 15: 423, 1960.
Choice of cholesterol-lowering drugs. Med Lett Drugs Ther 33 (835) 2, 1991.
Fraunfelder FW, Fraunfelder FT, Illingworth DR. Adverse ocular effects associated with niacin therapy. Br J Ophthalmol 79: 54–56, 1995.
Gass JDM. Nicotinic acid maculopathy. Am J Ophthalmol 76: 500–510, 1973.
Harris JL. Toxic amblyopia associated with administration of nicotinic acid. Am J Ophthalmol 55: 133, 1963.
Jampol LM. Niacin maculopathy. Author reply, Millay RH. Ophthalmology 95(12): 1704–1705, 1988.
Leske MC. The lens opacities case-control study. Risk factors for cataract. Arch Ophthalmol 109: 244–251, 1991.
Metelitsina TI, Grunwald JE, DuPont JC, et al. Effect of niacin on the choroidal circulation of patients with age related macular degeneration. Br J Ophthalmol 88: 1568–1572, 2004.
Millay RH, Klein ML, Illingworth DR. Niacin maculopathy. Ophthalmology 95(7): 930–936, 1988.
Parsons WB, Jr, Flinn JH. Reduction in elevated blood cholesterol levels by large doses of nicotinic acid. JAMA 165: 234–238, 1957.
Peczon JD, Grant WM, Lambert BW. Systemic vasodilator, intraocular pressure and chamber depth in glaucoma. Am J Ophthalmol 72: 74–78, 1971.
Spirn MJ, Warren FA, Guyer DR, et al. Optical coherence tomography findings in nicotinic acid maculopathy. Am J Ophthalmol 135: 913–914, 2003.
Zahn K. The effect of vasoactive drugs on the retinal circulation. Trans Ophth Soc UK 86: 529–536, 1966.

Herbal or supplement name: Retinol (Vitamin A).

Proprietary names: Aquasol-A, Palimitate-A, Pedi-Vit-A, Retinol A.

Primary use

Vitamin A is used as a dietary supplement, in the management of vitamin A-deficient states and in the treatment of acne.

Ocular side effects

Systemic administration
Certain
1. Eyelids or conjunctiva
   a. Conjunctivitis – non-specific
   b. Yellow or orange discoloration
   c. Loss of eyelashes or eyebrows
   d. Irritation
2. Exophthalmos
3. Intracranial hypertension
   a. Paresis or paralysis of extraocular muscles
   b. Papilledema
   c. Visual fields
      i. Scotomas
      ii. Enlarged blind spot
   d. Diplopia
   e. Nystagmus
   f. 6th nerve palsy
   g. Peripapillary hemorrhages
   h. Optic nerve atrophy
4. Problems with color vision
   a. Objects have yellow tinge
   b. Improves red dyschromatopsia

Probable
1. Increased intraocular pressure – minimal
2. Subconjunctival or retinal hemorrhages

Possible
1. Eyelids or conjunctiva – exfoliative dermatitis

Clinical significance

Vitamin A deficiency is the leading cause of blindness in the world. With increased interest in diet and popularization of vitamin therapy, an increased incidence of vitamin intoxication is occurring. Ocular manifestations from hypervitaminosis A are varied and dose-related. While some direct effects, such as loss of eyelashes, are evident, most are central effects due to increased intracranial pressure, such as diplopia and strabismus. Simultaneous use of vitamin A and tetracyclines, isotretinoin or other drugs causing pseudotumor may increase the incidence of intracranial hypertension. To date, it is not known how excess vitamin A causes intracranial hypertension. Ocular side effects due to hypervitaminosis A are much more frequent and extensive in infants and children than in adults. Nearly all ocular side effects are rapidly reversible if recognized early and the vitamin therapy discontinued. In some instances it may be several months before these effects are completely resolved. This prolonged effect of vitamin A probably occurs because of the extensive storage of vitamin A in the liver. Papilledema, if untreated, may progress to permanent optic atrophy. Berson et al (1993) suggested that vitamin A may have beneficial effects on retinitis pigmentosa. Other authors, including Clowes (1993a) and Massof and Finkelstein (1993) are not as enthusiastic. If exophthalmos is present, it may be secondary to thyroid changes since vitamin A has antithyroid activity. Hypercalcemia due to vitamin A is infrequent, and band keratopathy has not been reported in the literature or to the National Registry. Dryness and irritation of the eyes has been reported in patients on high dosages of vitamin A, probably since the vitamin has been found to be present in tears.

Evans and Hickey-Dwyer (1991) report an 'hour glass' cornea and iris in an infant after the mother took excessive vitamin A products during pregnancy.

REFERENCES AND FURTHER READING

Baadsgaard O, Thomsen NH. Chronic vitamin A intoxication. Danish Med Bull 30: 51, 1983.

Baxi SC, Dailey GE. Hypervitaminosis. A cause of hypercalcemia. West J Med 137: 429, 1982.

Berson EL, Rosner B, Sandberg MA, Hayes KC, Nicholson BW, et al. Vitamin A supplementation for retinitis pigmentosa (letter). Arch Ophthalmol 111(11): 1456–1459, 1993.

Clowes DD. A randomized trial of vitamin A and vitamin E supplementation for retinitis pigmentosa (letter). Arch Ophthalmol 111(6): 761–772, 1993a.

Clowes DD. A randomized trial of vitamin A and vitamin E supplementation for retinitis pigmentosa. Arch Ophthalmol 111(11): 1461–1462, 1993b.

Evans K, Hickey-Dwyer MU. Cleft anterior segment with maternal hypervitaminosis A. Br J Ophthalmol 75(11): 691–692, 1991.

LaMantia RS, Andrews CE. Acute vitamin A intoxication. South Med J 74: 1012, 1981.

Marcus DF, et al. Optic disk findings in hypervitaminosis A. Ann Ophthalmol 17: 397, 1985.

Massof RW, Finkelstein D. Supplemental vitamin A retards loss of ERG amplitude in retinitis pigmentosa. Arch Ophthalmol 111(6): 751–754, 1993.

Morrice G, Havener WH, Kapetansky F. Vitamin A intoxication as a cause of pseudotumor cerebri. JAMA 173: 1802–1805, 1960.

Ng EWM, Congdon NG, Sommer A. Acute sixth nerve palsy in vitamin A treatment of xerophthalmia. Br J Ophthalmol 84: 931–932, 2000.

Oliver TK, Havener WH. Eye manifestations of chronic vitamin A intoxication. Arch Ophthalmol 60: 19–22, 1958.

Pasquariello PS, Jr. Benign increased intracranial hypertension due to chronic vitamin A overdosage in a 26-month-old child. Clin Pediatr 16: 379–382, 1977.

Pearson MG, Littlewood SM, Bowden AN. Tetracycline and benign intracranial hypertension. BMJ 1: 292, 1981.

Stirling HF, Laing SC, Barr DGD. Hypercarotenaemia and vitamin A overdose from proprietary baby food. Lancet 1: 1089, 1986.

Ubels JL, MacRae SM. Vitamin A is present as retinol in the tears of humans and rabbits. Curr Eye Res 3: 815, 1984.

Van Dyk HJL, Swan KC. Drug-induced pseudotumor cerebri. In Symposium on ocular therapy 4: 71–77, 1969.

Wason S, Lovejoy FH, Jr. Vitamin A toxicity. Am J Dis Child 136: 174, 1982.

White JM. Vitamin-A-induced anaemia. Lancet 2: 573, 1984.

Herbal or supplement name: Vitamin D. The following preparations contain vitamin D as a single entity: calcifediol, calcitriol, dihydrotachysterol (DHT), doxercalciferol, ergocalciferol (calciferol), paricalcitol.

Proprietary names: Calcijex, Calderol, Delta-D, DHT, Drisdol, Hectorol, Hytakerol.

Primary use

Vitamin D is used as a dietary supplement and in the management of vitamin D-deficient states and hypoparathyroidism.

Ocular side effects

Systemic administration
Certain
1. Calcium deposits or band keratopathy
   a. Conjunctiva
   b. Cornea
   c. Sclera
2. Papilledema
3. Optic atrophy
4. Narrowed optic foramina
5. Subconjunctival or retinal hemorrhages secondary to drug-induced anemia
6. Photophobia (late)

Probable
1. Decreased pupillary reaction to light
2. Small optic discs

Possible
1. Strabismus
2. Epicanthus
3. Nystagmus
4. Visual hallucinations
5. Amblyopia

Clinical significance

Severe adverse ocular reactions due to vitamin D are caused by either a direct toxicity or an unusual sensitivity and are primarily seen in infants. Calcium deposits in or around the optic canal cause narrowing of the optic foramina, which may in turn cause papilledema. If the vitamin intake is not discontinued, optic atrophy may result. Children with these toxic effects often have elfin-like faces and prominent epicanthal folds. In adults, the toxic effects are few and the main adverse reaction appears to be the calcium deposits in ocular tissue. It is of interest that in addition to corneal calcification, white fleck-crystalline calcium deposits may also occur on the conjunctiva. One case of a presumed basilar artery insufficiency with hemianopsia due to vitamin D intake has been reported.

REFERENCES AND FURTHER READING

Baxi SC, Dailey GE. Hypervitaminosis. A cause of hypercalcemia. West J Med 137: 429, 1982.

Cogan DC, Albright F, Bartter FC. Hypercalcemia and band keratopathy. Arch Ophthalmol 40: 624, 1948.

Cohen HN, et al. Deafness due to hypervitaminosis D. Lancet 1: 973, 1978.

Dukes MNG (ed). Meyler's Side Effects of Drugs. Amsterdam Exceptra Medica, Vol. X, pp 721–723,1984.

Gartner S, Rubner K. Calcified scleral nodules in hypervitaminosis D. Am J Ophthalmol 39: 658, 1955.

Harley RD, et al. Idiopathic hypercalcemia of infancy: optic atrophy and other ocular changes. Trans Am Acad Ophthalmol Otolaryngol 69: 977, 1965.

Wagener HP. The ocular manifestations of hypercalcemia. Am J Med Sci 231: 218, 1956.

Anderson PC, AEM McLean. Comfrey and liver damage. Hum Toxicol 8: 68–69, 1989.

Arase Y, Ikeda K, Murashima N. The long term efficacy of glycyrrhizin in chronic hepatitis C patients. Cancer Lett 79: 1494–1500, 1997.

Benjamin JT, Muir T, Briggs K. A case of cerebral haemorrhage – can Ginkgo biloba be implicated? Postgrad Med J 77: 112–113, 2001.

Blumenthal M (ed.). The Complete German Commission E Monographs Therapeutic Guide to Herbal Medicines, American Botanical Council, Austin, Texas, 1988.

Coxeter PD, et al. Herb-drug interactions: An evidence based approach. Curr Med Chem 11: 1513–1525, 2004.

Dharmananda S. The nature of ginseng: traditional use, modern research and the question of dosage. Herbal Gram 54: 34–51, 2002.

Dobbins KR, Saul RF. Transient visual loss after licorice ingestion. J Neuro-Ophthalmol 20(1): 38–41, 2000.

Edwards R, Biriell C. Harmonisation in pharmacovigilance. Drug Saf 10(2): 93–102, 1994.

Eisenberg DM. Trends in alternative medicine use in the United States, 1990–1997: results of a follow-up national survey. JAMA 289(18): 1569–1575, 1998.

Espaillat A. Canthaxanthine retinopathy. Arch Ophthalmol 113(3): 412–413, 1999.

Fong KCS, Kinnear PE. Retrobulbar haemorrhage associated with chronic Gingko biloba ingestion. Postgrad Med J 79: 532–533, 2003.

Fraunfelder FW. Ocular side effects from herbal medicines and nutritional supplements. Am J Ophthalmol 138(4): 639–647, 2004.

Fraunfelder FW. Adverse ocular effects from lice shampoo. [comment]. Arch Ophthalmol 122(10): 1575, 2004.

Fraunfelder FT, Fraunfelder FW. Drug-Induced Ocular Side Effects, 5th edn. Butterworth-Heinemann, Woburn, MA, 824, 2001.

Fraunfelder FW, Fraunfelder FT. Evidence for a probable causal relationship between tretinoin, acitretin, and etretinate and intracranial hypertension. J Neuro-Ophthalmol 24(3): 214–216, 2004.

Fraunfelder FW, Fraunfelder FT, Illingworth DR. Adverse ocular effects associated with niacin therapy. Br J Ophthalmol 79(1): 54–56, 1995.

Fraunfelder FW, Fraunfelder FT, Goetsch RA. Adverse ocular effects from over-the-counter lice shampoo. Arch Ophthalmol 121(12): 1790–1791, 2003.

Fraunfelder FW, Fraunfelder FT, Corbett JJ. Isotretinoin-associated intra-cranial hypertension. Ophthalmology 111(6): 1248–1250, 2004.

Gass JDM. Nicotinic acid maculopathy. Am J Ophthalmol 76: 500–510, 1973.

Grimm W, Muller H. A randomized controlled trial of the effect of fluid extract of echinacea purpurea on the incidence and severity of colds and respiratory infections. Am J Med 106(2): 138–143, 1999.

Harnois C. Canthaxanthin retinopathy. Anatomic and functional reversibility. Arch Ophthalmol 107(4): 538–540, 1989.

Hayman J. Datura poisoning – the angel's trumpet. Pathology 17: 465–466, 1985.

Jampol LM. Niacin maculopathy. Ophthalmology 95: 1704–1705, 1988.

Knefeli U. The 247 most beneficial plants. Guia practica ilustrade de las plantas medicinales, Vol. 26, Qar T (ed), Barcelona, Blume, 1981.

Ling AM. FDA to ban sales of dietary supplements containing ephedra. J Law Med Ethics 32(1): 184–186, 2004.

Morrice G, Havener WH, Kapetansky F. Vitamin A intoxication as a cause of pseudotumor cerebri. JAMA 173: 1802–1805, 1960.

Morris CA, Avorn J. Internet marketing of herbal products. JAMA 290(11): 1505–1509, 2003.

Mullins RJ. Echinacea-associated anaphylaxis. Med J Aust 168(4): 170–171, 1998.

Nortier JLea. Urothelial carcinoma associated with the use of a Chinese herb. N Engl J Med 342: 1686–1692, 2000.

Oosterhuis JA. Canthaxanthin retinopathy without intake of canthaxan-thin. Klin Monatsbl Augenheilkd 194(2): 110–116, 1989.

Physicians' Desk Reference for Nutritional Supplements, 1st edn, Medical Economics Company, Inc., p 575, 2001.

Physicians' Desk Reference for Herbal Medicines, 3rd edn, Thomson Healthcare, Inc, Montvale, NJ, 2004.

Reader AL. Mydriasis from Datura Wrightii. Am J Ophthalmol 82(2): 263–264, 1977.

Rosenblatt M. Spontaneous hyphema associated with ingestion of Ginkgo biloba extract. N Engl J Med 336: 1108, 1997.

Subiza J. Allergic conjunctivitis to chamomile tea. Ann Allergy 65: 127–132, 1990.

WHO guidelines on good agricultural and collection practices for medicinal plants. In: Marketing and Dissemination, World Health Organization, Geneva, Switzerland, 2004.

Index of Side Effects

A

Accommodation – decreased or paralysis of

adrenal cortex injection, 169–173
alcohol, 291–292
alprazolam, 90
amfepramone, 89
amlptyline, 95–96
amoxapine, 96
atropine, 142–143
beclomethasone, 169–173
bendroflumethiazide, 161–162
benzathine benzylpenicillin, 53–54
benzatropine, 195–196
benzfetamine, 89
benzylpenicillin potassium, 53–54
betamethasone, 169–173
bethanechol, 144
biperiden, 195–196
carbachol, 145
carbamazepine, 97
carbinoxamine, 193
carbon dioxide, 137
carisoprodol, 91
cetirizine, 194
chloramphenicol, 55
chlordiazepoxide, 90
chloroquine, 73–75
chlorothiazide, 161–162
chlorpromazine, 101–103
chlortalidone, 161–162
clemastine fumarate, 193
clomipramine, 96
clonazepam, 90
clorazepate, 90
cocaine, 282–283
cortisone, 169–173
cyclopentolate, 271–272
desipramine, 95–96
desloratadine, 194
dexamethasone, 169–173
diacetylmorphine, 125
diazepam, 90
dicyclomine, 144
diethylstilbestrol, 177
diphenhydramine, 193
disopyramide, 152
doxepin, 96
doxylamine succinate, 193
dronabinol, 107
droperidol, 103
emetine, 47
ergometrine, 146
ergotamine tartrate, 146

Accommodation – decreased or paralysis of (Continued)

fexofenadine, 194
fludrocortisone, 169–173
fluorometholone, 169–173
fluorouracil, 210–211
fluphenazine, 101–103
flurazepam, 90
glibenclamide, 188–189
glycopyrrolate, 144
haloperidol, 103
hashish, 107
herbal medicines, 42
homatropine, 142–143
hydrochlorothiazide, 161–162
hydrocortisone, 169–173
hydroflumethiazide, 161–162
hydromorphone, 125–126
hydroxyamfetamine, 272
hydroxychloroquine, 73–75
hyoscine, 129–130
hyoscine methobromide, 129–130
indapamide, 161–162
iodide and iodine solutions and compounds, 174–175
ipratropium, 160
isoniazid, 82–83
lithium carbonate, 104
loratadine, 194
lorazepam, 90
loxapine, 105
LSD, 108–109
maprotiline, 99–100
marihuana, 107
medrysone, 169–173
mepenzolate, 144
meprobamate, 91
mescaline, 108–109
methacholine, 152
methylclothiazide, 161–162
methylene blue, 182–183
methylergometrine maleate, 146
methylphenidate, 100
methylprednisolone, 169–173
metolazone, 161–162
midazolam, 90
morphine, 126–127
nalidixic acid, 64
nortriptyline, 95–96
opium, 126–127
orphenadrine, 198
oxazepam, 90
oxprenolol, 153

Accommodation – decreased or paralysis of (Continued)

oxymorphone, 125–126
pentazocine, 128
perphenazine, 101–103
phendimetrazine, 89
phenoxymethylpenicillin, 53–54
phentermine, 89
phenytoin, 92–93
pilocarpine, 269–270
pimozide, 105–106
piperazine, 49
polythiazide, 161–162
pralidoxime, 197–198
prednisolone, 169–173
prednisone, 169–173
primidone, 110
procaine benzylpenicillin, 53–54
prochlorperazine, 101–103
procyclidine, 195–196
promethazine, 101–103
propantheline, 144
propranolol, 153
psilocybin, 108–109
radioactive iodides, 174–175
rimexolone, 169–173
telithromycin, 67–68
temazepam, 90
tetanus immune globulin, 244
tetanus toxoid, 244
thiethylperazine, 101–103
thioridazine, 101–103
tiotixene, 106–107
tolterodine, 144
triamcinolone, 169–173
triazolam, 90
trichlormethiazide, 161–162
trihexylphenidyl, 195–196
trimipramine, 96
tripelennamine, 194
vincristine, 221–222

Accommodative spasm

acetylcholine, 266–267
carbachol, 145
cyclophosphamide, 207
ecothiopate, 268
methylene blue, 182–183
morphine, 127
opium, 127
organophosphates, 303–304
physostigmine, 303–304
pilocarpine, 269–270
pyridostigmine, 303–304

Color code for categories of side effects: certain, probable, possible, conditional/unclassified.

Color code for categories of side effects: certain, probable, possible, conditional/unclassified.

Index of side effects

Color code for categories of side effects: certain, probable, possible, conditional/unclassified.

Color code for categories of side effects: certain, probable, possible, conditional/unclassified.

Color code for categories of side effects: certain, probable, possible, conditional/unclassified.

319

Index of side effects

Color code for categories of side effects: certain, probable, possible, conditional/unclassified.

Color code for categories of side effects: certain, probable, possible, conditional/unclassified.

Color code for categories of side effects: certain, probable, possible, conditional/unclassified.

Color code for categories of side effects: certain, probable, possible, conditional/unclassified.

Color code for categories of side effects: certain, probable, possible, conditional/unclassified.

Color code for categories of side effects: certain, probable, possible, conditional/unclassified.

Color code for categories of side effects: certain, probable, possible, conditional/unclassified.

Color code for categories of side effects: certain, probable, possible, conditional/unclassified.

Color code for categories of side effects: certain, probable, possible, conditional/unclassified.

Color code for categories of side effects: certain, probable, possible, conditional/unclassified.

Color code for categories of side effects: certain, probable, possible, conditional/unclassified.

Hyperpigmentation of eyelids or conjunctiva (Continued)
   travoprost, 252–253
   trimipramine, 96
   verapamil, 147–148
   zidovudine, 46
Hypertrichosis see Eyelashes – increased number
Hyphema
   alteplase, 183–184
   amphotericin B, 69–70
   ecothiopate, 268
   Ginkgo biloba, 42, 309–310
   reteplase, 183–184
   streptokinase, 185–186
   tenecteplase, 183–184
   warfarin, 187
Hypopyon
   cocaine, 282–283
   iodide and iodine solutions and
      compounds, 174–175
   proxymetacaine, 283–284
   radioactive iodides, 174–175
   rifabutin, 83–84
   tetracaine, 283–284
   urokinase, 281

Infection – decreased resistance to
   adrenal cortex injection, 169–173
   azathioprine, 231
   beclomethasone, 169–173
   betamethasone, 169–173
   cortisone, 169–173
   cytarabine, 208
   dexamethasone, 169–173
   fludrocortisone, 169–173
   fluorometholone, 169–173
   hydrocortisone, 169–173
   medrysone, 169–173
   methylprednisolone, 169–173
   prednisolone, 169–173
   prednisone, 169–173
   rimexolone, 169–173
   silicone, 277
   tacrolimus, 233–234
   triamcinolone, 169–173
   see also Herpes infections; Overgrowth of
      non-susceptible organisms
Internuclear ophthalmoplegia
   diacetylmorphine, 125
   penicillamine, 228–229
   tacrolimus, 233–234
Intracranial hypertension
   ciclosporin, 232
   cytarabine, 207–208
   OXPRENOLOL, 153
   pioglitazone, 190–191
   PROPRANOLOL, 153
   rosiglitazone, 190–191
   vitamin A, 42, 311–312
   see also Papilledema secondary to intracranial
      hypertension
Intraocular pressure – decreased
   acebutolol, 154–155
   acetylcholine, 266–267
   alcohol, 291–292
   alkalis, 297
   amyl nitrite, 147

Intraocular pressure – decreased (Continued)
   aspirin, 121–122
   atenolol, 154–155
   atorvastatin, 140–141
   bendroflumethiazide, 161–162
   betaxolol, 249–251
   bupivacaine, 135–136
   butyl nitrite, 147
   carbachol, 145
   carteolol, 257–258
   carvedilol, 154–155
   chlorothiazide, 161–162
   chlortalidone, 161–162
   cidofovir, 262
   clofibrate, 142
   clonidine, 156–157
   dipivefrine, 258–259
   dronabinol, 107
   droperidol, 103
   ecothiopate, 268
   ephedrine, 165
   epinephrine, 165–166
   ergometrine, 146
   ergotamine tartrate, 146
   fluvastatin, 140–141
   furosemide, 163
   glycerol, 163–164
   guanethidine, 157
   haloperidol, 103
   hashish, 107
   hydrochlorothiazide, 161–162
   hydroflumethiazide, 161–162
   indapamide, 161–162
   iotalamic acid, 230
   labetolol, 154–155
   levobunolol, 249–251
   lidocaine, 135–136
   lovastatin, 140–141
   mannitol, 164
   marihuana, 107
   mepivacaine, 135–136
   methacholine, 152
   methoxyflurane, 132
   methylclothiazide, 161–162
   methylergometrine maleate, 146
   metipranolol, 259–260
   metolazone, 161–162
   metoprolol, 154–155
   morphine, 126–127
   nadolol, 154–155
   nitrous oxide, 133
   norepinephrine, 165–166
   opium, 126–127
   oxprenolol, 153
   pethidine, 127
   phenoxybenzamine, 164
   pilocarpine, 269–270
   pindolol, 154–155
   polythiazide, 161–162
   pravastatin, 140–141
   procaine, 135–136
   propranolol, 153
   rescinnamine, 159–160
   reserpine, 159–160
   rosuvastatin, 140–141
   simvastatin, 140–141
   suxamethonium, 130–131
   timolol, 249–251

Intraocular pressure – decreased (Continued)
   trichlormethiazide, 161–162
   urokinase, 281
Intraocular pressure – increased, 12
   adrenal cortex injection, 169–173
   alkalis, 297
   amyl nitrite, 147
   atropine, 142–143
   beclomethasone, 169–173
   betamethasone, 169–173
   bevacizumab, 245–246
   bromfenac, 285
   bupivacaine, 135–136
   butyl nitrite, 147
   carbon dioxide, 137
   chloroprocaine, 135–136
   citalopram, 98
   clomifene, 179–180
   cortisone, 169–173
   cyclopentolate, 271–272
   dexamethasone, 169–173
   diclofenac, 285
   dicyclomine, 144
   ecothiopate, 268
   fludrocortisone, 169–173
   fluoromethotone, 169–173
   fluoxetine, 98
   fluvoxamine, 98
   glycopyrrolate, 144
   homatropine, 142–143
   hydralazine, 158
   hydrochloric acid, 289–290
   hydrocortisone, 169–173
   hydrofluoric acid, 289–290
   hyoscine, 129–130
   hyoscine methobromide, 129–130
   ketamine, 132
   ketorolac trometamol, 285
   lidocaine, 135–136
   medrysone, 169–173
   mepenzolate, 144
   mepivacaine, 135–136
   methyl ethyl ketone peroxide, 306
   methylprednisolone, 169–173
   morphine, 127
   naphazoline, 266
   nepafenac, 285
   nitrous oxide, 133
   opium, 127
   paroxetine, 98
   pegaptanib, 245–246
   phencyclidine, 109
   phenylephrine, 167–168
   pilocarpine, 269–270
   prednisolone, 169–173
   prednisone, 169–173
   prilocaine, 135–136
   procaine, 135–136
   propantheline, 144
   ranibizumab, 245–246
   rimexolone, 169–173
   sertraline, 98
   sodium chloride, 286
   sodium hyaluronate, 287
   sulfuric acid, 289–290
   suxamethonium, 130–131
   tetryzoline, 266
   tolterodine, 144

Color code for categories of side effects: certain, probable, possible, conditional/unclassified.

Color code for categories of side effects: certain, probable, possible, conditional/unclassified.

Color code for categories of side effects: certain, probable, possible, conditional/unclassified.

Color code for categories of side effects: certain, probable, possible, conditional/unclassified.

336

Index of side effects

Color code for categories of side effects: certain, probable, possible, conditional/unclassified.

Color code for categories of side effects: certain, probable, possible, conditional/unclassified.

Color code for categories of side effects: certain, probable, possible, conditional/unclassified.

Color code for categories of side effects: certain, probable, possible, conditional/unclassified.

Color code for categories of side effects: certain, probable, possible, conditional/unclassified.

341

Color code for categories of side effects: certain, probable, possible, conditional/unclassified.

Color code for categories of side effects: certain, probable, possible, conditional/unclassified.

Color code for categories of side effects: certain, probable, possible, conditional/unclassified.

Color code for categories of side effects: certain, probable, possible, conditional/unclassified.

Color code for categories of side effects: certain, probable, possible, conditional/unclassified.

Color code for categories of side effects: certain, probable, possible, conditional/unclassified.

Color code for categories of side effects: certain, probable, possible, conditional/unclassified.

Index of side effects

Color code for categories of side effects: certain, probable, possible, conditional/unclassified.

Color code for categories of side effects: certain, probable, possible, conditional/unclassified.

Color code for categories of side effects: certain, probable, possible, conditional/unclassified.

Color code for categories of side effects: certain, probable, possible, conditional/unclassified.

Color code for categories of side effects: certain, probable, possible, conditional/unclassified.

Color code for categories of side effects: certain, probable, possible, conditional/unclassified.

Index of side effects

355

Color code for categories of side effects: certain, probable, possible, conditional/unclassified.

Color code for categories of side effects: certain, probable, possible, conditional/unclassified.

Subject index